The Role of Selenium in Nutrition

Gerald F. Combs, Jr.

Department of Poultry and Avian Sciences
and Division of Nutritional Sciences
Cornell University
Ithaca, New York

Stephanie B. Combs

Department of Poultry and Avian Sciences
Cornell University
Ithaca, New York

1986

ACADEMIC PRESS, INC.

Harcourt Brace Jovanovich, Publishers

Orlando   San Diego   New York   Austin
Boston   London   Sydney   Tokyo   Toronto

ACADEMIC PRESS, INC.
Orlando, Florida 32887

United Kingdom Edition published by
ACADEMIC PRESS INC. (LONDON) LTD.
24–28 Oval Road, London NW1 7DX

Library of Congress Cataloging in Publication Data

Combs, Gerald F.
    The role of selenium in nutrition.

    Includes bibliographies and index.
    1. Selenium in human nutrition.   2. Selenium in
animal nutrition.   3. Selenium—Physiological effect.
4. Selenium—Metabolism.   I. Combs, Stephanie B.
II. Title.   [DNLM: 1. Nutrition.   2. Selenium—
metabolism.   QU 130 C731r]
QP535.S5C66   1986   612'.3924   85-26822
ISBN 0–12–183495–6 (alk. paper)

PRINTED IN THE UNITED STATES OF AMERICA

86 87 88 89   9 8 7 6 5 4 3 2 1

We dedicate this work to

the group of scientists around the world who, having undertaken during the last 40 years to learn about the biological activity of selenium, have produced collectively the information summarized in this volume, and to

those scientists from many countries and backgrounds who, each bringing a new perspective, are extending this information toward the full understanding of the roles of selenium in the nutrition and health of man and other animals, and to

a world that needs many such collaborations.

Contents

4. The Biological Availability of Selenium in Foods and Feeds

5. Absorption, Excretion, and Metabolism of Selenium

6. Biochemical Functions of Selenium

7. Selenium Deficiency Diseases of Animals

8. Selenium in Human Nutrition and Health

9. Selenium in Immunity and Infection

10. Selenium and Cancer

11. Effects of Selenium Excesses

Preface

One of the most important discoveries in nutrition in the last 30 years has been the recognition of the essentiality of the element selenium and the elucidation of the biochemical bases of its nutritional interrelationships with vitamin E and other factors. This area of inquiry first involved a new and apparently novel role of the element in the normal nutrition of experimental animals fed purified diets. Subsequently, it has included several applied areas of animal and human health ranging from the prevention of reproductive disorders in cattle to the modification of cancer risk in humans. Thus, despite the economic importance now attached to selenium in agriculture and the potential value now proposed for the element in certain aspects of medicine, our understanding of these roles of selenium is far less applied in nature. The beginning of the selenium story occurred in basic research laboratories and not in field situations; basic research produced answers before practical problems were identified.

Since the mid-1930s, selenium had been recognized as the toxic principle responsible for "alkali disease" and "blind staggers" in grazing livestock on the seleniferous prairies of the northern American Great Plains. Imagine the surprise of the late Klaus Schwarz and his colleagues at the National Institutes of Health 20 years later when they found that this little-known element was also the active principle in brewer's yeast responsible for the protection of vitamin E-deficient rats from necrotic liver degeneration. In his excitement, Schwarz telephoned Milton Scott at Cornell University and said, "Milt, try selenium!" Scott had recently found that brewer's yeast contained a factor (later shown to be niacin) that reduced leg weakness in turkey poults, and had become acquainted with Schwarz through their mutual interest in the nutritional attributes of that feedstuff. Scott had also found that brewer's yeast contained a factor that prevented exudative diathesis (the disease described in the 1930s by Heinrich Dam) in the vitamin E-deficient chick. "Try selenium!" Schwarz said, and Scott did. That year,

1957, Schwarz and Scott announced the discovery of the nutritional essentiality of selenium.

The discovery that exudative diathesis in the chick is a clinical sign of combined selenium and vitamin E deficiency in that species actually preceded the occurrence of that syndrome as a practical problem in the production of poultry. By the time that field cases of exudative diathesis in chicks and gizzard myopathy in turkeys were observed, basic research in several laboratories had generated information applicable to those practical problems. This central role of the basic investigator in selenium-related research has continued over the past three decades. This has resulted in the fortunate present situation wherein the human and veterinary health communities are able to consider the plausibility of apparent associations of selenium and disease in the light of an extensive and growing understanding of the biochemistry, metabolism, and nutrition of the element.

Our purpose in preparing this volume has been to assemble an extensive review of the most pertinent scientific literature dealing with these basic aspects of the present understanding of the roles of selenium in nutrition and health. We have sought, as best we could, to give our own perspectives where we felt that decisions must be made in the face of very limited information (e.g., identification of daily selenium allowances and the upper safe limits of selenium intake for humans). In those cases, we have tried to outline our logic to assist the reader in understanding our recommendations. We have made special efforts to discuss the subjects of selenium bioavailability and the two selenium-related diseases recently reported in China. We see these topics as of central importance to our considerations of the roles of selenium in nutrition and health, yet neither has previously been reviewed as extensively as the information on each deserves. We have also included collations of much experimental data (e.g., the exhaustive summary of the selenium contents of foods), which we believe will be useful to those interested in this field. It is our hope that this volume will serve as a useful reference and guide to the scientific literature for researchers, students, public health officers, and others whose interests relate to selenium in nutrition and health.

We approached the preparation of this volume as an effort of the truest kind of didactic scholarship. But, as Richard Bach wrote,* "You teach best what you most need to learn," we have found that the intellectual rewards of our effort, that is, the understanding that we have gained during the process of poring through the hundreds of papers and of trying to assemble their messages into a coherent story, have given us a perspective that we could not have acquired otherwise. To the extent that we will have been able to share that perspective in a fashion useful to others, our efforts will have been successful. That is our wish.

---

*Illusions. The Adventures of a Reluctant Messiah. Dell Publ., New York, 1977.

Acknowledgments

A review of this type, by its very nature, depends on the researchers whose ideas, experiments, and reports constitute the body of knowledge addressed. In that respect, we are indebted to literally hundreds of researchers throughout the world whose individual efforts have produced the approximately 1800 reports that we have considered in preparing this volume. To those many, often underheralded, scientists we offer our warmest appreciation.

We owe a special debt to several individuals who generously provided photographs and figures that we have included in this volume. We extend our sincere appreciation for that assistance to the following people: Dr. J. E. Oldfield, Oregon State University; Dr. J. H. Harrison and Dr. H. R. Conrad, Ohio State University; Dr. Liu Jinxu, Institute of Animal Science, Chinese Academy of Agricultural Sciences; Dr. M. L. Scott, Cornell University; Dr. J. F. Van Vleet, Purdue University; Dr. J. A. Marsh, Cornell University; Dr. Tan Jianan, Institute of Geography, Chinese Academy of Agricultural Sciences; and Dr. H. A. Poston, U.S. Fish and Wildlife Service.

We are particularly indebted to several individuals who lent their time and judgment in the review of draft versions of the manuscript. These include Dr. K. R. Mahaffey, National Institute of Occupational Safety and Health; Dr. J. A. Marsh, Cornell University; and Dr. L. C. Clark, Cornell University. Their thoughtful criticisms were valuable to us.

This project was absolutely dependent on two individuals in our research group whose tireless efforts made our tasks manageable. We offer our most sincere gratitude to Ms. Pamela Senter for her highly efficient and enthusiastic handling of the manuscript in its various draft stages and for the layout of the extensive tabular material. Without the dedicated assistance also of Jamie Saroka, we could not have produced this volume. The understanding of the other people in our research group (Lynne Deuschle, Steve Mercurio, Young Sook Kim, Bao-Ji Chen, Johnny Lü, Tom Grant, and Harlan Redder) and of our children (Jerry, Kiersten, and Matt) during the months in which we engaged in this project is a gift of which we are very much aware and thankful; we will not forget them.

It has been our personal pleasure to participate, over the last dozen or so years, in an intellectual endeavor of global proportions toward the elucidation of the role of selenium and related factors in nutrition and health. This participation has brought us together in various forums (over lecterns, laboratory benches and beer glasses) with many of the scientists whose work constitutes the greater part of the body of information on which our current understanding of the biology and nutrition of selenium now rests. To these scientists, who are too numerous to name, but who may recall some lively conversations into the night in Lubbock, Beijing, Washington, Boston, Helsinki, Chicago, Dallas, St. Louis, Cincinnati, Anaheim, Ithaca, Madison, Davis, Columbia, Saxton's River, or any number of other big and little places, we thank you.

1

CHEMICAL ASPECTS OF SELENIUM

I. FORMS OF SELENIUM

Selenium (Se) is classified in group VIA of the periodic table of elements. This group includes the nonmetals sulfur and oxygen in the periods above Se, and the metals tellurium and polonium in the periods below Se. By period, Se lies between the group VA metal arsenic and the group VIIA nonmetal bromine. Thus, Se is considered a metalloid, having both metallic and nonmetallic properties. Its atomic properties are summarized in Table 1.1.

Elemental Se, like its sister elements, sulfur and tellurium, shows allotropy; that is, it can exist in either an amorphous state or one of three crystalline states. Amorphous Se is a hard, brittle glass at temperatures below 31°C, is vitreous at 31°-230°C, and is a free-flowing liquid above 230°C. The increased viscosity of amorphous Se at temperatures less than 230°C results from the formation of polymeric chains at lower temperatures. Crytalline Se can take the form of flat hexagonal and polygonal crystals (called alpha-monoclinic or "red" Se), of prismatic or needle-like crystals (called beta-monoclinic or "dark red" Se), or of spiral polyatomic chains of the form Se_n (variously called hexagonal, trigonal, metallic, "gray" or "black" Se). The hexagonal crystalline form of Se is the most stable; both monoclinic forms convert to the hexagonal form at temperatures above 110°C, and amorphous Se converts spontaneously to the hexagonal crystalline form at 70°-210°C. The properties of the allotropic forms of Se are discussed in detail elsewhere.[1,2]

Elemental Se can be reduced to the -2 oxidation state (selenide), or oxidized to the +4 (selenite) or +6 (selenate) oxidation states. Hydrogen

1

Table 1.1

Atomic Properties of Selenium

Atomic number	34
Atomic weight	78.96
Electronic configuration	$Ar3d^{10}4s^24p^4$
Atomic radius	1.40 Å
Covalent radius	1.16 Å
Ionic radius	1.98 Å
Common oxidation states	-2, 0, +4, +6
Bond energy	
(M—M)	44 kcal/mole
(M—H)	67 kcal/mole
Ionization potential	9.75 eV
Electron affinity	-4.21 eV
Electronegativity	2.55 (Pauling's scale)

selenide (H_2Se) is a fairly strong acid with a pK_a of 3.8 in aqueous systems. The gas is colorless, has an unpleasant odor, and is highly toxic [the LC_{50} for 30-min exposure for guinea pigs is 6 ppm [3]]. It can be produced by heating elemental Se above 400° C in air, but it decomposes in air to form elemental Se and water. Hydrogen selenide is fairly soluble in water (270 ml per 100 ml water at 22.5° C). It reacts directly with most metals to form metal selenides, but these compounds are practically insoluble in water. Organic selenides are ready electron donors to their surrounding environments, thus oxidizing these forms of Se to higher oxidation states.

In the +4 oxidation state, Se can exist as selenium dioxide (SeO_2), as selenious acid (H_2SeO_3) or as selenite (SeO_3^{-2}). Selenium dioxide is formed by burning elemental Se in air or reacting it with nitric acid. It is readily reduced to the elemental state by ammonia, hydroxylamine, sulfur dioxide, and several organic compounds. It is soluble in water (38.4 g per 100 ml water at 14° C) and forms selenious acid (H_2SeO_3) when dissolved in hot water. Selenious acid is weakly dibasic, with a pK_a of 2.6; dissolved selenite salts exist as biselenite ions in aqueous solutions at pH 3.5 to 9. In contrast to the organic selenides, selenites readily accept electrons from their environments, their Se being easily reduced. At low pH, selenite is readily reduced to the elemental state by mild reducing agents such as ascorbic acid and sulfur dioxide. Selenites in soils are strongly bound by hydrous oxides of iron, forming insoluble complexes at moderate pH (4-8.5).

In its most oxidized (+6) state, Se can exist as selenic acid (H_2SeO_4) or as selenate (SeO_4^{-2}) salts. Selenic acid is a strong acid. It is formed by the oxidation of selenious acid or elemental Se by strong oxidizing agents in the presence of water. Selenic acid is very soluble in water; most selenate salts are soluble in water, in contrast to the corresponding selenite salts and metal selenides. Selenates tend to be rather inert and are very resistant to reduction.

Six stable isotopes of Se exist in nature. These are ^{74}Se (natural abundance 0.815 mass %), ^{76}Se (natural abundance 8.66 mass %), ^{77}Se (natural abundance 7.31 mass %), ^{78}Se (natural abundance 23.21 mass %), ^{80}Se (natural abundance 50.65 mass %), and ^{82}Se (natural abundance 8.35 mass %). These isotopes have been employed in study of the biological utilization of Se in foods, in which their quantitation has been achieved by neutron activation (for ^{74}Se, ^{76}Se, and ^{80}Se),[4] or by mass spectrometry (for ^{76}Se,^{80}Se, and ^{82}Se).[5] More than two dozen radioisotopes of Se can be produced by neutron activation or by radionuclear decay. These include such short-lived species as ^{77m}Se (half-life 17.5 sec) and ^{87}Se (half-life 16 sec), and such long-lived species as ^{75}Se (half-life 120 days). Of these, ^{75}Se and ^{77m}Se have been found to be suitable for the measurement of Se in biological materials by neutron activation analysis.[6,7] Due to its emission of gamma-radiation and to its relatively long half-life, ^{75}Se has been widely employed in biological experimentation and in medical diagnostic work.

Table 1.2
Selenium Compounds Important in Nutrition

Oxidation state of Se	Compound
Se^{-2}	H_2Se
	Na_2Se
	$(CH_3)_2Se$
	$(CH_3)_3Se^+$
	Selenomethionine
	Selenocysteine
	Se-methyl-selenocysteine
	Selenocystathionine
	Selenotaurine
Se^0	Selenodiglutathione
	Amorphous selenium
	Red selenium (alpha-monoclinic)
	Dark red selenium (beta-monoclinic)
	Gray selenium (hexagonal)
Se^{+4}	H_2SeO_3
	Na_2SeO_3
Se^{+6}	Na_2SeO_4

Selenium is a semiconductor with photoconductivity (i.e., excitation with electromagnetic radiation can markedly increase its conductivity).[2] This property has made Se compounds useful in photocells and in xerography. As a result of the utility conferred by these properties, the literature on the chemistry of inorganic and organic Se compounds is large. Because this area is outside of the scope of the present volume, the reader is referred to the comprehensive review edited by Klayman and Gunther[8] and the recent volume of Ihnat[9] for discussions of the chemical properties and analytical chemistry of Se.

The Se compounds of greatest interest in nutrition are presented in Table 1.2. It should be noted that whereas forms of Se available as supplements of foods and feeds are primarily compounds of the higher oxidation states of Se, the metabolites of chief concern in nutrition and biochemistry are compounds in which Se occurs in the reduced state.

II. CHEMISTRY OF SELENIUM

The chemical and physical properties of Se are very similar to those of sulfur (S). The two elements have similar outer-valence-shell electronic configurations and atomic sizes (in both covalent and ionic states), and their bond energies, ionization potentials, electron affinities, electronegativities, and polarizabilities are virtually the same.[9] Despite these similarities, the chemistry of Se and S differ in two respects that distinguish them in biological systems.

The first important difference in the chemistry of Se and sulfur is in the ease of reduction of their oxyanions.[10,11] Quadrivalent selenium in selenite tends to undergo reduction, but quadrivalent S in sulfite tends to undergo oxidation. This difference is demonstrated by the following reaction:

$$H_2SeO_3 + 2\ H_2SO_3 \longrightarrow Se + 2\ H_2SO_4 + H_2O$$

Thus, in biological systems, Se compounds tend to be metabolized to more reduced states, and S compounds tend to be metabolized to more oxidized states.

The second important difference in the chemical behaviors of these elements is in the acid strengths of their hydrides. Although the analogous oxyacids of Se and S have comparable acid strengths [$SeO(OH)_2$: pK_a 2.6 vs. $SO(OH)_2$: pK_a 1.9], the hydride H_2Se (pK_a 3.8) is much more acidic than is H_2S (pK_a 7.0). This difference in acidic strengths is reflected in the dissociation behaviors of the selenohydryl group (-SeH) of selenocysteine (pK_a 5.24) and the sulfhydryl (-SH) group on cysteine (pK_a 8.25).[12] Thus, while thiols such as cysteine are predominantly protonated at physiological pH, the selenohydryl groups of selenols such as selenocysteine are predominantly dissociated under the same conditions.

Selenite can react with nonprotein thiols and with protein sulfhydryls to undergo reduction of the Se^{+4} to Se^0. This reaction, originally postulated by Painter,[13] was confirmed by Ganther,[14] who demonstrated that selenite can react with either glutathione (reduced form), cysteine, or coenzyme A to form 1,3-dithio-2-selane products of the form RS—Se—SR, which are referred to as "selenotrisulfides." The reaction is represented as follows:

$$4 \, RSH + H_2SeO_3 \longrightarrow RS{-}Se{-}SR + RS{-}SR + 3 \, H_2O$$

In this reaction, four sulfhydryl sulfurs are oxidized from the -2 oxidation state to the -1 oxidation state of disulfide sulfurs. This is balanced by the concommitant reduction of a single Se atom from the selenite oxidation state of +4 to the zero oxidation state. However, because the electronegativities of Se and S are very similar, Martin[15] has suggested that the -2 charge may be rather evenly distributed across the selenotrisulfide bridge, yielding an effective oxidation number of -2/3 for each of its members.

A similar reaction, indicated by Jenkins[16,17] and confirmed by Ganther and Corcoran[18], can occur between selenite and the free sulfhydryls of proteins to yield selenotrisulfide types of products.

Thus, whereas the chemical and physical properties of Se and S are similar, important differences in their chemistries result in their having very different behaviors in biological systems.

III. ANALYSIS OF SELENIUM

The analysis of Se can be accomplished by a variety of techniques, some of which are applicable to biological materials. Because these methods are reviewed in detail elsewhere,[9] the following discussion is presented to provide the reader with a general orientation concerning the methods and problems of analysis of Se, particularly in foods, feeds, and animal tissues.

Several procedures for Se analysis that have been employed for industrial purposes do not lend themselves to biological applications due to low sensitivity. These methods have been discussed by Nazarenko and Ermakov[19] and include

(i) gravimetric measurement of Se after reduction and quantitative precipitation with acid
(ii) gravimetric measurement of Se after electrolytic deposition with Cu

(iii) colorimetric titration with oxidizing agents after reduction with thiocyanate or other reducing agents

(iv) colorimetric measurement of Se hydrosols after reduction by hydrazine, $SnCl_2$, or ascorbic acid, and stabilization of the hydrosols with hydroxylamine hydrochloride, gum arabic, or gelatin

(v) colorimetric measurement of azo compounds formed by the reaction of aromatic amines with diazonium salts, the latter being produced by the oxidation of organic compounds by Se^{+4}

(vi) colorimetric measurement of complexes of Se^{-2} with phenyl-substituted thiocarbazides or semicarbazide after reduction of Se to the Se^{-2} state.

The limits of detection of Se by these procedures are generally in excess of 0.5 ppm and, for the gravimetric methods, can be several ppm. These procedures are not free of interferences by elements that can co-precipitate in the case of gravimetric methods, or by oxidizing agents in the case of the chemical methods. Therefore, they are generally not suitable for analysis of Se in biological materials.

Other methods have been found to be useful for the determination of Se in plant and animal specimens. These are presented in Table 1.3.[20-67]

Of these procedures, the fluorometric method using diaminonaphthalene (DAN) has been the most popular. This method involves oxidation of sample selenium to Se^{+4}, and reaction with DAN to form benzopiazselenol. The product fluoresces intensely at 520 nm when excited at 390 nm and can be quantified using a fluorometer. The chief advantages of the DAN procedure are its good sensitivity (ca. 0.002 ppm) and its relatively low cost. Nevertheless, the method has two potential pitfalls that must be avoided.

The first involves the loss of Se during the acid digestion of samples containing large amounts of organic materials. Adequate acid digestion of selenium in biological materials requires the complete conversion of the native forms of the mineral to Se^{+4} and/or Se^{+6}, and the subsequent reduction of any Se^{+6} formed in the process to Se^{+4} without loss of total Se. Inorganic Se can be volatilized to an appreciable extent under the conditions of acidic digestion in the presence of such large amounts of organic materials that charring occurs, especially when sulfuric acid is used as an oxidant.[53,68] The volatilized Se, probably in the form of H_2Se, can result in significant errors in the analysis of fatty materials, such as egg yolks or adipose tissues. Because Se is volatilized from acid solutions by reducing agents,[69] this loss can be avoided by maintaining strongly oxidizing conditions during digestion and by using low heat such that the oxidation of Se^{+4} to Se^{+6} proceeds relatively slowly by gradually raising the temperature of the perchloric acid solution to 210°C.[55] When the nitric-perchloric acid digestion is controlled and carefully attended, it produces satisfactory conversion to Se^{+4} even

Table 1.3

Methods of Analysis of Selenium in Biological Materials

Method	Detection limit (ppm)	Sample preparation	Known interferences	References
Polarigraphic determination of piazselenol after reaction with diaminobenzidine	0.1	Perchloric-nitric acid digestion	—	20
Cathodic stripping voltametric determination following ion-exchange separation of Se	0.001	Nitric-sulfuric acid digestion	Preconcentration of Se on anion-exchange resin	21
Inductively coupled plasma atomic emission spectrometry with hydride generation	0.0005	HCl digestion	Hydride generation matrix effects	22
Direct current plasma atomic emission spectrometry	0.02	Acid digestion	Matrix effects	23
Atom-trapping atomic absorption spectrometry	0.025	O_2 combustion	Mineral cations	24
Electrothermal atomic absorption spectrometry	0.003	Thermal stabilization with Ni	Matrix effects	25-32
Atomic absorption spectrometry with hydride generation	0.01	Acid digestion; hydride generation	Matrix effects (particularly Cu, As, Sb)	33-37
Proton-induced X-ray emission analysis	0.01	Lyophilization: pelletization	—	38-41
X-ray fluorescence spectrometry	0.04	Lyophilization, pelletization	—	42, 43
Isotope dilution with detection by combined gas-liquid chromatography/mass spectrometry	0.0005	Nitric-phosphoric acid digestion; chelation with 4-nitro-o-phenylenediamine	—	5
Neutron activation analysis using [75]Se	0.02	—	—	44-46
"Fast" neutron activation analysis using [77m]Se	0.05	—	—	6,7,44,47,47-53
Fluorimetric determination of piazselenol after reaction of Se[+4] with 3,3'-diaminobenzidine	0.01	Nitric-perchloric acid digestion, or O_2 combustion	Loss of volatilized Se if digests char	54-57
Fluorimetric determination of piazselenol after reaction of Se[+4] with 2,3-diaminonaphthalene	0.002	Nitric-perchloric acid digestion, or O_2 combustion	Loss of volatilized Se if digests char	57-67

of such forms as trimethylselenonium (a major urinary metabolite) which are resistant to oxidation by nitric acid alone.[63,67,70] Comparisons of the nitric-perchloric digestion method with direct combustion in an oxygen environment have shown that both yield comparable results.[57]

The second potential problem involves interfering fluoresence due to apparent degradation products of DAN itself, which can produce fluoresence.[71] These can be avoided by purifying the DAN reagent by recrystallization from water in the presence of sodium sulfite and activated charcoal,[72] or by stabilizing the DAN reagent with HCl and extracting with hexane.[62] Several investigators have incorporated these procedures into methods using DAN that are very convenient for use in the routine analysis of Se in biological materials.[64-66]

Conventional atomic absorption spectroscopy (AAS) has not been suitable for the determination of Se in biological samples due to the generally high limit of detection (ca. 0.1 ppm) by that procedure. Variant AAS methods, however, have been developed with sensitivities adequate for biological use. One such method involves hydride generation of sample Se followed by quantitative detection by AAS.[36,37] This method requires only small sample sizes (e.g., 0.1 ml of serum), has adequate sensitivity (ca. 0.01 ppm), and the hydride generation step has been automated. However, it suffers from possible interferences due to other elements that can form hydrides (e.g., Cu, As, Sb). Of these, the most serious interference is due to Cu; steps must be taken to remove Cu by the use of HCl,[34] tellurite,[73] or thiourea.[37] Better sensitivity has been obtained using electrothermal AAS. This method avoids the problems associated with wet digestion by employing high temperature oxidation in a graphite furnace. Use of high temperature (e.g., atomization at 2400°C) reduces interferences due to nonspecific absorption of organic compounds and non-Se salts, but introduces the problem of volatility of Se under such conditions. This problem can be avoided by the use of salts for the thermal stabilization.[74] In practice, electrothermal AAS has sensitivity for Se at ca. 0.003 ppm[30,31]; with the use of a Zeeman-effect background correction system, sensitivities approaching 0.001 ppm have been reported.[32]

Plasma atomic emission spectrometry (PAES) has not been used widely for the analysis of Se in biological materials. Although very good sensitivity (ca. 0.001 ppm) has been reported using inductively coupled PAES,[22] matrix effects present such a great amount of interference that most laboratories are not able to obtain reasonable sensitivity by this method. Direct current PAES has not had adequate sensitivity for biological use.

Instrumental neutron activation analysis (INAA) of Se offers the advantages of applicability to small sample sizes and relative ease of sample preparation. Although the greatest sensitivity (ca. 0.02 ppm) by this method is obtained by measuring ^{75}Se, its use necessitates lengthy irradiation (100 hrs), and long periods of post-irradiation holding (60 days) and counting (2 hrs). Greater economy by increased sample throughput has been achieved, at the expense of sensitivity, by the use of the short-lived (17.38 sec half-life) [77m]Se. This isotope can be irradiated (5 sec), decayed (15 sec), and counted (25 sec) very quickly in an automated system.[51] Due to the ease of this procedure as well as to its nondestructive nature, some investigators with access to research reactors have found instrumental neutron activation analysis useful for the measurement of Se. Nevertheless, the utility of the "fast" method is limited at the present time by its relatively low sensitiviy, rendering it unsuitable for accurate quantitation of such low concentrations of Se as are found in tissues of animals chronically deficient in the element.

The measurement of Se by proton-induced X-ray emission (PIXE) offers the potential advantage of simultaneous elemental analysis of biological materials. This method involves proton bombardment of target atoms (the sample) to cause loss of inner shell electrons and their consequent replacement by electrons from the outer shell. The X-rays emitted during that transition are characteristic of the energy differences between electron shells and are, therefore, identifiable and quantifiable. At the present time, the sensitivity of this procedure for the determination of Se (ca. 0.01 ppm)[40] makes it useful for many biological purposes, especially when simultaneous elemental analysis may be needed; however, it is not sensitive enough for the accurate determination of very low tissue levels.

X-ray fluorescence spectrometry offers another nondestructive technique for multi-element analysis[42,43]; however, its sensitivity for Se does not compare favorably with other methods available for biological use.

A procedure for determining Se by double isotope dilution has been developed.[5] This method involves the use of two stable isotopes of Se as tracer ([76]Se) and internal standard ([82]Se). Samples spiked with a known quantity of the internal standard are digested in nitric-phosphoric acid, undigested lipids are removed with chloroform, and hydrochloric acid is used to reduce any Se^{+6} to Se^{+4}. Selenite is reacted with 4-nitro-o-phenylenediamine to form 5-nitropiazselenol, and the nitropiazselenonium ion cluster is determined by combined gas-liquid chromatography/mass spectrometry. The native Se in the sample is calculated from the measured isotope ratios, using the [80]Se naturally present in the sample. Reamer and Veillon[5] have carefully developed this technique and have reported a sensitivity of less than 0.001 ppm. Their method employs a rapid digestion, which avoids several of the problems associated with the use of perchloric acid, and is capable of fully oxidizing the often problematic trimethylselenonium.[5] It thus appears to be suitable for biologic measurements and has been put to such use already.[75]

A IUPAC interlaboratory (12 sites) comparison of the more widely used methods for the determination of Se in clinical materials[76] found statistically significant differences among the mean concentrations reported for Se in lyophilized human serum analyzed by either (a) acid-digestion/DAN-fluorometry, (b) electrothermal AAS, (c) acid-digestion/hydride generation AAS, or (d) acid-digestion/isotope dilution mass spectrometry, with slightly higher values reported by the first procedure. The four methods compared very favorably for the analysis of pooled lyophilized urine samples. However, only the fluorometric method showed homogeneity of variance among laboratories.

The DAN fluorometric procedure remains the most widely used method for the analysis of Se in biological materials due to its good sensitivity and good reliability. Despite the tedious nitric-perchloric acid digestion which it entails, the operating costs of the method are not great because the only instrumentation required is a good quality fluorometer. Therefore, this procedure is the method of choice for many biomedical laboratories. Newer methods, including electrothermal AAS, AAS with hydride generation, PIXE, "fast" INAA, and isotope dilution with gas-liquid chromatography/mass spectrometry, offer good options for biological investigations, but these methods generally require large amounts of background development with large start-up costs. As these methods improve, future investigations will probably employ them more extensively.

REFERENCES

1. Chizhikov, D. M., and Shchastlivyi., V. P., *Selenium and Selenides,* Collet Publ. Co., London, 1968.
2. Crystal, R. G., Elemental selenium: structure and properties, in *Organic Selenium Compounds: Their Chemistry and Biology,* Klayman, D. L., and Gunther, W. H. H., Eds., Wiley, New York, 1962, Chap. 2.
3. Spector, W. S., *Handbook of Toxicology,* Volume 1, W. B. Saunders Co., Philadelphia, 1956, 340.
4. Janghorbani, M., Ting, B. T. G., and Young, V., Use of stable isotopes of selenium in human metabolic studies: development of analytical methodology, Am. J. Clin. Nutr., 34, 2816, 1981.
5. Reamer, D. C., and Veillon, C., A double isotope dilution method for using stable selenium isotopes in metabolic tracer studies: analysis by gas chromatography/mass spectrometry (GC/MS), J. Nutr., 113, 786, 1983.
6. McKown, D. M., and Morris, J. S., Rapid measurement of selenium in biological samples using instrumental neutron activation analysis, J. Radioanal. Chem., 43, 411, 1978.
7. McKnown, D. M., and Morris, J. S., Selenium analysis methodology and applications, Trace Subs. Envir. Hlth., 11, 338, 1977.
8. Klayman, D. L., and Gunther, W. H. H., *Organic Selenium Compounds: Their Chemistry and Biology,* Wiley, New York, 1973.

9. Ihnat, M., *Occurrence and Distribution of Selenium,* CRC Press, Boca Raton, Florida, 1986 (in press).

10. Rosenfeld, I., and Beath, O.A., *Selenium: Geobotany, Biochemistry, Toxicity and Nutrition,* Academic Press, New York, 1964.

11. Levander, O.A., Selected aspects of the comparative metabolism and biochemistry of selenium and sulfur, Trace Elements Human Hlth., 2, 135, 1976.

12. Huber, R. E., and Criddle, R. S., Comparison of chemical properties of selenocysteine and selenocystine with their sulfur analogs, Arch Biochem. Biophys., 122, 164, 1967.

13. Painter, E. P., The chemistry and toxicity of selenium compounds with special reference to the selenium problem, Chem. Rev., 28, 179, 1941.

14. Ganther, H. E., Selenotrisulfides: formation by reaction of thiols with selenious acids, Biochemistry, 7, 2898m 1968.

15. Martin, J. L., Selenium assimilation in animals, in *Organic Selenium Compounds: Their Chemistry and Biology,* Klaymann, D. L., and Gunther, W. H. H., eds., Wiley, New York, 1973, 663.

16. Jenkins, K. J., Evidence for the absence of selenocysteine and selenomethionine in the serum proteins of chicks administered selenite, Can. J. Biochem., 46, 1417, 1968.

17. Jenkins, K. J., Hidiroglou, M., and Ryan, J. F., Intravascular transport of selenium by chick serum proteins, Can. J. Physiol. Pharmacol., 47, 459, 1969.

18. Ganther, H. E., and Corcoran, C., Selenotrisulfides II. Cross-linking of reduced pancreatic ribonuclease with selenium, Biochemistry, 8, 2557, 1969.

19. Nazarenko, I. I., and Ermakov, A. N., *Analytical Chemistry of Selenium and Tellurium,* Wiley, New York, 1972.

20. Christian, G. D., Knoblock, E. C., and Purdy, W. C., Polarigraphic determination of selenium in biological materials, J. Assoc. Offic. Anal. Chem., 48, 877, 1965.

21. Adelojiu, S. B., Bond, A. M., Briggs, M. H., and Hughes, H. C., Stripping voltametric determination of selenium in biological materials by direct calibration, Anal. Chem., 55, 2076, 1983.

22. deOliveira, E., McLaren, J. W., and Berman, S. S., Simultaneous determination of arsenic, antimony and selenium in marine samples by inductively coupled plasma atomic emission spectrometry, Anal. Chem., 55, 2047, 1983.

23. Urasa, I. T., Determination of arsenic, boron, carbon, phosphorus, selenium and silicon in natural waters by direct current plasma atomic emission spectrometry, Anal. Chem., 56, 904, 1984.

24. Lau, C. M., Ure, A. M., and West, T. A., The determination of selenium by atom-trapping atomic absorption spectrometry, Anal. Chim. Acta 141, 213, 1982.

25. Pierce, F. D., and Brown, H. R., Comparison of inorganic interferences in atomic absorption spectrometric determination of arsenic and selenium, Anal. Chem., 49, 1417, 1977.

26. Ihnat, M., and Thompson, B. K., Acid digestion, Hydride evolution atomic absorption spectrophotometric method for determining arsenic and selenium in foods: part II. Assessment of collaborative study, J. Assoc. Offic. Anal. Chem. 63, 814, 1980.

27. Varo, P., and Koivistoinen, P., An intercalibration of selenium analyses, Kemia Kemi, 8, 238, 1981.

28. Kumpulainen, J., and Koivistoinen, P., Interlaboratory comparison of selenium levels in human serum, Kemia, 8, 372, 1981.

29. Subramanian, K. S., and Meranger, J. C., Rapid hydride evolution-electrothermal atomisation atomic-absorption spectrophotometric method for determining arsenic and selenium in human kidney and liver, Analyst, 107, 157, 1982.

30. Alfthan, G., and Kumpalainen, J., Determination of selenium in small volumes of blood plasma and serum by electrothermal atomic absorption spectrometry, Anal. Chim. Acta, 140, 221, 1982.

31. Kumpalainen, J., Raittila, A. M., Lehto, J., and Koivistoinen, P., Electrothermal atomic absorption spectrometric determination of selenium in foods and diets, J. Assoc. Off. Anal. Chem., 66, 1129, 1983.

32. Carnick, G. R., Manning, D. C., and Slavin, W., Determination of selenium in biological materials with platform furnace atomic absorption spectroscopy with Zeeman background correction, Analyst, 108, 1297, 1983.

33. Van Loon, J. C., Metal speciation by chromatography/atomic spectrometry, Anal. Chem., 51, 1139, 1979.

34. Vijan, P. N., and Leung, D., Reduction of chemical interference and speciation studies in the hydride generation-atomic absorption method for selenium, Anal. Chim. Acta, 120, 141, 1980.

35. Uchida, H., Shimoishi, Y., and Toei, K., Gas chromatographic determination of selenium (II,0), -(IV), and -(VI) in natural waters, Environ. Sci. Technol., 14, 541, 1980.

36. Lloyd, B., Holt, P., and Delves, H. T., Determination of selenium in biological samples by hydride generation and atomic-absorption spectroscopy, Analyst, 107, 927, 1982.

37. Bye, R., Engvik, L., and Lund, W., Thiourea as a complexing agent for reduction of copper interference in the determination of selenium by hydride generation/atomic absorption spectrometry, Anal. Chem., 55, 2457, 1983.

38. Maenhart, W., DeRev, L., Tomza, U., and Versieck, J., The determination of trace elements in commercial human serum albumin solutions by proton-induced x-ray emission spectrometry and neutron activation analysis, Anal. Chim. Acta, 136, 301, 1982.

39. Lecomte, R., Landsberger, S., and Monaro, S., Evaluation of trace element sensitivities in PIXE analysis of ions—temperature-ashed serum samples, Int. J. Appl. Radiat. Isot., 33, 121, 1982.

40. Hyvoneu-Dabek, M., Nikkineu-Vilkki, P., and Dabek, J. T., Selenium and other elements in human maternal and umbilical serum, as determined simultaneously by proton-induced x-ray emission, Clin. Chem. 30, 529, 1984.

41. Berti, M., Buso, G., Colautti, P., Moschini, G., Stievano, B. M., and Tregnaghi, C., Determination of selenium in blood serum by proton-induced x-ray emission, Anal. Chem., 49, 1313, 1977.

42. Strausz, K. I., Purdham, J. J., and Strausz, O. P., X-ray fluorescence spectrometric determination of selenium in biological materials, Anal. Chem., 47, 2032, 1975.

43. Milman, N., Laursen, J., Podenphant, J., and Staun-Olsen, P., Iron, copper, zinc and selenium in human liver tissue measured by x-ray fluorescence spectrometry, Scand. J. Clin. Lab. Invest, 43, 691, 1983.

44. Bowen, H. J. M., and Cawse, P. A., The determination of selenium in biological material by radioactivation, Analyst, 88, 721, 1963.

45. Abbord, S., Schlesinger, T., Weingarten, R., Lavi, N., Sadeh, T., David, M., and Fuerman, E. J., Investigation of a possible correlation between level of selenium in the blood and skin disease by neutron activation analysis, in Selenium in Biology and Medicine, Spallholz, J. E., Martin, J. L., and Ganther, H. E., Eds., Avi Publ. Co., Westport, Conn, 1976, 541.

46. Noda, K., Taniguchi, H., Suzuki, S., and Hirai, S., Comparison of the selenium contents of vegetables of the genus Allivon measured by fluorometry and neutron activation analysis, Agric. Biol. Chem., 47,613,1983.

47. Filby, R. H., and Yakeley, W. L., Determination of selenium in eye-lenses by neutron activation analysis, Radiochem. Radioanal. Lett., 26, 89, 1976.

48. McConnell, K. P., Broghamer, W. L., Jr., Blotchy, A. J., and Hurt, O. H., Selenium levels in human blood and tissues in health and disease, J. Nutr., 105, 1026, 1975.

49. Diksic, M., and McGrady, M., Fast determination of selenium in biological materials by instrumental neutron activation analysis, Radiochem. Radioanal. Lett., 26, 89, 1976.

50. Primm, P., Anderson, H. D., and Morris, J. S., The effects of dialysis time on selenium loss from human blood sera, Trans. Mo. Acad. Sci., 13, 117, 1979.

51. Morris, J. S., McKown, D. M., Anderson, H. D., May, M., Primm, P., Cordts, M., Gebhardt, D., Crowson, S., and Spate, V., The determination of selenium in samples having medical and nutritional interest using a fast instrumental neutron activation analysis procedure, in *Selenium in Biology and Medicine,* Spallholz, J. E., Martin, J. L., and Ganther, H. E., Eds., Avi Publ. Co., Westport, Conn., 1981, 438.

52. Bem, H. E., Determination of selenium in the environment and in biological material, Envir. Hlth. Perspect., 37, 183, 1981.

53. Morris, J. S., Stampfer, M. J., and Willett, W., Dietary selenium in humans: toenails as an indicator, Biol. Trace Elem. Res., 5, 529, 1983.

54. Cousins, F. B., A fluorimetric microdetermination of selenium in biological material, Australian J. Exptl Biol. Med. Sci. 38, 11, 1960.

55. Dye, W. B., Bretthauer, E., Seim, H. J., and Blincoe, C., Fluorometric determination of selenium in plants and animals with 3,3′ prime-diaminobenzidine, Anal. Chem., 35, 1687, 1963.

56. Grant, A. B., Observations on analysis of selenium in plant and animal tissues and in soil samples, N. Zealand J. Sci., 6, 577, 1963.

57. Watkinson, J. H., Fluorometric determination of selenium in biological materials with 2,3-diaminonapthalene, Anal. Chem., 32, 981, 1966.

58. Allaway, W. H., and Cary, E. E., Determination of submicrogram amounts of selenium in biological materials, Anal. Chem., 36, 1359, 1964.

59. Cukor, P., Walzcyk, J., and Lott, P. F., The application of isotopic dilution analysis to the fluorometric determination of selenium in plant materials, Anal. Chim. Acta, 30, 473, 1946.

60. Cummins, L. M., Martin, J. L., and Magg, D. D., A rapid method for the determination of selenium in biological material, Anal. Chem., 37, 430, 1965.

61. Olson, O. E., Fluorometric analysis of selenium in plants, J. Assoc. Offic. Anal. Chem. 52, 627, 1969.

62. Wilkie, J. B., and Young, M., Improvement in the 2,3-diaminonaphthalene reagent for microfluorescent determination of selenium in biological materials, Agric. Food Chem., 18, 944, 1970.

63. Olson, O. E., Palmer, I. S., and Cary, E. E., Modification of the official fluorometric method for selenium in plants, J. Assoc. Offic. Anal Chem., 58, 117, 1975.

64. Brown, M. W., and Watkinson, J. H., An automated fluorometric method for the determination of nanogram quantities of selenium, Anal. Chim. Acta, 89, 29, 1977.

65. Spallholz, J. E., Collins, G. F., and Schwarz, K., A single test tube method for the fluorometric microdetermination of selenium, Bioinorganic Chem., 9, 435, 1978.

66. Whetter, P. A., and Ullrey, D. E., Improved fluorometric method for determining selenium, J. Assoc. Offic. Anal. Chem., 61, 927, 1978.

67. Lalonde, L., Jean, Y., Roberts, K. D., Chapdelaine, A., and Bleau, G., Fluorometry of selenium in serum and urine, Clin. Chem., 28, 172, 1982.

68. Gorsuch, T. T., Radiochemical investigation on the recovery for analysis of trace elements, Analyst, 84, 135, 1959.

69. Bock, R., and Jacob, D., Die bestimmung von selenspuren, Z. Anal. Chem., 200, 81, 1964.

70. Janghorbani, M., Ting, B. T. G., Nahapetian, A., and Young, V. R., Conversion of urinary selenium to selenium (IV) by wet oxidation, Anal. Chem. 54, 1188, 1982.
71. Cukor, P., and Lott, P. F., The kinetics of the reaction of selenium (IV) with 2, 3-diaminonaphthalene, J. Phys. Chem., 69, 3232, 1965.
72. Parker, C. A., and Harvey, L. G., Luminescence of some piazselenols, Analyst, 87, 558, 1962.
73. Kirkbright, G. F., and Taddia, M., Use of tellurium (IV) to reduce interferences from some metal ions in the determination of selenium by hydride generation and atomic absorption spectrometry, At. Absorpt. Newslett., 18, 68, 1979.
74. Ediger, R. D., Atomic absorption analysis with the graphite furnace using matrix modification, At. Absorpt Newslett., 14, 127, 1975.
75. Swanson, C. A., Reamer, D. C., Veillon, C., and Levander, O. A., Intrinsic labeling of chicken products with a stable isotope of selenium (76Se), J. Nutr., 113, 793, 1983.
76. Thomassen, Y., Ihnat, M., Veillon, C., and Wolynet, M. S., IUPAC interlaboratory trial for the detrmination of selenium in clinical materials, in *Proceedings of the Third International Symposium on Selenium in Biology and Medicine,* Combs, G. F., Jr., Spallholz, J. E., Levander, O. A., and Oldfield, J. E., Eds., Avi Publishing Co., Westport, Conn., 1986.

2

SELENIUM IN THE ENVIRONMENT

I. SELENIUM IN MINERAL DEPOSITS

Selenium is widely distributed in the earth's crust with an abundance that has been estimated to be approximately 0.09 ppm.[1,2] It is most frequently found in greatest abundance in igneous rock, particularly in mineral sulfide ores, where the Se contents may be in excess of 1000 ppm.[3-7] Selenium forms selenides or sulfoselenides with Cu, Ag, Pb, and Hg; in fact, the sulfidic copper ores of North America and the Soviet Union (some of which have been reported to contain as much as 24% Se[3]) are the principal commercial source of Se, which is obtained as a by-product of the electrolytic refining of copper.[8] More than 80% of the world's annual production of almost 1100 tons of Se comes from this source. Whereas copper sulfide ores represent point sources of Se in the environment, sources of greater agronomic significance are the sedimentary rocks, which comprise the principal parent material for cultivated soils. Sedimentary rocks generally contain lower levels of Se than do igneous formations, which obtained Se from volcanic discharges during earlier geological ages; however, the Se provided by sedimentary rocks is important in determining the concentrations of Se in soils. Shales, which comprise over half of all sedimentary rocks, have been found to contain in general a few ppm of Se. However, some, such as the Permian shales of Wyoming, USA, have been found to contain several hundred ppm of Se, and the Pierre and Niobrara shales of the seleniferous area of the United States Great Plains have been found to contain approximately 2 ppm.[5] Limestones and sandstones generally contain lower and more variable amounts of Se; however, some carbonaceous deposits of these materials may have as much as 30 ppm and 130 ppm, respectively, of Se.[5,9,10] Rock phosphates, particularly those from the western phosphate field of the USA, have been found to contain from a few to nearly 180 ppm Se[11]; the use of these materials as fertilizers may make them significant agricultural sources of Se.

Crude sulfur has been found to contain from a few ppm to as much as 8350 ppm Se.[86,87] Coal and oil can contain substantial amounts of Se, which are released into the environment when they are burned; samples of Texas crude oil contained less than 0.35 ppm Se, but coal from other parts of the United States has been found to contain 1-5 ppm Se.[9] Coal from Enshi County, Hubei Province, The People's Republic of China (P.R.C.), has been found to contain as much as 90,000 ppm Se.[12,13] This unusually concentrated source of Se is thought to be a factor in the frank selenosis of humans and animals that has been diagnosed in that locale (see Chapter 11).

II. SELENIUM IN SOILS

Selenium enters soils primarily as a result of the weathering of Se-containing rocks, although volcanic activity, dusts (e.g., in the vicinity of the burning of coal), some phosphate fertilizers, and some waters can also be sources of Se for soils. Therefore, soils in the vicinity of high-Se mineral deposits are generally, but not always, rich in Se. For example, soils derived from the Se-rich Niobara and Pierre shales of South Dakota tend to be seleniferous; however, soils derived from other Se-rich formations in the same state do not contain particulary high levels of Se.[3] Surveys in the USA[15-17] have shown that although some seleniferous soils contain as much as 90 ppm Se, most nonseleniferous soils contain appreciably less than 2 ppm. Therefore, factors in addition to the Se contents of parent rocks are important determinants of the concentration of Se in soils. These factors include soil pH, oxidation-reduction conditions, moisture level, and degree of aeration.[3,5,18]

Much of the Se that is released from rocks weathering under alkaline and well-aerated conditions is oxidized to form selenates. Selenates are highly soluble in water and do not form stable adsorption complexes. Therefore, they are readily taken up by plants or are easily leached into ground water. These types of soils are usually found in semi-arid or poorly drained areas; when they are irrigated, Se may be transported into, or leached out of, these soils depending upon the selenate content of the irrigation water. In contrast, Se released from rocks under acid and very moist (i.e., poorly aerated) conditions is present in insoluble reduced forms (elemental Se and selenides) and selenite, which can form stable adsorption complexes with ferric hydroxide. Therefore, Se released under the latter soil conditions is poorly available to plants and is not readily transported by ground water. In soils that are slightly acid to neutral, Se is present in organic compounds formed from the vegetation growing there. Harvesting of crops from such soils can result in depletion of soil Se by interrupting the replacement of these organic Se compounds into the soil.

Seleniferous soils can, therefore, be of two types with respect to the availability of their Se to plants. Those that are alkaline and fairly dry can support plant Se concentrations great enough to be toxic to animals. Such toxic seleniferous soils are found in much of the northern Great Plains (i.e., North Dakota, South Dakota, Wyoming, Montana, Nebraska, Kansas, Colorado) and the Southwest (Utah, Arizona, New Mexico) of the USA[3]; in Limerick, Mead, and Tipperary counties, Ireland[19-22]; in Enshi County, Hubei Province (P.R.C.)[13,14]; and in parts of Colombia,[23,24] Venezuela,* and Israel.[29] Many of these soils contain free calcium carbonate[3]; soil Se content averages about 4-5 ppm, but may be as great as 80 ppm in some places.[16] The predominant amount of Se in alkaline toxic seleniferous soils is water-soluble and is thought to be selenate.[30] Those soils that are produced from Se-rich rocks under acid and moist conditions can be seleniferous but not toxic. Such soils are found in Hawaii and Puerto Rico; they contain relatively high concentrations of Se (e.g., as much as 15 ppm) but with very low amounts that are water-soluble.[31] The consequent low availability of Se from such acid soils for plants does not support the uptake of toxic levels of Se by vegetation in these areas.

Selenium in soils is present in varying mixtures of insoluble selenides and elemental Se, insoluble pyritic selenite complexes, soluble selenates, and organic Se compounds. The latter forms, produced from soil microorganisms, have greatest solubility in alkaline soil conditions. Therefore, the amount of water-soluble Se in soils varies considerably and does not correlate with total soil Se. Studies by Byers et al.[15] and Olson et al.[32] demonstrated this lack of correlation in samples of soils that ranged in water-soluble Se from 0.2 to 41.4 ppm and 0.05 to 38 ppm, respectively, and in total Se from 3.7 to 90 ppm and 2.7 to 38 ppm, respectively. In those studies, the amounts of water-soluble Se in seleniferous soils ranged from less than 4% to more than 60% of total soil Se. Therefore, the Se available to plants can vary tremendously among soils from different locations, and the total soil Se level is a poor predictor of the availability of the element to plants.

*Although the Se contents of Venezuelan soils have not been reported, the findings of Jaffe et al.[25-28] of very high Se content of foods and feeds in that county indicate that it, too, has seleniferous soils.

Several regions of the world have soils that contain low concentrations (i.e., less than 0.5 ppm total Se) of Se. These include Denmark[33] and eastern Finland[34]; New Zealand[35-40]; a long belt extending from northeast to south central China (P.R.C.) and including parts of Heilongjiang, Jilin, Liaoning, Hebei, Shanxi, Shaanxi, Sichuan, and Zhejiang Provinces and Inner Mongolia, P.R.C.[41-47]; eastern British Columbia, west central Alberta, northern Ontario, southeastern Quebec, and the Atlantic Provinces of Canada[48-50];* and western Australia;* and the Pacific Northwest, Northeast, and Southeastern seaboard of the USA.[17,51,52] Most of these soils were formed from parent materials that were largely either recent low-Se volcanic deposits (e.g., U.S. Pacific Northwest); granites and very old metamorphic rocks (e.g., parts of Montana, USA); low-Se tertiary volcanic rocks (e.g., parts of Arizona and New Mexico, USA); very old sedimentary rocks (e.g., Northeastern USA); or coastal deposits from highly weathered land masses (e.g., U.S. South Atlantic seaboard).

III. SELENIUM IN WATER AND AIR

Selenium enters water as soluble selenites and selenates and as suspended particles of insoluble and organic forms of the element. Therefore, the greatest concentrations of Se are found in water systems that drain seleniferous soils. This is particularly true for alkaline aerated waters in which redox conditions favor selenate.[53] Such waters from wells in South Dakota, USA, have been found to contain as much as 330 ppb Se[54,55]; one well in Colorado, USA, was found to contain 9000 ppb Se.[56] Springs flowing from Niabarra shale in South Dakota, USA, contained 70-400 ppb Se[57]; Beath[58] reported one spring that contained 1600 ppb Se. More recent studies by Valentine et al.[59-61] have shown that the public water supplies of Jade Hills and Red Butte, Wyoming, and Grants, New Mexico, USA, contain 174-202, 363-560, and 26-1800 ppb Se, respectively.

Most water systems contain only very low concentrations of Se. This is due to the facts that most waters do not drain seleniferous soils, and that, in those that do so, a susbstantial amount of Se is removed from water by precipitation with basic oxides (e.g., hydrous ferric oxide). Therefore, it is not unusual to find lake[62] or well[54,55] waters in seleniferous areas with little or no detectable Se. Smith et al.[54,55] were unable to detect Se in 34 of a total of 44 wells sampled in a seleniferous area of South

---

*Although soil Se concentrations were not stated, the report of Gardiner et al.[51] indicated that the occurrence of Se-responsive myopathies in sheep was associated with particular soil types in western Australia that produced forage crops of low (e.g., 0.02-0.04 ppm) Se content, implicating that region as one with soil having a low level of water-soluble Se.

Dakota, USA. Surface water in Colorado, USA,[63] and well water in a low-Se area of Oregon, USA,[64] was found to contain ca. 1 ppb Se. Taylor[65] reported that U.S. public water supplies generally contain less than 8 ppb Se, and a survey of the major watersheds of the USA[66] found that all but two contained less than 10 ppb Se.

Irrigation of seleniferous soils can markedly increase the concentrations of Se in downstream water systems. Studies by Williams and Byers[67] demonstrate this phenomenon. They found that the Colorado River contained ca. 1 ppb Se at points upstream from tributaries that drained soils derived from the seleniferous Mancos shales. The tributary waters contained as much as 2700 ppb Se, the addition of which raised the Se content of the Colorado River to ca. 3 ppb when sampled downstream. Byers et al.[15] found similar increases of 8- to 80-fold in the Se content of the Gunnison River in Colorado, due to its receipt of irrigation waters from seleniferous soils. Su et al.[68] found that spring waters in the highly seleniferous area of Enshi County, Hubei Province, P.R.C., contained very low (e.g., 1-2 ppb) concentrations of Se at the highest elevations, but increased in Se content to ca. 200 ppb when sampled at low elevations, after having drained deposits of coal containing several thousand ppm Se.

Schutz and Turekian[69] found that the major oceans contain only low concentrations (average 0.09 ppb) of Se. This low level is thought to be due to the precipitation of Se with metal oxides.

Most of the Se found in air is in aerosol and large particulate forms that result from windblown dusts, volcanic action, and discharges from such human activities as the combustion of fossil fuels, the smelting and refining of nonferrous metals, and the manufacturing of glass and ceramics. These sources contribute to atmospheric concentrations of Se in the nanogram per cubic meter range in most samples of ambient air.[70-72] Of the human-made sources, the combustion of fossil fuels probably contributes the greatest share of Se to the air. While crude oil generally contains less than 0.35 ppm Se,[9] coal has been found to contain greater and more variable amounts. A survey by Pillay et al.[9] found coal from 20 U.S. states to contain 1-5 ppm Se, and coal in Enshi County, Hubei Province, P.R.C., has been found to contain as much as 90,000 ppm Se.[12,13] Although the combustion of coal and oil results in the release of Se as selenium dioxide (SeO_2), this form (which contains Se^{+4}) is generally reduced to elemental Se (Se^0) by sulfur dioxide produced concurrently. The predominant amount of elemental Se is carried in flyash, samples of which have been found to contain 1.2-16.5 ppm Se in the USA.[73] In plants which reduce the output of airborne particulates by electrostatic precipitation of flyash, the atmospheric discharge of Se from the combustion of fossil fuels is markedly reduced.

The annual discharge of Se to the atmosphere in the USA was estimated to be less than 900 tons in 1969-1971, 1240 tons in 1978, and 1560 tons in 1983.[74-76] Of the 986 tons that Davis[94] estimated were disharged in 1969, 65% was thought to result from the combustion of coal. Other major sources were discharges from the manufacture of glass and ceramics (21% of the total), discharges from metallurgical processing (9% of the total), and discharges from the combustion of other fuels (7% of the total). Other sources of atmospheric Se include discharges from the incineration of paper,[77,98] rubber tires,[79] garbage and trash[80,81]; however, these probably contribute no more than 1% of the total human-made atmospheric discharges of Se according to the estimates of Davis.[74]

Aerosol and large particulate forms of Se are generally not directly available for plants and animals. This is particularly true for Se discharged from combustions, most of which is rapidly reduced to Se^0 and cannot be used in biological systems. However, in addition to those forms of Se, air can also contain low levels of volatile Se compounds, which are produced by and can be utilized by biological systems. The predominant volatile Se compound which has been found in ambient air is dimethylselenide $[(CH_3)_2Se]$.[82,83] It is produced enzymically by soil microorganisms[84-88] and plants,[89-91] and is released by growing plants[89-91] and by drying plant materials.[92] Whereas most plant species release dimethylselenide, some Se-accumulator species have been found to release dimethyldiselenide $[(CH_3)_2SeSe(CH_3)_2]$.[89,91] Although dimethylselenide is normally produced at very low levels by animals, it is a major excretory metabolite of animals exposed to high levels of Se (see Chapter 4) and is responsible for the "garlic breath" of selenotic animals.

The volatile forms of Se in the atmosphere can be absorbed and assimilated, at least in part, by plants[93-96]; Zieve and Peterson[95] found that as much as 2% of the total Se retained in the shoots of barley, tomato, radish, and broad red clover can be derived from atmospheric dimethylselenide.

IV. UPTAKE OF SELENIUM BY PLANTS

Despite early reports that suggested that Se may be required for the growth of the Se-accumulator species *Astragalus beathii* and *A. racemosus*,[96,97] subsequent investigations[93,98,99] have failed to confirm the premise that Se may have essentiality in plant nutrition. Nevertheless, plants take up Se from the soil according to the amount and availability of the Se present. The availability of soil Se to plants is determined primarily by the soil characteristics which influence the water solubility of Se. Plant uptake of Se varies with soil pH; thus, the best utilization of soil Se is achieved by plants growing in alkaline soil conditions.[100-104] Soil clay content also influences the utilization of Se by plants; Se uptake is generally better from sandy soils than from loamy soils.[103,104] Poorest utilization of soil Se is observed among plants growing in soils that are acid to neutral, in which selenite and reduced forms of Se are favored, and that are loamy, thus fixing the otherwise soluble selenite and rendering it unavailable for uptake by plants. Cary and Allaway[103] showed that while the accumulation of Se by alfalfa was greater in soils of relatively high pH (i.e., pH 7.3-7.8 vs. pH 5.4-6.1), the positive effect of soil pH on Se uptake was greater in sandy soils than in loams.

Differences in soil conditions, which result from differences in both soil composition and climate, can markedly influence the utilization of soil Se by plants. In this regard, Gissel-Nielsen[105] contrasted the situations found in Scandinavia and India. The soils of both areas have been found to contain comparable levels of Se (0.01-0.04 ppm).[33,106] However, Indian soils tend to be alkaline with low precipitation, and Se is present mainly as selenate, which is not fixed in the soil. In contrast, Scandinavian soils are relatively acidic with great amounts of precipitation and leaching, rendering the remaining Se strongly fixed in the soil. Gissel-Nielsen[105] cited these differences in the availability of soil Se to plants in these regions as responsible for the accumulation of tissue concentrations of Se ten-fold greater in plants in India in comparison to plants in Scandinavia.

The uptake of Se by plants can be affected by altering soil chemistry. Cary and Gissel-Nielsen[107] found that the solubility (measured as extractability in 0.01 M $CaCl_2$) of native Se in both a sandy loam and a silt loam were not affected by additions of either phosphate, nitrate, or sulfate; however, the extractability of added selenite was enhanced by phosphate supplementation, and that of added selenate was enhanced by nitrate or sulfate supplementation. These findings appear to be in contrast to the antagonisms of Se uptake by plants due to fertilization with P, N, and S that have been reported[99,108-110]; however, they demonstrate that such antagonisms result from effects on the plant (e.g., interactions in absorption, differential stimulation of growth), rather than on the availability of Se from the soil. Davies and Watkinson[100] found that the application of superphosphate resulted in significant decreases (ca. 24%) in plant Se, but this effect was thought to have been due to the stimulatory effect of the fertilizer on plant growth which had a dilution effect on plant Se. Gissel-Nielsen[108] observed decreases in the Se content of barley due to phosphate as well as to nitrate. In later experiments with maize,[110] he found that application of nitrate resulted in increases in the Se content of roots, but real decreases (after correction for increased plant growth) in the Se content of the foliage. Nitrate application produced large (e.g., three- to five-fold) increases in the selenite content of roots and in the Se-containing amino acid content of leaves, both of which comprised more than one-third of the total Se in each organ, respectively, after treatment.

Sulfur can be antagonistic to the uptake of Se by plants by affecting absorption. Muth and co-workers[111,112] observed that the incidence of the Se-deficiency disease, "white muscle disease," in lambs in the low-Se area of Oregon, USA, increased after treating soils with gypsum ($CaSO_4 \cdot 2H_2O$). Such observations can be understood in view of the findings of several investigators that the uptake of Se by plants can be inhibited by S. Hurd-Karrer and Kennedy[113] showed that the Se content of winter wheat grown in a seleniferous area could be greatly reduced from toxic levels by the application of either gypsum or orthorhombic (elemental) sulfur. Gissel-Nielsen[114] also found that the addition of sulfate to the soil decreased the uptake of added Se by barley and red clover and that the antagonism was greater for selenate than for selenite. That the antagonism occurs at the level of absorption was demonstrated by Leggett and Epstein,[115] whose studies of the kinetics of sulfate absorption by barley roots showed competitive inhibition of sulfate absorption by selenate. Their results indicate that both ions show comparable affinities for theoretical binding sites on the absorptive membranes and that the antagonistic uptake is based on competition for these sites. Studies of the uptake of selenate by two species of Astragalus (including a nonconcentrator species) showed it to be an active transport process competitively inhibited by sulfate.[116,117] Other studies have shown that selenate and sulfate are mutually competitive for uptake by Chlorella vulgaris[118] and Penicillium chrysogenum.[119] Shrift and Ulrich[117] suggested that sulfate and selenate may compete at the level of binding with sulfate permease, i.e., that the enzyme could transport either compound indiscriminately.

In order to increase the Se contents of crops produced in low-Se areas, Se has been added to soils by the use of Se-enriched fertilizers, other Se-rich materials, and Se salts. Fertilizers contain variable amounts of Se depending upon the Se contents of the raw materials from which they were manufactured. Gissel-Nielsen[120] reported the following ranges for several types of fertilizers: superphosphate, 4.2-8.0 ppm Se; PK type, 3.6-5.5 ppm Se; NPK (based on sulfuric acid) type, 1.1-4.0 ppm Se; NPK (based on nitric acid) type, 0.02-0.19 ppm Se; KCl fertilizer, 0.04-0.09 ppm Se; lime, 0.033-0.037 ppm Se. The richest sources of Se in the raw materials used in fertilizer manufacture were pyrites (25-30 ppm Se), sulfuric acid made from pyrites (8.6 ppm Se), and rock phosphates (3.1-25.0 ppm Se). In studies of the utilization of the Se from NPK and PK fertilizers by barley, Gissel-Nielsen[120] found that less than 1% of the Se added to the soil was found in the tops of the plants harvested at maturity. Because Se uptake was estimated by the incorporation of ^{75}Se from fertilizer preparations labeled extrinsically with $Na_2^{75}SeO_3$, and because the Se intrinsic to the fertilizer was thought likely to be less soluble than the extrinsic label, the estimates of plant uptake were taken as maxima. Hence, the study demonstrated that the contribution of Se from such fertilizers to the total Se contents of plants is probably negligible.

The Se contents of crops and forages have been increased through the addition of seleniferous materials to the soil. Flyash, which has been used as a modifier of the physical characteristics of soils[121] and as a liming agent,[122] can also add significant amounts of Se to soils that are not rich in the element. In greenhouse experiments, Barrows and Swader[123] observed that the addition at the rate of 25% by weight to each of three types of New York State (low-Se) soils of flyash (containing 6.5 ppm Se) produced significant increases in the Se contents of several crops: corn grain, 11- to 20- fold; oats, 19- to 25-fold; alfalfa, second cutting, 2- to 12-fold; birdsfoot trefoil, first cutting, 30- to 32-fold; smooth bromegrass, first cutting, 9- to 18-fold; orchard grass, 10- to 19-fold. In field studies, Barrows and Swader[123] found that the Se contents of corn grain and of sorghum-sudangrass silage increased linearly with the amount of flyash added to the soil (corn grain Se, ppm = 0.0612 + (0.009248 × percentage flyash), r = 0.909; silage Se, ppm = 0.0564 + (0.008976 × percentage flyash), r = 0.7848), although corn yields declined at flyash levels greater than 12.5-25.0%. Studies by Furr et al.[124,125] have also demonstrated the direct relationship of plant Se content and the rate of flyash application for a number of vegetables, grains, and forages.

Selenium in flyash has very low availability to animals but can be transformed by plants into forms that animals can use. Combs et al.[126] determined that the Se present in soft coal flyash was only ca. 7% as effective as Na_2SeO_3 in preventing the Se-deficiency disease, exudative diathesis, in the chick. However, when the same flyash was used to amend soil, the Se contained in white sweet clover produced on it had biological availability for the chick of 20-25% of Na_2SeO_3. Other studies with guinea pigs,[127,128] pigs,[128,129] and chicks[126,130] have shown that volunteer plants grown on flyash or plants cultivated on flyash-amended soils can provide Se in forms which are assimilated by animals.

The Se contents of deficient soils can be increased by the application of selenite or selenate salts, and in many areas of livestock production, this practice has been found to be an effective means of preventing Se-deficiency diseases. Allaway et al.[131] traced the movement of Se, applied as Na_2SeO_3 to low-Se soil, to alfalfa grown on the soil, and then to sheep fed the alfalfa. They found that the application of Na_2SeO_3 to Se-deficient

Oregon soil at the rate of 1 ppm Se increased the Se content of alfalfa cut 2 months later from 0.01-0.04 ppm to 2.6-2.7 ppm. When it was fed to ewes, the Se-enriched alfalfa conferred protection to their lambs from the Se-responsive myopathy white muscle disease (WMD) and continued to do so for lambs born as late as 10 months after the feeding period. Residual effects were also noted on the Se content of alfalfa for up to 2 years after the application of Se to the soil. Nevertheless, less than 2% of the Se applied was taken up by alfalfa in the first five cuttings. Therefore, Allaway et al.[131] concluded that soil application was an inefficient means of providing Se- fortification for animals.

Cary and Gissel-Nielsen[107] compared the efficacies of selenite and selenate as means of fortifying plants. They found selenate to be more desirable for this purpose. A greater proportion (ca. 50%) would be expected to remain in water-soluble forms after application, thus showing better availability to plants than selenite, much of which would be fixed, especially in clay soils. They noted that, whereas selenate would be more efficiently taken up by plants (it is actively absorbed by roots in the manner of sulfate [115,116]), it also presented a greater threat of toxicity for that reason if application rates were not controlled. This conclusion is supported by the report of Fleming,[132] who found that selenate was more readily absorbed from Se-deficient soil than was selenite by red clover and perennial ryegrass, but that selenate depressed the growth of red clover at a level at which selenite was without effect on plant growth.

The topdressing of Se-deficient soils with Na_2SeO_3 was permitted by law in New Zealand in 1982. The approval of this technique for prevention of WMD in lambs, particularly on the north island, did not come without much research on efficacy and safety. Watkinson[133,134] has reviewed the recommended practices for Se topdressing. These involve the annual application of pellets containing 2.4% Na_2SeO_4 in a clay carrier. These are applied at the rate of 1 kg/ha (i.e., 10 g Se/ha) to pastures, and it has been suggested that this rate may be decreased after ca. 30 years of treatment. Farms with low stocking densities are treated on only those pastures in which ewes are grazed for 4 weeks at mating. Alternatively, application of Se (17 g/ha) to at least 5% of the pasture area has been shown to be adequate.[135] Watkinson[134] reported that these procedures result in the uptake of ca. 15% of the Se applied by pasture vegetation. He noted, however, that the concentration of pasture Se increases rapidly to peak levels within a month after topdressing, and decreases slowly thereafter reaching pretreatment levels at about 9 months. This rate of application is designed so that at peak pasture Se levels, grazing ewes should consume no more than 20 μg Se/kg body weight/day, a level that is nutritionally important and safe. Watkinson[134] has demonstrated that pasture Se content varies linearly with Se application rate, and that ewes' blood Se levels vary exponentially with peak pasture Se. Thus, a significant safety margin is inherent in Se-fortification by this topdressing method, which, at the recommended rate of 17 g Se/ha, does not affect the Se contents of streams draining treated pastures.[136] Other methods of soil Se application, including addition with superphosphate fertilizer and soil injection, have also proved effective.[137-139]

Plant Se fortification can also be accomplished by foliar application with Se salts; however, this approach has been less satisfactory due to more variable results.[42,140,141] Watkinson and Davies[140] compared the effects of foliar and soil application of Na_2SeO_3 on the uptake of Se by two common New Zealand pasture species, white clover and browntop. White clover readily absorbed Se by the foliar treatment and deposited more Se in tissues including roots than by the soil treatment. In contrast, browntop absorbed very little Se by foliar exposure and was able to utilize Se from the soil treatment much better. Gupta et al.[141] found that a single foliar application at exceptionally high levels (i.e., 1-4 kg Se as Na_2SeO_3 per hectare) to plants growing in slightly acid sandy loam was comparable to direct soil application of the same amount of Se, in terms of both the immediate increases in Se in alfalfa, timothy and barley grain, and the residual effects on subsequent croppings. However, Se applied at even the lowest rate (i.e., 1 kg/ha) produced significant decreases in the yields of each of these crops. The levels of Se that were applied by Gupta et al.[141] were 50-200 times that recommended by Watkinson[134] for annual application by topdressing; despite the beneficial residual effects that the former authors noted, such levels seem excessive and potentially hazardous.

Under normal conditions of plant exposure to Se (i.e., Se uptake from the soil), the greatest concentrations of Se are usually found in root tissues. Johnson et al.[142] measured the distribution of radioactivity from $Na_2{}^{75}SeO_3$ added to low-Se culture media of 12 species of vegetables, grains, and forages; they found that each species accumulated Se preferentially in the roots with ratios (root ^{75}Se/top ^{75}Se) that varied from 2.6 for onion to 23.4 for spinach. Similar results were reported by Broyer et al.,[93] and others[140,143,144] have shown the Se concentrations to be much greater in the roots of crop and pasture species than in the tops.

Plant species vary with respect to the Se that they can accumulate from the soil; in seleniferous soils, some species are capable of accumulating tremendous amounts of Se that would be toxic to other species. Rosenfeld and Beath[3] classified plants into three groups according to their abilities to accumulate Se when grown on seleniferous soils: (i) primary indicators, (ii) secondary absorbers, (iii) nonconcentrators. The geographic distribution of the primary indicators is restricted to seleniferous soils in which they grow naturally, often accumulating several thousand parts per million (air-dry basis) of Se. These include about two dozen species and cultivars of the genera *Astragalus, Machaeranthera* (section *Xylorhiza*), *Haplopapus* (section *Oonopsis*), and *Stanleya*. Accumulator species can attain levels of Se 100- to 10,000-fold those of most other native and crop species. One species, *A. bisulcatus*, can accumulate as much as 10,000 ppm Se (air-dry basis) and has been proposed as a potential means of biologically mining Se from seleniferous soils.*[145] Cattle and sheep grazing on pastures containing primary accumulators have long been known to suffer from the condition called "blind staggers," resulting, at least in part, from selenosis.[3]

Rosenfeld and Beath[3] classified as secondary absorbers those plants that accumulated in general 25-100 ppm Se (air-dry basis). This group includes species in the genera *Aster, Atriplex, Castilleja, Comandra, Gyria, Grindelia, Gutierrezia, Machaeranthera,* and *Mentzelia*. These species differ from the primary accumulators by having relatively more Se present as selenate, but can also be toxic to livestock. Rosenfeld and Beath[3] classified as nonconcentrators all species that ordinarily do not accumulate more than about 25 ppm Se (air-dry basis). This is the largest category, including most cultivated plant species. Selenosis in livestock from the consumption of nonconcentrator plants is possible (eg., after long-term consumption of "high-Se" grain, i.e., 5-10 ppm); however, such events are extremely rare due to the fact that, even in seleniferous areas, most nonconcentrator species do not accumulate hazardous levels.†

Table 2.1

Organic Se Compounds Reported in Plants[a]

Dimethyl selenide	Selenocysteine-selenic acid
Dimethyl diselenide	Se-methylselenocysteine
Selenomethionine	Se-methylselenomethione
Selenomethionine selenoxide	Se-propenylselenocysteine
Selenohomocysteine	selenoxide
Selenocystathionine	Se-containing peptides
Selenocysteine	Seleno-waxes

[a]From Shrift[146].

*Beath[145] calculated that, with good recovery of Se from the harvested plant, the cultivation of *A. bisulcatus* could yield as much as 6.8 kg Se/ha.

†Lakin and Byers[146] found that of wheat produced in seleniferous soils in the northern Great Plains, USA, more than 82% of samples contained 1 ppm or less of Se, and less than 8% contained more than 4 ppm Se.

Absorbed Se can be metabolized by species of all three classes to many different organic compounds. Table 2.1 presents a list of the organic forms of Se that have been reported in higher plants. Most of the seleno-compounds reported are analogs of sulfur compounds known in plant biochemistry; however, the ability to synthesize certain of these Se-containing compounds varies markedly between species that accumulate Se and those that do not. Studies by Shrift and associates[148-152] showed that the predominant Se-containing compound synthesized by Se-accumulators was Se-methylselenocysteine, whereas Se-methylselenomethionine was the predominant form synthesized by nonaccumulators. In comparative studies of the Se-containing amino acids in seven Se-accumulator species (including five species of *Astragalus*) and four nonaccumulator species of *Astragalus*, Se-methylselenomethionine was either not detected (four species) or found at low concentrations (two species) among the Se-accumulators, which instead contained high levels of Se-methylselenocysteine.[149] In contrast, the nonaccumulators contained either nondetectable or low levels of Se-methylselenocysteine, and high levels of Se-methylselenomethionine. The sulfur analog of the latter, *S*-methylmethionine, is known to occur as a natural plant metabolite[147]; the synthesis of the Se-methylselenomethionine, which occurs in several, if not most, nonaccumulator species exposed to high amounts of Se,[147,150] probably occurs by the *S*-methylmethionine pathway. In view of the fact that the nonaccumulator species, which produce Se-methylselenomethionine, show much greater sensitivity to the toxic effects of high levels of Se, it is thought that Se toxicity in plants may be due to antagonisms of Se-methylselenomethionine and normal sulfur-containing metabolites.[151] Consequently, the lack of sensitivity to Se toxicity of species that accumulate Se seems to be related to their lack of ability to produce Se- methylselenomethionine and to their ability to synthesize Se-methylselenocysteine instead. The latter compound is made initially from the metabolism of serine to form Se-cysteine, which is subsequently methylated.[153] This synthesis is stimulated by exposing the plant to selenate, but is inhibited by exposure to sulfate,[154] suggesting that it may occur by the pathway for the synthesis of *S*-methylcysteine.

Very little information is available concerning the chemical forms of Se in the tissues of nonconcentrator plants. This is indeed unfortunate because it is this category of plant species that includes the important forages and crops of importance in the Se nutrition of animals and humans. Studies of wheat indicate that, in contrast to the situation of Se-accumulators in which Se is present mainly in nonprotein forms, much of the Se in nonconcentrators is protein-bound. Early work by Franke[155] showed that the toxicant, later found to be Se, in samples of toxic (i.e., seleniferous) wheat and corn was associated with the protein fractions of those materials.

Later, Olson et al.[156] confirmed that much of the Se in naturally seleniferous wheat (i.e., 31 ppm) occurred in the gluten fraction and that almost one-half of that was in the form of selenomethionine. In studies of wheat radiolabeled by soil application of $Na_2^{75}SeO_4$, Olson et al.[156] did not detect selenocysteine either in the pronase hydrolysates of crude wheat gluten or in protein-free hot water extracts of the grain or straw. They concluded that, whereas the plant could metabolize selenate to selenomethionine, it did not metabolize it further to selenocysteine to any appreciable extent. Studies by Peterson and Butler[144] also found a Se-compound that co-chromatographed on paper with selenomethionine selenoxide.

The papers by Olson et al.[156] and Peterson and Butler[144] are frequently cited in support of the conclusion that most of the Se present in foods and feeds of plant origin is selenomethionine. While they do indicate that this is probably true for wheat, the generalization to other nonconcentrator species may be premature until further investigations of other species are made. The need for research to identify the major forms of Se in plants is greatest for those staple food and feed plants that normally contain only low levels (i.e., less than 0.1 ppm) of Se. These plants comprise major portions of diets and are, therefore, major determinants of the Se nutriture of humans and animals consuming them. When such plants contain low (i.e., less than 0.1 ppm) amounts of Se, as they usually do in most parts of the world, the efficiency with which that Se is utilized by the consuming individual can determine the nutritional adequacy with respect to Se. Differences in the typical Se contents among nonconcentrator species have been identified; these presumably relate to differences in the metabolism of Se and, therefore, to the distribution of Se among the products of its metabolism. Differences have also been demonstrated in the biological availabilities of Se in various foods and feeds; these differences are also presumed to relate, at least in part, to the major chemical forms of Se. Therefore, further studies to elucidate the identification of the major forms of Se in foods and feedstuffs will be necessary to understand and to predict the biological availability of Se in the mixed diets of humans and animals.

V. GEO-BOTANICAL MAPPING OF AREAS OF SELENIUM DEFICIENCY AND EXCESS

The toxicity of Se-accumulator plants was cause for the study of their geographic distribution. These plants were recognized to be toxic to grazing animals, and there was thus a practical need to learn where they were found. After Se was recognized to be one of the toxic factors in several of these species, it was possible to describe the distribution of both the primary indicator and the secondary absorber species with reference to the concentrations of Se in soils. Therefore, the distribution of seleniferous vegetation and, hence, the distribution of seleniferous soils in the USA was mapped.[3]

It was not until Se was recognized to be an essential nutrient for animals that the geographic distribution of Se-deficient soils and, hence, of Se-deficient forages and crops, was appreciated. Early reports described enzootic Se-responsive diseases of livestock. These included muscular dystrophies of sheep, cattle, horses, swine and poultry ("white muscle disease"), and exudative diathesis in poultry, which occurred in parts of New Zealand,[157] Great Britain,[158] and the USA [159] The occurrence of these diseases stimulated interest in mapping areas in which animals and, perhaps, people may be at high risk to nutritional Se deficiency. Muth and Allaway[159] produced such a map of the USA showing the noncoincidence of areas of white muscle diseases and of areas where soils were formed from seleniferous parent materials. Allaway and Hodgson[160] found that the Se contents of forages in areas of enzootic white muscle disease of the United States were consistently less than 0.1 ppm (air-dry basis). They noted that white muscle diseases were rare in areas in which forages contained more than that amount of Se. In view of this asssociation of low forage Se levels with the incidence of white muscle diseases in animals, Kubota *et al.*[161] surveyed the distribution of Se in more than 1000 samples of forages (primarily alfalfa) from different parts of the USA. They used the results of the survey to produce a generalized map of the distribution of Se in U.S. crops. Because their map was based upon crop Se data, it has greater relevance to considerations of nutritional aspects of Se than would one based upon geological data, inasmuch as it represents the distribution of Se in the particular terrain (i.e., valleys and plains) used for food and feed production. This map has been revised recently[162] by the incoporation of Canadian data to extend its coverage to both the USA and Canada (see Fig. 2.1). It shows that the areas of production of low-Se (i.e., less than 0.10 ppm) foods and feedstuffs of plant origin are located primarily in the east central, northeastern, Pacific northwestern, and southeastern portions of the USA; and in most of Canada. Many of these low-Se regions, already known for their enzootic muscular dystrophies of livestock, are areas of high densities of human populations. This observation has stimulated many questions concerning the public health implications of regional Se-deficiency. These are discussed at some length in Chapter 8.

A survey of the regional distribution of Se in feed and food crops in the P.R.C. was completed by scientists in that country.[163] In a massive undertaking, Liu *et al.*[163] measured the Se contents of 11,467 samples of a variety of plant foods produced in 1103 sites from among 28 of that

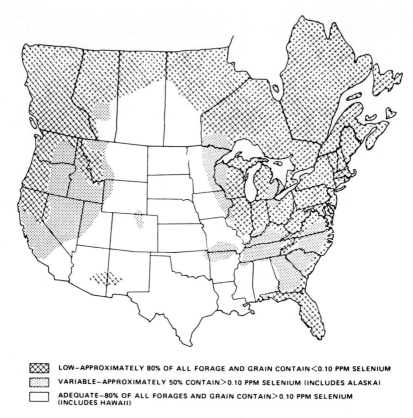

☒ LOW—APPROXIMATELY 80% OF ALL FORAGE AND GRAIN CONTAIN <0.10 PPM SELENIUM
▨ VARIABLE—APPROXIMATELY 50% CONTAIN >0.10 PPM SELENIUM (INCLUDES ALASKA)
☐ ADEQUATE—80% OF ALL FORAGES AND GRAIN CONTAIN >0.10 PPM SELENIUM
(INCLUDES HAWAII)

Fig. 2.1 Regional distribution of Se in food and feed plants in the USA and Canada as indicated by the Se contents of forages and cereal crops.[162] Reproduced with permission of the National Academy of Sciences Publishing Office.

country's provinces in 1980-1982. Almost 70% of the foods and feedstuffs surveyed contained less than 0.05 ppm Se (dry matter basis), and 25% contained less than 0.02 ppm Se. Their results (see Fig. 2.2) show that a belt of severe Se deficiency extends from the Northwest to the west central portions of China. This belt includes the provinces of Heilongjiang, Jilin, Qinghai, and Sichuan, as well as Tibet and Inner Mongolia, in which 47-93% of the foods and feedstuffs sampled contained less than 0.02 ppm Se (dry matter basis). Other areas (e.g., Zhejiang, Shanxi, Shaanxi and Gansu provinces) were found to have significantly high incidences (i.e., ca. 30%) of Se-deficiency. Each of these Se-deficient areas has large human populations and extensive livestock production. An extensive survey of the Se contents of pig livers throughout China[164] showed that the counties and provinces in which pig liver Se was lowest were those identified by

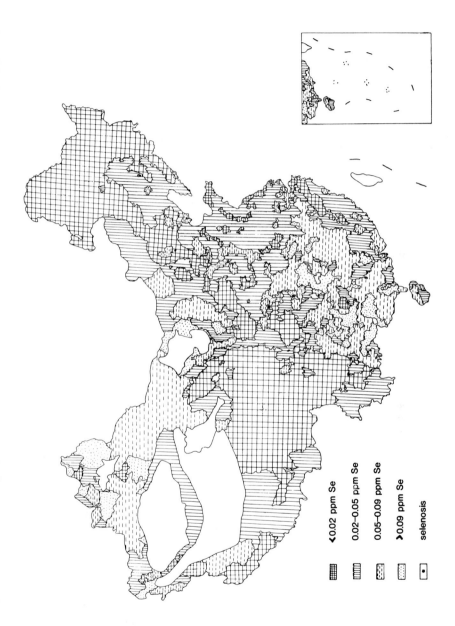

Fig. 2.2 Regional distribution of Se in food and feed plants in the People's Republic of China.[163] Reproduced from the authors' original report, with their permission.

< 0.02 ppm Se

0.02–0.05 ppm Se

0.05–0.09 ppm Se

> 0.09 ppm Se

selenosis

Liu *et al.*[163] as having the lowest levels of Se in food and feed crops. The correlated results of these two independent surveys are shown in Fig. 2.3.

The mapping of Se in food and feed crops has been very important in the development of understanding of the role of Se in the nutrition of animals and humans. Despite the fact that extensive geo-botanical mapping of Se has been conducted in only a few regions of the world, the knowledge gained has broad implications. These studies have demonstrated the importance of the available Se content of local soils as the primary determinant of the Se contents of foods and feedstuffs of plant origin. They have shown that areas of endemic soil Se deficiency can result in deficient intakes of Se, not only among the local residents consuming locally produced plant foods, but also among residents of nonendemic areas who consume foods imported from Se-deficient areas. For example, much of the feed grains used for livestock in the southeastern USA is produced in the relatively Se-deficient east central states. The result is that diets used for swine and poultry in the southeast require supplementation with Se to prevent Se-deficiency syndromes, even though that region is not classified as a Se-deficient one. The converse situation has been described by Watkinson[165] and Varo and Koivistoinen,[166] who documented the increases in Se in the food supplies of New Zealand and Finland as the result of importation of wheat from higher Se areas of Australia and Canada, respectively, into those countries. Therefore, the geo-botanical mapping of Se has served to focus attention on both the local and regional nutritional impacts of regional Se deficiency.

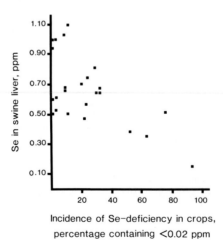

Fig. 2.3   Relationship of Se status of swine and incidence of Se deficiency in crops in the People's Republic of China. From data of Zhai *et al.*[164] and Liu *et al.*,[163] respectively.

REFERENCES

1. Lakin, H. W., Selenium accumulation in soils and its absorption by plants and animals, Geol. Soc. Am., Bull., 83, 181, 1972.
2. Frost, D. V., Significance of the symposium, in *Symposium on Selenium and Biomedicine,* Muth, O.H., Ed., Avi Publ. Co., Westport, Conn., 1967, 2.
3. Rosenfeld, I., and Beath, O.A., *Selenium: Geobotany, Biochemistry, Toxicity and Nutrition,* Academic Press, New York, 1964.
4. Hawlay, J. E., and Nichol, I., Selenium in some Canadian sulfides, Econ. Geol., 54, 608, 1959.
5. Lakin H. W., and Davidson, D. E., The relation of geochemistry of selenium to its occurrence in soils, in *Selenium in Biomedicine,* Muth, O. H., Ed., Avi Publ. Co., Westport, Conn., 1967, 27.
6. Coleman, R. G., and Delevaux, M. H., Occurrence of selenium in sulfides from some sedimentary rocks of the United States, Econ. Geol., 52, 499, 1957.
7. Takimoto, K., Minoto, T., and Hiroko, S., On the distribution of selenium in some sulfide minerals sharing the relations of intimate paragenesis, J. Japan Assn. Miner. Petrologists. Econ. Miner., 42, 161, 1958.
8. Louderback, T., Selenium in the environment, Colo. Sch. Mines Miner. Ind. Bull., 18, 1, 1975.
9. Pillay, K. K. S., Thomas, C. C., Jr., and Kaminski, J. W., Neutron activation analysis of selenium contest of fossil, Nucl. Appl. Technol., 7,478, 1969.
10. Gange, T. J.,Selenium, in *Diagnostic Criteria for Plants and Soils,* Chapman, H. D., Ed., Univ. Calif., Davis, 1966, 304.
11. Johnson, C. M., Selenium on soils and plants: contrasts in conditions providing safe but adequate amounts of selenium in the food chain, in *Trace Elements in Soil-Plant-Animal Systems,* Nicholas, D. J. D., and Egan, A. R., Eds., Academic Press, New York, 1975, 165.
12. Radler, L. F., Jr., and Hill, W. L., Occurrence of selenium in natural phosphate, superphosphates and phosphoric acid, J. Agr. Res., 51, 1071, 1935.
13. Yang, G. Q., Zhou, R., Sun, X., Wang X., and Li, S., Endemic selenium toxicosis in man in China, Yingyang Xuebao, 4, 81, 1982.
14. Levander, O. A., Clinical consequences of low selenium intake and its relationship to vitamin E, Ann. N.Y. Acad. Sci., 355, 870, 1982.
15. Byers, H. G., Miller, J. T., Williams, K. T., and Kalia, H. W., Selenium occurrence in certain soils in the United States with a discussion of related topics, 3rd report, USDA Tech. Bull., 601, 1938.
16. Trelease, S. F., Selenium in soils, plants and animals, Soil Sci., 60, 125, 1945.
17. Shacklette, T., Boerngen, J. G., and Keith, J. R., Selenium, fluorine and arsenic in surficial materials of the conterminous United States, in *Geol. Serv. Circ. 292, U.S. Geol. Survey, Reston, Va., 1974.*
18. *Allaway, W. H.,* The chemistry of selenium, *in Proc. Amer. Feed Manuf. Nutr. Council Mtg.,* December 2, 1968, 27.
19. Walsh, T., and Gleming, G. A., Selenium toxicity associated with an Irish soil series, Nature, 168, 881, 1951.
20. Walsh, T., and Fleming, G.A., Selenium levels in rocks, soils and herbage from a high selenium locality in Ireland, Int. Soc. Sci. Comm., 2, 178, 1952.
21. Fleming, G. A., and Walsh, T., Selenium occurrence in certain Irish soils and its toxic effect on animals, Roy. Irish Acad. Proc., 58, sec. b7, 151, 1957.
22. Fleming, G. A.., Selenium in Irish soils and plants, Soil Sci., 94, 28, 1962.

23. Ancizar-Sordo, J., Occurrence of selenium in soils and plants of Colombia, South America, Soil Sci. 63, 437, 1947.

24. Benavides, S. T., and Mojica, R. F. S., Selenosis: Occurrencia de selenio en rocas, suelosa y plautes, intoxicacion por selenio en animales y humanos, Inst. Geograf. Col. Publ. IT., 3. 1959.

25. Jaffe, W.G., Chavey, J.F., and Mondragon, M. C., Contenido de selenio en alimentos venezolanos, Arch. Latinoamer. Nutar., 17, 59, 1967.

26. Jaffe, W. G., Chavez, J. F., and Mondagon, M. C., Contenido de selenio en muestras de semillas de ajonjoli *(Sesamum indicum)* procedentes de varios paises, Arch. Latinoamer. Nutr., 19, 299, 1969.

27. Mondragon, M. C., and Jaffe, W. G., Selenio en alimentos y en orina de escolares de diferentes zenas de Venezuela, Arch. Latinoamer. Nutr., 21, 185, 1971.

28. Jaffe, W. G., Ruphael, M., Mondragon, M. C., and Cuevas, M. A., Estudio clinico y bioquimico en ninos escalares de una zona selenifera, Arch. Latinoamer. Nutr., 22, 570, 1972.

29. Ravikovitch, S., and Margolin, M., Selenium in soils and plants, Agr. Res. Sta. Rehovot, 7, 41, 1957.

30. Beath, O. A., Hagner, A.F., and Gilbert, C.S., Some soils of high selenium content, Wyoming Geol. Serv. Bull. No. 36, Univ. Wyoming, Laramie, 1946.

31. Lakin, H.W., *Selenium in Agriculture,* Agric. Handb. 200, USDA, Washington, D.C., 1961.

32. Olson, O. E., Whitehead, E. I., and Moxon, A. I., Occurrence of soluble selenium and its availability to plants, Soil Sci., 545, 47, 1942.

33. Gissel-Nielsen, G., Gupta, Y. C., Lamand, M., and Westermarck, T., Selenium in soils and plants and its importance in livestock and human nutrition, Adv. Agron., 37 (in press), 1984.

34. Koljoneu, T., The behavior of selenium in Finnish soils, Ann. Agric. Fenniae, 14, 240, 1975.

35. Watkinsi, J. H., Soil selenium and animal health, Trans. Int. Soc. Soil Sci., 5, 149, 1962.

36. Wells, N., Selenium in horizons of soil profiles, N. Zealand J. Sci., 10, 142, 1967.

37. Wells, N., Selenium content of soil forming rocks, N. Zealand J. Geol. Geophys., 10, 198, 1967.

38. Healy, W. B., McCabe, W. J., and Wilson, G. F., Ingested soil as a source of microelements for grazing animals, N. Zealand J. Agric. Res., 13, 503, 1970.

39. Andrews, E.D., Hogan, K. G., and Sheppard, A.D., Selenium in soils, pastures, and animals tissues in relation to the growth of young sheep in a marginaly selenium-deficient area, N. Zealand Vet. J., 24, 11, 1976.

40. Hodder, A. P. W., and Watkinson, J.H., Low selenium levels in Tephra-derived soil—inherent or pedogenetic?, N. Zealand J. Sci., 19, 397. 1976.

41. Watkinson, J.H., The New Zealand scene: soil and biological factors related to selenium deficiency in animals, in *Proc., N. Zealand Wkshp. Trace Elements,* 1981, 72.

42. Cheng, B., Ju, S., Yue, S., Sheng, S., He, R., and Zhang, G., The trace element selenium in the eco-environment and the Keshan Disease, Acta Ecol. Sinica, 1, 274, 1981.

43. Li, J. Y., Ren, S. X., and Cheng, D. Z., A study of selenium associated with Kaschin-Beck disease in different environments in Shaanxi, Acta Scientnae Circumstantiae, 2, 1, 1982.

44. Tan, J. A., Zeng, D. X., Hou, S. F., Zhu, W. Y., Li, R. B., Zhu, Z. Y., Wang, W. Y., Zhao, N. Q., Li, D. Z., Liu, Y. L., and Zhu, Z. Y., The relation of Keshan Disease

to the natural environment and the background of selenium nutrition, Acta Nutrimenta Sinica, 4, 175, 1982.

45. Tan, J.A., The Keshan Disease in China: a study of ecological chemico-geography, Nat. Geog. J. India, 28, 15, 1982.

46. Su, Y., and Yu, W. H., Nutritional bio-geochemical etiology of Keshan Disease, Chin. Med. J., 96, 594, 1983.

47. Yin, Z., Yue, S., and He, R., Characteristics of the environmental geochemistry and its relationship with "Keshan Disease" in the plataeau soil of Keshiketengqu, Inner Mongolia, J. Chin. Geog. Soc., 3, 182, 1983.

48. Cheng, B., Ju, S., Yue, S., He, R., and Sheng, S., Studies on the selenium in soils of northeastern China, Acta Ecol. Sinica, 1, 61, 1981.

49. Williams, K. T., Lakin H. W., and Byers, H. G., Selenium occurrence in certain soils in the United States with a discussion of related topics, 5th report, USDA Tech. Bull., 758, 1941.

50. Levesque, M., Selenium distribution in Canadian soil profiles, Can. J. Soil Sci. 54, 63, 1974.

51. Gardiner, W. R., and Gorman, R. C., Further observations on plant selenium levels in western Australia, Australia J. Exptl. Agr. Anim. Husb., 3, 284, 1963.

52. Slater, C. S., Holmes, R. S., and Byers, H. G., Trace elements in the soils from the erosion experiment stations, with supplementary data on other soils, USDA Tech. Bull., 552, 1937.

53. Cary, E. E., Wieczorek, G. A., and Allaway, W.H., Reactions of selenite-selenium added to soils that produce low selenium forages, Soil Sci. Soc. Am. Proc., 31, 21, 1967.

54. Smith, M. I., Frank, K. W., and Westfall, B. B., The selenium problem in relation to public health, U.S. Public Health Repts., 51, 1496, 1936.

55. Smith, M. I., and Westfall, B. B., Further field studies on the selenium problem in relation to public health, U.S. Public Health Repts., 52, 1375, 1937.

56. Beath, O. A., Selenium poisons Indians, Sci. Newslett., 81, 254, 1962.

57. Miller, J. T., and Byers, H. G., A selenium Spring, Ind. Eng. Chem. News Ed., 13, 456, 1935.

58. Beath, O. A., Toxic vegetation growing on the Salt Wash. Santstone Member of the Morrison Formation, Am. J. Botany, 30, 698, 1940.

59. Valentine, J. L., Kang, H. K., and Spirey, G. H., Selenium levels in human blood, urine, and hair in response to exposure via drinking water, Environ. Res., 17, 347, 1978.

60. Valentine, J. L., Kang, H. K., Dang. P. M., and Spirey, G., Selenium levels in humans as a result of drinking water exposure, in *Selenium in Biology and Medicine*, Spalholz, J. E., Martin, J. L., and Ganther, H. E., Eds., Avi Publ. Co., Westport, Conn., 1981, 345.

61. Valentine, J. L., Reisbord, L. S., Kang, H. K., and Schluchter, M.D., Effects on human health of exposure to selenium in drinking water, in *Proceedings of the Third International Symposium in Selenium in Biology and Medicine*, Combs, G. F., Jr., Spallholz, J. E., Levander, O. A., and Oldfield, J. E., Eds., Avi Publ. Co., Westport, Conn., 1986.

62. Beath, O. A., Eppson, H. G., and Gilbert, C. S., Selenium and other toxic minerals in soils and vegetation, Wyoming Exp. Sta. Bull. No. 206, 1935.

63. Scott, R. C., and Voegeli, P.T., Radiochemical analyses of ground and surface water in Colorado, Colo. Water Conserv. Bd. Basic Data Rep. 7, Denver, 1961.

64. Hadjimarkos, D. M., and Bonhorst, C. W., The selenium content of eggs, milk and water in relation to dental cavities in children, J. Pediatr., 59, 256, 1961.

65. Taylor, F. B., Significance of trace elements in the public, finished water supplies, J. Am. Water Works Assn., 55, 619, 1963.
66. U.S. Dept. Health Education and Welfare, National Water Quality Network Annual Compilation of Data, PUSPHS Public No. 663, USPHS, Washington, D.C., 1962.
67. Williams, K. T., and Byers, H. G., Occurrence of selenium in the Colorado River and some of its tributaries, Ind. Eng. Chem., Anal., Ed., 7, 431, 1935.
68. Su, Q., Lu, Z. H., and Liu, C. H., unpublished research, 1983.
69. Schutz, D. D., and Turekian, K. K., The investigation of the geographical and vertical distribution of several trace elements in the sea water using neutron activation analysis, Geochim. Cosmochim. Acta, 29, 259, 1965.
70. Harrison, P. R., Rahn, K. A., Dams, R., Robbins J.A., Winchester, J. W., Brar, S.S., and Nelson, D.M., Area wide trace metal concentrations measured by multielement neutron activation analysis—one-day study in northwest Indiana, J. Air Pollut. Control Assn., 21, 563, 1971.
71. John, W, Kaifer, R., Rahm, K., and Weslowski, J. J., Trace element concentrations in aerosols from the San Francisco Bay Area, Atmos. Environ., 7, 107, 1973.
72. Pierson, D. H., Cawse, P. A., Salmon, L., and Cambray, R. S., Trace elements in the atmospheric environment, Nature, 241, 252, 1973.
73. Gutenmann, W. H., Bache, C. A., Youngs, W. D., and Lisk, D. J., Selenium in fly ash, Science, 191, 966, 1976.
74. Davis, W. E., National inventory of sources and emissions; boron, copper, selenium and zinc, U.S. Nat. Tech. Inform. Serv. Rept. No. 219679, 1969.
75. Flinn, J. E., and Reimers, R. S., Development of predictions of future problems, E.P.A. Rept. No. 600/5-005, 1974, 36.
76. Lee, R. E., Jr., and Duffield, F. V., Sources of environmentally import metals in the atmosphere, Adv. Chem. Ser., 172, 146, 1977.
77. West, D. W., Selenium containing inorganics in paper may play cancer role, Chem. Eng. News, 45, 12, 1967.
78. Olson, O. E., and Frost, D. V., Selenium in papers and tobacco, Environ. Sci. Technol., 4, 686, 1970.
79. Hashimoto, Y., Hwang, J. T., and Yanagisawa, J., Possible source of atmospheric pollution of selenium, Environ. Sci. Technol., 4, 157, 1970.
80. Johnson, C. M., Selenium in the environment, Residue Rev., 62, 102, 1976.
81. Shendriker, A. D., and West, P. W., Determination of selenium in the smoke from trash burning, Environ. Lett., 5, 59, 1973.
82. Jiang, S., Robberecht, H., and Adams, F., Identification and determination of alkyl selenide compounds in environmental air, Atmosph. Environ., 17, 111, 1983.
83. Mosher, B., and Duce, R., Vapor phase selenium in the atmosphere, Searex Newslett., 4, 9, 1981.
84. Barkes, L., and Fleming, R. W., Production of dimethyl selenide gas from inorganic selenium by eleven soil fungi, Bull. Environ. Contam. Toxicol., 12, 308, 1974.
85. Francis, A. J., Duxbury, J. M., and Alexander, M., Evolution of dimethylselenide from soils, Appl. Microbiol., 28, 248, 1984.
86. Chau, Y. K., Wong, P. J. S., Silverberg B. A., Luxon, P. L., and Bengert, G. A., Methylation of selenium in the aquatic environment, Science, 192, 1130, 1976.
87. Hamdy, A. A., and Gissel-Nielsen, G., Volatilization of selenium from soils, Z. Pflanzer. Boden., 6, 671, 1976.
88. Zieve, R., and Peterson, P. J., Factors influencing the volatilization of selenium from soil, Sci. Total Environ., 19, 277, 1981.
89. Lewis, B. E., Johnson, C. M., and Delwiche, C. C., Release of volatile selenium compounds by plants: collection procedures and primary observations, Agr. Food Chem., 14, 638, 1966.

90. Lewis, B. G., Johnson, G. M., and Broyer, T. C., Cleavage of Se-methylselenomethionine selenonium salt by cabbage leaf enzyme fraction, Biochim. Biophys. Acta, 237, 603, 1971.

91. Zieve, R., and Peterson, P. J., Volatilization of selenium from plants and soils, Sci. Total Environ. 32, 197, 1984.

92. Asher, C. J., Evans, C. S., and Johnson, C. M., Collection and partial characterization of volatile selenium compounds from *Medicago Sativa* 1., Australian J. Biol. Sci., 20, 737, 1967.

93. Broyer, T. C., Lee, D. C., and Asher, C. J., Selenium nutrition of green plants: effect of selenite supply on growth and selenium content of alfalfa and subterranean clover, Plant Physiol., 41, 1425, 1966.

94. Zieve, R., and Peterson, P. J., The accumulation and assimilation of dimethylselenide by four plant species, Planta (Berlin), 160, 180, 1984.

95. Zieve, R., and Peterson, P. J., Selenium in plants: soil versus atmospheric origin, in *Proceedings of the Third International Symposium on Selenium in Biology and Medicine,* Combs, G. F., Jr., Spallholz, J. E., Levander, O. A., and Oldfield, J. E., Eds., Avi Publ. Co., Westport, Conn., 1986.

96. Trelease, S. F., and Trelease, H. M., Selenium as a stimulator and possibly essential element for indicator plants, Am. J. Botany, 25, 372, 1938.

97. Trelease, S. F., and Trelease, H. M., Physiological differentiation in *Astragalus* with reference to selenium, Am. J. Botany, 26, 530, 1939.

98. Broyer, T. C., Johnson C. M., and Huston, R. P., Selenium and Nutrition of *Astragalus.* I. Effects of selenite and selenate supply on growth and selenium content, Plant Soil, 36, 365, 1972.

99. Broyer, T. C., Johnson, C. M., and Huston, R. P., Selenium and nutrition of *Astragalus.* II. Ionic absorption interaction among selenium, phosphate, and the macro-and micro-nutrient ratios, Plant Soil, 36, 651, 1972.

100. Davies, E. B., and Watkinson, J. H., Uptake of native and applied selenium by pasture species. I. Uptake of Se by browntop, ryegrass, cocksfoot, and white clover from atiamuri sand, N. Zealand J. Agric. Res., 9, 641, 1966.

101. Kubota, J., Allaway, W. H., Carter, D. L., Cary, E. E., and Lazar, V. A., Selenium in crops in the United States in relation to selenium-responsive diseases of animals, Agr. Food Chem., 15, 448, 1967.

102. Geering, H. R., Cary, E. E., Jones, L. H. P., and Allaway, W. H., Solubility and redox criteria for the possible forms of selenium in soils, Soil Sci. Soc. Amer. Proc., 32, 35, 1968.

103. Cary, E. E., and Allaway, W. H., The stability of different forms of selenium applied to low selenium soils, Soil Sci. Soc. Amer., Proc., 33, 571, 1969,

104. Gissel-Nielsen, G., Influence of pH and texture of the soil on plant uptake of added selenium, J. Agr. Food Chem., 19, 1165, 1971.

105. Gissel-Nielson, G., Selenium in the soil-plant system, in *Proceedings of the Third International Symposium on Selenium in Biology and Medicine,* Combs, G. F., Jr., Spallholz, J. E., Levander, O. A., and Oldfield, J. E., Avi Publ. Co., Westport, Conn, 1986.

106. Patel, C.A., and Mehta, B. V., Selenium status of soils and common fodders of Gujarat, Ind. J. Agr. Sci., 40, 389, 1970.

107. Cary, E. E., and Gissel-Nielsen, G., Effect of fertilizer anions on the solubility of native and applied selenium in soil, Soil Sci. Soc. Amer. Proc., 37, 590, 1973.

108. Gissel-Nielsen, G., Effect of fertilization on uptake of selenium by plants, in *Plant Analysis an Fertilizer Problems,* Vol. 1, *Proceedings of the International Colloquium on Plant Analysis and Fertilizer Problems,* Hanover, W. Germany, 1974 111.

109. Singh, M., Effect of N-carriers, soil type and genetic variation on growth and accumulation of selenium, nitrogen, phosphorus and sulfur in sorghum and cow peas, Forage Res., 1, 68, 1975.
110. Gissel-Nielsen, G., Uptake and translocation of selenium -75, in *Zea Mayes, Symposium on Isotopes and Radiation in Research on Soil-Plant Relationships,* International Atomic Energy Agency, Vienna, Austria, 1979, 427.
111. Muth, O. H., White muscle disease (myopathy) in lambs and calves. I. Occurrence and nature of the disease under Oregon conditions. J. Am. Vet. Med. Assn., 126, 355, 1955.
112. Schubert, J. R., Muth, O. H., Oldfield, J. E., and Remment, L. F., Experimental results with selenium in white muscle disease of lambs and calves, Federation Proc., 20, 689, 1961.
113. Hurd-Karrer, A. M., and Kennedy, L., Inhibiting effect of sulphur in selenized soil on toxicity of wheat to rats, J. Agr. Res., 52, 933, 1936.
114. Gissel-Nielsen, G., Uptake and distribution of selenite and selenate by barley and red clover as influenced by sulfur, J. Sci. Food Agr., 24, 649, 1973.
115. Leggett, J. E., and Epstein, E, Kinetics of sulfate absorption by barley roots, Plant Physiol., 31, 222, 1956.
116. Ulrich, J. M., and Shrift, A., Selenium absorption by excised *Astragalus* roots, Plant Physiol., 43, 14, 1968.
117. Shrift, A., and Ulrich, J. M., Transport of selenate and selenite into *Astragalus* roots, Plant Physiol., 44, 893, 1969.
118. Shrift, A., Sulfur-selenium antagonism. I. Anti-metabolite action of selenate on the growth of *Chlorella vulgaris,* Am. J. Bot., 41, 223, 1954.
119. Yamamoto, L. A., and Segal, I. H., The inorganic sulfate transport system of *penicillium chrysogenum,* Arch. Biochem. Bioph., 114, 523, 1966.
120. Gissel-Nielsen, G., Selenium content of some fertilizers and their influence on uptake of selenium in plants, J. Agr. Food Chem., 19, 564, 1971.
121. Patterson, J. C., Henderlong, P. A., and Adams, L. M., Sintered flyash as a soil modifier, West Va. Acad. Sci. 40, 151, 1974.
122. Capp, J. P., and Gillmore, D. W., Flyash from coal-burning power plants: an aid to revegetating coal mine refuse and spoil banks, Paper presented at the Coal and the Environment Conference, Louisville, Ky, 1974.
123. Barrows, S. A., and Swader, F. N., Agricultural uses of flyash in the Northeast, final report to Empire State Electric Energy Research Corp., Cornell University, Ithaca, New York, 1978.
124. Furr, A. K., Kelly, W. C., Bache, C. A., Gutenmann, W. H., and Lisk, D. J.,Multielement uptake by vegetables and millet grown in pots in flyash amended soil, J. Agric. Food Chem., 24, 885, 1976.
125. Furr, A. K., Parkinson, T. F., Gutenmann, W. H., Pakkala, I. S., and Lisk, D. J., Elemental content of vegetables, grains and forages field-grown on flyash amended soil, J. Agric. Food Chem., 26, 357, 1978.
126. Combs, G. F., Jr., Mandisodza, K. T., Gutenmann, W. H., and Lisk, D. J., Utilization of selenium in flyash and in white sweet clover grown in flyash by the chick, J. Agr. Food Chem., 29, 149, 1981.
127. Furr, K., Stoewsand, G. S., Bache, C. A., Gutenmann, W. H., and Lisk, D. J., Multielement residues in tissues of guinea pigs fed sweet clover grown on flyash, Arch. Environ. Health, 30, 244, 1975.
128. Gutenmann, W. H., Bache, C. A., Youngs, W. D., and Lisk, D. J., Selenium in flyash, Science, 191, 966, 1976.
129. Mandisodza, K. T., Pond, W. G., Lisk, D. J., Hogue, D. E., Krook, L., Carey, E. E., and Gutenmann, W. H., Tissue retention of Se in growing pigs fed flyash or white sweet clover grown in flyash, J. Animal Sci., 49, 535, 1979.

130. Combs, G. F., Jr., Barrows, S. A., and Swader, F. N., Biologic availability of selenium in corn grains produced on soil amended with flyash. J. Agric. Food Chem. 28, 406, 1980.

131. Allaway, W. H., Moore, D. P., Oldfield, J. E., and Muth, O. H., Movement of physiological levels of selenium from soils through plants to animals, J. Nutr., 88, 411, 1966.

132. Fleming, G. A., Some factors affecting the uptake of selenium by plants, Irish J. Agric. Res., 1, 131, 1962.

133. Watkinson, J. H., Prevention of selenium deficiency in grazing animals by annual topdressing of pasture with sodium selenate, N. Zealand Vet. J., 31, 78, 1983.

134. Watkinson, J. H., Annual topdressing of pasture with selenate pellets to prevent selenium deficiency in grazing stock: research and farming practices in New Zealand, in *Proceedings of the Third International Symposium on Selenium in Biology and Medicine*, Combs, G. F., Jr., Spallholz, J. E., Levander, O. A., and Oldfield, J. E., eds., Avi Publ. Co., Westport, Conn., 1985.

135. Hupkens van der Elst, F. C. C. and Watkinson, J. H., Effects of topdressing pasture with selenium prills on selenium concentration in blood of stock, N. Zealand J. Exptl. Agr. 5, 79, 1976.

136. Watkinson, J. H., and Hupkens van der Elst, P. C. C., Selenium content of a stream in the central North Island after catchment topdressing with Se-prills, N. Zealand J. Sci., 23, 383, 1980.

137. Andrews, E. D., Hartley, W. J., and Grant, A. B., Selenium-responsive diseases of animals in New Zealand, N. Zealand Vet. J., 16, 3, 1968.

138. Grant, A. B., Selenium topdressing -- results of some preliminary trials, in *Proceedings of the Twelfth Technical Conference*, New Zealand Fertilizer Manufacturers Assn., Dunedin, 1969, 47.

139. Hupkens van der Elst, F. C. C. and Watkinson, J. H., Selenium deficiency on high moor peat soils in New Zealand, in *Proceedings 4th Int. Peat Conf.*, Helsinki, 1972, 149.

140. Watkinson, J. H., and Davies, E. B., Uptake of native and applied selenium by pasture species. IV. Relative uptake through foliage and roots by white clover and browntop: distribution of selenium in white clover, N. Zealand J. Agr. Res., 10, 122, 1967.

141. Gupta, U. C., Kunelius, H. T., and Winter, K. A., Effect of foliar applied selenium on yields and selenium concentration of alfalfa, timothy and barley, Can. J. Soil Sci., 63, 455, 1983.

142. Johnson, C. M., Asher, C. J., and Broyer, T. C., Distribution of selenium in plants, in *Symposium: Selenium in Biomedicine*, Muth, O. H., Ed., Avi Publ. Co., Westport, Conn., 1967, 57.

143. Moxon, A. L., Olson, O. E., and Searight, W. V., Selenium in rocks, soils and plants, South Dakota Agr. Expt. Sta. Tech. Bull. 2, 1, 1939.

144. Peterson, P. J., and Butler, G. W., The uptake and assimiliation of selenite by higher plants, Australian J. Biol. Sci. 15, 126, 1962.

145. Beath, O. A., Economic potential and botanical limitation of some selenium-bearing plants, Univ. Wyoming Agr. Expt. Sta. Bull. No. 360, Laramie, 1959.

146. Lakin, H. W., and Byers, H. G., Selenium in wheat and wheat products, Cereal Chem., 18, 73, 1941.

147. Shrift, A., Aspects of selenium metabolism in higher animals, Ann. Rev. Plant Physiol. 20, 475, 1969.

148. Shrift, A. and Virupaksha, T. K., Biosynthesis of Se-methylselenocysteine from selenite in selenium-accumulating plants, Biochim. Biophys. Acta, 71, 483, 1963.

149. Virupaksha, T. K. and Shrift, A., Biosynthesis of selenocystathionine from selenite in *Stankya pinnata*, Biochim. Biophys. Acta, 74, 791, 1963.

150. Shrift, A., and Virupaksha, T. K., Seleno-amino acids in selenium-accumulating plants, Biochim. Biophys. Acta, 100, 65, 1965.
151. Virupaksha, T. K., and Shrift, A., Biochemical differences between selenium accumulator and non-accumulator *Astragalus* species, Biochim. Biophys. Acta, 107, 69, 1965.
152. Martin, J. L., Shrift, A., and Gerlach, M. L., Use of s75sSe-selenite for the study of selenium metabolism in *Astragalus*, Phytochem., 10, 945, 1971.
153. Chen, D. M., Nigam, S. N., and McConnell, W. B., Biosynthesis of Se-methylselenocysteine and S-methylcysteine in *Astragalus bisulcatus*, Can. J. Biochem., 48, 1278, 1970.
154. Chow, C. M., Nigam, S. N., and McConnell, W. B., Biosynthesis of Se-methylselenocysteine and S-methylcysteine in *Astragalus bisulcatus*: effect of selenium and sulfur concentrations in the growth medium, Phytochem., 10, 2693, 1971.
155. Franke, K. W., A new toxicant occurring naturally in certain samples of plant foodstuffs. II. The occurrence of the toxicant in the protein fraction, J. Nutr., 8, 609, 1934.
156. Olson, O. E., Novacek, E. J., Whitehead, E. I., and Palmer, I. S., Investigations on selenium in wheat, Phytochem., 9, 1181, 1970.
157. Hartley, W. J., and Grant, A. B., A review of selenium responsive diseases of New Zealand livestock, Federation Proc., 20, 679, 1961.
158. Blaxter, K. L., Muscular dystrophy in farm animals: its cause and prevention, Proc. Nutr. Soc., 21, 211, 1962.
159. Muth, O. H., and Allaway, W. A., The relationship of white muscle disease to the distribution of naturally occurring selenium, J. Am. Vet. Med. Assn., 142, 1379, 1963.
160. Allaway, W. H., and Hodgson, J. F., Symposium on nutrition, forage and pastures: selenium in forages as related to the geographic distribution of muscular dystrophy in livestock, J. Anim. Sci. 23, 271, 1964.
161. Kubota, J., Allaway, W. H., Carter, D. L., Cary, E. E., and Lazar, V. A., Selenium in crops in the United States in relation to selenium-responsive diseases of animals, Agr. Food. Chem., 15, 448, 1967.
162. Subcommittee on Selenium, Committee on Animal Nutrition, Board on Agriculture, National Research Council, *Selenium in Nutrition*, revised edition, National Academy Press, Washington, D.C., 174 pp., 1983.
163. Liu, C. H., Lu, Z. H., Su, Q., and Duan, Y. Q., Regional selenium deficiency of feeds in China, in *Proceedings of the Third International Symposium on Selenium in Biology and Medicine*, Combs, G. F., Jr., Spallholz, J. E., Levander, O. A., and Oldfield, J. E., Eds., Avi Publ. Co., Westport, Conn., 1986.
164. Zhai, X. J., Cheng, Y. H., Wang, Y. W., Yan, X. F., Cai, Y., Qi, Z. M., and Gao, T., Selenium content of swine liver in PRC, in *Proceedings of the Third International Symosium on Selenium in Biology and Medicine*, Combs, G. F., Jr., Spallholz, J. E., Levander, O. A., and Oldfield, J. E., Eds., Avi Publ. Co., Westport, Conn., 1986.
165. Watkinson, J. H., Changes in blood selenium in New Zealand adults with time and importation of Australian wheat, Am. J. Clin. Nutr., 34, 936, 1981.
166. Varo, P., and Koivistoinen, P., Selenium in Finnish Food, in *Proceedings of the Third International Symosium on Selenium in Biology and Medicine*, Combs, G. F., Jr., Spallholz, J. E., Levander, O. A., and Oldfield, J. E., Eds., Avi Publ. Co., Westport, Conn., 1986.

3

SELENIUM IN FOODS
AND FEEDS

The Se contents of human foods and animal feedstuffs vary widely due to such factors as the type (i.e., species or product), the particular variety or cultivar, the methods of preparation and/or processing, the climatic conditions during the growing season, and the amount of biologically available Se in the particular nutrient environment (e.g., the soluble Se content of the soil for plant species, the biologically available Se content of the diet for animal species). Of these factors, the most important by far in determining the Se contents of foods and feeds is the last. Due to the intimate relationship between plants and animals in food chains, the Se contents of foods from both plant and animal origins tend to be greatly influenced by the local soil Se environment. Thus, all types of foods and feedstuffs tend to show strong geographic patterns of variation in Se content, reflecting in general the local soil Se conditions. It is of interest to know something of the Se contents of human foods and animal feedstuffs, so that reasonable estimates of the Se intakes of populations of people and classes of animals can be made.

I. SELENIUM IN FOODS

Table 3.1 presents a summary of the results of many analyses of the Se contents of human foods. Despite the great number of foods that have been examined in this regard, the reader should note that current knowledge is restricted to the foods of only a small number of countries, and that for most of the world there is no information available to describe the

Table 3.1

Selenium Contents of Foods (ppm, Fresh Weight Basis) Reported from Various Countries

Food	USA			Canada	England	Italy	W. Germany	Sweden
	Low Se	Moderate Se	High Se					
Cereals								
Barley	.24(1)[a]	.66(11)	.32(18) .38(96)	.29(21)				.005–.018(3)
Buckwheat, flour	.57(2)							
Corn								
Grain								
Meal	n.d.[a](1) .08(3) .067(2)		.22(1) .07(18)	.05(21)				
Starch	.22(2)		.031(18)					
Millet	n.d.(1)							
Oats	.56(1) .50(2)			.10–.45(21)				<.005–.039(3)
Rye flour								
Rye, whole	.07(3)	.357(2)					.026(4)	.043(4) .06(3)
Rice, polished	.27(4) .387(2)	.319(11) .38(12) .210(13)	.20(96) .23(18)	.24(21)	.10(23)		.11(24)	
Rice, brown		.389(11)	.028(18) .04(96)					

(continues)

Table 3.1 (Continued)

Food	Finland	New Zealand	China			Japan	Venezuela	Other countries
			Se-deficient	Moderate Se	Seleniferous			
Cereals								
Barley	0.010(28) 0.005-0.009(29)					.08(45)	.132(73)	
Buckwheat, flour			.017(37)	.039(37)				
Corn								
Grain	.040(28)		.016(37) .005(38) .004(39)	.049(37) .053(37) .036(39)	6.9(39)			Yugoslavia: <.01(46)
Meal		.004(98)					.305(72)	
Starch								
Millet	.020(28) .006-.009(29)		.018(37)	.097(37)				
Oats	.010(28) .010(28)	.013(36) .020(69)	.005(40)	.040(40)			.322(72)	
Rye flour	.017(4)							
Rye, whole	005-.011(29)							France: .021(4); USSR: .068(4); Argentina: .043(4), .06(3)
Rice, polished	.02-13(31) .02(28)	.073(69)	.008(40) .020(37) .008(41) .006(39)	.030(39) .020(40) .064(37) .087(37) .043(41)	1.48-6.08(39)	.02-12(45)	.464(72)	
Rice, brown	.020(28)	.043(69)						

(continues)

43

Table 3.1 (Continued)

Food	USA			Canada	England	Italy	W. Germany	Sweden
	Low Se	Moderate Se	High Se					
Wheat, whole	.63(1)	.32(3)	2.66-21.34(1)	.61(4)			.88(24)	.026(4)
	.05-.12(65)	.61(3)	3.5(19)	1.13(3)			.34(4)	<.01-.02(3)
	.065(95)	.50(12)	.64-.85(65)	.58-1.09(65)				
		.24-.46(4)						
		.20-.53(65)						
Wheat flour, white	.46-.62(1)	.192(11)	.39(18)	.28(21)	.42(23)			
	.331(2)	.18-.52(65)	.57-.78(65)	.35-.64(65)				
	.03-.09(65)		.36(96)					
Wheat flour, whole wheat	.615(2)	.636(11)	.87(18)	.61(21)	.53(23)			
			.45(96)					
Wheat flour, cake	.03-.06(65)	.05-.07(65)	.09(18)	.01-.02(65)	.04(23)			
	.050(2)							
Wheat bran	.63(1)		5.4(19)	.87(21)				.023(3)
Wheat germ	1.11(1)							
	.792(2)							
Breads								
White	.329(2)	.277(11)	.30(18)	.54(21)		.012(70)		
		.093(13)	.28(96)					
		.665(11)						
Whole wheat			.41(18)	.68(21)				
			3.5(19)					
Rye			.33(18)	.59(21)				
			.28(96)					

(continues)

44

Table 3.1 (*Continued*)

Food	Finland	New Zealand	China			Japan	Venezuela	Other countries
			Se-deficient	Moderate Se	Seleniferous			
Wheat, whole	.005-.011(29) .017(4) .01-.17(31)	007(98) .011-.086(36)	.006(41) .007-.009(42) .018(37) .005(38) .005(40)	.038(41) .019-.063(42) .017(38) .106(37) .052(37) .020(40)	1.057(42)		.248(72)	Denmark: .043(4); France: .012(4); USSR: .094(4); Argentina: .043 (4), .05(3); Yugoslavia: <.01-.018 (46); Australia: .048-.224(36)
Wheat flour, white	.010(28)	.011-.148(36) .014(69)	.005(38)	.035(38)		.03-.17(45)		
Wheat flour, whole wheat	.115(4)	.022(69)						
Wheat flour, cake								
Wheat bran	.020(28)							Argentina: .067(3)
Wheat germ	.030(28)	.025(69)						
Breads White	.010(28)	.011(69) .011-.086(36)				.12-.87(45)		Norway: .17(18)
Whole wheat	<.010-.020(28)	.021(69) .011(36)					.506(72)	
Rye	.010(28)	.062(36) .012(36)						

(*continues*)

Table 3.1 *(Continued)*

Food	USA			Canada	England	Italy	W. Germany	Sweden
	Low Se	Moderate Se	High Se					
Oatmeal				.60(21)				
White rolls			.29(18)	.51(21)				
Bagels			.32(18)					
Pasta(dry)								
Lasagna	.529(2)		.96(96)	.81(21)				
Macaroni	.502(2)		.61(96)	1.35(21)	.16(23)			
			.63(18)					
Egg noodles	.571(2)	.623(11)	.59(18)	.94(21)				
			.59(96)					
Spaghetti	.741(2)	.555(13)	.62(18)	.84(21)				
			.61(96)					
Crackers								
Graham	.061(2)	.11(18)	.06(18)					
Wheat	.040(2)		.14(96)					
Rye	.677(2)		.019(18)					
Soda	.061(2)		.11(18)	.11(21)				
Breakfast cereals								
Cream of wheat			.20(18)					
Corn flakes		.026(11)	.047-100(18)	.04-12(21)	.02(23)			
			.10(96)					
Oat meal	.444(2)	.110(11)	.28(18)	.10-45(21)	.03(23)	.074(24)		
Wheat flakes	.09(1)	.105(11)	.55(18)	.08(21)				
	.081(2)							

(continues)

Table 3.1 *(Continued)*

Food	Finland	New Zealand	China			Japan	Venezuela	Other countries
			Se-deficient	Moderate Se	Seleniferous			
Oatmeal	.010(28)							
White rolls	<.010(28)							
Bagels								
Pasta (dry)								
Lasagna								
Macaroni	.010(28)							
Egg noodles				.04(45)				
Spaghetti	.010(28)							
Crackers								
Graham								
Wheat	<.01(28)							
Rye								
Soda								
Breakfast Cereals								
Cream of wheat								
Corn flakes	.020(28)	.025(36)						
Oat meal	.010(28)	.013(36)						
	.010(28)	017(36)						

47

(continues)

Table 3.1 *(Continued)*

Food	USA			Canada	England	Italy	W. Germany	Sweden
	Low Se	Moderate Se	High Se					
Shredded wheat	.05(1)		.05(18)	.04(21)				
Wheat bran	.04(1) .58(2)		.10(18)	.07-.30(21)				
Puffed rice	.02(1)	.029(11)	.12(18)	.07(21)				
Vegetables								
Asparagus	.004(2)	.006(11)	.023(18)	.005(21)				
Beans, green fresh	n.d.-.02(1) .004(2)	.008(13)	.015(18)	.005(21)				
Beans, black, dry								
Beans, broad, dry							.022(24)	
Beans, wax. fresh	n.d.(1)							
Beans, wax, canned	.009(2)							
Beans, red kidney	.02(1)			.055(21)				
Beans, lima	.014(2) .005(2)		.072(18)					
Beans, great northern, dry	.129(2)							
Beans, navy, dry			.11(18) .13(96)					
Beans, soy		.08-.48(14) .07(15)	1.18(1)	.090(21)				
Bean curds (tofu)								

(continues)

48

Table 3.1 *(Continued)*

Food	Finland	New Zealand	China			Japan	Venezuela	Other countries
			Se-deficient	Moderate Se	Seleniferous			
Shredded wheat								
Wheat bran		.020(69)						
Puffed rice	.020(28)	.013,.016(98)						
Vegetables								
Asparagus	.002(30)							
Beans, green fresh	<.002(30)							
Beans, black, dry					2.82(39)		2.978(72)	
Beans, broad, dry								
Beans, wax, fresh			.021(37)	.051(37)	33.2(39)			
Beans, wax, canned								
Beans, red kidney								
Beans, lima							.065(72)	
Beans, great northern, dry								
Beans, navy, dry								
Beans, soy			.010(39)	.069(39)	.34–11.9(39)	.02(45)		
			.008(40)	.063(41)				
			.019(37)	.059(37)				
			.022(40)	.041–.081(40)				
Bean curds (tofu)						.02(45)		

(continues)

49

Table 3.1 (*Continued*)

Food	USA			Canada	England	Italy	W. Germany	Sweden
	Low Se	Moderate Se	High Se					
Beets, tuber	n.d.(1)		.009(18) .006(96)	.004(21)			.009(24)	
Beets, greens	n.d.(1)		.024(18)					
Broccoli			.017(18)	.002(21)			.017(24)	
Brussel sprouts							.027(24)	
Cabbage		.023(11)	.011(96)	.030(21)	<.01(23)	n.d.(70)	.014(24)	
Carrots, fresh	n.d.(1)	.022(11)	.019(96)	.006(21)		n.d.(70)	.004(24)	
Carrots, canned		.013(11)	.009(18)					
Carrots, greens		.001(13)						
Cauliflower	n.d.(1)	.007(11)	.004(96) .032(18)	.004(21)		n.d.(70)	.014(24)	
Cassava (tapioca)			.003(96)					
Celery			.011(18)			n.d.(71)	.006(24)	
Cow peas, fresh	n.d.(1)							
Cucumbers			.006(18)	.119(21)				
Egg plant								
Endive							.009(24)	
Horseradish								
Kohlrabi							.008(24)	
Leeks	n.d.(1)						.021(24)	

(*continues*)

Table 3.1 (*Continued*)

Food	Finland	New Zealand	China			Japan	Venezuela	Other countries
			Se-deficient	Moderate Se	Seleniferous			
Beets, tuber	<.002(30)							
Beets, greens								
Broccoli	<.002(30)							
Brussel sprouts		.001(98)						
Cabbage	<.002-.010(30) <.001(31)	<.001(69)		.002-.038(43)	2.91(39)	.01(45)	.010(72)	
Carrots, fresh	<.002(30) <.001(31)				1.06(39)	.01(45)	.019(72)	
Carrots, canned								
Carrots, greens					3.06(39)			
Cauliflower	<.002(30)	.003(69)					.010(72)	
Cassava (tapioca)							.006(72)	
Celery		<.001(98)					.095(72)	
Cow peas, fresh					7.85(39)			
Cucumbers	<.002(30)					.002(45)		
Egg plant					3.06(39)			
Endive								
Horse radish	.002(30)							
Kohlrabi								
Leeks	<.002(30)				9.45(39)	.03(45)		

(continues)

51

Table 3.1 *(Continued)*

Food	USA Low Se	USA Moderate Se	USA High Se	Canada	England	Italy	W. Germany	Sweden
Lentils							.098(24)	
Lettuce	n.d.(1)	.132(11)	.008(18)	.008(21)			.006(24)	
Mushrooms, fresh			.07(96) .11(18)	.060(21)	.09(23)	.13(70)		
Mushrooms, canned		.105(11)	.054(18)					
Onions, mature	.01-.04(1)	.015(11)	.034(96) .031(18)	.013(21)			.011(24)	
Parsley	n.d.(1)			.005(21)		n.d.(70)		
Parsnips				.027(21)				
Peas	.003(2)	.009(13)	.015(96) .011(18)	.005(21) .015(21)			.054(24)	
Peppers, green	n.d.(1)	.007(11)	.022(18) .048(96)			n.d.(70)		
Peppers, red								
Potatoes, fresh. peeled	n.d.(1) .008(2)	.006(11) .004(13) .009(11)	.016(18)	.023(21)	<.01(23)		.017(24)	
Potatoes, canned								
Potatoes, dried flakes	.02(1) .263(2)		.028(18)	.043(21)				
Pumpkins								
Radishes		.039(11)	.02(18) .10(18)	.022(21)			.015(24)	
Rhubarb								

(continues)

Table 3.1 (*Continued*)

Food	Finland	New Zealand	China Se-deficient	China Moderate Se	China Seleniferous	Japan	Venezuela	Other countries
Lentils								
Lettuce	<.001(31)						.014(72)	
Mushrooms, fresh	.004–.99(30)			.014(43)		.02(45)		
Mushrooms, canned								
Onions, mature	<.002(30) <.001(31)	.002(69) .021(69)			2.52(39)	.01(45)	.003(72)	
Parsley	<.002(30)							
Parsnips	<.002(30)							
Peas	.002(30)	.004(69)	.003(37)	.011(37)			.044(72)	
Peppers, green								
Peppers, red	<.002(30)				5.93(39)	.01(45)	.014(72)	
Potatoes, fresh, peeled	<.002(30) .002(31)	.003(69)	003(37)	.006(37)	.40(39)	.02(45)	.016(72)	
Potatoes, canned								
Potatoes, dried flakes								
Pumpkins	<.002(30)				2.66(39)	.01(45)		
Radishes	<.002(30)							
Rhubarb	<.002(30)							

(continues)

Table 3.1 (*Continued*)

Food	USA			Canada	England	Italy	W. Germany	Sweden
	Low Se	Moderate Se	High Se					
Sauerkraut							.036(24)	
Seaweed								
Spinach			.012(18)				.018(24)	
Squash, yellow	n.d.(1)		.013(18) .032(96)					
Squash, zucchini			.030(18)					
Sweet corn	.007(2) n.d.(1)	.004(11)	.012(18) .096(96)	.004(21)				
Sweet potato	.26–.57(1)							
Swiss chard								
Tomatoes, fresh	n.d.(1)	.005(11)	.013(18) .008(96)	.001(21)		n.d.(70)	.007(24)	
Tomatoes, canned		.010(11) .009(13)						
Turnips, root	.27(1)	.007(11)	.009(18)	.025(21)				
Turnips, greens								
Soy meat analogs								
Beef		.517(15)						
Ham		.368(15)						
Turkey		.327(15)						
Chicken		.375(15)						
Soy protein isolate		.10–.18(15)						

(continues)

54

Table 3.1 (*Continued*)

Food	Finland	New Zealand	China			Japan	Venezuela	Other countries
			Se-deficient	Moderate Se	Seleniferous			
Sauerkraut	<.002-.003(30)							
Seaweed						.02-.09(45)		
Spinach	<.002(30)			.03-.10(43)		.01(45)		
Squash, yellow							.075(72)	
Squash, zucchini								
Sweet corn								
Sweet potato			.003-.005(40) .003(37)	.075-.089(40) .007(37)	2.76(39)	.02(45)	.002(72)	
Swiss chard								
Tomatoes, fresh	<.002(30)	<.001-.001(69)					.014(72)	
Tomatoes, canned					.96(39)			
Turnips, root	<.002(30)				45.7(39)			
Turnips, greens								
Soy meat analogs								
Beef								
Ham								
Turkey								
Chicken								
Soy protein isolate								

(continues)

Table 3.1 (Continued)

Food	USA			Canada	England	Italy	W. Germany	Sweden
	Low Se	Moderate Se	High Se					
Fruits								
Apples, peeled	.006(2)	.005(11)	.003(18) .002(96)	.004(21)	<.01(23)		.010(24)	
Applesauce		.002(13) .002(11) .004(13)		.001(21)				
Apricots								
Bananas	n.d.(1)	.010(11)	.011(18)	.004(21)			.041(24)	
Bilberries								
Blackberries						n.d.(70)		
Blueberries	n.d.(1)							
Cantaloupe				.004(96)				
Cloudberries								
Cranberries								
Currents, red and black				.012(21)				
Dates, dried				.019(21)				
Figs				.023(21)				
Gooseberries								
Grapefruits				.009(21)				
Grapes				.002(96)			.030(24)	
Lemons, peeled							.012(24)	
Oranges, peeled		.013(11)	.002(18)	.015(21)	<.01(23)		.029(24)	
Papaya								

(continues)

56

Table 3.1 (*Continued*)

| Food | Finland | New Zealand | China | | | Japan | Venezuela | Other countries |
			Se-deficient	Moderate Se	Seleniferous			
Fruits								
Apples, peeled	<.002(30)	.004(69) .001(98)					.006(72)	
Applesauce								
Apricots	.002(30)							
Bananas	.005(30)						.005(72) .064(72)	
Bilberries	<.002(30)							
Blackberries								
Blueberries								
Cantaloupe								
Cloudberries	<.002(30)							
Cranberries	<.002(30)							
Currents, red and black	<.002(30)							
Dates, dried	.030(30)							
Figs								
Gooseberries	<.002(30)							
Grapefruits	.002(30)							
Grapes								
Lemons, peeled						.004(45)		
Oranges, peeled	<.002(30)						.008(72)	
Papaya							.032(72)	

(continues)

Table 3.1 (*Continued*)

	USA								
Food	Low Se	Moderate Se	High Se	Canada	England	Italy	W. Germany	Sweden
Peaches, fresh, peeled		.004(11)		.004(21)				
		.006(13)						
Peaches, canned		.003(11)		.001(21)				
Pears, fresh, peeled		.008(13)		.004(21)			.014(24)	
		.006(11)						
Pears, canned		<.002(11)		.002(21)				
Plums				.002(21)				
Pineapples, fresh		.006(11)		.002(21)				
Pineapples, canned		.010(11)						
Prunes								
Raisins	.005(2)			.010(21)				
	n.d.(1)							
Raspberries								
Strawberries								
Nuts and seeds								
Almonds	.02(1)		.047(18)		.04(23)			
Brazil	1.03(1)	29.6(16)	29.6(18)		2.3-53(23)			
Cashews	.027(2)		.20(18)		.34(23)			
Chestnuts					<.01(23)	n.d.(70)		
Coconuts			.14(18)					
Hazel	.072(2)		.032(18)					
	.02(1)							

(continues)

58

Table 3.1 *(Continued)*

Food	Finland	New Zealand	Se-deficient	Moderate Se	Seleniferous	Japan	Venezuela	Other countries
				China				
Peaches, fresh, peeled	<.002(30)							
Peaches, canned	<.002(30)							
Pears, fresh, peeled	<.002(30)	002(69)						
Pears, canned								
Plums	<.002(30)							
Pineapples, fresh							.007(72)	
Pineapples, canned	<.002(30)							
Prunes	.005(30)							
Raisins	<.005(30) <.002(30)					.004(45)		
Raspberries	<.002(30)							
Strawberries	<.002(30)							
Nuts and seeds								
Almonds	.020(30)							
Brazil								
Cashews								
Chestnuts								
Coconuts								
Hazel	.030(30)							

(continues)

59

Table 3.1 *(Continued)*

Food	USA			Canada	England	Italy	W. Germany	Sweden
	Low Se	Moderate Se	High Se					
Hickory	.081(2)				<.01(23)			
Peanuts	n.d.(1) .078(2)	.03-.04(15)	.07(18)		.03(23)		.37(24)	
Peanut butter	.085(2)		.10(18) .12(96)					
Pecans	.03(1)		.051(18)					
Soybeans, roasted		.04-.07(15)	.59(18)			.43(3)		
Sunflower seeds	.847(2)		.61(18)					
Walnuts	.026(2)		.122(18)		.19(23)			
Meats								
Beef								
Muscle (steaks)	.36(1) .023(2)	.058-.084(13) .270(11) .25(12)	.24(96) .29(18)	.03-.15(21)	.03(23)		.28(25) .13(24)	.15(27)
Tongue			.18(18)					
Heart			.38(96) .38(18)		.03(23)		.12(24)	
Liver	.18(1) .630-.880(2)	.432(11)	.63(18) .62(96)	.50(21)	.20(23)		.09(24)	
Kidney	1.70(1)	1.55(11)	1.45(96) 1.48(18)	2.31(21)	1.06(23)		.95(24)	
Horse, muscle								

(continues)

60

Table 3.1 (*Continued*)

Food	Finland	New Zealand	China			Japan	Venezuela	Other countries
			Se-deficient	Moderate Se	Seleniferous			
Hickory								
Peanuts	.020(30)							
Peanut butter								
Pecans								
Soybean, roasted								
Sunflower seeds								USSR: .24(3)
Walnuts								
Meats								
Beef								
Muscle (steaks)	.01-02(32)	.04(103)				.08(45)	.171(72)	Norway: .09(47), .036(74)
	.02-07(31)	.011(73)						
		.012(98)						
Tongue	.020(32)							
Heart	.05(32)							
Liver	.07-08(32)	.09(98)					.685(72)	
		.089(73)						
		.05(103)						
Kidney	.700(32)	.84, .92(98)						
		.088(73)						
		.87(103)						
Horse, muscle	.02-03(32)							

(*continues*)

Table 3.1 (*Continued*)

Food	USA			Canada	England	Italy	W. Germany	Sweden
	Low Se	Moderate Se	High Se					
Lamb								
Muscle (chops)	.30(1)	.178(11)	.31(18)		<.01(23)		.23(24)	
	.045-.069(2)	.25(12)	.32(96)					
	.05(5)	.14(5)	.28(5)					
			.76(5)					
Heart			.48(18)					
			.49(96)					
Liver	.10(5)	.27(5)	.76(5)		.06(23)			
			.90(18)					
			.98(96)					
			3.26(5)					
Kidney	1.20(5)	1.43(11)	1.38(18)		.93(23)			
			2.41(5)					
			1.34(96)					
			.52(18)					
Pancreas								
Mutton								
Pork								
Muscle (chops)	.039-.082(2)	.239(11)	.31(96)	.31(21)	.14(23)		.19(24)	
		.24(12)	.31(18)					
			.35(96)					
			.35(18)					
Heart							.20(24)	
Liver	.64(1)		.70(18)	.36(21)			.17(24)	
			.70(96)					

(continues)

Table 3.1 *(Continued)*

Food	Finland	New Zealand	China			Japan	Venezuela	Other countries
			Se-deficient	Moderate Se	Seleniferous			
Lamb								
Muscle (chops)		.04(103)						Norway: .083(74)
Heart	.030(32)							
Liver	.090(32)	.10(103)						
		.056(69)						
Kidney	.660(32)	.08, .31(98)						
		.059(69)						
		.55, .63(98)						
		.70(103)						
Pancreas	.060(32)	.014(69)						
Mutton	.01-.02(32)							
Pork								
Muscle (chops)		.09(101)				.16(45)	.833(72)	Norway: .092(74)
		.057(69)						
Heart	.220(32)	.42(103)				.48(44)	.36(45)	
Liver	.470(32)	.093(69)						

(continues)

Table 3.1 *(Continued)*

Food	USA			Canada	England	Italy	W. Germany	Sweden
	Low Se	Moderate Se	High Se					
Kidney	4.17(1)	1.90(11)	2.21(18)	3.22(21)	2.46(23)		.78(24)	
			2.10(96)					
Bacon			.25(18)					
Chicken								
Breast		.116(11)	.38(96)	.16(21)		.06(70)		
		.13(12)	.60(18)					
		.039(17)						
Leg		.136(11)	.40(96)	.15(21)				
Skin		.150(11)				.08(70)		
Liver		.081(17)	.71(18)			.21(70)		
			.71(96)			.21(70)		
Kidney						.21(70)		
Turkey								
Breast	.038–.053(2)	.08(6)	.34(18)					
	.056(6)		.35(6)					
Skin	.07(6)	.13(6)	.36(6)					
Liver	.15(6)	.54(6)	1.06(6)					
Pheasant			.51(96)					
Moose, muscle								
Rabbit, muscle								
Reindeer, muscle								
Whale								
Processed meats								
Beef jerky			.54(96)					
			.76(18)					

(continues)

Table 3.1 *(Continued)*

Food	Finland	New Zealand	China Se-deficient	Moderate Se	Seleniferous	Japan	Venezuela	Other countries
Kidney	1.71(32)	.87, .97(98) 2.03(103)						
Bacon								
Chicken								
Breast	.100(32)					.18(45)	.702(72)	Norway: .22(74)
Leg								
Skin								
Liver								
Kidney							1.658(72)	
Turkey								
Breast	.050(32)							Norway: .18(74)
Skin								
Liver								
Pheasant								
Moose, muscle	.040(32)							
Rabbit, muscle	.100(32)							
Reindeer, muscle	.250(32)							
Whale						.13(45)		
Processed meats								
Beef jerkey								

(continues)

65

Table 3.1 (Continued)

Food	USA			Canada	England	Italy	W. Germany	Sweden
	Low Se	Moderate Se	High Se					
Bologna	.082(2)		.30(18)					
Bratwurst			.30(18)					
Braunschweiger	.220(2)		.29(96)					
Corned beef			.19(18)					
			.25(96)					
Frankfurters, pork			.23(18)					
			.23(96)					
Bacon			.26(96)					
Ham			.51(18)					
			.47(96)					
Head cheese			.38(18)					
Liverwurst	.22(2)		.58(18)					
Salami			.35(96)					
			.33(18)					
Sausage, Polish			.25(18)					
			.31(96)					
Sausage, pork			.32(18)			.03(70)		
			.33(96)					
Fish								
Anchovy								
Braem								
Carp							.30(24)	

(continues)

Table 3.1 *(Continued)*

| Food | Finland | New Zealand | China | | | | Japan | Venezuela | Other countries |
			Se-deficient	Moderate Se	Seleniferous				
Bologna									
Bratwurst									
Braunschweiger									
Corned beef									
Frankfurters, pork	.020(32)								
Bacon	.080(32)	.03(98)							
Ham	.10-.17(31)	.032(69)							
Head cheese	.120(32)								
Liverwurst									
Salami									
Sausage, Polish	.02-.05(32)								
Sausage, pork	.020(32)								
	.02-.05(31)								
Fish									
Anchovy	.200(33)								
Braem	.310(33)								
Carp									

(continues)

67

Table 3.1 (*Continued*)

Food	USA			Canada	England	Italy	W. Germany	Sweden
	Low Se	Moderate Se	High Se					
Cod	.12(1)	.428(11)	.27(18)	.86(21) .42(22) .51(22)	.10(23)		.24(24)	
Eel								
Flounder		.337(11)		.046(22)				
Haddock			.19(18)	.51(22) 1.01(21)				
Halibut				.60(22) 1.36(21)				
Herring	1.41(1)		.27(18)		.61(23)		.44(24)	
Lutefisk			.20(18)					
Mackerel					.35(23)			
Octopus								
Perch	.368(1)		.34(18)				.41(24)	
Pike							.38(24)	
Rainbow trout			.34(18)	.59(21)		.06(70)	.50(24)	
Roe								
Salmon			.31(18)	.75-1.48(21)			.53(24)	
Sardines								
Smelt	1.23(1) .321(2)							
Sole				.95(22) 1.57(21)				
Sunfish	.36(1)						.50(24)	
Tuna	1.6(19)		.95(18) 1.15(96)	1.42(22)			.53(24)	

(continues)

Table 3.1 (*Continued*)

| | | | China | | | | | |
Food	Finland	New Zealand	Se-deficient	Moderate Se	Seleniferous	Japan	Venezuela	Other countries
Cod	.270(33)	.034-.046(69)						
		.31(98)						
Eel	.570(33)	.050(69)						
Flounder	.240(33)	.27(98)						
		.027(69)						
Haddock								
Halibut								
Herring	.18-.24(32)							
	.18(31)							
Lutefish								
Mackerel							.932(72)	
Octopus						.09(45)		
Perch	.280(33)							
Pike	.220(33)							
Rainbow trout	.260(33)							
Roe	.27-.98(33)							
Salmon	.260(33)					.25(45)		
Sardines	.350(33)					.78(45)		
Smelt								
Sole		.047(69)					.318(72)	
Sunfish								
Tuna	.420(33)					1.36(45)		

(continues)

Table 3.1 *(Continued)*

Food	USA			Canada	England	Italy	W. Germany	Sweden
	Low Se	Moderate Se	High Se					
Fish flour	1.93(1)							
Shell fish								
Clams	.55(1)							
Crabs	.51(1)			.92(22)				
Lobster	1.04(1)	.658(11)		1.22(21)				
Mussels								
Oysters	.49(1)	.653(11)	.49(18)	91(21)				
Scallops	.77(1)							
Shrimp	1.88(1)	.588(11)	.21(18)	1.61(21)				
Dairy products								
Milk, whole	.005(7)	.058(7)	.061(18)	.15(21)	<.01(23)	.008(70)	.200(26)	
	.009-.014(2)	.012(11)	.046(8)				.018(24)	
	.013-.018(8)	01(12)	.05(20)					
		.022-.03(8)	.069(96)					
Milk, low fat	.009(2)	.048(11)	.059(18)					
Milk, dried	06(1)	.096(11)		.093(21)				.16(3)
skimmed	.276(2)	.241(11)						
		.08(12)						
Milk, condensed,		.013(11)		.035(21)				
canned								
Cream			.05(18)	.004(21)				

(continues)

70

Table 3.1 *(Continued)*

Food	Finland	New Zealand	China			Japan	Venezuela	Other countries
			Se-deficient	Moderate Se	Seleniferous			
Fish flour				1.47-1.96(43)				
Shell fish								
Clams						.18(45)		
Crabs								
Lobster								
Mussels	.56(33)							
Oysters		.056(69) .46(98)						
Scallops						.15(45)	.197(72)	
Shrimp	.21(33)							
Dairy Products								
Milk, whole	.07(4) .004-.008(31) .002-.003(34)	.006-.008(56) .004(69) .003-.010(99)				.03(45)	.115(72)	Norway: .008-.012(74)
Milk, low fat	.08(4) .002(34)							
Milk dried skimmed	.08(4) .020(4)						.417(72)	
Milk, condensed, canned								
Cream	.002(34)							

(continues)

Table 3.1 (*Continued*)

Food	USA			Canada	England	Italy	W. Germany	Sweden
	Low Se	Moderate Se	High Se					
Cheese								
American processed		.090(11)	.23(96)	.056(21)				
			.13(18)					
Blue								
Brick	.106(2)		.11(18)					
Camembert							.03(24)	
Cheddar	.132(2)		.71(18)		.115(21)	.12(23)		
			.18(18)					
			.14(96)					
Colby			.56(18)					
Cottage	.034(2)	.052(11)	.14(18)	.068(21)				
			.19(18)					
			.23(96)					
Edam								
Emmenthal								
Gouda								
Gruyere						.010(70)		
Monterey jack			.14(18)					
			.76(18)					
			.20(18)					
Parmesan						.030(70)		
Swiss	.074(2)	.105(11)	.13(18)					
			.34(18)					
Ice cream			.070(18)					

(continues)

72

Table 3.1 (*Continued*)

Food	Finland	New Zealand	China Se-deficient	China Moderate Se	China Seleniferous	Japan	Venezuela	Other countries
Cheese								
American								
processed	.010(34)							
Blue	.020(34)							.425(72)	
Brick								
Camembert								
Cheddar								
Colby								
Cottage	.020(34)							
Edam	.040(34)							
Emmenthal	.040(34)							
Gouda	.010(34)							.384(72)	
Gruyere	.030(34)							
Monterey jack								
Parmesan								
Swiss								.382(72)	
Ice cream	<.005(34)							

(continues)

Table 3.1 (*Continued*)

Food	USA			Canada	England	Italy	W. Germany	Sweden
	Low Se	Moderate Se	High Se					
Yogurt			.050(18)					
Sweeteners								
Sugar, refined, white	n.d.(1) .010(2)	.003(11)			<.01(23)			
Sugar, raw. brown	n.d.(1)	.011(11)	.029(18)		<.01(23)			
Corn syrup	.14(1)							
Maple syrup	n.d.(1)							
Honey			.008(18)					
Molasses, cane	.26(1) .276(2)		.94(18) 1.28(96)					
Molasses, sorghum	.017(2)							
Saccharin		.005(11)						
Jams, fruit								
Jellies, fruit		.009-.012(13)						
Eggs								
Whole	.056(7) .065(2)	.098(11) .470(7)	.45(18) .47(96)	.39(21)			.18(24)	
Yolks	.08-.26(9) .140(2)	.183(11) .130(17)	.62(18)	.69(21) .127(10)	.20(23)	.068(70)		
Whites	.053(2) .048(9)	.051(11) .028(17)	.35(18)	.15(21) .123(10)	.06(23)	.036(70)		

(continues)

Table 3.1 (*Continued*)

Food	Finland	New Zealand	China			Japan	Venezuela	Other countries
			Se-deficient	Moderate Se	Seleniferous			
Yogurt	.003(34)							
Sweeteners								
sugar, refined, white	<.010(35)							
Sugar, raw, brown								
Corn syrup	.010(35)							
Maple syrup								
Honey	<.010(35)							
Molasses, cane								
Molasses, sorghum								
Saccharin								
Jams, fruit	.003(30)							
Jellies, fruit	.003(30)							
Eggs								
Whole	.11-.18(31) .110(34)	.31(98) .24(69) .98(69)				.24(45)	1.52(72)	Norway: .25(74)
Yolks	.300(34)	.055(69) .63(98)						
Whites		.08(98)						

(continues)

Table 3.1 *(Continued)*

Food	USA			Canada	England	Italy	W. Germany	Sweden
	Low Se	Moderate Se	High Se					
Fats								
Butter	.006(11)	.03(12)	.016(18)	.003(21)	<.01(23)			
Margarine								
Lard	.42(1)		.016(18)		<.01(23)			
Condiments								
Alspice	.03(1)							
Caraway seeds	.02(1)							
Chili powder	.25(1)							
	.348(2)							
Cinnamon	.25(1)							
	.048(2)							
Dill								
Garlic	.014(1)	.249(11)	.26(18)	.069(21)	.02(23)			
	.380(2)							
Ginger								
Mustard, prepared								
Nutmeg	.019(1)							
	.034(2)							
Paprika	.11(1)							
Pepper, black	.01(1)							
Salt	.04(1)							
Soy sauce			.008(18)					

(continues)

Table 3.1 (*Continued*)

| Food | Finland | New Zealand | China | | | Japan | Venezuela | Other countries |
			Se-deficient	Moderate Se	Seleniferous			
Fats								
Butter	.005(34)							
Margarine	<.010(34)							
Lard								
Condiments								
Allspice								
Caraway seeds								
Chili powder								
Cinnamon								
Dill	<.002(30)							
Garlic					17.47(39)	.02(45)	.047(72)	
Ginger					1.01(30)	.01(45)		
Mustard, prepared	.060(35)							
Nutmeg								
Paprika								Spain: .006(45)
Pepper, black								
Salt	<.010(35)							
Soy sauce								

(continues)

77

Table 3.1 (Continued)

Food	USA			Canada	England	Italy	W. Germany	Sweden
	Low Se	Moderate Se	High Se					
Vinegar, apple cider	.89(1)							
Snack foods								
Corn tortilla chips	.090(2)		.068(18)					
Potato chips	.032(2)		.12(18)					
Pretzels				.15(21)				
Candy								
Chocolate			.038(18)					
Licorice, black			.35(18)					
Licorice, red			.022(18)					
Sugar			.003(18)					
Beverages								
Coffee								
Ground, dry	.090(2)		.069(18)					
Instant, dry	n.d.-.11(1)	.391(13)	.130(18)					
Decaffeinated, instant, dry	.05-.25(1)	.459(13)	.04(96)					
Tea, black. dry	.062(2) .01(1)							
Tea, green, dry			.05(96)					
Tea, instant, dry	n.d.-.06(1)		.049(18)					

(continues)

Table 3.1 (*Continued*)

Food	Finland	New Zealand	China			Japan	Venezuela	Other countries
			Se-deficient	Moderate Se	Seleniferous			
Vinegar, apple cider								
Snack foods								
Corn tortilla chips								
Potato chips								
Pretzels								
Candy								
Chocolate	.020(35)							
Licorice, black	.010(35)							
Licorice, red								
Sugar	.010(35)							
Beverages								
Coffee								
Ground, dry								
Instant, dry	.030(35)							
Decaffeinated instant, dry								
Tea, black, dry								
Tea, green, dry								.04(45)	
Tea, instant, dry								

(continues)

79

Table 3.1 *(Continued)*

Food	USA			Canada	England	Italy	W. Germany	Sweden
	Low Se	Moderate Se	High Se					
Apple juice	.04(1)	.006(13)						
Grape juice		.004(13)						
Grapefruit juice	.06(1)	.006(13)						
Orange juice								
Beer	.19(1)				<.01(23)			
Wine	.05(1)							
Sodas, fruit flavored								
Sodas, cola flavored								
Miscellaneous foods								
Cocoa powder	.205(2)							
Gelatin	.19(1)							
	.395(2)							
Gelatin dessert, with fruit	.067(2)							
Beef broth		.101(13)						

(continues)

80

Table 3.1 (*Continued*)

Food	Finland	New Zealand	China Se-deficient	China Moderate Se	China Seleniferous	Japan	Venezuela	Other countries
Apple juice								
Grape juice	<.002(30)							
Grapefruit juice								
Orange juice	<.002(30)							
Beer	<.001(35)							
Wine	.001(35)							Hungary: .0005(35); France: .0008(35); Spain: .00025(35)
Sodas, fruit flavored	<.001(35)							
Sodas, cola flavored	.001(35)							
Miscellaneous foods								
Cocoa powder								
Gelatin								
Gelatin dessert, with fruit								
Beef broth								

[a]References are shown in parentheses.
[b]n.d., None detected.

Se contents of food supplies. Nevertheless, the great geographic variation in Se contents of related foods is apparent from the available work. For example, two countries, Finland and New Zealand, in which interest in the Se status of the food supply was stimulated by local experiences with Se-deficiency syndromes in livestock, have been found to have foods with relatively low Se levels in comparison to many other countries. Within the USA, the low and high-Se areas that have been identified on the basis of their relative soil Se conditions have been found to have foods which also differ appreciably in Se content. This is best seen in comparing the Se contents of locally produced foods in the relatively high-Se area of the Dakotas with those of comparable foods produced in the relatively low-Se areas of Ohio and Indiana. On a global basis, foods with the lowest Se contents have been found in parts of the low-Se regions of China, in particular the provinces of Heilongjiang, northern Shaanxi, and Sichuan. Ironically, foods containing the greatest concentrations of Se have also been found in China, in two areas of endemic selenosis of animals and people in Enshi County, Hubei Province, and in Ziyang County in the southern part of Shaanxi Province. Although the Se contents of Chinese foods have not been characterized extensively, that work is presently in progress in several institutes in that country.

The Se contents of prepared liquid infant formulas have been reported for the USA,[48] West Germany,[26] and Finland[34]; those for solid infant foods have been reported for the United States[11] and Canada.[21] These data are presented in Table 3.2. It is not surprising that the Se contents of solid foods prepared for infant use correlate with those of the corresponding foods shown in Table 3.1. It is noteworthy that, of the prepared liquid formulas, those based on meat or casein contain approximately an order of magnitude more Se (i.e., 0.073 ppm, fresh weight basis) than those based on milk or soy protein (i.e., 0.011 ppm, fresh weight basis). The Se contents of human breast milk, in contrast, are generally between these levels. The results of several analyses of breast milk Se (see Table 3.3) show that this source of Se nutriture for the infant generally contains approximately 0.020 ppm Se (fresh weight basis), and that the level is two to four times greater in colostrum (less than 4-day milk).[26,48,55,56] The Se contents of breast milk in the low-Se countries of Finland[34,54,55] and New Zealand[57] have been found to be only about 0.010 ppm, fresh weight basis, ranking as low as milk- and soy-based liquid infant formulas in the USA. It is of great scientific and medical interest to know something of the Se contents of breast milk of residents of the low-Se regions of China, especially as this may relate to the incidence of the Se-responsive cardiomyopathy of post-weaning children, Keshan Disease, which has been described there. The available data are discussed on pages 106-107.

Table 3.2

Selenium Contents (ppm, Fresh Weight Basis)
Reported for Infant Foods in Several Countries

Item	USA	Canada	W. Germany	Finland
Prepared liquid formulas				
Milk-based	.005, .009, .010, .023(48)[a] .005, .008 (49)		.007, .008, .008 .014, .011 (26) .013 (104)	.020 (34)
Milk-based, with Fe	.006, .024 (48) .006, .009(49)			
Soy-based	.006, .008, .013, .024 (48) .006, .008 (49)			
Casein-based	.053, .097, .098 (48)			
Meat-based	.052, .067 (48)			
Cereals				
Barley		.31, .59 (21)		
Oatmeal	.030(11)	.74, 1.09 (21)		
Rice	.021(11)	.21, .39 (21)		
Strained vegetables				
Beans, green	.005 (11)	.003, .005 (21)	.002 (104)	
Beans, wax		.003, .007 (21)		
Carrots	.002 (11)	.001, .002 (21)	.003 (104)	
Peas		.004, .010 (21)		
Potatoes		.003, .004 (21)	.016 (105)	
Squash		.003, .004 (21)		
Cucumbers			.003 (105)	
Mixed vetables		.033 (21)		
Vegetable soup		.039 (21)		
Strained fruits				
Applesauce		.001, .002 (21)	.005 (105)	
Apricots		.001, .002 (21)	.003 (105)	
Bananas		.004 (21)	.032 (105)	
Peaches	.004 (11)	.001, .002 (21)		
Pears	.004 (11)	n.d. (21)		
Plums		.003 (21)		
Oranges			.002 (105)	
Meats				
Beef	.116(11)	.026, .040 (21)		
Chicken	.107 (11)	.150, .207 (21)		
Ham		.110 (21)		
Lamb	.131 (11)	.045, .057 (21)		
Liver, source unspecified	.258 (11)			
Pork	124 (11)			
Turkey		.136, 1.68 (21)		
Veal		.055 (21)		
Miscellaneous				
Vanilla custard	.016 (11)			

[a]References are shown in parentheses.

Table 3.3

Selenium Contents (ppm, Fresh Weight Basis)
Reported for Human Milk in Various Countries

Country	Colostrum (<4 days)[a]	Transitory milk (4-10 days)[a]	Mature milk (>10 days)[a]
USA	.041 (49)[b]		.014 -.016 (49)
			.021 (50)
			.020 (51)
			.013-.028 (52)
			.024 (51)
			.015-.020 (53)
England			.01 -.02 (23)
West Germany	.086 (26)	.031 (26)	.028 (26)
Finland			.010 (34)
			.006-.011 (54)
			.010-.012 (55)
Greece			.020 (51)
Japan	.080 (55)		.017 -.018 (56)
New Zealand	.012-.035 (56)	.010-.022 (56)	.012-.015 (57)
			.008 (100)
China			
Low-Se areas			.003[c] (41)
			.004[d] (41)
Moderate-Se area[e]			.021 (41)
High-Se area[f]			.283 (41)

[a]Days post partum.
[b]References are shown in parentheses.
[c]From area of endemic Keshan Disease.
[d]From area without endemic Keshan Disease (so-called "safety island").
[e]Beijing.
[f]Enshi, Hubei Province, average of three samples.

The Se contents of several medical food supplements and tube feeding formulas were determined by Zabel et al.[48] and are presented in summary in Table 3.4. Zabel et al.[48] found differences in the Se contents of casein hydrolysate-based solutions used for total parenteral nutrition (TPN) and TPN solutions based on mixtures of recrystallized amino acids. Whereas the latter type provided less than 5 μg Se/1000 kcal of diet, the former type provided at least three times that amount and as much as 95 μg Se per 1000 kcal by virtue of the Se inherent in casein.

II. SOURCES OF VARIATION IN THE SELENIUM CONTENTS OF FOODS AND FEEDS

Much of the variation in the Se content of foods and feeds is due to large scale geographical differences in environmental Se. Variation due to

Table 3.4

Selenium Contents Reported for Various Medical Food Supplements and
Tube Feeding Formulas in the USA[a]

Item	Se content		
	ppm, Wet weight basis	ppm, Dry weight basis	μg Se/1000 kcal
Milk-based supplements	.011-.039	.064-.178	13-42
Soy-casein based supplements	.014-.015	.068	14-15
Blended foods	043-.050	.205-.264	46-52
Chemically defined diets	—		
Egg albumen based	—	.292-.620	78-147
Casein hydrolysate	—	.062	14
Amino acid mixture	—	.002-.005	< 1 to 1
Parenteral feeding solutions (TPN)			
Casein hydrolysates	.019-.037	.093-.324	16-95
Amino acid mixtures	< .001-.001	Trace to .010	Trace to 5

[a]From Zabel et al.[48]

these geochemical differences are readily seen in comparisons of the Se contents of like foods from different countries. Wheat suitably illustrates this point; whole wheat grain may contain more than 2 ppm Se (air-dry basis) if produced in the Dakotas,[1] but as little as 0.11 ppm Se if produced in New Zealand,[36] and only 0.005 ppm Se if produced in Shaanxi Province, China.[37] The geographic variation in the Se contents of several different foods produced within the same country (i.e., the USA) and with similar technologies is shown in Table 3.5. It shows that certain regions (e.g., Colorado, parts of Iowa, North and South Dakota) produce several foods that are relatively rich in Se.

The Se contents of foods of plant origin can vary according to climatic conditions during the growing season that may affect crop yield, maturity at harvest, etc. For this reason, annual variations are to be expected in the Se contents of such foods as the cereal grains, with those of grains produced in high-yield seasons to be somewhat lower than those of grains produced in low-yield ones. This effect was apparent in the report of Varo et al.,[29] who found that the Se contents of wheat, rye, barley, and oats produced in Finland were low in 1975, which had an exceptionally favorable growing season (i.e., above average temperatures, relatively low humidity) and good harvesting (i.e., fast ripening, low humidity) conditions. This combination of conditions resulted in the production of mature grain with relatively high starch content, but with Se (and other mineral) contents that were only about two-thirds of those of the previous year in which average yields were realized. In contrast, grains produced in Finland in

Table 3.5

Geographic Variation in Se Contents (ppm) of Selected Foods Produced in the USA

State of origin	Hard winter wheat[a]	Hard spring wheat[a]	Soft winter wheat[a]	Soybeans[b]	Lamb muscle[c]	Lamb liver[c]	Lamb kidney	Cow's milk[d]	Human milk[e]
Arizona	.05								.020
Arkansas				.16					
California									.018
Colorado					.28	.74	1.64		.015
Connecticut									.015
Florida				<.07					.018
Georgia									.018
Idaho	.10	.12	.06						
Illinois			.05		.16	.27	.84	.013	
Indiana			.13	<.07					
Iowa				.28					
Kansas	.20–.30								
Maryland				<.07					
Minnesota	.83	.53–.70		.90	.28	.57	1.48		
Mississippi			.05						
Missouri			.12						
Montana	.79–.85							.018–.044	.020
New York								.012–.015	.021
									.015

(continues)

Table 3.5 *(Continued)*

State of origin	Hard winter wheat[a]	Hard spring wheat[a]	Soft winter wheat[a]	Soybeans[b]	Lamb muscle[c]	Lamb liver[c]	Lamb kidney	Cow's milk[d]	Human milk[e]
North Carolina				<.07					
North Dakota									.013
Ohio		.43–.54	.04–.09						.016
Oklahoma									.021
Oregon								.014	.021
Pennsylvania									.028
South Dakota		.68			.44	.73	1.66	.047	
Tennessee			.03–.08						.016
Texas	.25								.022
Utah		.64	.07						
Washington					.09	.18	1.12		
West Virginia					.70	.60	1.30		
Wyoming									.016

[a] 14% Moisture basis, from Lorenz.[66]
[b] Air-dry basis, from Wauchope.[14]
[c] Fresh weight basis, from Paulson *et al.*[5]
[d] Fresh weight basis, from Shamberger and Willis.[8]
[e] Fresh weight basis, from Shearer and Hadjimarkos.[52]

1973 were generally higher in Se content due to conditions that resulted in relatively low yields during that year. These data are presented in Table 3.6.

On a larger scale, the importation of foods or feedstuffs from regions of different geochemical Se status can introduce variation in the Se contents of food supplies. Studies in New Zealand[36] and Finland[4] have documented the effects of the importation of relatively high-Se wheat into those countries which naturally produce foods low in the mineral. Watkinson[36] found that the importation of wheat containing ca. 0.150 ppm Se (air-dry basis) from Australia to New Zealand during the relatively poor harvest years of 1973-1975 and 1978-1980 in the latter country produced marked increases in the Se content of the New Zealand food supply. According to Watkinson's calculations,[36] the consumption of Australian wheat by New Zealanders in partial substitution for locally produced wheat containing only 0.011 ppm Se (air-dry basis) resulted in an approximate 50% increase in the average Se intake of the New Zealand population. This increase in consumption was reflected in increases in the blood Se concentrations of New Zealand residents by as much as 50% during the years of greatest wheat importation (e.g., 1975). Varo and Koivistoinen[4] found a similar effect of the importation of relatively high-Se grains from the USA and Canada on the Se content of the Finnish food supply. Their studies showed that the importation of large quantities of North American wheat (containing at least 0.400 ppm Se, air-dry basis) in 1979-1980 had significant effects on increasing the Se contents not only of wheat-based food products, but also of food products derived from animals fed the higher-Se feed grains. The cumulative effects of the importation of high-Se North American grains, as well as the increasing use of sodium selenite as a nutritional supplement to livestock feeds, was that the average Se intake of residents of Finland was estimated to have increased from ca. 30 μg per person per day before 1980[68] to 50-60 μg per person per day in 1980.[4] Table 3.6 presents summaries of these reports documenting the annual variations in the Se contents of the food supplies of Finland and New Zealand.

The Se contents of foods of animal origin depend in large part on the Se intakes of livestock. Food animals raised in regions with feeds of low-Se content will thus deposit relatively low concentrations of the mineral in their edible tissues and products (e.g., milk, eggs), while animals raised with relatively high-Se nutriture will produce foods with much greater Se concentrations. Due to the needs of livestock for Se to prevent debilitating deficiency syndromes, Se (usually as sodium selenite) is used as a nutritional supplement in animal agriculture in many parts of the world. This practice, which has become widespread in North America and Europe only within the last 10-15 years, has had the effect of reducing what would otherwise

Table 3.6

Annual Variations in Se Contents of Foods in New Zealand and Finland

Country	Foods	Se concentration (ppm, fresh weight basis)								
		Sept. 1973	Feb. 1976[d]	Feb. 1977	Aug. 1977	Feb. 1978	Aug. 1978	Feb. 1979[d]	Aug. 1979[d]	Feb. 1980[d]
New Zealand[a]										
	Wheat bread, white	.012	.086	.012	.011	.011	.011	.074	.010	.097
	Wheat/rye bread	—	.062	.012	—	—	—	—	—	—
	Wheat flour, white	.015	.089	.011	.011	.011	.011	.148	.012	.011
	Wheat biscuits	.017	.072	.011	.014	.011	.019	.016	.017	.083
Finland[b]		1975–1977	Fall 1981[d]		Spring 1982		Spring 1983		Fall 1983	
	Wheat bread, whole	.068	.054		.129		.034		.024	
	Wheat/rye bread	.013	.016		.036		.091		.016	
	Beef	.018	.053		.041		.059		.069	
	Ham	.077	.130		.116		.116		.126	
	Pork sausage	.016	.034		.030		—		—	
	Whole milk	.004	.006		.008		.008		.008	
	Whole eggs	.108	.176		.137		.159		.182	
	Baltic herring	.257	—		.225		—		—	
Finland[c]		1972	1973[f]		1974		1975[e]		1976	
	Spring wheat	.008	.008		.008		.005		.009	
	Winter wheat	.008	.008		.009		.011		.007	
	Rye	.011	.008		.007		.005		.006	
	Barley	.007	.009		.008		.005		.006	
	Oats	.007	.006		.009		.006		.008	

[a]From Watkinson.[36]
[b]Calculated from the data of Varo and Koivistoinen.[4]
[c]From Varo et al.[29]
[d]Year of importation of relatively high-Se wheat.
[e]Good harvest year.
[f]Poor harvest year.

be strong geographic variation in the Se contents of animal food products over many different parts of the world.

In general, increases in dietary Se produce increases in the Se contents of animal meats, milk, and eggs (see Table 3.7). However, this relationship, while direct, is not linear. Within the ranges of normal levels of Se intakes, muscle meats from most species tend to plateau in Se concentration at 0.3-0.4 ppm (fresh weight basis). Organ meats usually accrue greater concentrations of Se; the livers of several species have been found to accumulate about four times as much Se as skeletal muscle, and the kidneys of steers, lambs, and swine have been found to accumulate 10-16 times the amounts in muscle (see Table 3.7). Poultry do not accumulate such great renal concentrations of Se. Thompson and Scott[62] found that the concentrations of Se in kidneys from young broiler chickens and turkey poults averaged only 4.8 and 1.4 times those of livers, respectively. Because of the property of most species to accumulate relatively great concentrations of Se in liver and kidney, foods made from these organ meats tend to be rich sources of Se in human diets.

Varietal differences can be the sources of significant variation in the Se contents of some plant species. Although there have been few extensive varietal comparisons of Se content, the work of Wauchope[14] has nicely demonstrated the phenomenon in the case of the soybean [*Glycine max* (L.) Merr.]. That study compared the Se contents of 18 varieties of soybeans grown on adjacent plots either in Ames, Iowa, USA, or in Stoneville, Mississippi, USA (see Table 3.8). The six varieties grown in Iowa varied in Se content by 600% (i.e., 0.08-0.48 ppm, air-dry weight). The 12 varieties in Mississippi varied in Se content by ca. 550% (i.e., 0.24-1.57 ppm) when grown in clay soil, and by ca. 145% (i.e., 0.53-1.28 ppm) when grown in loamy soil. The significant interactive effect of variety and soil type shows that varietal differences in the Se contents of foods and feedstuffs of plant origin can vary between different geographic regions according to the local agronomic conditions.

The processing of cereal grains and oil seeds can produce food products with Se concentrations less than those of the parent materials due to the removal of relatively Se-rich components. Selenium in soybeans is strongly associated with the protein fraction of the bean. Ferretti and Levander[15] found that the processing of soybeans for the production of isolated soy protein resulted in an almost two-fold increase in Se concentration of the product compared to that of the full-fat starting material (see Table 3.9). In general, the germ and outer layers of cereal kernels are richer in Se than the endosperm. Therefore, milling products based on germ, bran, and shorts (e.g., wheat screenings, corn mill germ, rice bran) tend to contain higher levels of Se than the parent whole grains, and products based primarily

Table 3.7

Influence of the Se Concentrations of Livestock Feeds on the Se Contents of Meats, Milk, and Eggs

Animals	Type of diet	Dietary Se[a], (ppm, fresh weight basis)	Se content of food product (ppm, fresh weight basis)			Reference
			Muscle	Liver	Kidney	
Steers	Practical, low-Se	.085	.070	.258	1.483	(58)
		.206	.086	.384	1.372	
		.294	.100	.435	1.366	
Steers	Practical, high-Se	.199	.135	.498	1.458	(58)
		.255	.136	.499	1.578	
		.328	.158	.524	1.544	
Lambs	Practical, low-Se	.085	.088	.242	1.207	(58)
		.206	.092	.380	1.261	
		.294	.110	.533	1.233	
Lambs	Practical, high-Se	.199	.167	.618	1.301	(58)
		.255	.159	.656	1.351	
		.328	.167	.756	1.211	
Lambs	Practical, low-Se (<.2 ppm Se)	.02 in salt lick	.032	.132	.741	(59)
		31 in salt lick	.065	.298	.807	
		65 in salt lick	.057	.398	.796	
		170 in salt lick	.096	.653	.903	
Lambs	Practical, high-Se (.19-.78 ppm Se)	.02 in salt lick	.245	.617	1.036	(59)
		31 in salt lick	.240	.578	.990	
		65 in salt lick	.182	.580	.932	
		170 in salt lick	.239	.770	.903	
Pigs	Semi-purified, Se-deficient	<.02	.070	.084	1.25	(60)
		.05	.308	1.381	7.50	

(continues)

Table 3.7 (*Continued*)

Animals	Type of diet	Dietary Se[a], (ppm, fresh weight basis)	Se content of food product (ppm, fresh weight basis)			Reference
			Muscle	Liver	Kidney	
Pigs	Practical, low-Se	+.10 as Na_2SeO_3	.062	.233	1.129	(61)
		+.40 as Na_2SeO_3	.094	.464	1.218	
		+.10 as fish meal	.058	.167	.904	
		+.40 as fish meal	.122	.436	1.339	
		+.10 as browen's grains	.093	.276	1.038	
		+.40 as browen's grains	.116	.554	1.458	
Chickens	Practical, low-Se (.07ppm)	.07	.061	.25	.39	(62)
		.17	.071	.48	.34	
		.27	.103	.53	.80	
		.47	.114	.59	.56	
		.67	.126	.80	.62	
		.87	.157	.77	.71	
Chickens	Practical, high Se (.67ppm)	.67	.293	.80	1.08	(62)
		.87	.423	1.05	.98	
Turkeys	Practical, low-Se (.07ppm)	.07	.056	.15	.07	(62)
		.17	.07	.33	.14	
		.27	.08	.54	.13	
		.47	.11	.56	.12	
		.67	.10	.78	.16	
		.87	.10	.94	.17	
Turkeys	Practical, high-Se (.68 ppm)	.68	.32	1.03	.36	(62)
		.88	.35	1.06	.31	

Hens	Practical, low-Se (.10ppm)	.10	Whole egg	Hen muscle	
Hens	Practical, low-Se (.10ppm)	.10	.086	.099	(63)
Hens	Practical, high-Se (.42 pm)	.42	.202	.123	(63)
		.42	.338	.337	
Hens	Practical, low-Se (.04ppm)	.04	.136	—	(64)
		.09	.252	—	
		.14	.260	—	
		.24	.295	—	
Hens	Practical, high-Se (.45)	.45	.325	—	(64)
		.50	.355	—	
		.55	.376	—	
		.65	.391	—	

			Milk		
Cows	Practical, low-Se	+0	.010		(65)
		+.094	.017		
		+.225	.017		
Cows	Practical, high-Se	+0	.029		(65)
		+.572	.037		
Cows	Practical, high-Se	.334	.040		(66)
		.385	.047		
		.450	.050		
		.772	.064		

[a]Supplemental Se was added as Na_2SeO_3 in all cases, unless otherwise indicated.

Table 3.8

Varietal Differences in Se Contents of Soybeans Grown in the Same Locales[a]

Locale	Soybean variety	Se content (ppm, air-dry basis)
Ames, Iowa	Wells	.08
	Beeson	.17
	Amsoy 71	.24
	Corsoy	.30
	Hark	.39
	Chippewa	.48
Stoneville, Mississippi	Hood 75	.24
(clay soil)	Lee 68	.31
	Hill	.39
	Bragg	.47
	Lee 74	.56
	Davis	.58
	Mack	.67
	Traoy	.98
	Cajeme	1.06
	Pickett 71	1.07
	Forrest	1.09
	Ransom	1.57
Stoneville, Mississippi	Cajeme	.53
(loamy soil)	Lee 74	.84
	Davis	.96
	Forrest	.96
	Hood 75	.98
	Mack	1.00
	Lee 68	1.08
	Pickett 71	1.18
	Hill	1.20
	Bragg	1.29

[a]Data from Wauchope.[14]

on endosperm (e.g., wheat patent flour, corn flour, polished rice) tend to contain lower levels of Se than the parent whole grains (see Table 3.9). Nevertheless, the reductions in Se concentrations due to milling of cereal grains are generally only of low magnitude inasmuch as the differences in Se content of the various fractions of the kernel tend to be small. For example, Ferretti and Levander[67] found that the Se contents of wheat flour, white corn flour, yellow corn flour, and polished rice were approximately 87, 86, 70, and 92%, respectively, of the corresponding whole grain. The Se contents of wheat flours are affected by the blend of wheat milling fractions used to make them. Lorenz[66] studied the Se contents of seven types of wheats milled in several locations and the flours produced from

Table 3.9

Effects of Milling and Processing on Se Contents of Grain and Soybean Products[a]

Parent material	Fractions	Se content (ppm, dry matter basis)
Wheat	Raw wheat	.376
	Wheat flour	.326
	Farina	.272
	Screenings	.406
	Ground wheat feed	.490
White corn	Raw corn	.219
	Corn flour	.188
	Corn meal	.193
	Grits, degerminated	.208
	Hominy mill feed	.294
	Mill germ	.254
	Screenings	.185
Yellow corn	Raw corn	.267
	Corn flour	.186
	Corn meal	.173
	Grits, degerminated	.178
	Hominy mill feed	.158
	Mill germ	.373
	Screenings	.131
Oats	Green oats	.643
	Regular oat flakes	.725
	Quick oat flakes	.666
	Oat flour	.774
	Miniature oat flakes	.891
	North star	.712
	Light oats	.558
	Oat hulls	.221
Rice	Rough rice	.082
	Brown rice	.091
	Milled rice	.084
	Rice hulls	.032
	Rice bran	.170
Soybeans	Full-fat soybean meal	.052
	Solvent extracted soybean meal	.069
	Ethanol (70%) concentrate	.100
	pH 4.5 precipitated protein isolate	.138

[a]Calculated from the data of Ferretti and Levander for grain[67] and soy[15] products.

them at each mill. His results (see Table 3.10) showed that the apparent decrease in Se content due to the milling of flour varied enormously (i.e., from –5 to 68%). Although Lorenz[66] concluded that the Se content of flour decreased as the extraction percentage of the patent decreased, a close examination of those data reveals that the apparent decreases were not

Table 3.10

Effect of Milling on the Se Content of Wheat Flours[a]

Type of wheat	Se content of grain[b] (ppm)	Extraction percentage of patent (%)	Se content of flour[b] (ppm)	Decrease in Se due to milling flour (%)
Hard red winter	.05	100.0	.03	40
	.10	100.0	.09	10
	.20	96.0	.18	10
	.25	95.0	.21	16
	.27	95.0	.22	19
	.30	94.0	.21	30
	.31	96.0	.31	0
	.83	96.8	.68	18
	.85	94.8	.60	29
Hard red spring	.43	98.0	.37	14
	.53	100.0	.52	2
	.53	98.0	.52	2
	.54	76.0	.30	44
	.58	—	.59	−2
	.61	74.0	.53	13
	.61	52.0	.57	7
	.64	96.0	.57	11
	.68	100.0	.61	10
	.70	100.0	.60	14
	.74	71.5	.61	18
	.74	—	.78	−5
	.79	80.0	.64	19
	.79	81.0	.60	24
	1.09	59.0	.35	68
Durum	.12	71.6	.07	42
Soft red winter	.03	20.0	.02	33
	.04	100.0	.03	25
	.05	35.0	.03	40
	.05	65.0	.04	20
	.08	49.6	.06	25
	.08	82.0	.05	38
	.09	100.0	.05	44
	.12	100.0	.06	50
	.13	—	.12	8
Soft white	.05	100.0	.05	0
	.06	50.3	.05	17
White club	.07	58.5	.07	0
Ontario soft winter	.02	10.0	.01	50
	.03	100.0	.02	33

[a]From Lorenz.[66]

[b]14% Moisture basis.

related either to the extraction percentage of the patent or to the Se content of the whole grain. The apparent decreases were greatest for soft red winter and Ontario soft winter wheats (i.e., 31 and 42%, respectively) in comparison to the other wheats studied (e.g., hard red winter: 19%; hard red spring: 16%).

Higgs et al.[68] have examined the effects of several cooking procedures on the Se contents of a variety of foods typically found in American diets. Their results (see Table 3.11) show that most of the techniques used in Western-style cooking (e.g., boiling, baking, broiling) do not cause appreciable losses of Se from most foods. In fact, some cooking methods, such as those that resulted in the loss of fats from meats, resulted in apparent increases in Se in the cooked food. However, heat drying of breakfast cereals and boiling of asparagus and mushrooms (both of which are relatively high in Se) resulted in significant losses of Se (see Table 3.11).

Table 3.11

Effects of Cooking Procedures on the Se Contents of Foods[a]

| | | Se content, (ppm dry matter basis) | | |
| | | | | Apparent Se |
Cooking procedure	Food	Fresh	Processed	loss (%)
Heat drying (100°C, overnight)	Wheat breakfast cereal	.039	.030	23
	Oat breakfast cereal	.051	.047	8
Boiling, 5 min	Oatmeal	.078	.084	−8
	Wheat cereal	.047	.051	−8
Boiling, 20 min	Oatmeal	.078	.067	14
	Wheat cereal	.047	.053	−9
	Polished rice	.023	.023	0
	Egg noodles	.065	.061	6
	Mushrooms	1.40	.78	44
	Asparagus	.96	.68	29
Boiling, 45 min	Egg noodles	.065	.066	−2
Baking (175°C), 45 min	Chicken breast	.48	.49	−2
Baking (175°C), 60 min	Flounder fillet	1.38	1.51	−9
Broiling, 20 min	Lamb chops	.34	.34	0
	T-bone steak	.70	.60	14
Broiling, 45 min	Pork chops	.22	.20	9

[a] From Higgs et al.[68]

III. SELENIUM IN HUMAN DIETS

Differences in geography, agronomic practices, food availability and preferences, and methods of food preparation result in differences in the dietary contents of Se among human populations. Because many of these differences are difficult to quantify, evaluations of Se intakes of specific human population groups are often not precise. General comparisons can be made, however, of the Se contents of different food supplies by using the average Se concentrations determined within specific major classes of foods in different locales. Table 3.12 presents the typical Se contents of the major classes of foods from 11 countries. These values are, for the most part, based on actual analyses of foods from each country; where it was considered reasonable to do so, estimates have been given by the present authors in the absence of analytical data. Information has been listed for different regions within the USA, Canada, and the P.R.C. to demonstrate the marked differences in the Se contents of foods within each of those countries.

Table 3.12 can be used for comparing the Se contents of individual classes of foods among the various countries for which such information is available. It can also be used to estimate the Se contents of typical diets of residents of those countries. For example, the hypothetical Western-style menu shown in Table 3.13 would be expected to provide different amounts of Se were it to be prepared in different parts of the world. Table 3.14 shows that its projected Se contents vary from as little as 13 μg Se, based on foods from the region of endemic Se-deficiency of China, to more than 300 times that amount, based on foods from the local areas of endemic selenosis in the same country. Although this menu would be expected to provide 100-200 μg Se in most of the USA and Canada, it would provide only about 30 μg Se in Finland and New Zealand. By this comparison, great differences in relative dietary exposure to Se are evident among the residents of these countries.

Several authors have estimated the average per capita daily Se intakes of adults in various countries of the world (see Table 3.15). Certain of these estimates must be questioned at the present time due to the relatively limited information on which they are based (e.g., the estimate for Italy by Bombace et al.[71] may be too low). However, most correlate very well with the amounts of Se projected in the hypothetical menu calculated with the analytical data available from each country (see Table 3.14). The estimates presented in Table 3.15 show that the Se intakes of residents of different regions is highly variable and can be as low as 7-11 μg Se per person per day in the areas of Se-responsive human disorders in China. The residents of two countries with well recognized endemic Se-deficiency

Table 3.12

Typical Se Contents (ppm, Fresh Weight Basis) of Foods in Various Countries

Food	USA			Canada[b]		England[c]	Italy[d]	West Germany
	Low-Se	Moderate-Se	High-Se	East	West, north			
Cereal products	.300	.330	.560	.390	.410	.110	.012	.290
Vegetables	.010	.040	.070	.020	.025	.010	.002	.020
Fruits	.004	.006	.006	.005	.010	.005	.005[g]	.010
Nuts and seeds	.190	.190	.200	.20[g]	.20[g]	.15[g]	.20[g]	.20[g]
Red muscle meats	.195	.210	.370	.150	.390	.120	.05[g]	.210
Organ meats	1.070	1.020	1.335	1.15[g]	1.30[g]	.60[g]	.50[g]	.500
Processed meats	.350	.350	.375	.35[g]	.375[g]	.30[g]	.30[g]	.25[g]
Poultry	.100	.120	.410	.150	.390	.120	.060	.20[g]
Fish	.665	.665	.665	.150	.390	.120	.060	.425
Shellfish	.710	.710	.710	.70[g]	.70[g]	.320	—	
Milk	.010	.030	.055	.010	.050	.010	.010	.010
Cheeses	.085	.100	.300	.085[g]	.25[g]	.085[g]	.020	.100
Butter, cream	.006	.006	.016	.006[g]	.01[g]	.010	.006[g]	.01[g]
Eggs	.060	.100	.450	.06[g]	.16[g]	.15[g]	.050	.180
Sweeteners, condiments	.010	.010	.010	.005[g]	.01[g]	.01[g]	.01[g]	.01[g]

(continues)

Table 3.12 (*Continued*)

Food	Finland	New Zealand[a]	People's Republic of China			Japan[a]	Venezuela[e]	Ukranian SSR[f]
			Se-deficient	Moderate-Se	Seleniferous			
Cereal products	.020	.035	.010	.050	3.880	.070	.340	.280
Vegetables	.002	.003	.010	.050	5.680	.015	.030	.125
Fruits	.002	.003	.001[g]	.005[g]	—	.003	.020	.004
Nuts and seeds	.025	.10[g]	.05[g]	.20[g]	—	.15[g]	.40[g]	.20[g]
Red muscle meats	.050	.030	.025[g]	.10[g]	—	.120	.500	.292
Organ meats	.480	.075	.075[g]	.480	—	—	1.170	.16[g]
Processed meats	.065	.030[g]	—	—	—	.120	—	—
Poultry	.075	.075[g]	.050[g]	.10[g]	—	.180	.700	.50[g]
Fish	.325	.040	.150[g]	.40[g]	—	.350	.535	.10[g]
Shellfish	.385	—	—	—	—	—	.200	—
Milk	.025	.004	.002[g]	.02[g]	—	.03	.115	.100
Cheeses	.025	.06[g]	—	—	—	.03	.465	.300
Butter, cream	.002	.002[g]	—	—	—	.03	.01[g]	.01[g]
Eggs	.135	.240	.05[g]	.16[g]	—	.240	1.520	.020
Sweeteners, condiments	.005	.01[g]	.002[g]	.01[g]	—	.020	.01[g]	.01[g]

[a]Estimates derived from Table 3.1.
[b]Estimates from Thompson et al.[10]
[c]Estimates from Thorn et al.[23]
[d]Estimates from Bombace et al.[71]
[e]Estimates derived from Table 3.1 and Mondragon and Jaffee.[73]
[f]Estimates from Suchkov.[74]
[g]Estimates by the present authors.

Table 3.13

Hypothetical Western-Style Menu[a] Used to Compare Se Contents of Food Supplies
of Several Countries

Meal	Item
Breakfast	Oatmeal (240 g, cooked) with butter or margarine (14 g) and honey (20g)
	Bacon, fried (16 g)
	Orange (1 medium)
	Whole milk (230 ml)
	Coffee, black (230 ml)
Lunch	Roll, white (35 g) with butter or margarine (14 g)
	Salad: lettuce (50 g), carrot (100 g), tomato (150 g), hard-boiled egg (54 g) and dressing (14 g)
	Apples (150 g) and raisins (80 g)
	Whole milk (230 ml)
Dinner	Chicken breast, baked (85 g)
	Fried rice (190 g, cooked) with green onions (23 g)
	Boiled carrots (145 g) with butter or margarine (14 g)
	Spinach (80 g) with tofu (50 g)
	Fig bars (50 g)
	Tea (230 ml)

[a]This menu provides approximately 2460 kcal (10.11 MJ) and 83 g protein.

Table 3.14

Comparison of Se Contents of a Hypothetical
Western-Style Menu[a] Prepared in Several Countries

Country	Se provided (μg)
USA: Se-deficient area	85
USA: moderate-Se area	122
USA: seleniferous area	241
Canada: east	116
Canada: west, north	169
England	51
Italy	42
West Germany	129
Finland	32
New Zealand	32
China: low-Se area	13
China: moderate-Se area	63
China: high-Se area	>3945
Japan	66
Venezuela	291
Ukrainian SSR	221

[a]Menu is presented in Table 3.13.

Table 3.15

Estimated Average per Capita Daily Intakes of Se by Adults in Several Countries

Country	Estimated intake (μg)	Reference
USA, low-Se areas	60-150	(1)
	147, 154, 198	(77)[a]
	82[b], 86[c], 93	(76)
USA, moderate-Se areas	132	(78)
	90-168	(80)
	150	(81)
	81[d]	(79)
USA, high-Se areas	191, 216	(77)[a]
	216	(97)
Canada, eastern	98, 149	(10)
Canada, west and north	181, 224	(10)[a]
	197	(21)
England	60	(23)
	70	(82)
Italy[e]	13	(71)
Finland	30	(69)
	50-60	(83)[f]
	33[g]	(54)
New Zealand	6-33[h], 34-70	(84)
	28	(70)
	32	(36)
China, Se-deficient area	7-11	(41)
China, moderate-Se area	92	(41)
China, seleniferous area	750-4990	(41)
Japan	88	(85)
	203	(86)
Venezuela	326	(73)

[a] Based on surveys conducted in different states.
[b] Ovo-lacto vegetarian diet.
[c] Vegetarian diet.
[d] Estimate made by duplicate plate analysis.
[e] Amiata Mountain region.
[f] This estimate was made in 1979 after the importation of wheat from North America resulted in a significant increase in Se in the Finnish food supply. This increase is seen by contrasting this estimated Se intake to that made by the same authors in 1973 (i.e., 30 μg/person/day).
[g] Estimated average intake of Se by lactating women in 1982.
[h] Diets with no fish or organ meats.

disorders of livestock, Finland and New Zealand, have estimated Se intakes at least three-fold those of people in the Se-deficient regions of China; and persons in the so-called low-Se portions of the USA have estimated Se intakes approximately two- to five-fold those of Finns or New Zealanders.

The most important sources of Se in the diets for most people are cereals, meats, and fish. This is shown by the relative contributions of each class of food to the total Se intakes of residents of several countries, as estimated by several authors (see Table 3.16). In the eight countries for which data is presented, meats and fish appear to make rather stable contributions of Se, generally around 40-50% of the total, regardless of the level of total Se consumed. The Se contributions of cereals, in contrast, varied with the total Se intake, indicating that the relative availability of this class of foods may also be an important factor in determining the total Se intakes of populations. Table 3.16 shows that, whereas cereals provide from about one-quarter to two-thirds of the dietary Se in countries with total Se intakes greater than about 40 μg per person per day, they appear to contribute only one-tenth to one-quarter of the total dietary Se in countries with intakes lower than that level (e.g., Finland, New Zealand, Italy). Dairy products and eggs contribute small amounts (i.e., up to 12 μg per person per day) of Se to the total intakes in most countries, although such levels can represent large percentages of the total Se intakes in countries where the balance

Table 3.16

Contributions of Major Classes of Foods to the Se Intakes (μg Se/Person/Day) of Adults in Several Countries[a]

Class (reference)	U.S.A			Canada	
	Moderate-Se area		High-Se area	East	West, North
	(77)	(80)	(97)	(10)[b]	(10)
Cereals	45 (34%)	93 (62%)	57 (26%)	90 (66%)	97 (48%)
Vegetables, fruits	5 (4%)	1 (0.6%)	10 (5%)	6 (4%)	8 (4%)
Meats, fish	69 (52%)	56 (37%)	101 (47%)	28 (21%)	76 (38%)
Dairy products, eggs	13 (10%)	0 (0%)	48 (22%)	12 (9%)	20 (10%)
Total	132	150	216	136	201

Class (reference)	England	Finland	New Zealand		Japan	Venezuela
	(23)	(69)	(70)	(36)	(85)	(73)
Cereals	30 (50%)	3 (10%)	4 (14%)	3 (9%)	24 (27%)	88 (27%)
Vegetables, fruits	3 (5%)	1 (4%)	1 (4%)	2 (7%)	6 (7%)	15 (5%)
Meats, fish	23 (37%)	19 (63%)	12 (43%)	16 (50%)	46 (52%)	153 (47%)
Dairy products, eggs	5 (8%)	7 (23%)	11 (39%)	11 (34%)	12 (14%)	70 (21%)
Total	60	30	28	32	88	326

[a]Numbers in parentheses show the percentage of the total intakes contributed by each class of foods.

[b]Averages from two surveys in Toronto: see Thompson et al.10

of the diet provides little Se (e.g., Finland, New Zealand, Italy). Vegetables and fruits, uniformly low in Se (when expressed on a fresh weight basis), provide only small amounts (less than 8% of the total intake) of the mineral in most human diets.

Due to the current shortage of information concerning the Se contents of foods and food consumption patterns in the low-Se areas of China, it is not possible to estimate the relative contributions of the major classes of foods to the total Se intakes of residents of those areas. However, it is important to make such evaluations in view of the finding that people in those areas have lower natural levels of Se consumption (which, according to Yang,[41] are only 7-11 μg per person per day) than have been reported anywhere else. In consideration of what is known to be the low consumption of meats and fish and the reliance on wheat, corn, and rice as major dietary staples in those areas, it can be inferred that cereals constitute the major and, perhaps, the only natural source of dietary Se in those areas of endemic Keshan Disease.

Differences in patterns of food consumption, whether general ones due to cultural influences or specific ones due to personal preferences and food availability, can significantly affect Se intake. An example is shown in Table 3.17. It presents a comparison of the projected Se intakes in several countries (based upon food analyses in those countries) for individuals consuming either of two general patterns of food consumption. The "American" pattern is based on the results of the 1973 Total Diet Survey of the United States Food and Drug Administration as presented by Mahaffey et al.[81]; the "Japanese" pattern is that reported by Sakurai and Tsuchiya.[85] Whereas the Japanese-type pattern is relatively rich in cereals, the American-type pattern contains appreciably more meats, dairy products, and eggs, as well as total food. Table 3.17 shows that when these two patterns of food consumption are compared within each country, the predicted Se intakes for the Japanese-type pattern were substantially lower that those for the American-type pattern. Although the Se intakes for each pattern were fairly similar (i.e., within 7-16%) when calculated for foods in the USA, Canada, and West Germany, projected Se intakes varied by 22-54% when calculated for the other countries. Thus, while residents in Japan or England would be expected to have similar daily intakes of 91-94 μg Se per person when following an American-type dietary pattern, these intakes might easily differ by as much as one-third for residents of one of these countries consuming an American-type diet compared to residents consuming a Japanese-type diet or a Western-style vegetarian diet.[105,106]

In view of this potential for variation in Se intake with different dietary habits, it is not surprising to find this actually to be the case for individuals able to select their own patterns of food consumption from a variety of

Table 3.17

Comparison of Two General Patterns of Food Consumption on the Predicted Intakes
of Se (μg/Person/Day) of Adults in Several Countries[a]

Food consumption pattern	USA (moderate-Se area)	Canada (east)	England	West Germany	Finland	New Zealand
American-type[b]:						
Cereals (369 g/day)	122	144	41	107	7	13
Vegetables, fruits (676 g/day)	27	14	7	14	1	2
Meats, fish (290 g/day)	61	44	35	61	15	9
Dairy products, eggs (756 g/day)	23	8	8	8	19	3
Total	233	210	91	190	42	27
Japanese-type[c]:						
Cereals (426 g/day)	141	166	47	124	21	15
Vegetables, fruits (489 g/day)	20	10	5	10	1	1
Meats, fish (119 g/day)	25	18	14	25	6	4
Dairy products, eggs (127 g/day)	4	1	1	1	1	1
Total	190	195	67	160	29	21

Food consumption pattern	China (Se-deficient area)	China (moderate-Se area)	Japan	Venezuela	Ukrainian SSR
American-type[b]:					
Cereals (369 g/day)	4	18	26	125	103
Vegetables, fruits (676 g/day)	7	34	10	20	85
Meats, fish (290 g/day)	7	29	35	145	85
Dairy products, eggs (756 g/day)	2	15	23	87	76
Total	20	96	94	377	349
Japanese-type[c]:					
Cereals (426 g/day)	4	21	30	145	119
Vegetables, fruits (489 g/day)	5	24	7	15	61
Meats, fish (119 g/day)	3	12	14	60	35
Dairy products, eggs (127 g/day)	<1	3	4	15	13
Total	12	51	55	235	228

[a]Based on typical Se contents presented in Table 3.12.
[b]From 1973 total diet survey data, U.S. Food and Drug Administration, as presented by Mahaffey *et al.*[81]
[c]From pattern of intake reported by Sakurai and Tsuchiya.[85]

foods. In a study of the Se intakes of such individuals in Maryland, USA,
Welsh *et al.*[78] found that individual variation was great (see Table 3.18).
Although the mean daily intake of Se by the 22 subjects in their study
was 81 μg per person, approximately 17% of a sampling of 132 diets selected
by those subjects were found to contain less than 50 μg Se per person

Table 3.18

Variation in the Se Contents of Self-Selected
Diets of Individuals in Beltsville, Maryland,
USA, in 1976[a]

Daily Se intake (μg/person)	Percentage of diets[b]
0-25	2
>25-50	15
>50-75	35
>75-100	27
>100-125	8
>125-150	7
>150-175	2
>175-200	1
>200-225	2
>225-250	0
>250-275	0
>275-300	1

[a]From Welsh et al.[79]
[b]Based on 132 daily diet composites from 22 subjects. The mean and median daily intakes were 81.0 and 74.0 μg Se/person, respectively.

per day, and 5% of the diets provided more than 150 μg Se per person per day.

Differences in Se consumption by adults in different parts of the world are reflected in differences in the Se contents of human milk and, therefore, in the Se intakes of breast-fed infants. Table 3.19 presents the daily intakes of Se by 3-month-old breast-fed infants in seven different countries, estimated on the basis of the Se concentrations of human milk reported in those countries as presented earlier in Table 3.3. Here large differences in the Se nutriture (i.e., estimated intakes from 7.5 to 212 μg per infant per day) can be seen. However, with the exception of the selenosis area (Enshi, Hubei) of China, it is apparent that the differences in estimated infant Se intakes between different countries (which show a range of 180%) are much less than those of the estimated intakes of adults in the same countries (see Table 3.16). At the present time, there have been only limited analyses of the Se contents of human milk in the areas of China with endemic Se deficiency and Keshan Disease in young children. That report[41] indicates that the Se intakes of nursing infants, particularly in areas of endemic Keshan Disease, may be as little as 33-40% of those of breast-fed infants in other low-Se countries (e.g., Finland, New Zealand) where Se deficiency-related disorders have not been reported.

Table 3.19

Estimated Average Daily Intakes of Se by 3-Month-Old (4.8 kg) Breast-Fed Infants in Several Countries

Country	Average breast milk Se[a] (μg/ml)	Daily Se intake[b] (μg/child)
USA	.019	14.3
England	.015	11.3
West Germany	.028	21.0
Finland	.010	7.5
Greece	.020	15.0
Japan	.018	13.5
New Zealand	.012	9.0
China, low-Se areas	.003	2.3
China, moderate-Se areas	.021	15.8
China, high-Se area	.283	212.3

[a]Based on values presented in Table 3.3.

[b]This estimate is based on the consumption of ca. 750 ml (i.e., 530 kcal) per child per day and an average caloric density of breast milk of 71 kcal/100 ml.

IV. SELENIUM IN FEEDSTUFFS FOR ANIMALS

Many edible products of plants and animals are consumed by both humans and livestock. Therefore, the Se contents of many feedstuffs for animals are very similar to those of analogous human foods. Examples are found in comparing the Se contents of feed grains (e.g., wheat, oats, barley) to food products based on the same grains. Many other livestock feedstuffs, while obtained from the same species as human foods, are derived from different portions of the original plant or food animal (e.g., wheat middlings vs. wheat grain; rice bran vs. polished rice; meat scraps and bone meals vs. steaks and chops). Such materials can differ considerably in Se content. Other animal feedstuffs are produced from materials not generally used for human consumption (e.g., grass silage, oyster shells). These feedstuffs have no correlates among human foods; their Se contents must be measured independently. Thus, although information concerning the Se contents of foods can be of some value in estimating the Se contents of animal feeds, considerations of the Se nutrition of animals requires an independent base of information describing the Se contents of the ingredients used in animal feeds.

At the present time, this information base is extensive for feedstuffs used in animal agriculture in the USA, Canada, and West Germany, but is very incomplete with regard to most other countries. These data are presented in Table 3.20. Of the feedstuffs shown, two, corn and soybean meal, are particularly important as major components in diets for monogastrics in

Table 3.20

The Se Contents of Livestock Feedstuffs (ppm, air-dry basis)[a]

Feedstuff	USA			Canada	
	Low-Se	Moderate-Se	High-Se	East, central	West, north
Alfalfa hay	.04-.11 (94)	.03-.57 (94) .295 (87)	.15-.69 (94)		
Alfalfa meal	.10 (62)	.38 (62)		.06 (88)	
Bahiagrass		.061 (87)			
Bakery by-product		.4 (62)			
Barley	.1 (62)	.3, .4 (62)		.04 (88)	.211 (95) .35 (87)
Beet pulp					
Bermuda grass		.173 (87)		.69 (88)	
Blood meal					
Bone meal					
Brewers' dried grains		.7 (62)		.94 (88)	
Buckwheat					
Buttermilk, dried				.12 (88)	
Casein				.17 (88)	
Cassava meal					
Clover, red					
Copra meal					

(continues)

108

Table 3.20 (*Continued*)

Feedstuff	USA			Canada	
	Low-Se	Moderate-Se	High-Se	East, central	West, north
Corn	.025 (62) .038 (62) .03, .04, .05 (90)	.010 (5) .08 (3) .05 (62) .05, .09 (90)	.38 (62) .38, .40, .99 (90)	.04 (88) .04 (89)	
Corn silage	.01-.04 (94)	.059 (87) .09 (20)			
Corn and cob meal		.04 (62)			
Corn distiller's dried grains				.35 (88)	
Corn distiller's dried solubles		.5 (62)		.33 (88)	
Corn fermentation solubles, dried	10.9 (62)				
Corn gluten feed	.2 (62)			.17 (88)	
Corn gulten meal, 60% protein		1.15 (62)		.31 (88)	
Cottonseed meal					
Crab meal	1.3 (62)				
Feather meal				.72 (88)	
Fish meals, excluding tuna	1.3-1.5 (62)	1.7 (62) 2.22 (91)		1.83-2.84 (88)	1.8 (62)
Fish meals, tuna		6.2 (62)			
Fish solubles, dried		2.0 (62) 2.22 (92) 2.59 (92)			
Hays, grass or trefoil	.06 (62) .02, .09 (94)	.029 (5)			.176 (95)
Hominy feed		.1 (62)			

(*continues*)

Table 3.20 *(Continued)*

Feedstuff	USA			Canada	
	Low-Se	Moderate-Se	High-Se	East, central	West, north
Limestone			.07 (88)		
Linseed meal		1.0 (62)		1.05 (88)	
Meat and bone scraps, 50% protein		.29 (62)		.40 (88)	
Millet					
Oats	.05 (62)	.22, .25 (62)		.06 (88)	.30 (88)
Oyster shells		.01 (62)			
Palm kernel meal					
Peanut meal		.28 (62)			
Phosphates, diclcium		.2 (62)		.65 (88)	
Phosphates, defluorinated rock		1.2 (62)		64 (88)	
Phosphates, Curacao Island		1.2 (62)			
Potato meal	.06 (62)				
Poultry by-product meal	1.2 (62)				
Rapeseed meal				.98 (88)	
Rice		.071 (3)			
Rye		.272 (4)			
Shrimp meal		1.8 (62)			

(continues)

Table 3.20 *(Continued)*

Feedstuff	USA			Canada	
	Low-Se	Moderate-Se	High-Se	East, central	West, north
Skim milk, dried				.12 (88)	
Sorghum silage	.07 (62)	.057 (87)			
Soybean meal		.1.54 (61)		.12 (88)	
Sunflower seed meal				.12 (89)	
Wheat	.05 (62)	.32, .28, .54 (4) .61 (3)	.8 (62)	.06 (88)	.61 (4) 1.13 (3)
Wheat bran		.63 (62)		.32 (88)	.51 (88)
Wheat middlings		.50 (62)		.22 (88)	.95 (88)
Wheat shorts	.28 (62)	.57 (62)		.20 (88)	.70 (88)
Whey, dried		.08 (62)		.06 (88)	.81 (88)
Yeast, dried brewers'		1.1 (62)		1.23 (88)	
Yeast, dried torula		.04 (62)			

(continues)

111

Table 3.20 (Continued)

Feedstuff	West Germany	Sweden	China			Other countries
			Se-deficient	Moderate-Se	Seleniferous	
Alfalfa hay	.06 (24)					
Alfalfa meal	.09 (24)	.07 (3)				
Bahiagrass						
Bakery by-product						
Barley	.19 (24)	.005-.018 (3)				Finland: .005-.009 (29)
Beet pulp		.04-.27 (3)				England: .29 (3)
Bermuda grass						
Blood meal	.07 (24)	.28 (3)				
Bone meal	.01 (24)					
Brewers' dried grains						
Buckwheat			.017 (37)	.039 (37)		
Buttermilk, dried						
Casein						
Cassava meal	.10 (24)					
Clover, red	.11 (24)					Africa: 1.29 (3)
Copra meal						

(continues)

112

Table 3.20 (*Continued*)

Feedstuff	West Germany	Sweden	China Se-deficient	China Moderate-Se	China Seleniferous	Other countries
Corn	.11 (24)		.016 (37) .007 (92) .003, .004, .010 (39) .005-.009 (42) .003-.005 (38)	.049, .053 (37) .023 (39) .010-.027 (42) .004 (38)	.325 (39) 6.33 (39) .128 (42)	Finland: .04 (28) Yugoslavia: < .01 (46)
Corn silage			.004-.006 (41)	.029 (41)		
Corn and cob meal						
Corn distiller's dried grains						
Corn distiller's dried solubles						
Corn fermentation solubles, dried						
Corn gluten feed						
Corn gluten meal, 60% protein						
Cottonseed meal	.06 (24)					
Crab meal						
Feather meal						
Fish meals, excluding tuna	1.61 (24)	1.28, 2.21 (3)				England: 2.01 (3) Peru (anchovy): 1.36 (3), 1.39 (91) Norway (herring): 2.78 (91)
Fish meals, tuna						
Fish solubles, dried						
Hays, grass or trefoil		.010-.030 (3)				
Hominy feed	.1 (24)					

113

(*continues*)

Table 3.20 (*Continued*)

Feedstuff	West Germany	Sweden	China			Other countries
			Se-deficient	Moderate-Se	Seleniferous	
Limestone	.17 (24)					Argentina: .07 (3)
Linseed meal		.06 (3)				
Meat and bone scraps, 50% protein		.18 (3)				
Millet				.097 (37)		
Oats	.08 (24)	.005-.039 (3)	.018 (37)			Finland .006-.009 (29
Oyster shells						
Palm kernel meal	.12 (24)					
Peanut meal	.28 (24)					
Phosphatges, dicalcium	.21 (24)					
Phosphates, defluorinated rock	1.67 (24)					
Phosphates, Curacao Island						
Potato meal						
Poultry by-product meal						
Rapeseed meal		.08 (3)				
Rice			.020 (37)	.043 (41)	1.483 (39)	
			.008 (41)	.064, .087 (37)		
			.006, .023 (39)	.030, .041 (39)		
Rye	.20 (24)	.006 (3)				
	.043 (4)	.005 (4)				
Shrimp meal						USSR: .070 (4)
						France: .025 (4)
						Argentina: .063 (3), .05 (4)
						Turkey: .053 (3)
						Finland: .005-.0511 (29),
						.02 (4)

114

(continues)

Table 3.20 *(Continued)*

Feedstuff	West Germany	Sweden	China			Other countries
			Se-deficient	Moderate-Se	Seleniferous	
Skim milk, dried	.08 (2)					
Sorghum silage						
Soybean meal	.43 (3)	.51 (3)	.016 (93)	.035, .076 (39)	.052 (93)	Yugoslavia: < .01 (46)
	.20 (24)		.006, .007, .026 (39)	.063 (41)		
			.008–.014 (41)			
Sunflower seed meal	.10 (24)					
Wheat	.34 (4)	.026 (4)	.007–.009 (42)	.019–.063 (42)	1.057 (42)	USSR: .24 (3)
		.015 (3)	.018 (37)	.052, .106 (37)	.099, .301 (93)	USSR: .09 (4)
			.006, .013 (39)	.038, .061 (39)		Denmark: .04 (4)
			.005 (38)	.016 (38)		France: .021 (4)
			.006–.008 (41)	.038 (41)		Yugoslavia: .012–.018 (46)
						Argentina: .045 (3), .04 (4)
						Finland: .005–.011 (29),
						.017 (4)
Wheat bran	.44 (24)	.023 (3)				Australia: .048 (36)
Wheat middlings		.026 (3)				Argentina: .067 (3)
Wheat shorts						Argentina: .074 (3)
Whey, dried	.18 (3)	.06 (3)				
Yeast, dried brewers'	.11 (24)	.48 (3)				Austria: .08 (3)
Yeast, dried torula	.08 (24)	.63 (3)				

[a]Original references are cited in parentheses.

115

much of North America; they are also exported from the USA and Canada to many other countries for such use. These feedstuffs generally contain ca. 0.05 and 0.10 ppm Se (air-dry basis), respectively. Because many mixed feeds for poultry, swine, and other animals may contain two-thirds or more of both of these ingredients, many corn-soy type diets can be naturally low in Se. The calculated amounts of Se inherent (i.e., occurring naturally in the ingredients) in several practical livestock feeds is presented in Table 3.21 to demonstrate this point. It shows that typical diets based on corn and soybean meal produced in the United States would be expected to contain as little as 0.04-0.06 ppm Se (air-dry basis) if produced in the low-Se parts of the country, but as much as 0.25 ppm or more if produced in high-Se areas. Because large amounts of feedstuffs for animals are produced in low- to moderate-Se areas of North America, many diets based on these feedstuffs do not satisfy the nutritional demands of many animals. For example, before the widespread practice in the USA of supplementing livestock feeds with sodium selenite, Thompson and Scott[102] found many diets of young poultry flocks in New York State to contain only ca. 0.07 ppm Se (air-dry basis).

Because the requirements of most animals for Se are greater than those frequently obtainable by simple blends of corn or wheat and soybean or other oil seed meals, the use of high-Se ingredients or supplements of Se salts is often necessary to ensure adequate Se concentrations in animal feeds. Feedstuffs such as marine fish meals and condensed fish solubles generally contain several parts per million of Se and can, therefore, be important sources of the mineral when they are included in blended diets. Fish meals are often used in diets for dogs and are routinely used to varying degrees in diets for cats and cultured food fishes. Table 3.22 shows the typical amounts of Se inherent in examples of these kinds of diets in which fish meals contribute 60-90% of the total Se. Because fish meals are frequently not economical to use in the formulation of practical feeds for poultry or swine in many parts of the world,* these feeds generally must be supplemented directly with Se to avoid Se-deficiency-related disorders. Depending on the combination of feedstuffs used and on their respective Se contents, and depending on whether Se supplements are used, practical feeds can vary considerably in total Se content. Scott[103] demonstrated this in a survey of the Se contents of 22 different poultry feeds used for the commercial production of broilers, pullets, laying hens, turkey poults, and breeding turkeys in 16 states of the USA and in one province in Canada.

---

*It is not generally economical to use fish meals in soybean meal-based diets for monogastrics unless their prices are less than 1.5 times the price of dehulled (49% protein) soybean meal, in which case fish meal can be used to replace some of the soybean meal. In many parts of the world, the price of fish meal may be 1.6-2.3 times the local price of soybean meal.

Table 3.21

Typical Amounts of Se (Air-Dry Basis) Inherent in Several
Practical Livestock Feeds in Low-, Moderate-, and High-Se Regions of the USA

Parameter	Broiler chicks (to 4 weeks)	Laying hens (24-42 weeks)	Pigs (weanling)	Rabbits (to 4 kg)
Feed formula (% of diet)				
Corn meal	52.0	66.3	73.5	23.5
Corn silage	—	—	—	23.5
Soybean meal (49% protein)	31.5	10.0	13.9	10.0
Ground barley	—	—	—	11.0
Ground oats	—	—	—	—
Alfalfa hay	—	—	—	50.0
Alfalfa meal (17% protein)	2.5	1.5	5.0	—
Wheat bran	—	—	—	5.0
Wheat middlings	—	—	—	—
Meat and bone meal (50% protein)	4.0	7.5	5.0	—
Corn distillers grains with solubles	3.0	6.5	—	—
Molasses	—	—	—	—
Stabilized grease	3.5	—	—	—
Dicalcium phosphate	2.0	—	1.6	—
Limestone	0.75	7.0	—	—
Salt	0.25	0.25	0.5	—
Vitamins, trace elements, [b] amino acid supplement	0.5	0.5	0.5	0.5
Se contents (ppm)				
Low-Se area	0.06	0.07	0.05	0.07
Moderate-Se area	0.16	0.12	0.12	0.26
High-Se area	0.25	0.16	0.17	0.37

(continues)

Table 3.21 *(Continued)*

Parameter	Lambs (creep feed)	Calves (nursing)	650 kg Lactating cow (producing 27 kg milk/day)
Feed formula (% of diet)			
Corn meal	12.0	32.5	13.2
Corn silage	—	—	61.2
Soybean meal (49% protein)	10.0	5.5	5.0
Ground barley	—	20.0	—
Ground oats	9.0	—	—
Alfalfa hay	65.0	—	20.4
Alfalfa meal (17% protein)	—	—	—
Wheat bran	—	—	—
Wheat middlings	—	15.0	—
Meat and bone meal (50% protein)	—	—	—
Corn distillers grains with solubles	—	20.0	—
Molasses	3.0	5.0	—
Stabilized grease	—	—	0.2
Dicalcium phosphate	—	1.0	—
Limestone	—	0.5	—
Salt	—	0.5	—
Vitamins, trace elements, [b] amino acid supplement	1.0		
Se contents (ppm)			
Low-Se area	0.06	0.16	0.04
Moderate-Se area	0.25	0.25	0.12
High-Se area	0.38	0.35	0.17

[a]Creep feed is provided as a supplement to nursing lambs at about 2 weeks of age.
[b]Se in trace element supplements was not counted in these calculations.

Table 3.22

Typical Amounts of Se Inherent in Several Practical Diets for Dogs, Cats and Warm Water Fish in Moderate-Se Areas of the USA

Parameter	Dogs	Cats	Channel Catfish
Feed formulas (% of diet):			
Corn meal	51.2	—	29.2
Soybean meal (49% protein)	12.0	—	48.2
Rolled oats	—	20.0	—
Potatoes, cooked	—	15.0	—
Meat scraps	—	20.0	—
Meat and bone meal (50% protein)	8.0	—	—
Bone meal, steamed	2.0	2.0	—
Wheat germ	8.0	—	—
Wheat bran	4.0	—	—
Wheat middlings	—	—	10.0
Crude casein	—	10.0	—
Dried skimmed milk	4.0	—	—
Fish meal	5.0	20.0	8.0
Brewers' yeast	2.0	—	—
Distillers' grains	1.0	—	—
Animal fat	2.0	10.0	1.5
Cod liver oil	—	3.0	—
Dicalcium phosphate	—	—	1.0
Salt	0.5	—	—
Vitamins, trace elements[a]	0.3	—	0.1
Pellet binder	—	—	2.0
Se contents (ppm):	0.49	1.33	0.70

[a]Se in trace element supplements was not counted.

He found the total Se contents of those feeds to range from 0.02 to 0.27 ppm (15% moisture basis), with 15 of those feeds from 10 states and Canada to contain less than 0.10 ppm Se.

The semi-purified or purified diets used in laboratory animal experimentation are usually low in Se by virtue of the fact that the major ingredients available for use in such diets (e.g., isolated soy protein, casein, recrystallized sugars, corn starch) are usually low in Se. Table 3.23 presents formulations of semipurified diets for use in rearing several laboratory animal species. It shows that the concentrations of Se inherent in those diets are projected to be only 0.03-0.05 ppm (air-dry basis). Therefore, it is necessary to supplement these types of diets with Se in order to prevent Se-deficiency syndromes in experimental animals.

Selenium can be added to animal feeds in the form of sodium selenite. This compound is readily soluble in water and can be applied as an aqueous solution by spraying on to the feed, or it can be dried on a carrier and handled in dry form as part of a direct premix or of a vitamin-trace mineral

Table 3.23

Typical Amounts of Se Inherent in Semi-Purified Diets for Several Laboratory Animal Species

Parameter	Rats, mice	Hamsters	Guinea pigs	Chicks	Chicks	Baby pigs
Feed formulas (% of diet)						
Casein	20.0	18.0	30.0	25.0	—	20.0
Isolated soy protein	—	—	—	—	25.0	—
Corn starch	15.0	35.5	43.1	—	—	—
Sucrose	50.0	28.0	43.1	—	—	—
Glucose monohydrate	—	—	—	57.5	60.2	71.9
Vegetable oil	5.0	6.0	4.0	4.0	4.0	—
Cellulose	5.0	5.0	13.0	3.0	3.0	—
Agar	—	—	2.0	—	—	—
Vitamins, minerals,[a] amino acid supplement	5.0	7.5	7.9	10.5	7.8	8.1
Se contents (ppm):	0.04	0.03	0.05	0.04	0.04	0.03

[a]Includes macro-minerals and trace elements, but Se was not counted.

premix. Several products based on Se-enriched yeasts are also available as feed supplements. These vary with respect to the proportions of their Se actually incorporated into yeast protein and those that are simply adsorbed to the yeast carrier. Those products in which Se occurs predominantly in protein-bound form appear to be very well utilized (i.e., nearly equal to that of sodium selenite) by animals. Due to the known toxicity of high levels of Se and to the inherent risks involved in handling Se premixes, it is prudent to exercise great care while using Se supplements. The addition of Se to livestock feeds in the USA is regulated by the U.S. Food and Drug Administration, which permits the addition of 0.1 mg Se/ kg finished feed for most classes of livestock.

REFERENCES

1. Schroeder. H. A., Frost. D. V., and Valassa. J. J., Essential trace elements in man: selenium, J. Chron. Dis., 23, 227, 1970.
2. Moxon, A. L., and Palmquist, D. L., Selenium content of foods grown and sold in Ohio, Ohio Rept., 65, 13, 1980.
3. Lindberg, P., Selenium determination in plant and animal material and in water, Acta Vet. Scand., Suppl. 23, 5, 1968.
4. Varo, P., and Koivistoinen. P., Annual variations in the average selenium intake in Finland: cereal products and milk as sources of selenium in 1978/80. Int. J. Vit. Nutr. Res. 51, 62, 1981.
5. Paulson, G. D., Broderick, G. A.. Bauman, C. A., and Pope, A. L., Effect of feeding sheep selenium fortified trace mineralized salt: effect of tocopherol, J. Anim. Sci. 27, 195, 1968.
6. Scott, M. L., Selenium compounds in nature and medicine. A. Nutritional importance of selenium, in *Organic Selenium Compounds: Their Chemistry and Biology*, Klayman, D. L., and Gunther, W. H. H., eds., Wiley-Interscience, New York, 1973, 648.
7. Hadjimarkos, D. M., and Bonhorst, C. W., The selenium content of eggs, milk, and water in relation to dental caries in children, J. Pediat., 59, 256, 1961.
8. Shamberger, R. J., and Willis, C. E., Selenium distribution and human cancer mortality, in *C.R.C. Critical Reviews in Clinical Laboratory Sciences*, Chemical Rubber Publishing Co., Boca Raton, Florida, 1971, 211.
9. Whitacre, M., and Latshaw, J. D., Selenium utilization from menhaden fish meal as affected by processing, Poultry Sci., 61, 2520, 1982.
10. Thompson, J.N., Erdody, P., and Smith, D. C., Selenium content of food consumed by Canadians, J. Nutr., 112, 274, 1975.
11. Morris, V. C., and Levander, O. A., Selenium content of foods, J. Nutr. 100, 1383, 1970.
12. Schrauzer, G. N., White, D. A., and Schneider, C. J., Cancer mortality correlation studies. IV. Associations with dietary intakes and blood levels of certain trace elements, notably Se-antagonists, Bioinorg. Chem., 7, 35, 1977.
13. Combs, G. F., Jr., and Spencer, H., unpublished research, 1984.
14. Wauchope, R. D., Selenium and arsenic levels in soybeans from different production regions of the United States, J. Agric. Food Chem., 26, 266, 1978.

15. Ferretti, R. J., and Levander, O. A., Selenium content of soybean foods, J. Agric. Food Chem., 24, 54, 1976.
16. Palmer, I. S., Herr, A., and Nelson, T., Toxicity of selenium in Brazil nuts to rats, J. Food Sci. 47, 1595, 1982.
17. Swanson. C. A., Reamer. D. C.. Veillon, C., and Levander. O. A., Intrinsic labeling of chicken products with a stable isotope of selenium ([76]Se): J. Nutr., 113, 793, 1983.
18. Olson, O. E., and Palmer, I. S., Selenium in foods purchased or produced in South Dakota, J. Food Sci., 49, 446, 1984.
19. Alexander, A. R., Whanger, P. D., and Miller, L. T., Bioavailability to rats of selenium in various tuna and wheat products, J. Nutr., 113, 196, 1983.
20. Maus, R. W., Martz, F. A., Belyea, R. L., and Weiss, M. F., Relationship of dietary selenium to selenium in plasma and milk from dairy cows, J. Dairy Sci., 63, 532, 1980.
21. Arthur. D., Selenium content of Canadian foods, Can. Inst. Food Sci. Technol. J., 5, 165, 1972.
22. Lo, M. -T., and Sandi, E., Selenium: occurrence in foods and its toxicological significance — a review, J. Environ. Pathol. Toxicol., 4, 193, 1980.
23. Thorn. J., Robertson, J., Buss, D. H., and Bunton, N. G., Trace nutrients. Selenium in British food, Br. J. Nutr., 39, 391, 1978.
24. Oelschlaeger, W., and Menke, K. H., Uber selengehalte pflanzlicher, tierischer und stoffe 2. Mitteilung, Selen- und schwefelgebalte in nahrungsmitten, Z. Ernahrungwissen., 9, 216, 1968.
25. Hecht, H., Der Gehalt des fleisches an toxischen elementen, Ber. Landw., 55, 976, 1977.
26. Lombeck, I., Kasperek, K., Bonnermann, B., Feinendageu, L. E., and Bremer, H. J., Selenium content of human milk, cow's milk and cow's milk infant formulas, Eur. J. Pediatr., 129, 139, 1978.
27. Kolar, K., and Widell, A., Untersuchung veber den selengehalt in fleisch, leber und nieren von schwein, rind and kalk., Mitt. Gebeite Lebensm. Hyg., 68, 259, 1977.
28. Varo, P., Nuurtamo, M., Saari, E., and Koivistoinen, P., Mineral element composition of Finnish foods. IV. Flours and bakery products, Acta Agric., Scand., Suppl. 22, 37, 1980.
29. Varo, P., Nuurtamo, M., Saari, E., and Koivistoinen, P., Mineral element composition of Finnish foods. III. Annual variations in the mineral element composition of cereal grains, Acta Agric. Scand., Suppl. 22, 27, 1980.
30. Varo, P., Lahelma, O., Nuurtamo, M., Saari, E., and Koivistoinen, P., Mineral element composition of Finnish foods. VII. Potato, vegetables, fruits, berries, nuts and mushrooms, Acta Agric. Scand., Suppl., 22, 89, 1980.
31. Varo, P., and Koivistoinen, P., Selenium in Finnish food, in *Proceedings of the Third International Symposium on Selenium in Biology and Medicine*, Combs, G.F., Jr., Spallholz, J.E., Levander, O.A., and Oldfield, J.E., eds., Avi Publ. Co., Westport, Conn., 1986.
32. Nuurtamo, M., Varo, P., Saari, E., and Koivistoinen, P., Mineral element composition of Finnish foods. V. Meat and meat products, Acta Agric. Scand., Suppl. 22, 57, 1980.
33. Nuurtamo, M., Varo, P., Saari, E., and Koivistoinen, P., Mineral element composition of Finnish foods. VI. Fish and fish products, Acta Agric. Scand., Suppl. 22, 77, 1980.
34. Varo, P., Nuurtamo, M., Saari, E., and Koivistoinen, P., Mineral element composition of Finnish foods. VIII. Dairy products, eggs and margarine, Acta Agric. Scand., Suppl. 2, 115, 1980.
35. Varo, P., Nuurtamo, M., Saari, E., and Koivistoinen, P., Mineral element composition of Finnish foods, IX. Beverages, confectionaries, sugar and condiments, Acta Agric. Scand., Suppl. 22, 127, 1980.

36. Watkinson, J. H., Changes in blood selenium in New Zealand adults with the importation of Australian wheat, Amer. J. Clin. Nutr., 34, 836, 1981.

37. Tan, J., Zheng, D., Hov, S., Zhu, W., Li, R., Zhu, Z., and Wang, W., Selenium ecological and chemico-geography and endemic Keshan Disease and Kaschin Beck's Disease in China, in *Proceedings of the Third International Symposium on Selenium in Biology and Medicine*, Combs, G. F., Jr., Spallholz, J. E., Levander, O. A., and Oldfield, J. E., eds., Avi Publ. Co., Westport, Conn., 1986.

38. Li, J., Ren, S., Cheng, D., and Wan, H., The distribution of selenium in micro-environment related to Kaschin Beck Disease, in *Proceedings of the Third International Symposium on Selenium in Biology and Medicine*, Combs, G. F., Jr., Spallholz, J. E., Levander, O. A., and Oldfield, J. E., eds., Avi Publ. Co., Westport, Conn., 1986.

39. Yang, G., Wang, S., Zhou, R., and Sun, S., Endemic selenium intoxication of humans in China, Amer. J. Clin. Nutr. 37, 872, 1983.

40. Chen, X., Yang, G., Chen, J., Chen, X., Wen, Z., and Ge, K., Studies on the relations of selenium and Keshan Disease, Biol. Trace Element Res., 2, 91, 1980.

41. Yang, G., Research on Se-related problems in human health in China, in *Proceedings of the Third International symposium on Selenium in Biology and Medicine*, Combs, G. F., Jr., Spallholz, J. E., Levander, O. A., and Oldfield, J. E., eds., Avi Publ. Co., Westport, Conn., 1986.

42. Li, J., Ren, S., Cheng, D., A study of selenium associated with Kaschin-Beck Disease in different environments in Shaanxi, Acta Scientnae Circumstantiae, 2, 1, 1982.

43. Huang, W., Yan, L., and Wang, P., Selenium in foods and the method for is determination, Shopin Kexue (Beijing), 33, 37, 1982.

44. Zhai, X. J., Chang, Y. H., Wang, Y. W., Yan, X. F., Cai, Y., Zi, Z. M., and Cao, T., Selenium content of swine liver in P.R.C., in *Proceedings of the Third International Symposium on Selenium in Biology and Medicine*, Combs, G. F., Jr., Spallholz, J. E., Levander, O. A., and Oldfield, J. E., eds., Avi Publ. Co., Westport, Conn., 1986.

45. Suzuki, S., Koizumi, S., Harada, H., Ito, K., and Totani, T., Hygenic chemical studies on harmful elements (II). Selenium content of foods, soil and water, Ann. Rept. Tokyo Metropol. Res. Lab. Publ. Hlth., 22, 153, 1970.

46. Gavrilovic, B., and Matesic, D., Importance of selenium quantity in soil and fodder in regard to some diseases occurring in cattle, pigs, sheep and poultry, in *Proceedings of the Third International Symposium on Selenium in Biology and Medicine*, Combs, G. F., Jr., Spallholz, J. E., Levander, O. A., and Oldfield, J. E., eds., Avi Publ. Co., Westport, Conn., 1986.

47. Hellesnes, I., Underal, R., Lunde, G., and Haire, G. N., Selenium and zinc concentrations in kidney, liver and muscle of cattle from different parts of Norway, Acta Vet. Scand., 16, 481, 1975.

48. Zabel, N. Z., Harland, J., Gormican, A. T., and Ganther, H. E., Selenium contents of commerical formula diets, Amer. J. Clin. Nutr. 31, 850, 1978.

49. Smith, A. M., Picciano, M. F., and Milner, J. A., Selenium intakes and status of human milk and formula fed infants, Amer. J. Clin. Nutr., 35, 521, 1982.

50. Hadjimarkos, D. M., Selenium content of human milk: possible effect on dental caries, J. Pediatr., 63, 273, 1963.

51. Hadjimarkos, D. M., and Shearer, T. R., Selenium in mature human milk, Amer. J. Clin. Nutr., 26, 583, 1973.

52. Shearer, T. R., and Hadjimarkos, D. M., Geographic distribution of selenium in human milk, Arch. Environ. Hlth., 30, 230, 1975.

53. Levander, O. A., Morris, V. C., and Moser, P. B., Dietary selenium (Se) intake and Se content of breast milk and plasma of lactating and non-lactating women, Federation Proc., 40, 890 (abstract #3749), 1981.

54. Kumpulainen, J., Vuori, E., Kuitunem, P., Makinen, S., and Kara, R., Longitudinal study on the dietary selenium intake of exclusively breast-fed infants and their mothers in Finland, Int. J. Vit. Nutr. Res., 53, 420, 1983.

55. Kumpulainan, J., Vuori, E., and Siimes, M. A., Effect of maternal dietary selenium intake on selenium levels in breast milk, Int. J. Vit. Nutr. Res., 54, 251, 1984.

56. Higashi, A., Tamari, H., Kuroki, Y., and Matsuda, I., Longitudinal changes in the selenum content of breast milk, Acta Pediatr. Scand., 72, 433, 1983.

57. Millar, R. R., and Sheppard, A. D., α-Tocopherol and selenium levels in human and cows' milk, New Z. J. Sci., 15, 3, 1972.

58. Ullrey, D. E., Brady, P. S., Whetter, P. A., Fu, P. K., and Magee, W. T., Selenium supplementation of diets for sheep and beef cattle, J. Anim. Sci., 46, 559, 1977.

59. Ullrey, D. E., Light, M. R., Brady, P. S., Whetter, P. A., Tilton, J. E., Henneman, H. A., and Magee, W. T., Selenium supplements in salt for sheep, J. Anim. Sci., 46, 1515, 1978.

60. Ewan, R. C., Effect of vitamin E and selenium on tissue composition of young pigs, J. Anim. Sci., 32, 883, 1971.

61. Mahan, D. C., and Moxon, A. L., Effects of adding inorganic or organic selenium sources to the diets of young swine, J. Anim. Sci., 47, 456, 1978.

62. Scott, M. L., and Thompson, J. N., Selenium content of feedstuffs and effects of dietary selenium levels upon tissue selenium in chicks and poults, Poultry Sci., 50, 1742, 1971.

63. Latshaw, J. D., Natural and selenite selenium in the hen and egg, J. Nutr., 105, 32, 1975.

64. Combs, G. F., Jr., and Scott, M. L., The selenium needs of laying and breeding hens, Poultry Sci., 58, 871, 1979.

65. Conrad, H. R., and Moxon, A. L., Transfer of dietary selenium to milk, J. Dairy Sci., 62, 404, 1979.

66. Lorenz, K., Selenium in wheat and commercial wheat flours, Cereal Chem., 55, 287, 1978.

67. Ferretti, R. J., and Levander, O. A., Effect of milling and processing on the selenium content of grains and cereal products, J. Agric. Food Chem., 22, 1049, 1974.

68. Higgs, D. J., Morris, V. C., and Levander, O. A., Effect of cooking on selenium content of foods, J. Agric. Food Chem., 20, 678, 1972.

69. Varo, P., and Koivistoinen, P., Mineral element composition of Finnish foods. XII. General discussion and nutritional evaluation, Acta Agric. Scand., 22, 165, 1980.

70. Thomson, C. D., and Robinson, M. F., Selenium in human health and disease with emphasis on those aspects peculiar to New Zealand, Amer. J. Clin. Nutr., 33, 303, 1980.

71. Bombace, M. A., Rossi, L. C., and Clemente, G. F., Selenium content of some foodstuffs and environmental samples in an area of Italy rich in minerals, in *Comparative Studies of Food and Environmental Contaminants, Proceedings of a Symposium*, Intern. Atomic Energy Agency, Vienna, 1974, 341.

72. Mondragon, M. C., and Jaffe, W. G., Selenio en alimentos y en orina de escolares de diferentes zenas de Venezuela, Arch. Latinamer. Nutr., 21, 185, 1971.

73. Mondragon, M. C., and Jaffe, W. G., Consumo de selenio en la cividad de Caracas en comparacion con el de otras cividades del mundo, Arch. Latinamer. Nutr., 26, 31, 1976.

74. Suchkov, B. P., Selenium content in major nutrients consumed by the population of the Ukranian SSR, Vopr. Pitan., 30, 72, 1971.

75. Karlsen, J. T., Norheim, G., and Froslie, A., Selenium content of Norwegian milk, eggs and meat, Acta Agric. Scand., 31, 165, 1981.

76. Ganapathy, S. N., Joyner, B. J., Sawyer, D. R., and Hafner, K. M., Selenium content of selected foods, in *Trace Element Metabolism in Man and Animals III*, Kirchgessner, M., ed., Technische Univ., Munich, 1978, 332.

77. U.S. Food and Drug Administration, *Bureau of Foods Compliance Program* Evaluation Report: Total Diet, Studies fiscal year 1974, U.S. Gov't. Print. Off., Washington, D.C., 1975.

78. Watkinson, J. H., The selenium status of New Zealanders, N.Z. Med. J., 80, 202, 1974.

79. Welsh, S. O., Holden, J. M., Wolf, W. R., and Levander, O. A., Selenium in self-selected diets of Maryland residents, J. Amer. Diet. Assn., 79, 277, 1981.

80. Schrauzer, G. N., and White, D. A., Selenium in human nutrition. Dietary intakes and effects of supplementation, Bioinorganic. Chem., 8, 303, 1978.

81. Mahaffey, K. R., Corneliussen, P. E., Jelinek, C. F., and Fiorina, J. A., Heavy metal exposure from foods, Environ. Health Perspect., 12, 63, 1975.

82. Bennet, B. G., Exposure of man to environmental selenium - an exposure commitment assessment, Sci. Total Environ., 31, 117, 1983.

83. Varo, P. and Koivistoinen, P., Annual variations in the average selenium intake in Finland: cereal products and milk as sources of selenium in 1979/80, Int. J. Vit. Nutr. Res., 51, 62, 1981.

84. Robinson, M. F., The moonstone: more about selenium, J. Hum. Nutr., 30, 79, 1976.

85. Sakurai, H. and Tsuchiya, K., A tentative recommendation for maximum daily intake of selenium, Environ. Physiol. Biochem., 5, 107, 1975.

86. Yasumoto, K., Iwami, K., Yoshida, M., and Mitsuda, H., Selenium content of foods and its average daily intake in Japan, Eiyo To Shokuryo, 29, 511, 1976.

87. Kappel, L. C., Ingraham, R. H., Morgan, E. B., Dixon, J. M., Zeringue, L., Wilson, D., and Babcock, D. K., Selenium concentrations in feeds and effects of treating pregnant Holstein cows with selenium and vitamin E on blood selenium values and reproductive performance, Am. J. Vet. Res., 45, 691, 1984.

88. Arthur, D., Selenium content of some feed ingredients available in Canada, Can. J. Anim. Sci., 51, 71, 1971.

89. Young, L. G., Jenkins, K. J., and Edmeades, D. M., Selenium content of feedstuffs grown in Ontario, Can. J. Anim. Sci., 57, 793, 1977.

90. Patrias, G. and Olson, O. E., Selenium contents of samples of corn from midwestern states, Feedstuffs, 41, 29, 1969.

91. Kifer, R. R., and Payne, W. L., Selenium contents of fish meal, Feedstuffs, 40, 32, 1968.

92. Soares, J. H., Jr. and Miller, D., Selenium contents of Atlantic, gulf menhaden fish solubles, Feedstuffs, 42, 22, 1970.

93. Combs, G. F., Jr., Liu, C. H., Lu, Z. H., and Su, Q., unpublished research, 1983.

94. Allaway, W. H., and Hodgson, J. F., Symposium on nutrition, forage and pastures: selenium in forages as related to the geographic distribution of muscular dystrophy in livestock, J. Anim. Sci., 23, 271, 1964.

95. Redshaw, E. S., Martin, P. J., and Laverty, D. H., Iron, manganese, copper, zinc and selenium concentrations in Alberta grains and roughages, Can. J. Anim. Sci., 58, 553, 1978.

96. Davis, K. R., Peters, L. J., Cain, R. F., LeTourneau, D., and McGinnis, J., Evaluation of the nutrient composition of wheat. III. Minerals, Cereal Foods World, 29, 256, 1984.

97. Olson, O. E., Palmer, I. S., and Howe, S. M., Selenium in foods consumed by South Dakotans, Proc. S. Dakota Acad. Sci., 5, 113, 1978.

98. Lorenz, K., and Reuter, F. W., Mineral composition of developing wheat, rye and triticale, Cereal Chem., 53, 683, 1976.

99. Robinson, M., personal communication.

100. Millar, K. R., Craig, J., and Dawe, L., α-Tocopherol and selenium levels in pasteurized cows' milk for different areas of New Zealand, N.Z.J. Agric. Res., 16, 301, 1973.

101. Williams, M. M. F., Selenium and glutathione peroxidase in mature human milk, Proc. Univ. Otago Med. Sch., 61, 20, 1983.

102. Thompson, J. N., and Scott, M. L., Selenium in practical chicken feeds, Proc. 1968 Cornell Nutr. Conf., 121, 1968.

103. Scott, M. L., Selenium and vitamin E in poultry rations, Proc. 9th Nutr. Conf. Feed Mfgrs., Nottingham, Engl. 117, 1975.

104. Ebert, K. H., Lombeck, I., Kasperek, K., Feinendegen, L. E., and Bremer, H. J., The selenium content of infant food, Z. Ernahrungwiss., 23, 230, 1984.

105. Abdulla, M., Andersson, I., Asp, N. G., Berthelsen, K., Birkhed, D., Dencker, I., Johansson, C. G., Jagerstad, M., Kolar, K., Nair, B. M., Nilsson-Ehle, P., Norden, A., Rassner, S., Akesson, B., and Ockerman, P. A., Nutrient intake and health status of vegetarians. Chemical analyses of diets using the duplicate portion sampling technique. Am. J. Clin. Nutr., 34, 2464, 1981.

106. Abdulla, M., Aly, K. O., Andersson, I., Asp, N. G., Birkhed, D., Denker, I., Johansson, C. G., Jagerstad, M., Kolar, K., Nair, B. M., Nilsson-Ehle, P., Nordon, A., Rassner, S., Svenson, S., Akesson, B., and Ockerman, P. A., Nutrient intake and health status of lactovegetarians: chemical analyses of diets using the duplicate portion sampling technique, Am. J. Clin. Nutr., 40, 325, 1984.

4

THE BIOLOGICAL AVAILABILITY OF SELENIUM IN FOODS AND FEEDS

Shortly after the recognition of the nutritional essentiality of selenium for animals,[1-3] Schwarz and Foltz[4] found that the utilization of Se by the rat varied greatly depending upon the chemical form in which the Se was fed. These observations were extended by Schwarz et al.,[5-7] who demonstrated that Se in many organic and inorganic compounds was utilized with very different efficiencies by the vitamin E- deficient rat for the prevention of dietary liver necrosis. In 1972, Scott and Cantor[8] observed that field cases of exudative diathesis in chicks and of gizzard and cardiac myopathies in turkeys frequently occurred in flocks fed theoretically adequate levels of Se. They suggested that Se in practical feedstuffs may not always be well utilized by these species, as had been demonstrated for the rat. Therefore, the question of how to determine and predict the biological utilization of dietary Se took focus as a problem with immediate relevance in livestock feeding and with obvious implications in human nutrition.

I. DEFINING SELENIUM BIOAVAILABILITY

The utilization of dietary Se is the net result of several physiological and metabolic processes that convert a portion of ingested Se to certain metabolically critical forms that are necessary for normal physiological

127

function. As shown schematically in Fig. 4.1., ingested Se (normally in the form of Se-containing proteins and inorganic compounds) is subject to several potential losses en route to the metabolic production of critical Se-protein(s) and, perhaps, other critical low molecular weight species. These losses include those associated with the digestion and enteric absorption of ingested Se; thus, Se compounds that are insoluble under conditions of the lumenal environment of the small intestine, as well as Se-containing proteins of low digestibility, will pass through the animal to be eliminated in the feces. It is probable that, under normal circumstances, there is only a small entero-hepatic circulation of absorbed Se and that, therefore, fecal Se represents only that amount of ingested Se which was not absorbed. Table 4.1[9-26] summarizes the results of studies of the apparent absorption of Se in humans and experimental animals as determined by several different methods. It shows that, in general, the apparent absorption of Se in foods, inorganic compounds, and Se-amino acids is good (ca. 70%); however, the apparent absorption is highly variable both between and within single sources.

Not all absorbed Se is physiologically important. Some is metabolized to methylated forms that are readily excreted. For example, trimethyl selenonium cation comprises a major portion of urinary Se, and the volatile dimethyl selenide is readily excreted across the lung in expired air, although the production of the latter species is probably only important under conditions of high intakes of Se. In addition to these forms, Se is normally metabolized to several species, most notably the Se-analogs of the S-containing amino acids and, hence, to Se-containing polypeptides and proteins. Of these, the Se-dependent glutathione peroxidase (SeGSHpx) is the only physiologically critical species known. However, several other Se-proteins with undefined function have been identified. One or more of these may prove to be physiologically important; however, because Se is metabolized in many cases nondiscriminately as an analog of S, it is likely that at least some of these Se-proteins are physiologically inert, serving only as reserves of Se to be made available for metabolism to critical forms only as they turn over.*

Thus, it can be seen that the biological utilization of dietary Se is the integrated response of several physiologic and metabolic processes of varying complexity. The quantitative description of biological utilization of Se has come to be called its "bioavailability" (i.e., biological availability). While the concept of Se bioavailability is very useful in facilitating the prediction

---

*This superficial discussion of Se metabolism is presented for the purpose of reference for subsequent considerations of methods of assessing the biological utilization of Se; for a detailed discussion of Se metabolism and biological functions, the reader is directed to Chapters 5 and 6 of this volume.

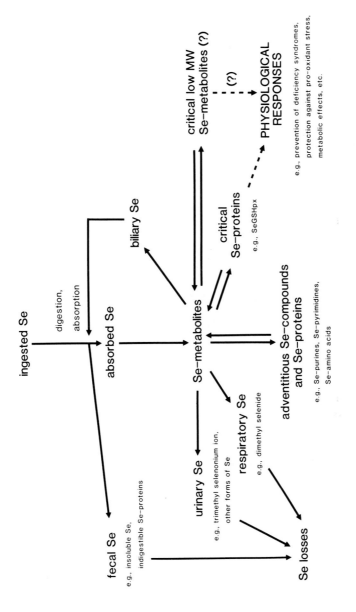

Fig. 4.1 Schematic representation of the utilization of dietary Se. MW, Molecular weight.

Table 4.1

Apparent Absorption of Orally-Ingested Se in Foods and Several Se-Compounds

Source of Se	Species	Se intake per subject	Method[a]	Apparent absorption (% intake)	Reference
Egg yolk	Human	—	A	75-82	(9)
Egg albumen	Human	—	A	52-55	(9)
Egg albumen	Human	150 μg/day	A	78-84	(10)
Egg albumen	Human	150 μg/day	B	78-82	(10)
Chicken meat	Human	231 μg/day	A	71, 72	(11)
Pork	Human	—	C	76-100	(12)
Formula diet with wheat	Human	217 μg/day	B	70,[b] 50[c]	(13)
Formula diet with wheat and tuna	Human	235 μg/day	B	64,[b] 49[c]	(13)
Low-Se formula diet	Human	34.5 μg/day	B	37[d]	(13)
Corn	Rat	Varied[e]	B	80-86	(14)
Fish muscle	Rat	4-6 μg dose[f]	C	64-77	(15)
Rabbit kidney	Rat	4 μg dose[f]	C	87	(16)
Soy bean	Rat	—	A	>90	(17)
Soy flour	Rat	—	A	ca. 75	(17)
Astragalus leaves and food	Hen	17.8 μg/day	B	65	(18)
Seleniferous wheat and food	Hen	18.5 μg/day	B	60	(18)
Fish meal and food	Hen	17.9 μg/day	B	58	(18)
Selenite	Human	249 μg/day	A	35, 38	(11)

(continues)

Table 4.1 (*Continued*)

Source of Se	Species	Se intake per subject	Method[a]	Apparent absorption (% intake)	Reference
Selenite	Human	—	D	59	(19)
Selenite and food	Human	23 μg/day	B	57	(20)
Selenite and corn	Rat	Varied[e]	B	75-78	(14)
Selenite	Rat	5 μg dose[f]	E	91	(21)
Selenite	Rat	5 μg dose[f]	F	93	(21)
Selenite	Rat	5 μg dose[f]	G	92	(21)
Selenite	Rat	Varied[e]	D	89-96	(22)
Selenite	Rat	Supranutritional[g]	D	84	(23)
Selenite and food	Hen	20.9 - 34.3 μg/day	B	68, 62	(18)
Selenite and food	Lamb	400 μg/day[h]	C	60-62	(24)
Selenite	Dog	50 μg/l infusion	E	8	(25)
Selenomethionine	Human	—	F	97	(21)
Selenomethionine and food	Human	24.2 μg/day	B	55	(20)
Selenomethionine	Rat	5 μg dose[f]	D	86	(25)
Selenomethionine	Rat	4 μg dose[f]	D	91	(16)
Selenomethionine and corn	Rat	Varied[e]	B	83-87	(14)

(continues)

131

Table 4.1 (*Continued*)

Source of Se	Species	Se intake per subject	Method[a]	Apparent absorption (% intake)	Reference
Selenomethionine	Rat	—	F	95	(21)
Selenomethionine	Rat	—	G	97	(21)
Selenomethionine	Rat	—	H	95	(21)
Selenomethionine and food	Lamb	400 μg/day[h]	C	63-67	(24)
Selenomethionine and food	Hen	21.1 μg/day	B	75	(18)
Selenomethionine	Dog	50 μg/l infusion	E	30	(25)
Selenocystine	Rat	5 μg dose[f]	D	81	(26)
Selenocystine	Dog	50 μg/l infusion	E	17	(25)
Selenocystine and food	Hen	20.4 μg/day	B	63	(18)

[a]Methods coded as follows: A, balance method using food intrinsically labeled with a stable isotope of Se; B, balance method using chemical analysis of Se; C, balance method using food labeled intrinsically with radioisotopic Se; D, balance method using radioisotopic Se; E, balance method from infusion of Se through external jejunal fistula; F, extrapolation from fecal excretion of radioisotopic Se; G, comparison of fecal excretion of radioisotopic Se from orally and intravenously treated individuals; H, comparison of whole body retention of radioisotopic Se in orally and intravenously treated individuals.

[b]Determined during 0-11 days of Se repletion after a 45-day depletion period.

[c]Determined during 11-22 days of Se repletion after a 45-day depletion period.

[d]Average of 45-day period of Se depletion.

[e]More than one level of Se used.

[f]Rats were fed a low-Se basal diet.

[g]Dietary concentration was 1 ppm Se.

[h]Diet contained .30 ppm Se.

of the adequacy of the Se associated with particular diets, patterns of food intake, etc., it is important to remember that estimates of Se bioavailability are experimentally derived values and, as such, must be considered in the context of the biological response(s) upon which they are based.

II. APPROACHES TO THE ESTIMATION OF SELENIUM BIOAVAILABILITY

Three approaches have been taken in the estimation of the bioavailability of Se; these have been discussed by Levander in two recent reviews.[27,28] They have involved the use of different types of biological response criteria. The first is the "preventative" approach. It involves the evaluation of the relative efficacy of known amounts of Se in reducing the incidence and/ or severity of a particular Se-deficiency syndrome in an experimental animal species. The candidate bioassays for this approach are (i) prevention of hepatic necrosis in the vitamin E- and Se-deficient rat; (ii) prevention of exudative diathesis in the vitamin E- and Se-deficient chick; (iii) prevention of pancreatic atrophy in the severely Se-deficient and vitamin E-fed chick;* and (iv) prevention of myopathies in vitamin E- and Se-deficient lambs, calves, or turkey poults. Of these, the first three have been employed most widely for this purpose. The second approach is the "tissue residue level" approach. It involves the evaluation of the relative efficacy of known amounts of Se in supporting the concentrations of Se in various tissues. This approach can be taken with any species, including those that do not show discrete pathological signs of nutritional Se deficiency and can employ such readily obtained tissues as blood plasma, cells, or platelets, rendering it applicable to human studies. The third approach is that of the "functional assay." It involves the evaluation of the relative efficacy of known amounts of Se in supporting the activities of SeGSHpx (which remains the only metabolically critical Se-dependent factor of current knowledge) in various tissues. Like the tissue residue level approach, this approach can be taken with any species that can be depleted of Se in advance, and, with the use of plasma or platelets as a source of SeGSHpx activity, it is suitable for human studies. With any approach to the estimation of the bioavailability of Se in discrete Se- compounds, foods, or feedstuffs, it has been conventional to use sodium selenite as a reference standard. Therefore, Se bioavailability estimates are expressed in terms of efficacies of the test Se sources for the elicitation of the particular biological response in comparison to that of sodium selenite; results are expressed on a percentage basis, with sodium selenite arbitrarily assigned the value of 100%.

*The diet for this assay must contain 100-200 IU vitamin E/kg.

III. SELENIUM BIOAVAILABILITY ESTIMATED BY THE
DISEASE PREVENTATIVE APPROACH

Estimating the bioavailability of Se via the disease preventative approach was pioneered by Schwarz and colleagues.[4,7,29-31] In a mammoth undertaking, those researchers evaluated 291 different inorganic and organic Se compounds on the basis of their abilities to prevent hepatic necrosis in the vitamin E-deficient rat.* Their results, which were expressed as ED_{50} values (i.e., the effective dietary concentration that provided protection of 50% of the population of rats from hepatic necrosis), have been recalculated by comparison to Se in sodium selenite selected as the standard for the estimation of Se bioavailability (see Table 4.2). Several important points emerge from those results: (i) of the common inorganic forms of Se, elemental Se is not biologically available, and sodium selenate is somewhat better utilized than sodium selenite; (ii) the common selenoamino acids have bioavailabilities comparable to sodium selenite; (iii) of the 281 organic Se-compounds tested, 16 had bioavailabilites appreciably greater (i.e., more than 150%) than that of sodium selenite, while 63 had little or no significant bioavailability (i.e., less than 20%). It is particularly important to note that none of the vast number of Se compounds tested was found to have activity in prevention of dietary liver necrosis in the rat comparable to that of the "Factor 3" preparation of hog kidney powder (the bioavailability of which was 306%). This finding was interpreted at the time to indicate that the hog kidney contained a form of Se, the so-called Factor 3, which, owing to its chemistry, was particularly biologically active; however, it is likely that the hog kidney powder preparation may have contained another factor(s) that potentiated the biological utilization of that Se, thus increasing its bioavailability.

Studies conducted almost exclusively by researchers at Cornell University[32-37] have estimated the bioavailability of Se on the basis of protection of the vitamin E- and Se-deficient chick from exudative diathesis, a debilitating and ultimately fatal disease characterized by subcutaneous edema and hemorrhaging. The results are summarized in Table 4.3.[38] They show that most forms of Se tested have bioavailabilites less than that of sodium selenite; in general, Se in animal by-product feedstuffs had rather low bioavailability (i.e., 9-25%), and Se in feedstuffs of plant origin had bioavailability of only ca. 79% that of sodium selenite. Although Cantor et al.[32] found Se in dehydrated alfalfa meal to have a bioavailability of 210%, this value appears suspiciously high in light of the results of Mathias

---

*This work was reported over the period of 1958-1974 and involved bioassays with a total of more than 16,000 rats.

Table 4.2

Biological Availability of Selenium in a "Factor 3" Preparation and Various
Se-Compounds Determined by Prevention of Liver Necrosis in Vitamin E-Deficient Rats

Se source	ED_{50}[a] (ppm Se)	Biologic availability (%)
"Factor 3" from pork kidney powder	7.7	306
Inorganic Se compounds[b]		
Selenium (elemental)	3200	Negligible
Sodium selenite	22	100[c]
Selenium dioxide	32	69
Sodium selenate	18	122
Selenic acid	27	81
Potassium selenocyanate	21	105
Se-containing amino acids[b]		
DL-Selenocysteine	24	92
DL-Selenocystine hydrochloride	23	96
Selenocystathionine	20	110
DL-Selenomethionine	23	96
Phenylselenocysteine	65	34
Miscellaneous organic Se compounds[b]		
Phenylselenide	1340	2
Dibenzyl diselenide	30	73
Bis(2—nitro—4—methylphenyl) triselenide	29	76
Bis(2—nitro—5—methylphenylselenenzyl) sulfide	16	138
Benzeneselenenic acid	67	33
4-Nitrobenzene seleninic acid	41	54
2,4-Dinitrobenzeneseleninic acid	22	100
4-Carboxybenzeneseleninic acid	Inactive	0
2-Selenouracil	Inactive, ca. 600	<4
6-Selenopurine	29	76
Actafluoroselenophane	Inactive	0
3,6-Dicarboxy-1,2-diselenane	Inactive	0
Symmetric monoseleno-dicarboxylic acids[d]		
HOOC—$(CH_2)_n$—Se—$(CH_2)_n$—COOH		
Seleno-diacetic acid	226	10
Seleno-2,2'-dipropionic acid, racemic	2780	<1
Seleno-2,2'-dipropionic acid, meso	1760	1
Seleno-2,2'-di-n-butyric acid, racemic	2750	<1
Seleno-2,2'-di-n-butyric acid, meso	2340	<1
Seleno-2,2'-diphenylacetic acid, racemic	260	8
Seleno-2,2'-diphenylacetic acid, meso	270	8
Seleno-3,3'-di-n-propionic acid	500	4
Seleno-4,4'-di-n-butyric acid	508	4
Seleno-5,5'-di-n-valeric acid	27	81
Seleno-6,6'-di-n-caproic acid	190	12

(continues)

Table 4.2 *(Continued)*

Se source	$ED_{50}{}^a$ (ppm Se)	Biologic availability (%)
Seleno-7,7'-di-*n*-oenanthic acid	40	55
Seleno-8,8'-di-*n*-caprylic acid	148	15
Seleno-9,9'-di-*n*-pelargonic acid	17	129
Seleno-10,10'-di-*n*-capric acid	115	19
Seleno-11,11'-di-*n*-undecanoic acid	13	169
Asymmetric monoseleno-dicarboxylic acids[d] R_1 — Se — R_2		
Seleno-acetic-4-*n*-butyric acid	820	3
Seleno-acetic-2-isobutyric acid	1310	2
Seleno-acetic-2-phenylacetic acid	540	4
Seleno-2-propionic-3'-propionic acid	150	15
Seleno-3-propionic-4-*n*-butyric acid	230	10
Seleno-3-propionic-4-*n*-valeric acid	380	6
Seleno-3-propionic-2-phenylacetic acid	73	30
Seleno-4-*n*-butyric-2-phenylacetic acid	240	9
Seleno-2-isobutyric-2-phenylacetic acid	370	6
Seleno-5-*n*-valeric-2-phenylacetic acid	82	27
Seleno-6-*n*-caproic-2-phelnylacetic acid	310	7
Symmetric diseleno-dicarboxylic acids[c]: HOOC—$(CH_2)_n$—Se—Se—$(CH_2)_n$-COOH		
Diseleno-diacetic acid	23	96
Diseleno-3,3'-di-*n*-propionic acid	18	122
Diseleno-4,4'-di-*n*-butyric acid	20	11
Diseleno-5,5'-di-*n*-valeric acid	23	96
Diseleno-6,6'-di-*n*-caproic acid	40	55
Diseleno-7,7'-di-*n*-oenanthic acid	64	34
Diseleno-8,8'-di-*n*-caprylic acid	32	69
Diseleno-9,9'-di-*n*-pelargonic acid	24	92
Diseleno-10,10'-di-*n*-capric acid	20	110
Diseleno-11,11'-di-*n*-undecanoic acid	28	79
Diseleno-12,12'-di-*n*-dodecanoic acid	40	55
Diseleno-2,2'-di-*n*-butyric acid	31	71
Diseleno-3,3'-di-*n*-butyric acid	34	65
Diseleno-4,4'-di-*n*-butyric acid	20	110
Diseleno-4,4'-di-*n*-valeric acid	16	138
Diseleno-5,5'-di-*n*-valeric acid	23	96
Diseleno-2,2'-diisobutyric acid	49	45
Diseleno-3,3'-diisobutyric acid	22	100
Diseleno-3,3'-diisovaleric acid	38	58
Diseleno-4,4'-di(2,2-dimethylbutyric) acid	850	3
Diseleno-4,4-di(3,3-dimethylbutyric) acid	560	4
Diseleno-4,4'-(2-hydroxy-3,3-dimethylbutyric) acid	470	5
Diseleno-5,5'-di-(3,3-dimethylvaleric) acid	820	3
Diseleno-2,2'-diphenylaceticacid	20	110
Diseleno-2,2'-di-(3-phenylpropionic) acid	130	17
Diseleno-3,3'-(3-phenylpropionic) acid	70	31

(continues)

Table 4.2 *(Continued)*

Se source	ED_{50}^{a} (ppm Se)	Biologic availability (%)
Symmetric diseleno-dicarboxylic acid amides[d]: $H_2N—CO—(CH_2)_n—Se—Se—(CH_2)_2—CO—NH_2$		
Diseleno-3,3′-di-*n*-propionamide	300	7
Diseleno-4,4′-di-*n*-butyramide	300	7
Diseleno-5,5′-di-*n*-valeramide	22	100
Diseleno-11,11′-di-*n*-undecanamide	12	183
Selena-carboxylic acids[e]: $R—Se—(CH_2)_2—COOH$		
3-Selena-butanoic acid	21	105
3-Selena-*n*-pentanoic acid	20	110
5-Selena-hexanoic acid	18	122
6-Selena-heptanoic acid	18	122
4-Selena-*n*-heptanoic acid	220	10
5-Selena-*n*-nonanoic acid	200	11
6-Selena-*n*-undecanoic acid	33	67
7-Selena-*n*-tridecanoic acid	90	24
8-Selena-*n*-pentadecanoic acid	16	138
9-Selena-*n*-heptadecanoic acid	89	25
10-Selena-*n*-nonadecanoic acid	51	43
11-Selena-*n*-heneicosanoic acid	82	27
12-Selena-*n*-tricosanoic acid	34	65
13-Selena-*n*-pentacosanoic acid	84	26
4-Selena-*n*-pentadecanoic acid	30	73
5-Selena-*n*-pentadecanoic acid	22	100
6-Selena-*n*-pentadecanoic acid	32	69
7-Selena-*n*-pentadecanoic acid	41	54
9-Selena-*n*-pentadecanoic acid	39	56
10-Selena-*n*-pentadecanoic acid	20	110
11-Selena-*n*-pentadecanoic acid	116	19
12-Selena-*n*-pentadecanoic acid	1040	2
13-Selena-*n*-pentadecanoic acid	40	55
14-Selena-*n*-pentadecanoic acid	26	85
3-Selena-*n*-hexadecanoic acid	39	56
4-Selena-*n*-hexadecanoic acid	29	76
5-Selena-*n*-hexadecanoic acid	41	54
6-Selena-*n*-hexadecanoic acid	20	110
7-Selena-*n*-hexadecanoic acid	43	51
8-Selena-*n*-hexadecanoic acid	20	110
9-Selena-*n*-hexadecanoic acid	91	24
10-Selena-*n*-hexadecanoic acid	21	105
11-Selena-*n*-hexadecanoic acid	14	157
12-Selena-*n*-hexadecanoic acid	132	17
13-Selena-*n*-hexadecanoic acid	82	27
4-Selena-*n*-hexadecanoic acid	31	71
12-Selena-*n*-reidecanoic acid	23	96
12-Selena-*n*-tetradecanoic acid	34	65

(continues)

Table 4.2 *(Continued)*

Se source	$ED_{50}{}^a$ (ppm Se)	Biologic availability (%)
12-Selena-*n*-pentadecanoic acid	84	91
12-Selena-*n*-heptadecanoic acid	16	138
12-Selena-*n*-octadecanoic acid	32	69
12-Selena-*n*-nonadecanoic acid	24	92
12-Selena-*n*-eicosanoic acid	19	116
12-Selena-*n*-heneicosanoic acid	31	71
12-Selena-*n*-docosanoic acid	25	88
12-Selena-*n*-tetracosanoic acid	25	88
12-Selena-*n*-pentacosanoic acid	29	76
12-Selena-*n*-hexacosanoic acid	29	76
12-Selena-*n*-heptacosanoic acid	32	69
12-Selena-*n*-octacosanoic acid	31	71
12-Selena-*n*-nonacosanoic acid	38	58
12-Selena-*n*-tritriacontanoic acid	27	36
Selena-carboxylic acid amides[e]: R—Se—$(CH_2)^n$-$CONH_2$		
12-Selena-*n*-reidecanoamide	9	244
12-Selena-*n*-tetradecanoamide	17	129
12-Selena-*n*-pentadecanoamide	62	32
12-Selena-*n*-hexadecanoamide	51	43
12-Selena-*n*-heptadeconamide	16	138
12-Selena-*n*-octadecanoamide	16	138
12-Selena-*n*-nonadecanoamide	12	183
12-Selena-*n*-eicosanoamide	12	183
12-Selena-*n*-heneicosanoamide	12	183
12-Selena-*n*-docosanomide	16	138
12-Selena-*n*-tricosanoamide	11	200
3-Selena-capramide	32	69
4-Selena-capramide	23, 21	96, 105
5-Selena-capramide	19	116
6-Selena-capramide	57	39
7-Selena-capramide	230	10
8-Selena-capramide	43	51
9-Selena-capramide	30	73
4-Selena-undecanamide	20	110
7-Selena-undecanamide	55	40
8-Selena-undecanamide	68	32
4-Selena-valeramide	16	138
4-Selena-capronamide	23	96
4-Selena-oenanthamide	83	27
4-Selena-caprylamide	109	20
4-Selena-pelargonamide	19	116
Other long-chain or branched selena acids or acid amides[e]		
10-Methyl-3-selena-octadecanoic acid	22	100
10-Methyl-9-selena-octadecanoic acid	31	71

(continues)

Table 4.2 *(Continued)*

Se source	$ED_{50}{}^{a}$ (ppm Se)	Biologic availability (%)
14-Hydroxyl-12-selena-tetradecanoic acid	31	71
12,16-Diselena-octadecanoic acid	77	29
12,16-Diselena-octadecanoamide	54	41
12,16-Diselena-docosanoic acid	35	63
12,16-Diselena-docosanoamide	47	47
12,16,20-Triselena-docosanoic acid	28	79
12,16,20-Triselena-docosonoamide	43	52
Diseleno-15.15′-di-(12-selena-pentadecanoic) acid	25	88
Dithio-15,15′-di(12-selena-pentadecanoic) acid	87	25
2-Carboxy-13-selena-hexadecanoic acid	229	10
2,4-Dinitrophenylselenocarboxylic acids[f]: $(NO_2)_2 — O — Se — R$		
2,4-Dinitrophenyl-seleno-acetic acid	78	28
2,4-Dinitrophenyl-seleno-3-*n*-propionic acid	20	110
2,4-Dinitrophenyl-seleno-4-*n*-butyric acid	47	47
2,4-Dinitrophenyl-seleno-5-*n*-valeric acid	18	122
2,4-Dinitrophenyl-seleno-6-*n*-caproic acid	62	15
2,4-Dinitrophenyl-seleno-7-*n*-oenanthic acid	23	96
2,4-Dinitrophenyl-seleno-8-*n*-caprylic acid	25	88
2,4-Dinitrophenyl-seleno-9-*n*-pelargonic acid	19	116
2,4-Dinitrophenyl-seleno-10-*n*-capric acid	37	59
2,4-Dinitrophenyl-seleno-11-*n*-undecanoic acid	18	122
2,4-Dinitrophenyl-seleno-2-propionic acid	75	29
2,4-Dinitrophenyl-seleno-3-*n*-butyric acid	27	81
2,4-Dinitrophenyl-seleno-4-*n*-valeric acid	23	96
Benzylseleno-*n*-carboxylic acid[f]: $O — CH_2 — Se — (CH_2)_n — COOH$		
Benzylseleno-acetic acid	19	116
Benzylseleno-2-*n*-propionic acid	24	92
Benzylseleno-3-*n*-propionic acid	24	92
Benzylseleno-2-isobutyric acid	130	17
Benzylseleno-4-*n*-butyric acid	20	110
Benzylseleno-3-isobutyric acid	20	110
Benzylseleno-3-*n*-butyric acid	28	79
Benzylseleno-3-isovaleric acid	68	32
Benzylseleno-5-*n*-valeric acid	13	169
Benzylseleno-6-*n*-caproic acid	29	76
Benzylseleno-7-*n*-oenanthic acid	11	200
Benzylseleno-8-*n*-caprylic acid	23	96
Benzylseleno-9-*n*-pelargonic acid	12	185
Benzylseleno-10-*n*-capric acid	21	106
Benzylseleno-11-*n*-undecanoic acid	12	183
Benzylseleno-4-(2,2-dimethylbutyric) acid	94	23
Benzylseleno-4-(3,3-dimethylbutyric) acid	910	2
Benzylseleno-5-(methylvaleric) acid	330	7

(continues)

Table 4.2 *(Continued)*

Se source	$ED_{50}{}^a$ (ppm Se)	Biologic availability (%)
Substituted benzylselenyl-carboxylic acids[f]: X — Θ — CH_2 — Se — $(CH_2)_n$ — COOH		
4-Nitrobenzylselenoacetic acid	41	54
4-Bromobenzylselenoacetic acid	23	96
4-Nitrobenzylseleno-2-propionic acid	370	7
4-Bromobenzylseleno-2-propionic acid	160	14
4-Methylbenzylseleno-3-*n*-propionic acid	230	10
4-Nitrobenzylseleno-3-*n*-propionic acid	30	73
4-Bromobenzylseleno-3-*n*-propionic acid	20	110
4-Nitrobenzylseleno-2-*n*-butyric acid	400	6
4-Bromobenzylseleno-2-*n*-butyric acid	580	4
4-Nitrobenzylseleno-2-isobutyric acid	20	110
4-Bromobenzylseleno-2-isobutyric acid	20	110
4-Nitrobenzylseleno-3-*n*-butyric acid	180	12
4-Bromobenzylseleno-3-*n*-butyric acid	92	24
4-Methylbenzylseleno-4-*n*-butyric acid	380	6
4-Nitrobenzylseleno-4-*n*-butyric acid	42	52
4-Bromobenzylseleno-4-*n*-butyric acid	16	138
4-Nitrobenzylseleno-4-*n*-valeric acid	83	27
4-Methylbenzylseleno-5-*n*-valeric acid	190	12
4-Nitrobenzylseleno-5-*n*-valeric acid	30, 42	73, 52
4-Bromobenzylseleno-5-*n*-valeric acid	16, 22	138, 100
4-Nitrobenzylseleno-6-*n*-caproic acid	42	52
4-Bromobenzylseleno-6-*n*-caproic acid	23	96
4-Nitrobenzylseleno-7-*n*-oenanthic acid	22	100
4-Bromobenzylseleno-7-*n*-oenanthic acid	23	96
4-Methylbenzylseleno-8-*n*-caprylic acid	370	6
4-Nitrobenzylseleno-8-*n*-caprylic acid	50	44
4-Bromobenzylseleno-8-*n*-caprylic acid	21	105
4-Nitrobenzylseleno-9-*n*-pelargonic acid	23	96
4-Bromobenzylseleno-9-*n*-pelargonic acid	17	129
4-Nitrobenzylseleno-10-*n*-caproic acid	42	52
4-Bromobenzylseleno-10-*n*-caproic acid	14	157
4-Nitrobenzylseleno-11-*n*-undecanoic acid	28	79
4-Bromobenzylseleno-11-*n*-undecanoic acid	20	110
4-Bromobenzylseleno-5-(3-methylvaleric) acid	20	110
Substituted phenylethylseleno-*n*-carboxylic acids[f]: X—Θ—$(CH_2)_2$—Se—$(CH_2)_n$—COOH		
Phenylethylseleno-3-propionic acid	43	51
Phenylethylseleno-5-*n*-valeric acid	45	49
4-Nitrophenylethylseleno-acetic acid	32	69
4-Nitrophenylethylseleno-3-propionic acid	20	110
4-Nitrophenylethylseleno-4-*n*-butyric acid	24	92
4-Nitrophenylethylseleno-5-*n*-valeric acid	32	69
4-Nitrophenylethylseleno-6-*n*-caproic acid	32	69

(continues)

Table 4.2 *(Continued)*

Se source	$ED_{50}{}^a$ (ppm Se)	Biologic availability (%)
Symmetric straight-chain dialkylmonoselenides[g]: CH_3—$(CH_2)_n$—Se—$CH_2)_n$—CH_3		
Diethyl monoselenide	860	3
Dipropyl monoselenide	1360	2
Dibutyl monoselenide	310	7
Dipentyl monoselenide	53	42
Dihexyl monoselenide	92	24
Diheptyl monoselenide	32	69
Dioctyl monoselenide	85	26
Dionyl monoselenide	21	105
Didecyl monoselenide	31	71
Diundecyl monoselenide	24	92
Symmetric straight-chain dialkyl diselenides[g]: CH_3—$(CH_2)_n$—Se—Se—$(CH_2)_n$—CH_3		
Dipropyl diselenide	61	36
Dibutyl diselenide	87	25
Dipentyl diselenide	19	116
Dihexyl diselenide	25	88
Diheptyl diselenide	28	79
Dioctyl diselenide	31	71
Diononyl diselenide	14.4	153
Didecyl diselenide	19	116
Diundecyl diselenide	10	220
Didodecyl diselenide	13	169
Ditridecyl diselenide	64	34
Ditetradecyl diselenide	48	46
Dipentadecyl diselenide	28	79
Dihexadecyl diselenide	37	59
Diheptadecyl diselenide	59	37
Dioctadecyl diselenide	68	32
Diheneicosyl diselenide	170	13
Dihydroxyalkyl-diselenides and acetyl derivatives[h]: R — Se — Se — R		
Di-(2-hydroxyethyl)-diselenide	14	157
Di-(3-hydroxyethyl)-diselenide	30	73
Di-(4-hydroxyethyl)-diselenide	20	110
Di-(5-acetoxypentyl)-diselenide	20	110
Di-(4-acetoxy-1-methyl-butyl)-diselenide	43	51
Di-(3-hydroxy-1-methyl-propyl)-diselenide	46	48
Di-(3-hydroxy-2-methyl-propyl)-diselenide	23	96
Di-(3-hydroxy-2,2-dimethyl-propyl)-diselenide	610	4
Diselenides of aliphatic and heterocyclic amines[h]: R — Se — Se — R		
Di-(3-aminopropyl)-diselenide	46	48
Di-(2-dimethylaminoethyl)-diselenide dipicrate	244	9
Di-(3-dimethylaminopropyl)-diselenide dihydrobromide	223	10
Di-(3-dimethylaminopropyl)-diselenide dipicrate	324	7

(continues)

Table 4.2 *(Continued)*

Se source	ED$_{50}$[a] (ppm Se)	Biologic availability (%)
Di-(2-diethylaminoethyl)-diselenide dipicrate	184	12
Di-(2-N-piperidylethyl)-diselenide dipicrate	109	20
Di-(3-N-piperidylpropyl)-diselenide dipicrate	103	21
Di-(2-N-morpholinylethyl)-diselenide dipicrate	358	6
Di-(3-N-morpholinylpropyl)-diselenide dipicrate	100	22
Se-containing ketones and an acetal[h]		
4-Selena-hexanone-2	35	63
4-Benzylseleno-butanone-2	28	79
ω-(4-Chloro-2-nitrophenylseleno)-acetophenone	14	157
Benzylseleno-acetaldehyde-dimethyl acetal	11	200
6-Selenoctic acid[i]	38	58

[a] ED$_{50}$, Effective dietary concentration that provides protection of 50% of the population from liver necrosis.
[b] Data from Schwarz and Foltz.[4]
[c] Arbitrarily set as the standard.
[d] Data from Schwarz and Fredga.[5]
[e] Data from Schwarz and Fredga.[6]
[f] Data from Schwarz and Fredga.[7]
[g] Data from Schwarz et al.[29]
[h] Data from Schwarz and Fredga.[30]
[i] Data from Schwarz et al.[31]

et al.,[33] which, when recalculated according to the method of Cantor *et al.*,[32] indicate the bioavailability of alfalfa to be in the range of 75-96%. In contrast to the results of the rat hepatic necrosis prevention bioassay, results of the chick exudative diathesis prevention assay show that the bioavailabilities of sodium selenate and the common selenoamino acids are only ca. 74% and 78% (using the authors' data recalculated according to the method of Cantor *et al.*[32]), respectively.

Cantor *et al.*[39] evaluated the bioavailabilities of five sources of Se on the basis of their efficacies in preventing pancreatic atrophy in chicks (see Table 4.4). This bioassay system would appear to offer certain advantages for the study of the utilization of dietary Se, inasmuch as the prevention of nutritional pancreatic atrophy of the vitamin E-fed chick is strictly dependent upon Se. This marked specificity for Se differentiates this bioassay from the others mentioned above, which each respond to small changes in the vitamin E nutriture of the experimental animal. Therefore, the pancreatic atrophy prevention assay does not necessitate the removal of vitamin E by extraction with hexane for the testing of Se bioavailability of practical foods and feedstuffs. Also, because nutritional pancreatic atrophy in the chick is prevented by very low dietary levels of Se, the

Table 4.3

Biological Availability of Se in Feedstuffs and Se Compounds as Determined by Prevention of Exudative Diathesis in the Vitamin E-Deficient Chick[a]

Source of Se	Biological availability (%)
Dehydrated alfalfa meal	210[b]
Brewers' yeast	89
Cottonseed meal	86
Corn meal	86[c]
Brewers' grains	80
Wheat	71
Distillers' dried grains and solubles	65
Soybean meal, dehulled	60
Herring meal	25
Tuna meal	22
Menhaden meal	16
Dried fish solubles	9
Poultry by-product meal	18
Meat and bone meal	15
High-Se yeast	106[d]
Elemental (gray) selenium	7[e]
Sodium selenide	42
Sodium selenate	58, 89
Sodium selenite	100[f]
Selenomethionine	18, 32, 61, (101)[g]
	(57, 90)[h]
Selenocystine	69, 78 (63)[g]
6-Selenopurine	20
Selenoethionine	44

[a]Data from Cantor et al.[32] unless otherwise indicated.

[b]This estimate is suspiciously high in light of the results of Mathias et al.,[32] which, when recalculated by the method of Cantor et al.,[32] indicate the biological activity of alfalfa to be 75-96%.

[c]Combs et al.[34] found that high-Se (i.e., 0.296 ppm Se) corn produced on soil amended with 50% coal flyash (containing 6.5 ppm Se) had a biological availability for prevention of exudative diathesis of 46%.

[d]Data from Combs et al.[31] calculated by the method of Cantor et al.[32]

[e]Se in coal flyash was found to have similarly low biological availability for prevention of exudative diathesis.[36]

[f]Arbitrarily set as the standard.

[g]Value shown in parentheses was calculated from the data of Osman and Latshaw[38] by the method of Cantor et al.[32]

[h]Values shown in parentheses were calculated from the data of Zhou and Combs[37] by the method of Cantor et al.[32] for chicks fed a normal level (22.5%) or a low level (16.9%) of total protein, respectively.

sensitivity of this bioassay makes it suitable for the evaluation of foods and feedstuffs of only moderate Se content. However, the great sensitivity of the pancreas disorder also means that it can be difficult or impossible to establish the bioassay, depending on the feasibility of producing a nutritionally balanced basal diet containing no more than 0.01 ppm Se. This has been feasible for researchers at Cornell University, who have employed a highly purified basal diet based on crystalline amino acids as the sole sources of nitrogen,[39-44] or an unusually low- Se practical diet based on corn meal and soybean meal produced in areas of endemic Se- deficiency in Heilongjiang Province, China.[45] Using the pancreatic atrophy prevention bioassay, Cantor et al.[39] found that the Se present in selenomethionine, selenocystine, or a sample of seleniferous wheat had bioavailability susbstantially greater than that of sodium selenite. The Se in tuna, which had been found by Cantor et al.[32] to have a low bioavailability for the prevention of exudative diathesis (see Table 4.3), was also found to have relatively low bioavailability for the prevention of nutritional pancreatic atrophy (see Table 4.4), although the value determined by the latter bioassay method was approximately twice that determined by the former bioassay method (i.e., 47% vs. 22%). Comparison of the general results of these two bioassay methods indicates that Se is better utilized by the chick for the prevention of nutritional pancreatic atrophy than for prevention of exudative diathesis.

Cantor et al.[46] took the preventative approach to estimating the bioavailability of Se in selenomethionine for turkey poults on the basis of its efficacy in preventing the myopathy of the gizzard that occurs in that species due to vitamin E- and Se- deficiency. Their results indicate that the Se in that selenoamino acid has a bioavailability of ca. 84% of that of sodium selenite.

A novel bioassay of the preventative approach type was that used by Combs[47] to evaluate the efficacy of Se in selenomethionine or a high-Se yeast to protect against the acute toxicity of paraquat in the chick. Those results indicate the bioavailabilities of these sources of Se to be ca. 112% and 124%, respectively.

Table 4.4

Biologic Availability of Se in Feedstuffs and Se-Compounds Determined by Prevention of Nutritional Pancreatic Atrophy in the Vitamin E-Fed Chick

Source of selenium	Biological availability (%)[a]
Sodium selenite	100[b]
Selenomethionine	348-377
Selenocystine	121-133
Tuna meal	47
Wheat	360

[a]Estimated from the data of Cantor et al.[39] on the basis of slope ratio comparisons of chick pancreas histological scores as function of dietary Se level.

[b]Arbitrarily set as the standard.

IV. SELENIUM BIOAVAILABILITY ESTIMATED BY THE TISSUE RESIDUE LEVEL APPROACH

The estimation of Se bioavailability by the tissue residue level approach has the disadvantage of considering the total amount of Se in particular tissues without regard for that portion which is present in noncritical forms (i.e., without biological activity). These forms are indicated as "adventitious" Se-compounds and Se-proteins in Fig. 4.1. Thus, implicit in the use of the tissue residue level approach is the assumption that the metabolism of absorbed and retained Se to such adventitious forms correlates with the metabolism of that Se to such physiologically critical forms as SeGSHpx. Although this assumption is largely untested experimentally, it seems plausible under conditions of suboptimal (as defined by manifestation of specific deficiency syndromes and/or reduced SeGSHpx activities) dietary intakes of Se. Indeed, support for this premise comes from the finding by Thomson et al.[48] that when blood total Se concentration was less than ca. 120 ng/l, blood Se correlated positively with blood SeGSHpx activity in samples from New Zealand residents. However, the lack of such a correlation for blood samples containing greater concentrations of Se indicates that the tissue residue level approach may not be useful when experimental subjects are not markedly depleted in Se. Because it can be assumed that the adventitious Se pool is released upon the turning over of noncritical Se-containing proteins for possible incorporation into critical Se form(s), tissue residue levels can also be indicative of the total body Se including these kinds of tissue reserves. As such, the tissues of main interest are liver and skeletal muscle, as these comprise the greatest body stores of Se, containing approximately 30% and 40%, respectively, of total body Se.[49]

Table 4.5 presents estimates of the bioavailability of Se from several sources recalculated from nine reports selected for having fed graded levels of Se as supplements to low-Se basal diets and for having employed sodium selenite as a control treatment series.[50-54] Despite a couple of widely discrepant estimates of bioavailability for the same Se source (e.g., 809% for poult muscle[46] vs. 138% for rat muscle[14]), the results of these evaluations show remarkable consistency within Se sources and between tissues. These collective results show that, for the support of tissue Se levels, the selenoamino acids and Se in foods of plant origin have bioavailabilities comparable to or somewhat greater than that of sodium selenite, but that Se in foods or feedstuffs of animal (in this case fish) origin has bioavailability appreciably less (e.g., 50-80%) than that of sodium selenite.

Other estimates of Se bioavailability have been made on the basis of single-point (i.e., experiments comparing the responses of different sources

Table 4.5

Biological Availability of Se in Se-Compounds and Natural Products as Estimated by Tissue Accumulation of Se in Response to Graded Intakes of Se

Se Source	Species	Dietary level, (ppm)	Relative accumulation rates in various tissues (%)[a]					
			Blood	Plasma	Liver	Kidney	Heart	Muscle
Selenomethionine	Chick	0-.500[b]						
Selenomethionine	Chick	.01-.05[b]						
Selenomethionine	Hen	0-.4[b]						
Selenomethionine	Poult	0-.12[b]		121	105	121	116	809
Selenomethionine	Rat	.024-.12[c]	110		112			138
Selenocystine	Chick	.01-.05[c]						
Selenodicysteine	Chick	.035-.205[c]	90		83	91		92
High-Se yeast	Rat	.05-.20[b]	132 (138)[c]		116 (147)[c]			
"Chelated" Se	Rat	.05-.20[b]	61 (60)[c]			70 (88)[c]		
Coal flyash	Chick	.02-.14[c]	80		82	65		
High-Se clover	Chick	.32-1.22[d]	167		124	122		
Fish meal	Chick	0-.222[b]						
Fish solubles	Chick	0-.234[b]						
Raw tuna	Rat	.05-.15[b]	57 (60)[c]		47 (70)[c]	74 (75)[c]		79 (100)[c]
Precooked tuna	Rat	.05-.15[b]	72 (60)[c]		41 (70)[c]	94 (88)[c]		75 (100)[c]
Canned tuna	Rat	.05-.15[b]	120 (80)[c]		121 (100)[c,f]	83 (100)[c]		136 (200)[c]
Whole wheat flour	Rat	.05-.15[b]	105 (100)[c]		121 (100)[c,g]	208 (138)[c]		182 (200)[c]
Whole wheat bread	Rat	.05-.15[b]	112 (80)[c]		121 (100)[c]	148 (100)[c]		200 (200)[c]
Wheat bran	Rat	.05-.15[b]	123 (80)[c]		103 (100)[c]	215 (125)[c]		161 (100)[c]
Mixed diet	Hen	.10-.30[c]						

(continues)

Table 4.5 (Continued)

Se Source	Species	Dietary level, (ppm)	Relative accumulation rates in various tissues (%)[a]						Reference
			Gizzard	Pancreas	Spleen	Skin, hair	Whole body	Egg	
Selenomethionine	Chick	0-.500[b]					200		(50)
Selenomethonine	Chick	.01-.05[b]		370					(38)
Selenomethionine	Hen	0-.4[b]						199	(51)
Selenomethionine	Poult	0-.12[b]	193	445					(46)
Selenomethionine	Rat	.024-.12[c]			119	128			(14)
Selenocystine	Chick	.01-.05[c]		115					(38)
Selenodicysteine	Chick	.035-.205[c]							(52)
High-Se yeast	Rat	.05-.20[b]							(53)
"Chelated" Se	Rat	.05-.20[b]							(53)
Coal flyash	Chick	.02-.14[c]							(36)
High-Se clover	Chick	.32-1.22[d]							(36)
Fish meal	Chick	0-.222[b]					232		(50)
Fish solubles	Chick	0-.234[b]					211		(50)
Raw tuna	Rat	.05-.15[b]							(54)
Precooked tuna	Rat	.05-.15[b]							(54)
Canned tuna	Rat	.05-.15[b]							(54)
Whole wheat flour	Rat	.05-.15[b]							(54)
Whole wheat bread	Rat	.05-.15[b]							(54)
Wheat bran	Rat	.05-.15[b]							(54)
Mixed diet	Hen	.10-.30[c]						597	(38)

[a] Compared to rate observed for Na_2SeO_3 (arbitrarily set at 100%) by slope (m) ratio analysis of accumulation regressions fitted to the general equation, tissue Se = m [log (dietary Se level)] + constant.

[b] Indicates level of Se added to a basal diet, which probably contained ca. 0.02 ppm Se.

[c] Value in parentheses is original authors' estimate of bioavailability determined by slope (m) ratio analyses of the linear function: tissue Se = m(diet Se) + constant.

[d] Levels include Se inherent in the basal diet.

[e] Se levels were obtained by blending high- and low-Se diets of the same formula.

[f] Douglass et al.[55] estimated, in rats fed a single level of Se, the bioavailability of Se in tuna to be 73 ± 17% compared to selenite.

[g] Douglass et al.[55] estimated, in rats fed a single level of Se, the bioavailability of Se in wheat to be 86 ± 2% compared to selenite.

147

of Se each fed at a single dietary concentration) determinations. These methods, although inherently less reliable than estimations based upon slope ratio comparisons of dose-response regressions, have yielded similar results (see Table 4.6).[55-57]

V. SELENIUM BIOAVAILABILITY ESTIMATED BY THE FUNCTIONAL ASSAY APPROACH

Subsequent to the discovery in 1973 by Rotruck et al.[58] of the biochemical role of Se as an essential constituent of SeGSHpx, it has been possible to employ the assay of this enzyme activity as a biological response parameter in the evaluation of Se bioavailability. In the absence of any other known critical physiological form of Se, SeGSHpx remains the only appropriate response parameter for estimating Se bioavailability via the functional approach. Therefore, it has been employed for this purpose in several studies, the results of which are summarized in Tables 4.7[59-61] and 4.8.[62-65]

The best estimates of Se bioavailability based upon the support of tissue SeGSHpx activities have been derived from studies employing graded low levels of Se in both the test and reference (sodium selenite) forms. Such studies have demonstrated that the SeGSHpx response to increasing amounts of dietary Se is best described by the general equation:

$$\text{SeGSHpx specific activity}^* = m[\log (\text{dietary Se})] + k$$

where m and k are constants, the latter being the y intercept of the regression. Because tissue SeGSHpx activities will be comparably low in Se-deficient subjects without any Se-supplementation, regressions of this form will have common intercepts for animals fed graded levels of test or reference forms of Se. Therefore, the efficacy of two forms of dietary Se can be estimated by slope (m) ratio comparisons of the individual regressions.

This approach has been employed in recalculating the data of several authors, the results of which are presented in Table 4.7. These results indicate that, by this functional bioassay, the bioavailabilities of the common selenoamino acids are generally comparable to estimates for those forms of Se derived from the exudative diathesis prevention bioassay (e.g., ca. 81% for SeGSHpx vs. ca. 78% for exudative diathesis) but are somewhat lower than those derived from the other preventative bioassays or from the tissue residue level bioassay. In addition, the variation in estimates

---

*Specific activity = units of enzyme activity (usually nano moles NADPH oxidized per minute) per milligram total protein.

Table 4.6

Biological Availability of Se in Selected Se-Compounds and Natural Products as Estimated by Tissue Accumulation of Se in Single-Point (i.e., Single Level Feeding) Bioassays

Se source	Species	Se intake	Relative accumulation rates in various tissues (%)[a]				Reference
			Blood	Plasma	Erythrocytes	Liver	
Sodium selenate	Poult	0.1 ppm[b]		134			(56)
Selenomethionine	Poult	0.1 ppm[b]		119			(56)
Selenomethionine	Human	100 µg/day, 4 wks[c]	242	215	218		(48)
Selenocystine	Poult	0.1 ppm[b]		117			(56)
Selenoethionine	Poult	0.1 ppm[b]		83			(56)
Wheat	Rat	0.2 ppm[b]			92 (216)[d]	68	(55)
Wheat	Human	200 µg/day, 11 wks[c]		260	754		(57)
Tuna	Rat	0.2 ppm[b]			55(134)[d]	54	(55)
Menhaden meal	Poult	0.1 ppm[b]		51			(56)
Beef kidney	Rat	0.2 ppm[b]			71 (134)[d]	60	(55)
High-Se yeast	Human	200 µg/day, 11 wks[c]		283	785		(57)

[a] Compared to response to Na_2SeO_3 (arbitrarily set at 100%).

[b] Indicates level of Se added to basal diet, which probably contained ca. 0.02 ppm Se.

[c] Indicates level of Se supplemented to free-choice diets low in Se (probably < 0.50 µg Se/day).

[d] Value in parentheses is calculated biavailability based on Se accumulation in only "young" (i.e., low-density) erythrocytes.

Table 4.7

Biological Availability of Se in Se Compounds and Several Natural Products as Determined by Support of Se-dependent Glutathione Peroxidase (SeGSHpx) Activities in Response to Graded Intakes of Se

Se source	Species	Dietary levels (ppm)	Relative biological availability (%)[a] by GSHpx in various tissues			Reference
			Plasma	Liver	Kidney	
Selenomethionine	Chicks	0–.06[b]	53			(32)
Selenomethionine	Chicks	0–.12[b]	78			(59)
Selenomethionine	Chicks	0–.09[b]	76			(34)
Selenomethionine	Chicks	.02–.18	93			(47)
Selenomethionine	Poults	0–.12[b]	94			(46)
Selenomethionine	Rats	0–.5[b]		66,[c] 86[d]		(60)
Selenodicysteine	Chicks	.035–.205	98			(52)
High-Se corn	Chicks	0–.09[b]	32			(34)
Corn gluten meal	Chicks	0–.12[b]	26			(59)
Soybean meal	Chicks	0–.12[b]	18			(59)
Fish meals	Chicks	0–.12[b]	42[e]			(61)
Cepalin fish meals	Chicks	0–.12[b]	60[f]			(59)
Mackerel fish meals	Chicks	0–.12[b]	34[g]			(59)
Tuna	Rats	.05–.15[b]		39	41	(54)
Wheat	Rats	.05–.15[b]		191	184	(54)
High-Se yeast	Chicks	.02–.18[b]	128			(47)
High-Se yeast	Chicks	.03–.14[b]	107	107		(35)
Coal flyash	Chicks	0–.12[b]	95			(36)

[a] Estimated by slope (m) ratio comparisons with Na_2SeO_3 using the general equation: SeGSHpx activity = m[log (diet Se)] + constant.

[b] Level of Se added to low-Se basal diets presumed to contain ca. 0.02 ppm Se.

[c] Value obtained with rats fed methionine-free diet; this estimate compares to that of original authors of 49% based on the dietary level of Se calculated to support half-maximal SeGSHpx activity in rat liver.

[d] Value obtained with rats fed diet containing 0.4% methionine; this estimate compares to that of original authors of 80% based on the dietary level of Se calculated to support half-maximal SeGSHpx activity in rat liver.

[e] Average value for four samples of fish meals (i.e., 41%, 60%, 36%, 32%).

[f] Average value for seven samples of fish meals (i.e., 41%, 60%, 50%, 40%, 39%, 59%, 48%).

[g] Average value for two samples of fish meals (i.e., 36%, 32%).

of Se bioavailability for selenomethionine (e.g., 53-94%) suggests that other factors may affect the SeGSHpx response. Estimates of the bioavailability of Se in plant materials (with the exception of wheat, found by Alexander et al.[54] to be nearly twice as bioavailable as sodium selenite to the rat) are generally much lower by the SeGSHpx bioassay method than by the other methods (e.g., ca. 25% by SeGSHpx vs. ca. 79% by exudative diathesis and ca. 100% by tissue Se). The bioavailability of Se in fish products is comparable when estimated by the SeGSHpx support (ca. 44%) or pancreatic atrophy prevention (ca. 47%) bioassays, both of which yield estimates that are substantially greater than that of the exudative diathesis prevention method (ca. 22%). Estimates of the bioavailability of Se in high-Se yeast products by the SeGSHpx support method (ca. 114%) compare very favorably with those obtained by other methods (e.g., ca. 124% by tissue Se accumulation; 106% by prevention of exudative diathesis).

Estimates of Se bioavailability based on single-point determinations (i.e., use of a single level of Se-supplementation) are inherently less accurate due to the incorrect assumption implicit in this approach that the SeGSHpx response from the basal to the tested levels of Se is linear. Thus, the comparison of the SeGSHpx activity in response to a particular level of Se fed as the test source to that fed as the reference standard is, in effect, a comparison to the slopes of the implied linear equations [general form: SeGSHpx specific activity = m(dietary Se level) + k]. Because observations from multiple-point experiments do not substantiate this linear relationship (in fact, they show the exponential relationship discussed above), estimations of this type, while often useful, are necessarily associated with relatively great error. This can be seen in Table 4.8, which presents a summary of the single- point experiments for which estimations of Se bioavailability of this type can be made. Another factor that undoubtedly contributes to the error of such single-point determinations is the use of levels of Se-supplementation that are great enough to be outside of the range of near linearity of the SeGSHpx response (i.e., 0.02-0.08 ppm Se).

VI. COMPARISON OF THE DIFFERENT APPROACHES TO THE ESTIMATION OF SELENIUM BIOAVAILABILITY

Different approaches to the determination of the bioavailability of Se in Se- compounds and in natural products have produced different quantitative estimates. These differences are apparent in Table 4.9, which presents a summary of the bioavailability estimates for several of the more frequently studied sources of Se. Of the five methods summarized, the greatest consistencies appear to be, within single Se sources, between the

Table 4.8

Biological Activity of Se in Se Compounds and Natural Products as Estimated by Support of Se-Dependent Glutathione Peroxidase (SeGSHpx) Activities by Single-Level Intakes or Limited Temporal Exposure to Se

Source of Se	Species	Se exposure	Relative Biological Availability(%)[a] by SeGSHpx in various tissues						Reference
			Plasma	Erythrocytes	Lymphocytes[b]	Platelets	Liver	Kidney	
Sodium selenate	Poult	.2 ppm in diet[c]	231[j]						(56)
Sodium selenate	Human	$10^{-7}M$ in cell culture			30[j]				(62)
Selenomethionine	Human	$10^{-7}M$ in cell culture			197[j]				(62)
Selenomethionine	Rat	2 ppm in diet[c]		29,[e,j] 98[f,i]			57[e,j]	104[f,j]	(63)
Selenomethionine	Poult	.2 ppm in diet[c]		72[j]					(56)
Selenomethionine	Human	100 μg/day, 4 wks[d]	68[j]						(48)
Selenomethionine	Rat	3.37 mg/kg dose	143[j]				93[j]	111[i,j]	(64)
Selenocysteine	Poult	.2 ppm in diet[c]						(62)	(56)
Selenocysteine	Human	$10^{-7}M$ in cell culture			197[j]				(56)
Selenoethionine	Poult	.2 ppm in diet[c]	72[j]						(56)
Menhaden meal	Poult	.1 ppm in diet[c]	65[j]						(56)
Tuna	Rat	.20 ppm in diet[c]		37 (40)[g,k]			39[k]		(55)
Beef kidney	Rat	.20 ppm in diet[c]		74 (54)[g,k]			104[k]		(55)
Wheat	Rat	.20 ppm in diet[c]		61 (66)[g,k]			75[k]		(55)
Wheat	Human	200 μg/day, 11 wks[d]	425[j]			128[j]			(57)
High-Se yeast	Human	200 μg/day, 11 wks	425[j]			134[j]			(57)
Infant formula, whey	Rat	.070 ppm[b]	115[k]				58[k]		(65)
Infant formula, casein	Rat	.086 ppm[b]	94[k]				77[k]		(65)
Infant formula, soy isolate	Rat	.104 ppm[b]	45[k]				18[k]		(65)

(continues)

Table 4.8 (Continued)

Source of Se	Species	Se exposure	Relative Biological Availability(%)[a] by SeGSHpx in various tissues						Reference
			Plasma	Erythrocytes	Lymphocytes[b]	Platelets	Liver	Kidney	
Infant formula, casein hydrolysate	Rat	.100 ppm[b]	111[k]				116[k]		(65)
Enteral formula, casein hydrolysate	Rat	.064 ppm[b]	46[k]				42[k]		(65)
Enteral formula, casein/soy	Rat	.044 ppm[b]	70[k]				42[k]		(65)
Enteral formula, casein/low MET	Rat	.080 ppm[b]	45[k]				37[k]		(65)
Enteral formula, casein/high MET	Rat	.080 ppm[b]	17[k]				19[k]		(65)
Enteral formula, milk-based	Rat	.064[b]	173[k]				90[k]		(65)

[a]Based on Na_2SeO_3 standard arbitrarily set at 100%.

[b]Phytohemagglutinin-transformed in vitro.

[c]Air-dry basis, added to based diet presumed to contain ca. 0.02 inherent Se.

[d]Supplemented to undefined, but probably low-Se (i.e., < 50 μg Se/ day), diet.

[e]Pyridoxine-deficient animals.

[f]Pyridoxine-fed animals.

[g]Value shown in parentheses based on "young" (i.e., low-density) erythrocytes only.

[h]Dry-matter basis, fed as sole sources of nutriture.

[i]Biological availability estimated by SeGSHpx in small intestine was 200%, in stomach it was 110%.

[j]Estimated by comparison of test response to that of single level/dose of Na_2SeO_3.

[k]Estimated by comparison of test response to that of graded levels of Na_2SeO_3.

153

Table 4.9

Comparison of the Bioavailabilities (%) of Several Sources of Se as Determined by Different Bioassy Methods

Bioassay method	Na_2SeO_3	Na_2SeO_4	Selenomethionine	Selenocysteine
Preventative approach				
Prevention of liver necrosis in vitamin E-deficient rats	100[a]	122[41]	96[4]	92[4]
Prevention of exudative diathesis in vitamin E-deficient chicks	100[a]	74[33]	71[b]	74,[33] 63[40]
Prevention of pancreatic atrophy in vitamin E-fed chicks	100[a]	—	363[41]	127[41]
Tissue residue level approach				
Accumulation of tissue Se	100[a]	—	109[c]	83[54]
Functional approach				
Support of tissue SeGSHpx	100[a]	231[58]	79[f]	121[g]

(continues)

154

Table 4.9 (*Continued*)

Bioassay method	High-Se yeast	Corn	Wheat	Soybean meal	Fish/fish meals
Preventative approach					
Prevention of liver necrosis in vitamin E-deficient rats	—	—	—	—	—
Prevention of exudative diathesis in vitamin E-deficient chicks	106[39]	86[33]	71[33]	60[33]	16[33]
Prevention of pancreatic atrophy in vitamin E-fed chicks	—	—	360[41]	—	47[4]
Tissue residue level approach					
Accumulation of tissue Se	116[d]	—	121[c]	—	69[e]
Functional approach					
Support of tissue SeGSHpx	121[h]	32[i]	128[i]	18[61]	46[k]

[a] Arbitrarily selected as standard.

[b] Average based on estimates of 37%,[31] 101%,[38] and 74%.[37]

[c] Average based on estimates using liver Se of 105%[46] and 112%.[14]

[d] Estimate calculated from liver Se data reported by Vinson and Bose.[53]

[e] Estimate calculated from liver Se data reported by Alexander et al.[54]

[f] Average based on estimated using plasma SeGSHpx of 68%,[48] 53%,[33] 78%,[59] 76%,[34] 93%,[47] 94%,[51], erythrocyte SeGSHpx of 29%,[63] 98%,[63] 72%,[56] liver SeGSHpx of 57%,[63] 104%,[63] 93%,[64] 66%,[60] 86%,[60] kidney SeGSHpx of 111%.[64]

[g] Average based on estimates using plasma SeGSHpx of 143%[56] and 98%.[46]

[h] Average based on estimates using plasma SeGSHpx of 107%[35] and platelet SeGSHpx of 134%.[57]

[i] Estimate derived from high-Se corn.[34]

[j] Average based on estimates using erythrocyte SeGSHpx of 61%[55]; platelet SeGSHpx of 128%[57]; liver SeGSHpx of 75%,[55] 191%[54]; kidney SeGSHpx of 75%,[55] 191%[54]; liver SeGSHpx of 184%.[54]

[k] Average based on estimates using erythrocyte SeGSHpx of 37%[55]; plasma SeGSHpx of 65%,[56] 42%,[60] 60%,[59] 34%,[59]; liver SeGSHpx of 39%.[55]

[l] Numerical superscripts in table and footnotes cite original references.)

155

bioavailabilities estimated by prevention of rat hepatic necrosis and support of tissue SeGSHpx, between prevention of chick pancreatic atrophy and accumulation of tissue Se, and between prevention of exudative diathesis in the chick and accumulation of tissue Se. In general, however, there is relatively poor agreement among estimates of Se bioavailability determined by these several methods. A notable exception is for the high-Se yeast products, which have shown remarkable consistency of bioavailability estimates (e.g., 106% by prevention of exudative diathesis, 116% by accumulation of tissue Se, and 121% by support of SeGSHpx).

Why should different bioassay systems yield different estimates of the bioavailability of Se from the same or similar sources? One reasonable hypothesis is that Se is utilized with different efficiencies by different species and, within a species, for different physiological purposes. Thus, the variation observed in the Se bioavailability as measured by such diverse responses as are included in the bioassays discussed above may evidence the utilization of Se in different ways and with different efficiencies for support of normal liver function in the rat, of normal capillary permeability or exocrine pancreatic function in the chick, or of SeGSHpx activities in various organs and different species. A particular Se-compound (e.g., selenomethionine) or Se-containing food (e.g., wheat) may be very useful in preventing a particular Se- deficiency syndrome (e.g., pancreatic atrophy in the chick), but may be of more limited use in preventing another syndrome (e.g., exudative diathesis in the chick).

It is clear that one determinant of bioavailability of Se is the chemical form in which it is presented, whether in purified form or in practical foods or feedstuffs. The following generalizations can be made: (i) the more reduced (and insoluble) inorganic forms of Se have very low bioavailabilities; (ii) the common selenoamino acids (i.e., selenomethionine, selenocysteine) and Se in most plant materials have reasonably good bioavailabilities (i.e., approaching that of sodium selenite); and (iii) Se in most animal products has low to moderate bioavailability. The variations in bioavailability that have been observed for discrete chemical forms of Se, as well as for Se in particular foods and feedstuffs, indicates that other factors can influence significantly the bioavailability of Se.

VII. FACTORS AFFECTING THE BIOAVAILABILITY OF DIETARY SELENIUM

Several factors associated with Se-containing foods or with other foods in mixed diets can affect the bioavailability of dietary Se by influencing the utilization of ingested Se in either the digestion/absorption, or the metabolism/excretion phases (see Fig 4.1). In principle, factors that increase the enteric absorption of Se and/or increase the metabolism of absorbed Se to the physiologically critical forms (e.g., SeGSHpx) will positively affect Se bioavailability. Alternatively, factors that decrease the enteric absorption of Se and/or increase the metabolism of Se to more readily excreted forms (e.g., the methylated forms) will negatively affect Se bioavailability. Experimental observations in several laboratories confirm that other dietary factors can influence the bioavailability of Se.

Table 4.10[66-90] presents a summary of the studies in which factors affecting the bioavailability of Se have been identified. These findings show that the bioavailability of particular sources of Se can be positively or negatively influenced by alterations in the composition and/or rate of feeding of the diet. Comparisons of diets of very different fundamental composition have shown the significant influence of diet composition on the utilization of supplements of sodium selenite.[45,66,67] Studies by Ganther et al.[66] and by Lane et al.[67] have shown that selenite is better retained and utilized for SeGSHpx by rats fed semi-purified diets in comparison to practical-type (corn-soy based) diets. Combs et al.[47] found that Se from selenite was used with comparable efficiency by chicks fed either a low-Se (0.009 ppm) purified diet based on crystalline amino acids or a low-Se (0.007 ppm) practical diet composed of Se-deficient corn and soybean meal produced in a low-Se region of China. Their results, however, indicated that the practical diet may have contained a factor other than Se that acted to reduce the severity of nutritional pancreatic atrophy in chicks. A complicating factor in these and other types of studies in which biological responses to Se is measured is the potential for change in the rate of food intake between either test and reference treatment groups, or within a treatment series of animals fed different levels of a test Se-source. Zhou and Combs[37] demonstrated that reduction in rate of feed intake of chicks can increase the utilization of ingested Se (from either sodium selenite or selenomethionine) such that both tissue Se levels and SeGSHpx activities are increased and that the incidence of exudative diathesis is decreased. These responses to reduced food intake are probably mediated by metabolic changes resulting from reduced rate of growth, the net result of which is increased Se bioavailability. In view of this finding, bioassays of Se bioavailability should be designed to produce equivalent rates of feed consumption and gain between animals of test and reference groups during the experimental period. Otherwise, estimates of Se bioavailability may be positively biased in treatments in which growth is depressed due to poor feed acceptability, nutritional deficiency or imbalance, etc.

Changes in the macronutrient composition of experimental diets have had variable effects on the biological utilization of Se. Mutanen and

Table 4.10

Dietary Factors Affecting the Biological Utilization of Se

Dietary factor	Species	Effect	Reference
General composition of diet Casein-based semipurified diet *vs.* practical-type diet	Rat	Semipurified diet resulted in increased retention (+36%), blood (+48%) and liver (+14%) levels; but decreased kidney levels (−25%) and respiratory (−48%) and urinary (−12%) losses of Na_2 $^{75}SeO_3$ tracer dose.	(66)
Torula yeast-based semipurified diet *vs.* corn-soybean meal-based practical-type diet	Rat	Semipurified diet supported greater responses[a] of SeGSHpx in small intestine (+30%), liver (+247%) and colon (+253%), and of total Se in liver (+275%) of rats fed low-S diets with graded levels of Na_2SeO_3.	(67)
Amino acid-based purified diet *vs.* corn-soybean meal-based practical-type diet	Chick	Purified diet produced increased frequency and severity of Se-responsive pancreatic atrophy with more rapid onset of signs.	(45)
Level of feed intake	Chick	Feed restriction (25% below ad libitum level) reduced incidence of exudative diathesis over a range of Se intakes, and increased the responses of SeGSHpx in plasma (+428%) and liver (+39%) and of Se in liver (87%) in vitamin E-deficient chicks.	(37)

(continues)

158

Table 4.10 (*Continued*)

Dietary factor	Species	Effect	Reference
Level and type of fat	Chick	Low-fat (4%) diets varied little in enteric absorption of Se (ca. 73%); this was reduced by ca. 5% in high-fat (20%) diets. At the 4% level, plasma SeGSHpx was reduced by diets with 0.5 ppm Se containing butter (−59%), olive oil (−37%), or rapeseed oil (−17%) vs. corn oil or sunflower oil. Increased levels of all fats increased plasma SeGSHpx by 109-333%.	(68)
Level of total protein	Chick	The efficacies[a] of both Na_2SeO_3 and Se-methionine for protection from exudative diathesis in the vitamin E-deficient chick was superior with a 16.9% protein diet vs. a 22.5% protein diet.	(37)
	Rat	Low protein diet (5.3% vs. 13.4%) increased tissue Se levels and SeGSHpx in blood and liver when the diet contained 0.03 ppm Se. No effects due to protein restriction were seen when the diet contained 0.3 ppm Se.	(69, 70)
Level of methionine	Rat	A suboptimal level of methionine (e.g., 0% vs. 0.4%) reduced the efficacy[a] of Se-methionine for SeGSHpx in plasma (−42%), liver (−30 to −44%) and heart (−29%); but affected the response[a] of SeGSHpx to Na_2SeO_3 only in plasma (−42%).	(60)

(*continues*)

159

Table 4.10 *(Continued)*

Dietary factor	Species	Effect	Reference
	Rat	Addition of methionine to a low-methionine, low-Se (0.01 ppm) rice-soy flour-based diet increased Se in whole blood (+14%) and liver (+19%), and increased SeGSHpx in blood (+14%) and liver (+31%). The same supplement to a moderate-Se diet (0.005 ppm) of the same formula produced slight increases in Se in tissues (+3-4%), and increased SeGSHpx only in liver (+12%).	(71)
Level of sulfur	Rat	A diet containing high-S alfalfa produced a 36% increase in liver Se deposition *vs.* a low-S alfalfa diet when the source of dietary Se was Na_2SeO_3.	(33)
	Rat	Sodium sulfate treatment resulted in decreased whole body retention (−14%) and increased urinary excretion (+60%) of Se from Na_2SeO_4; and increased urinary loss of Se from Na_2SeO_3 by only 32%, producing no change in apparent body retention of Se from the latter source.	(72)
	Rat	High levels of S (e.g., in excess of 3600 ppm) reduced the efficacy[a] with which Na_2SeO_3 was used in a *Torula* yeast-based semipurified diet for supporting duodenal SeGSHpx and liver Se; but increased the efficacy of that Se form supporting colonic SeGSHpx with the *Torula* diet or a corn-soy diet and for liver Se on the corn-soy diet.	(67)

(continues)

Table 4.10 (Continued)

Dietary factor	Species	Effect	Reference
	Chick	A diet containing high-S alfalfa reduced the efficacy (−21%) of Se in high-Se alfalfa for protection against exudative diathesis in vitamin E-deficient chicks, but did not affect the utilization of Se from Na_2SeO_3.	(33)
	Lambs	The addition of 0.33% S (as Na_2SO_4) reduced the apparent efficacy of 0.17 ppm Se (as Na_2SeO_3) to reduce muscular dystrophy, as indicated by a 58% increase in serum glutamic-oxaloacetic transaminase to a level equivalent to the Se-deficient control.[b]	(73)
	Lambs/ calves	Addition of Na_2SO_4 to diets of lambs and calves reduced effectiveness of Na_2SeO_3 in preventing white muscle disease.	(88)
	Sheep	Incidence of white muscle disease in sheep was higher after alfalfa was treated with gypsum.	(89)
	Lambs	Neither sulfate nor methionine treatments affect the incidence of white muscle disease in lambs, or the protection effect of organically bound Se (as high-Se alfalfa).	(90)
Level of pyridoxine (vitamin B_6)	Rat	A vitamin B_6-deficient diet reduced the utilization[a] of Se-methionine for SeGSHpx in liver (−45%) and erythrocytes (−71%), and of Na_2SeO_3 for SeGSHpx in erythrocytes (−27%).[c]	(63)

(continues)

161

Table 4.10 *(Continued)*

Dietary factor	Species	Effect	Reference
Level of riboflavin (vitamin B$_2$)	Pig	Severe riboflavin deficiency reduced SeGSHpx in liver (−82%) and muscle (−65%), and Se in liver (−59%) and muscle (−15%).	(74)
Level of vitamin E	Rat	A vitamin E-deficient Torula yeast-based diet (vs. one supplemented with 330 IU vitamin E/kg) reduced the rate of utilization of dietary Na$_2$SeO$_3$ for SeGSHpx in small intestine (−34%) and Se in liver (−48%). A high-level supplement (490 IU/kg) of vitamin E to a corn-soy-based diet (with 11 IU/kg) also increased SeGSHpx in small intestine, colon, and liver, and Se in liver in rats fed the 0.03 ppm Se.	(67)
	Chick	Vitamin E deficiency reduced plasma SeGSHpx (−46%) in chicks fed diets containing 0.04 ppm Se.	(75)
	Chick	Vitamin E deficiency reduced the rate of apparent absorption of a tracer dose of Na$_2$SeO$_3$ from duodenal segments *in situ*.[d]	(76)
	Chick	Incubation with alpha-tocopherol increased the utilization of Na$_2$SeO$_3$ from the medium for increasing SeGSHpx in cultured embryonic duodenal segments.	(77)
	Chick	Se-deficient chicks fed 500 IU all-*rac*-alpha-tocopheryl acetate per kg showed an increased rise (+17%) over vitamin E-deficient controls in hepatic SeGSHpx 12 hrs after a single oral dose of Na$_2$SeO$_3$ (6 µg Se/100 g body weight); vitamin E did not affect this response when high-Se yeast was the source of Se.	(35)

(continues)

162

Table 4.10 *(Continued)*

Dietary factor	Species	Effect	Reference
	Ewe	Oral supplements of alpha-tocopheryl acetate (e.g., 1000 IU/week) reduced the rate of utilization of Na_2SeO_3 for supporting total Se in blood (−12%) and milk (−49%).	(78)
	Lamb	Daily oral supplements of alpha-tocopheryl acetate (110 IU) increased Se contents of tongues (+83%) of lambs fed Na_2SeO_3 (0.4 mg Se/day), but did not affect Se contents of other tissues, Se contents of any tissues in animals given Se-methionine, or apparent absorption of Se from either source.[e,f]	(24)
Level of vitamin A	Chick	A supplement of vitamin A (10^6 IU/kg) increased the protective effect of Na_2SeO_3 against exudative diathesis in vitamin E-deficient chicks, and increased plasma SeGSHpx (+192%) in chicks fed a marginal level (0.06 ppm^g) of Se.	(79)
	Chick	Supplemental all-*trans*-retinyl acetate reduced the incidence of exudative diathesis (ED) in vitamin E-deficient chicks fed a diet with 0.04 ppm Se according to the equation ED(%) = 128 − 18.1 (log vitamin A level, IU/kg); high-level supplements (10^6 IU/kg diet) increased by 18% the rate of utilization of dietary Na_2SeO_3 for protection against ED, and increased the efficacy of a single level (0.04 ppm) of Se from various sources for prevention of ED (Na_2Se; +328%; Na_2SeO_3; +74%; Na_2SeO_4; +62%; cotton seed meal;: +301%; herring meal; +234%; menhaden meal: +499%; fish solubles; increased from nonavailable).	(80)

(continues)

163

Table 4.10 (*Continued*)

Dietary factor	Species	Effect	Reference
	Chick	A high-level supplement (106 IU/kg) of all -*trans*-retinyl acetate reduced the incidence of exudative diathesis (−79%) and increased plasma SeGSHpx (+240%) in chicks fed a vitamin E-deficient diet containing 0.03 ppm Se. The same level of supplemental vitamin A increased the 1-hr uptake of orally administered Se into the blood (+69%), and the rate of absorption of $Na_2{}^{75}SeO_3$ from duodenal segments *in situ* (+23%).	(75)
Level of ascorbic acid	Chick	Supplemental ascorbic acid increased the protective effect of Na2SeO3 against exudative diathesis in vitamin E-deficient chicks, and increased plasma SeGSHpx (+41%) in chicks fed a marginal level (0.06 ppm^g) of Se.	(79)
	Chick	Ascorbic acid produced dose-dependent protection from exudative diathesis and increases in glutathione peroxidase in vitamin E-deficient chicks fed a marginal level (0.04 ppm) of Se, but had no such effects at low levels of dietary Se. Ascorbic acid supplements increased the 1-hr uptake of orally administered Se in the blood (+142%), and the absorption of $Na_2{}^{75}SeO_3$ from duodenal segments *in situ*.	(76)

(continues)

164

Table 4.10 *(Continued)*

Dietary factor	Species	Effect	Reference
	Chick	Ascorbic acid supplemented to the diet at 500 ppm increased the efficacy of a single level (0.04 ppm) of Se from various sources for prevention of exudative diathesis in vitamin E-deficient chicks (Na_2Se, +328%; Na_2SeO_3, +82%; Na_2SeO_4, +137%; cotton seed meal, +234%; herring meal, +234%; menhaden meal,: +698%; fish solubles, increased from nonavailable).	(80)
	Chick	Ascorbic acid (500 ppm in the diet) reduced the incidence of exudative diathesis in vitamin E-deficient chicks fed 0.04 ppm Se as either Na_2SeO_3 or Se-methionine, and increased plasma SeGSHpx by more than two-fold at 14 days of age. Ascorbic acid levels $\geq$ 500 ppm increased the utilization[a] of dietary Na_2SeO_3 for hepatic SeGSHpx (+29 to +82%). *In vitro* incubation of duodenal epithelial cells with 500 ppm ascorbic acid increased the uptake of $^{75}SeO_3^{-2}$ by ca. 46%. *In vitro* incubation of duodenal segments with ascorbic acid increased the uptake of $^{75}SeO_3^{-2}$ and subsequent rise in SeGSHpx.	(77)
	Chick	Se-deficient chicks fed ascorbic acid (1000 ppm) showed enhanced rises in SeGSHpx in plasma (+21%) and liver (+382%) 12 hrs after a single oral dose of Na_2SeO_3 (6 μg Se/100 g body weight); ascorbic acid treatment did not affect the short-term utilization of Se from high Se-yeast.	(35)

(continues)

165

Table 4.10 *(Continued)*

Dietary factor	Species	Effect	Reference
Levels of synthetic antioxidant	Chick	The efficacy of supplemental Na_2SeO_3 in preventing exudative diathesis in vitamin E-deficient chicks was enhanced by dietary supplements of ethoxyquin,[h] DPPD,[i] BHT,[j] or DAH.[k]	(81)
	Chick	Dietary ethoxyquin[h] (500 ppm) increased the protective effect of Na_2SeO_3 against exudative diathesis in vitamin E-deficient chicks and increased plasma SeGSHpx (+97%) in chicks fed a marginal level (0.06 ppm[g]) of Se.	(79)
	Chick	Supplemental ethoxyquin[h] reduced the incidence of exudative diathesis (ED) in vitamin E-deficient chicks fed a marginal level of Se (0.06 pm[g]) according to the equation $ED(\%) = 64.4 - 21.3$ (log dietary ethoxyquin level, ppm). Supplemental ethoxyquin reduced the apparent requirement of the vitamin E-deficient chick for Se for prevention of ED according to the equation log (Se requirement) = −.0011 (dietary ethoxyquin level, ppm) − .7741.	(82)
	Chick	Supplemental ethoxyquin[h] (500 ppm) increased the utilization[a] of dietary Se for protection against exudative diathesis (ED) in the vitamin E-deficient chick. It also increased the efficacy of a single level (0.04 ppm) of supplemental Se from various sources for prevention of ED (Na_2Se, +567%; Na_2SeO_3, +136%; Na_2SeO_4, +225%; cotton seed meal, +434%; herring meal, +167%; menhaden meal, +1055%; fish solubles, increased from nonavailable).	(80)

(continues)

166

Table 4.10 *(Continued)*

Dietary factor	Species	Effect	Reference
	Chick	Se-deficient chicks fed BHT[j] (500 ppm) showed enhanced rises in SeGSHpx in plasma (+98%) and liver (+29%) 12 hrs after a single oral dose of Na_2SeO_3 (6 μg Se/100 g body weight). Similar treatment with Se as high-Se yeast resulted in increases in plasma (+65%) and liver (+10%) due to BHT.[j]	(35)
Level of heavy metals As	Rat	Injected As (2.9 mg/kg body weight, i.p., as Na_2AsO_3) reduced the 10-hr retention of injected $H_2{}^{75}SeO_3$ (2.4 mg Se/kg body weight, i.p.) by 36% in rats fed a casein-based, semi-purified diet and by 20% in rats fed a practical-type diet. As treatment of rats fed both diets, respectively, reduced Se in expired air (−47%, −71%) in blood (−39%, −41%) and in liver (−47%, −41%), increased Se in feces (+270%, +286%) and kidney (+223%, +84%), but did not affect urinary Se concentration.	(66)
Cd	Rat	Injected Cd (2.5 mg/kg body weight, i.p., as $CdCl_2$) increased the 10-hr retention of injected $H_2{}^{75}SeO_3$ (2.4 mg Se/kg body weight, i.p.) by 29% in rats fed a casein-based semi-purified diet, and by 48% in rats fed a practical-type diet. Cd treatment of rats fed both diets, respectively, reduced Se in expired air (−93%, −84%), feces (−34%, −23%), urine (−56%, −39%) and increased Se in blood (+80%, +116%) and liver (+41%, +47%).	(96)

(continues)

167

Table 4.10 (*Continued*)

Dietary factor	Species	Effect	Reference
Hg	Rat	Injections of $HgCl_2$ (10 or 20 μmol Hg/kg body weight) to pregnant rats increased the retention of a tracer dose of $Na_2{}^{75}SeO_3$ in maternal blood (+286% or +382%) and liver (+38% or +34%), but decreased ^{75}Se in fetal blood (-47% or -57%) and liver (-64% or -76%).	(83)

[a]Rates of responses were were calculated from slope (m) ratios using the general equation: dependent variable = m [log (diet Se level)] + constant.

[b]However, Smith et al.[85] found supplemental S not to affect the Se status of steers, as indicated by blood Se level.

[c]However, Sunde et al.[84] and Gu et al.[71] found vitamin B_6 deficiency not to affect the utilization of Se (fed as either Na_2SeO_3, Se-methionine or Se-cysteine) for supporting hepatic SeGSHpx in rats.

[d]However, Gu et al.[71] found that altered vitamin E status of rats did not affect the Se contents of blood, liver or kidney, or SeGSHpx in blood or liver in animals fed a low-Se (0.01 ppm Se) or moderate-Se (0.055 ppm) diet.

[e]However, Paulsen et al.[78] found an oral supplement (1000 IU/wk) of vitamin E not to affect blood Se levels in lambs.

[f]However, Jensen et al.[86] found dietary supplements of vitamin E (50 IU/kg) not to affect the utilization of Se as indicated by a spot test for plasma SeGSHpx in pigs.

[g]Includes 0.02 ppm Se inherent in the basal diet.

[h]1,2-Dihydro-6-ethoxy-2,54-trimethylquinoline.

[i]N,N'-Diphenyl-p-phenylenediamine.

[j]2,6-Di-tert-butyl-p-cresol.

[k]2,5-bis(1,1-Dimethylpropyl) hydroquinone.

Mykkanen[68] found that while the enteric absorption of Se in the chick is affected only slightly by dietary fat level (4% vs. 20%), the type and level of dietary fat greatly influenced the SeGSHpx response in plasma (corn oil or sunflower seed oil producing the greatest responses at the 4% level, and fats of any type increasing the response at the 20% level). Studies by Zhou and Combs,[37] Zhou et al.[69] and Sun et al.[70] have shown that chicks or rats fed diets with reduced protein (e.g., 25% below the level required for optimal growth) each show improved utilization of dietary Se as evidenced by increased tissue Se and SeGSHpx and, in chicks, by decreased incidence of exudative diathesis. The basis of the effect of reduced protein intake probably involves the effect of reduced growth rate as discussed previously. It may also involve correlated reductions in protein-associated factors (e.g., methionine) in the diet. Suboptimal levels of the sulfur-containing amino acid methionine have been shown to reduce the utilization of Se from selenomethionine[60] or Se inherent in soybean meal and/or rice flour[71] for the support of tissue SeGSHpx in the rat. High levels of sulfur (in the form of high-S alfalfa or sodium sulfite), however, have been shown to decrease the utilization of Se for tissue SeGSHpx in the rat[67] and for prevention of exudative diathesis in the chick[33] and skeletal myopathies in the lamb.[73] Mathias et al.[33] reported that a diet containing high-S alfalfa increased hepatic Se levels in rats; however, Ganther and Bauman[72] showed that sodium sulfate treatment significantly reduced whole body retention of Se by increasing its urinary excretion in the same species.

The micronutrient content of the diet can also significantly affect the biological utilization of Se. Yasumoto et al.[63] reported that the utilization of Se for supporting SeGSHpx by the rat was reduced by a dietary deficiency of pyridoxine (vitamin B6). Brady et al.[74] found that tissue levels of both SeGSHpx and Se were reduced in riboflavin-deficient baby pigs vs. pair-fed controls. Several studies have shown that vitamin E nutriture can affect the biological utilization of Se as measured by the responses of SeGSHpx in rats[67] and chicks[35,75] and of tissue Se levels of sheep.[24,78] Vitamin E appears to increase the utilization of Se by promoting its enteric absorption,[76] although recent studies by Cupp,[77] which employed the cultured embryonic chick duodenum, have indicated that vitamin E increases the post-absorptive incorporation of Se into SeGSHpx, perhaps thus causing a "sink" for intracellular Se, which thus drives the enteric absorption of the element by passive diffusion. Similar effects on the utilization of Se have been demonstrated for high-level supplements of vitamin A[77,79,80] and ascorbic acid.[35,76,77,79,80] Extensive studies by Cupp[77] using the isolated chick duodenum in organ culture have demonstrated that, like vitamin E, ascorbic acid treatment increases the post-absorptive incorporation of Se into SeGSHpx.

Cupp's[77] data suggested that the "sink" resulting from this incorporation drove the enteric absorption of Se, as experiments using isolated dissociated enterocytes showed that ascorbic acid did not have any direct effects on the passive uptake of Se. Cupp[77] proposed that, because structurally related compounds with antioxidant activities (e.g., ascorbic acid, all-*rac*-alpha-tocopherol, propyl gallate) each had similar effects on the utilization of Se, this effect was one due to general antioxidant activity; her data suggested that antioxidants that increase intracellular ratios of reduced : oxidized glutathione (i.e., GSH : GSSG) increase the intracellular utilization of Se.

If Cupp's hypothesis is true, then other antioxidants may be able to affect Se bioavailability. In fact, several studies[35,79-82] have demonstrated that the utilization of Se by the chick can be increased by dietary treatment with a variety of synthetic antioxidants including ethoxyquin (1,2-Dihydro-6-ethoxy-2,3,4-trimethylquinoline), DPPD (N,N'-diphenyl-*p*-phenyldiamine), BHT (2,6-di-*tert*-butyl-*p*-cresol), and DPH [2,5—Bis(1,1—dimethylpropyl)hydroquinone]. Combs[82] developed prediction equations that described the relationship of the dietary requirement of the chick for Se as a function of the amount of ethoxyquin supplemented to the diet.

The "antioxidant effect" on the utilization of dietary Se has been difficult to understand in view of the potential for such reducing agents as ascorbic acid to reduce biologically active forms of Se (e.g., selenite and selenate) to elemental Se, which has little or no biological activity. Certainly, if mixed together prior to addition to the diet, the amounts of ascorbic acid (500-2000 mg/kg diet) are sufficient to reduce completely the Se usually added to the diet (ca. 20-100 +g/kg diet), thus rendering that Se completely unavailable.[87] That this reduction and consequent loss of biological activity does not occur when each compound is added separately either to mixed solid diets[35,76,77,79,80] or to aqueous organ culture media[77] indicates that the local concentrations of the potential reactants in these circumstances are insufficient to effect the reduction of a significant amount of Se. Thus, while antioxidants may be expected to reduce the bioavailability of Se if added in concentrated solutions, experience shows that this effect is not significant in mixed diets in which stimulation of Se bioavailability by the "antioxidant effect" is observed. The finding of Choe et al.[91] that ascorbic acid reduces the urinary excretion of Se in humans indicates that the antioxidant effect may be important in human nutrition.

Heavy metals have been shown to affect the biological utilization of dietary Se. The retention of Se has been found to be reduced by treatment with As,[66] which increased the apparent enterohepatic circulation of Se; Se retention is increased by treatment with Cd[66] or Hg.[83] Morris et al.[92] found that dietary phytate can increase the fecal excretion of Se in young men, presumably reducing Se bioavailability to them.

VIII. SUMMARY OF FACTORS AFFECTING THE
BIOAVAILABILITY OF SELENIUM

Many factors can affect the biological utilization of Se and, hence, the estimation of Se bioavailability. These are summarized in Table 4.11. At the present time, there are abundant data supporting the roles of the chemical form of Se as a primary determinant of its biological utilization; and, in spite of the fairly large body of analytical data for the Se contents of foods and feedstuffs (see Chapter 3), there remains a paucity of information concerning the chemical forms in which that Se is present. Thus, much

Table 4.11

Summary of Factors Affecting the Bioavailability of Dietary Se

Bioavailability varies with the chemical form of Se in Se compounds
    Highly available forms
        Selenate
        Seleno-amino acids
    Poorly available forms
        Reduced forms of Se

Foods/feedstuffs vary with respect to Se bioavailability
    Highly available sources
        High-Se yeast
        Wheat
        Alfalfa
    Moderately available sources
        Most plant materials
    Poorly available sources
        Most meat and fish products
        Soybean
Other dietary factors can affect Se bioavailability
    Availability enhancers
        Restricted food intake
        Methionine/protein
        Vitamin E
        Vitamin A (high levels)
        Ascorbic acid
        Synthetic antioxidants
    Availability decreasers
        Heavy metals
        Pyridoxine (vitamin B_6) deficiency
        Riboflavin (vitamin B_2) deficiency
        Vitamin E deficiency
        Methionine deficiency
        Sulfur

of the current knowledge of the bioavailabilities of discrete Se-compounds and the factors affecting the utilization of Se from those compounds is applicable more to situations wherein they are used as nutritional supplements rather than to situations of feeding practical plant- and/or animal-derived materials as sources of Se.

Studies with practical foods and feedstuffs have indicated that, despite variations between bioassay methods, species, etc., some materials (e.g., high-Se yeasts, wheat, alfalfa) are generally highly available sources of Se, while Se in most other plant- derived foods and feedstuffs is generally of moderate bioavailability, and Se in materials of animal origin is generally poorly available. Despite these general differences, other dietary factors can have overwhelming significance in affecting Se bioavailability such that materials that otherwise are relatively poorly utilized sources of Se (e.g., fish meals) can have bioavailability exceeding that of sodium selenite[80] when fed with them. Present understanding of the dietary and, perhaps, physiological factors that can determine the utilization of dietary Se by animals and people is not complete enough to enable the description of their individual and interactive effects in mathematical terms. This achievement will be necessary in order to predict with accuracy the biological value of Se in practical diets, or the therapeutic value of Se supplements in medical and and/or veterinary practice, or to evaluate fairly the Se status of food supplies or of particular food or feed items.

REFERENCES

1. Schwarz, K., and Foltz, C. M., Selenium as an integral part of Factor 3 against dietary necrotic liver degeneration, J. Am. Chem. Soc. 79, 3292, 1957.
2. Patterson, E. L., Milstrey, H., and Stokstad, E. L. R., Effect of selenium in preventing exudative diathesis in chicks, Proc. Soc. Exp. Biol. Med., 95, 617, 1957.
3. Schwarz, K., Bieri, J. G., Briggs, G. M., and Scott, M. L., Prevention of exudative diathesis in chicks by Factor 3 and selenium, Proc. Soc. Exp. Biol. Med., 95, 621, 1957.
4. Schwarz, K. and Foltz, C. M., Factor 3 activity of selenium compounds, J. Biol. Chem., 233, 245, 1958.
5. Schwarz, K. and Fredga, A., Biological potency of organic selenium compounds. Aliphatic monoseleno- and diseleno-dicarboxylic acids, J. Biol. Chem, 244, 2103, 1969.
6. Schwarz, K. and Fredga, A., Biological potency of organic selenium compounds. II. Aliphatic selena-carboxylic acids and acid amides, Bioinorg. Chem., 2, 47, 1972.
7. Schwarz, K., and Fredga, A., Biological potency of organic selenium compounds. III. Phenyl-, benzyl-, and phenylethylseleno-carboxylic acids, and related compounds, Bioinorg. Chem., 2, 171, 1972.
8. Scott, M. L., and Cantor, H. A., Selenium availability in feedstuffs, Proc., Cornell Nutr. Conf., 66, 1972..
9. Sirichakwal, P. P., Young, V. R., and Janghorbani, M., Absorption and urine excretion of selenium from doubly labeled eggs, in *Proceedings of the Third International*

Symposium on Selenium in Biology and Medicine, Combs, G. F., Jr., Spallholz, J. E., Levander, O. A., and Oldfield, J. E., eds., Avi Publ. Co., Westport, Conn., 1986.

10. Swanson, C. A., Reamer, D. C., Veillon, C., King, J. C., and Levander, O. A., Quantitative and qualitative aspects of selenium utilization in pregnant and nonpregnant women: an application of stable isotope methodology, Amer. J. Clin. Nutr., 38, 169, 1983.

11. Christensen, M. J., Janghorbani, M., Steinke, F. H., Istfan, N., and Young, V. R., Simultaneous determination of absorption of selenium from poultry meat and selenite in young men: application of a triple stable-isotope method, Br. J. Nutr., 50, 43, 1980.

12. Heinrich, H. C., Gabbe, E. E., Bartels, H., Oppitz, K. H., Bender-Gotze, C., and Pfau, A. A., Bioavailability of food iron-(^{59}Fe), vitamin B_{12}-(^{60}Co), and protein-bound selenomethionine-(^{75}Se) in pancreatic exocrine insufficiency due to cystic fibrosis, Klin. Wochenschr., 55, 595, 1977.

13. Levander, O. A., Sutherland, B., Morris, V. C., and King, J. C., Selenium balance in young men during selenium depletion and repletion, Amer. J. Clin. Nutr. 34, 2662, 1981.

14. Cary, E. E., Allaway, W. H., and Miller, M., Utilization of different forms of dietary selenium, J. Anim. Sci., 36, 285, 1973.

15. Richold, M., Robinson, M. F., and Stewart, R. D. H., Metabolic studies in rats of ^{75}Se incorporated *in vivo* into fish muscle, Br. J. Nutr., 38, 19, 1977.

16. Thomson, C. D., Stewart, R. D. H., and Robinson, M. F., Metabolic studies in rats of (^{75}Se) selenomethionine and of ^{75}Se incorporated *in vivo* into rat kidney, Br. J. Nutr., 33, 45, 1975.

17. Mason, A. C., and Weaver, C. M., Selenium absorption from extrinsically and intrinsically labeled soy products, in *Proceedings of the Third International Symposium on Selenium in Biology and Medicin* Combs, G. F., Jr., Spallholz, J. E., Levander, O. A., and Oldfield, J. E., eds., Avi Publ. Co., Westport, Conn., 1986.

18. Latshaw, J. D., and Osman, M., Distribution of selenium in eggwhite and yolk after feeding natural and synthetic selenium compounds, Poultry Sci., 54, 1244, 1975.

19. Thomson, C. D., and Stewart, D. R. H., The metabolism of (^{75}Se) selenite in young women, Br. J. Nutr., 32, 47, 1974.

20. Stewart, R. D. H., Griffiths, N. M., Thomson, C. D., and Robinson, M. F., Quantitative selenium metabolism in normal New Zealand women, Br. J. Nutr., 40, 45, 1978.

21. Thomson, C. D., and Stewart, R. D. H., Metabolic studies of (^{75}Se) selenomethionine and (^{75}Se) selenite in the rat, Br. J. Nutr., 30, 139, 1973.

22. Amiot, J., Janghorbani, M., and Young, V. R., Absorption and retention of ^{75}SeO$_3$ in relation to soybean protein intake in the rat, Nutr. Res., 2, 491, 1982.

23. Griffiths, N. M., Stewart, R. D. H., and Robinson, M. F., The metabolism of (^{75}Se) selenomethionine in four women, Br. J. Nutr., 35, 373, 1975.

24. Ehlig, C. F., Hogue, D. E., Allaway, W. H., and Hamm, D. J., Fate of selenium from selenite or selenomethionine, with or without vitamin E, in lambs, J. Nutr., 92, 121, 1967.

25. Reasbeck, P. G., Barbezat, G. O., Robinson, M. F., and Thomson, C. D., Direct measurement of selenium absorption *in vivo*: triple-lumen gut perfusion in the conscious dog, Proc. N. Zealand Workshop Trace Elements, Univ. Otago, Dunedin, N.Z., 20, 1981.

26. Thomson, C. D., Robinson, B. A., Stewart, R. D. H., and Robinson, M. F., Metabolic studies of (^{75}Se) selenocystine and (^{75}Se) selenomethionine in the rat, Br. J. Nutr., 34, 501, 1975.

27. Levander, O. A., Considerations in the design of selenium bioavailability studies, Federation Proc., 42, 1721, 1983.

28. Levander, O. A., Assessing the bioavailability of selenium in foods, in *Proceedings of the Third International Symposium on Selenium in Biology and Medicine*, Combs, G. F., Jr., Spallholz, J. E., Levander, O. A., and Oldfield, J. E., eds., Avi Publ. Co., Westport, Conn., 1986.

29. Schwarz, K., Porter, L. A., and Fredga, A., Biological potency of organic selenium compounds. IV. Straight-chain dialkylmono- and diselenides, Bioinorg. Chem., 3, 145,1974.

30. Schwarz, K., and Fredga, A., Biological potency of organic selenium compounds. V. Diselenides of alcohols and amines, and some selenium-containing ketones, Bioinorg. Chem., 3, 153, 1974.

31. Schwarz, K., Foltz, C. M., and Bergson, G., Factor 3 and 6-selenoctic acid, Acta Chem. Scand., 12, 1330, 1958.

32. Cantor, A. H., Scott, M. L., and Noguchi, T., Biological availability of selenium in feedstuffs and selenium compounds for prevention of exudative diathesis in chicks, J. Nutr., 105, 96, 1975.

33. Mathias, M. M., Allaway, W. H., Hogue, D. E., Marion, M. V., and Gardner, R. W., Value of selenium in alfalfa for the prevention of selenium deficiencies in chicks and rats, J. Nutr., 86, 213, 1965.

34. Combs, G. F., Jr., Barrows, S. A., and Swader, F. N., Biologic availability of selenium in corn grain produced on soil amended with flyash, Agr. Food Chem., 28, 406, 1980.

35. Combs, G. F., Jr., Su, Q., and Wu, K. Q., Use of the short-term glutathione peroxidase response in selenium-deficient chicks for assessment of bioavailability of dietary selenium, Federation Proc., 43, 473 (abstract #1100), 1984.

36. Combs, G. F., Jr., Mandisodza, K. T., Gutenmann, W. H., and Lisk, D. J., Utilization of selenium in flyash and in white sweet clover grown on flyash by the chick, Agr. Food Chem., 29, 149, 1981.

37. Zhou, Y. P., and Combs, G. F., Jr., Effects of dietary protein level and level of feed intake on the apparent bioavailability of selenium for the chick, Poultry Sci. 63, 294, 1984.

38. Osman, M., and Latshaw, J. F., Biological potency of selenium from sodium selenite, selenomethionine and selenocystine in the chick, Poultry Sci., 55, 987, 1976.

39. Cantor, A. H., Langevin, M. L., Noguchi, T., and Scott, M. L., Efficacy of selenium in selenium compounds and feedstuffs for prevention of pancreatic fibrosis in chicks, J. Nutr., 105, 106, 1975.

40. Thompson, J. N., and Scott, M. L., Impaired lipid and vitamin E absorption related to atrophy of the pancreas in selenium-deficient chick, J. Nutr., 100, 797, 1970.

41. Gries, C. L., and Scott, M. L., Pathology of selenium deficiency in the chick, J. Nutr., 102, 1287, 1972.

42. Noguchi, T., Langevin, M. L., Combs, G. F., Jr., and Scott, M. L., Biochemical and histochemical studies of the selenium-deficient pancreas in chicks, J. Nutr., 103, 444, 1973.

43. Bunk, M. J., and Combs, G. F., Jr., Relationship of selenium-dependent glutathione peroxidase activity and nutritional pancreatic atrophy in selenium-deficient chicks, J.Nutr., 111, 1611, 1981.

44. Whitacre, M. E., and Combs, G. F., Jr., Selenium and mitochondrial integrity in the pancreas of the chick, J. Nutr., 113, 1972, 1983.

45. Combs, G. F., Jr., Liu, C. H., Lu, Z. H., and Su, Q., Uncomplicated selenium deficiency produced in chicks fed a corn-soy based diet, J. Nutr., 114, 964, 1984.

46. Cantor, A. H., Moorhead, P. D., and Musser, M. A., Comparative effects of sodium selenite and selenomethionine upon nutritional muscular dystrophy, selenium- dependent

glutathione peroxidase, and tissue selenium concentration of turkey poults, Poultry Sci., 61, 478, 1982.

47. Combs, G. F., Jr., Liu, C. H., Su, Q., and Lu, Z. H., unpublished research, 1984.

48. Thomson, C. D., Robinson, M. F., Campbell, D. R., and Rea, H. M., Effect of prolonged supplementation with daily supplements of selenomethionine and sodium selenite on glutathione peroxidase activity in blood of New Zealand residents, Am. J. Clin. Nutr., 36, 24, 1982.

49. Behne, D., and Wolters, W., Distribution of selenium and glutathione peroxidase in the rat, J. Nutr., 113, 456, 1983.

50. Miller, D., Soares, J. H., Jr., Baversfeld, P., Jr., and Cuppett, S. L., Comparative selenium retention by chicks fed sodium selenite, selenomethionine, fish meal and fish solubles, Poultry Sci., 51, 1669, 1972.

51. Latshaw, J. D., and Biggert, M. D., Incorporation of selenium into egg proteins after feeding selenomethionine or sodium selenite, Poultry Sci., 60, 1309, 1981.

52. Cantor, A. H., Sutton, C. D., and Johnson, T. H., Biological availability of selenodicysteine in chicks, Poultry Sci., 62, 2429, 1983.

53. Vinson, J. A., and Bose, P., Relative bioavailability of inorganic and natural selenium, in *Proceedings of the Third International Symposium on Selenium in Biology and Medicine*, Combs, G. F., Jr., Spallholz, J. E., Levander, O. A., and Oldfield, J. E., eds., Avi Publ. Co., Westport, Conn., 1986.

54. Alexander, A. R., Whanger, P. D., and Miller, L. T., Bioavailability to rats of selenium in various tuna and wheat products, J. Nutr., 113, 196, 1983.

55. Douglass, J. S., Morris, V. C., Soares, J. H., and Levander, O. A., Nutritional availability to rats of selenium in tuna, beef kidney and wheat, J. Nutr., 111, 2180, 1981.

56. Cantor, A. H., and Tarino, J. Z., Comparative effects of inorganic and organic dietary sources of selenium on selenium levels and selenium-dependent glutathione peroxidase activity in blood of young turkeys, J. Nutr., 112, 2187, 1982.

57. Levander, O. A., Alfthan, G., Arvilommi, H., Gref, C. G., Huttunen, J. K., Kataja, M., Koivistoinen, P., and Pikkarainen, J., Bioavailability of selenium to Finnish men as assesed by platelet glutathione peroxidase activity and other blood parameters, Am. J. Clin. Nutr., 37, 887, 1983.

58. Rotruck, J. T., Pope, A. L., Ganther, H. E., Swanson, A. D., Hafeman, D. G., and Hoekstra, W. G., Selenium: biochemical role as a component of glutathione peroxidase, Science, 179, 588, 1973.

59. Gabrielsen, B. O., and Opstvedt, J., Availability of selenium in fish meal in comparison with soybean meal, corn gluten meal and selenomethionine relative to selenium in sodium selenite for restoring glutathione peroxidase activity in selenium-depleted chicks, J. Nutr., 110, 1096, 1980.

60. Sunde, R. A., Gutzke, G. E., and Hoekstra, W. G., Effect of dietary methionine on the biopotency of selenite and selenomethionine in the rat, J. Nutr., 111, 76, 1981.

61. Gabrielsen, B. O., and Opstrvedt, J., A biological assay for determination of availability of selenium for restoring blood plasma glutathione peroxidase activity in selenium-depleted chicks, J. Nutr., 110, 1089, 1980.

62. Karle, J. A., Kull, F. J., and Shrift, A., Uptake of selenium-75 by PHA-stimulated lymphocytes. Effect on glutathione peroxidase, Biol. Tr. Elem. Res., 5, 17, 1983.

63. Yasumoto, K., Iwami, K., and Yoshida, M., Vitamin B_6 dependence of selenomethionine and selenite utilization for glutathione peroxidase in the rat, J. Nutr., 109, 760, 1979.

64. Pierce, S., and Tappel, A. L., Effects of selenite and selenomethionine on glutathione peroxidase in the rat, J. Nutr., 107, 475, 1977.

65. Litov, R. E., Evaluating the bioavailability of selenium from nutritional formulas for

enteral use, in *Proceedings of the Third International Symposium on Selenium in Biology and Medicine*, Combs, G. F., Jr., Spallholz, J. E., Levander, O. A., and Oldfield, J. E., eds., Avi Publ. Co., Westport, Conn., 1986.

66. Ganther, H. E., and Bauman, C. A., Selenium metabolism. I. Effects of diet, arsenic and cadmium, J. Nutr., 77, 210, 1962.

67. Lane, H. W., Shirley, R. L., and Cerda, J. J., Glutathione peroxidase activity in intestinal and liver tissues of rats fed various levels of selenium, sulfur and alpha- tocopherol, J. Nutr., 109, 444, 1979.

68. Mutanen, M. L., and Mykkanen, H. M., Effect of dietary fat on plasma glutathione peroxidase levels and intestinal absorption of ^{75}Se-labeled sodium selenite in chicks, J. Nutr., 114, 829, 1984.

69. Zhou, R., Sun, S., Zhai, F., Man, R., Guo, S., Wang, H., and Yang, G., Effect of dietary protein level on the availability of selenium. I. Effect of dietary protein level on the selenium contents and glutathione peroxidase activities of blood and tissues of rats, Yingyang Xuebao, 5, 137, 1983.

70. Sun, S., Zhou, R., Gu, L., Man, R., Guo, S., Wang, H., and Yang, G., Effect of dietary protein level on the availability of selenium. II. A study on the effect of dietary protein level on the selenium contents and glutathione peroxidase activities in blood and tissues of rats, Yingyang Xuebao, 5, 145, 1983.

71. Gu, L., Zhou, R., Yin, S., and Yang, Q., Influence of dietary constituents on the bioavailability of selenium, in *Proceedings of the Third International Symposium on Selenium in Biology and Medicine*, Combs, G. F., Jr., Spallholz, J. E., Levander, O. A., and Oldfield, J. E., eds., Avi Publ. Co., Westport, Conn., 1986.

72. Ganther, H. E., and Bauman, C. A., Selenium metabolism. II. Modifying effects of sulfate, J. Nutr., 77, 408, 1962.

73. Hintz, H. F., and Hogue, D. E., Effect of selenium, sulfur and sulfur amino acids on nutritional muscular dystrophy in the lamb, J. Nutr., 82, 495, 1964.

74. Brady, P. S., Brady, L. J., Parsons, M. J., Ullrey, D. E., and Miller, E. R., Effects of riboflavin deficiency on growth and glutathione peroxidase system enzymes on the baby pig, J. Nutr., 109, 1615, 1979.

75. Combs, G. F., Jr., Differential effects of high dietary levels of vitamin A on the vitamin E-selenium nutrition of young and adult chickens, J. Nutr., 106, 967, 1976.

76. Combs, G. F., Jr., and Pesti, G. M., Influence of ascorbic acid on selenium nutrition in the chick, J. Nutr., 106, 958, 1970.

77. Cupp, M. S., Studies of the nutritional-biochemical interactions of selenium and ascorbic acid in the chick, PhD Thesis, Cornell Univ., Ithaca, New York, 1984.

78. Paulsen, G. D., Broderick, G. A., Baumann, C. A., and Pope, A. L., Effect of feeding sheep selenium-fortified trace mineralized salt: effect of tocopherol, J. An. Sci., 27, 195, 1968.

79. Combs, G. F., Jr., and Scott, M. L., Antioxidant effects on selenium and vitamin E function in the chick, J. Nutr., 104, 1297, 1974.

80. Combs, G. F., Jr., Influences of vitamin A and other reducing compounds on the selenium-vitamin E nutrition of the chicken, Proc. Distillers Feed Res. Conf., 31, 40, 1976.

81. Bieri, J. G., Synergistic effects between antioxidants and selenium or vitamin E, Biochem. Pharmacol., 13, 1465, 1964.

82. Combs, G. F., Jr., Influence of ethoxyquin on the utilization of selenium by the chick, Poultry Sci., 57, 210, 1978.

83. Parizek, J., Ostadalova, I., Kalouskova, J., Babicky, A., Pavlik, L., and Bibr, B., Effect of mercuric compounds on the maternal transmission of selenium in the pregnant and lactating rat, J. Reprod. Fert., 25, 157, 1971.

84. Sunde, R. A., Sonnenburg, W.K., Gutzke, G. E., and Hoekstra, W. G., Biopotency of selenium for glutathione peroxidase synthesis, in *Trace Element Metabolism in Man and Animals*, Gawthorne, J. M., Howell, J. M., and White, C. L., eds., Springer- Verlag, New York, 1982.

85. Smith, S. I., Boling, J. A., Gay, N., and Cantor, A. H., Selenium and sulfur supplementation to steers grazing tall fescue, Biol. Trace Elements Res., 6, 347, 1984.

86. Jensen, P. T., Danielsen, V., and Nielsen, H. E., Glutathione peroxidase activity and erythrocyte lipid peroxidation as indices of selenium and vitamin E status in young pigs, Acta Vet. Scand., 20, 92, 1979.

87. Combs, G. F., Jr., unpublished research, 1973.

88. Muth, O. H., Schubert, J. R., and Oldfield, J. E., White muscle disease (myopathy) in lambs and calves. VII. Etiology and prophylaxis. Am. J. Vet. Res., 22, 466, 1961.

89. Schubert, J. R., Muth, O. H., Oldfield, J. E., and Remment, L. F., Experimental results with selenium in white muscle disease of lambs and calves. Federation Proc., 20, 689, 1961.

90. Whanger, P. D., Muth, O. W., Oldfield, J. E., and Weswig, P. H., Influence of sulfur on incidence of white muscle disease in lambs, J. Nutr., 97, 553, 1969.

91. Choe, M., Kies, C., and Fox, H. M., Selenium utilization of human adults as affected by ascorbic acid and selected mineral interactions, Federation Proc., 44, 1510 (abstract #6431), 1985.

92. Morris, V. C., Turnland, J. R., King, J. C., and Levander, O. A., Effect of sodiumphytate and alpha-cellulose on selenium (Se) balance in young men, Federation Proc., 44, 1670 (abstract #7367), 1985.

5

ABSORPTION, EXCRETION, AND METABOLISM OF SELENIUM

I. ABSORPTION AND TRANSFER

A. Intestinal Absorption of Selenium

The manner in which Se is absorbed by the intestine appears to depend on its form. McConnell and Cho,[1] using everted intestinal sacs of hamsters, showed that L-selenomethionine is transported against a gradient from the mucosal to the serosal side and also that its transport is inhibited by L-methionine. This, plus the fact that the transport rate of DL-selenomethionine was about half that of L-selenomethionine, suggests that L-selenomethionine is transported by the same carrier as L-methionine. Spencer and Blau[2] also showed that ^{35}S-methionine and ^{75}Se-selenomethionine accumulate identically on the serosal side of everted hamster intestinal sacs. Furthermore, chromatographic studies of the mucosal and serosal fluids showed only one gamma-emitting peak, suggesting that ^{75}Se-selenomethionine is not degraded in transport.

Selenite, on the other hand, showed no net exchange across the intestinal mucosa when concentrations were the same on both sides.[1] More recent studies with *in situ* intestinal loops, everted gut sacs, and isolated intestinal epithelial cells of rats,[3] however, suggest that intestinal cells can concentrate Se from selenite and that reduced glutathione (GSH) in the gut lumen plays a role in selenite absorption. Pre-treatment of animals with the GSH-depleting agent diethylmaleate reduced the rate of disappearance of ^{75}Se-selenite from the lumenal fluid of isolated loops, and addition of the agent to the incubation medium for intestinal cells reduced the accumulation of ^{75}Se from selenite in the cells. Addition of GSH enhanced the transfer. Furthermore, inhibition of gamma-glutamyl transferase reduced accumulation of ^{75}Se in cells. The authors proposed that GSH, presented to the intestinal lumen in bile,[4,5] combines with Se to form selenodiglutathione (GSSeSG) in a nonenzymic reaction elucidated by Ganther.[6] Selenodiglutathione may serve as a substrate for gamma-glutamyltransferase and thereby be transported across the cellular membranes. Unfortunately, these authors based the conclusion, that their isolated cells concentrated Se, upon estimates of concentrations and volumes, which are subject to large error. The evidence would be more convincing had they demonstrated net transfer of ^{75}Se in an experiment similar to McConnell's[1] with equal concentrations of selenite on both sides of the mucosa of an everted gut sac, with GSH on the mucosal side.

In an *in vivo* experiment using triple lumen gut perfusion in dogs, Reasbeck et al.[7] reported that the amount of selenomethionine absorbed was nearly twice that of selenocystine and about 4 times that of selenite during a 2-hour test period. This is consistent with the hypothesis that amino acid-bound Se is absorbed through specific amino acid active transport mechanisms. However, no information was given about the intestinal contents of the dogs and whether bile was present. If GSH from bile is important for the absorption of selenite, the comparison reported may underestimate the relative availability of selenite.

The enteric absorption of selenate and selenite were investigated by Wolffram et al.[98] using *in vivo* gut perfusion in rats. They found the greatest site of selenate absorption to be the ileum where it was absorbed by a carrier-mediated process. The absorption mechanism was not inhibited by selenite, but one would expect it to be inhibited by sulfate.

Without explaining mechanisms of absorption, many studies have quantified the amount of absorption of various forms of Se. Using three independent methods of calculating intestinal absorption in rats, Thomson and Stewart[8] found absorption of Se from ^{75}Se-selenite to average 91-93% and that from ^{75}Se-selenomethionine to be 95-97%. (Their methods allowed them to correct for Se absorbed and returned to the intestine. Hence, their estimates are of total absorption.) A subsequent publication from the same laboratory[9] reported the average intestinal absorption of an oral dose of ^{75}Se-selenomethionine to be 86% and that of ^{75}Se-selenocystine to be 81%. The same research group also labeled rabbit kidney[10] and fish muscle[11] with ^{75}Se and fed homogenates of the labeled tissues to rats. Absorption of Se from kidneys of rabbits fed ^{75}Se-selenomethionine was 87%, compared to 91% from ^{75}Se-selenomethionine mixed with unlabeled kidney homogenate. The Se from fish labeled by feeding ^{75}Se-selenomethionine was less well absorbed, about 74%, although absorption of ^{75}Se-selenomethionine in the presence of unlabeled fish homogenate was 96%.

Selenite appears to be less well absorbed by humans than by rats. In three young women given ^{75}Se-selenite, absorption was 70, 64, and 44% of the oral dose.[12] Using [74]Se, a stable isotope, Janghorbani et al.[13] measured net absorption in four male subjects with two different doses of selenite. These measurements did not include labeled Se that was absorbed into the blood and then returned to the intestine. With the smaller doses net absorption ranged from 55 to 99% (ave. ± SD: 76 ± 9%). With twice the dose, average net absorption was reduced to 68 ± 6%. However, the difference in these averages was due primarily to a change in one subject and does not provide sufficient evidence to conclude that percentage absorption is dose-dependent.

The Se status of an animal appears to have little or no effect on the intestinal absorption of selenite. Brown et al.[14] fed rats different levels of Se (0, 0.5, 4 ppm supplemented to a low-Se Torula yeast-based diet) as Na_2SeO_3 for 33 days before administering $Na_2{}^{75}SeO_3$, either by stomach tube or intraperitoneal injection. Absorption throughout the dosage range was 95-100% of the dose. This indicates the absence of a regulatory mechanism for absorption of selenite.

Although the Se status of an animal may not affect Se absorption,[14] status with respect to other elements may. Mykkanen and Humaloja[15] reported that feeding chickens 1000 ppm Pb for 3 weeks prior to measurement of absorption of ^{75}Se-selenite caused a reduction in transfer of selenite into the body by increasing retention in intestinal tissue. Increasing the dietary Se alleviated the inhibition. The authors proposed that long-term exposure to Pb may cause synthesis of proteins that can bind Se and that these binding sites may become saturated as Se intake is increased.

The type (i.e., saturated or unsaturated) or amount of dietary fat does not appear to affect the absorption of selenite.[16]

Relatively little work has been reported on the site of intestinal absorption of Se. Whanger et al.[17] reported that virtually no selenite or selenomethionine is absorbed from the stomach of the rat. Wright and Bell[18] also found no absorption from the rumen of sheep or the stomach of swine. Using ligated intestinal segments in rats, Whanger et al.[17] showed that selenite and selenomethionine are absorbed from all segments of the small intestine, with absorption from the duodenum being slightly greater than from other segments. Pesti and Combs[19] measured accumulation of ^{75}Se in segments of intestine of chicks administered $Na_2{}^{75}SeO_3$ by crop intubation and found a progressive decrease in accumulated radioactivity from the anterior to posterior regions of the gut. The importance of the upper intestine in Se absorption was verified by infecting chicks with various species of *Eimeria*, parasite organisms that cause intestinal coccidiosis and that are known to infect the chick intestine at specific sites. Those species that specifically infect the duodenum and upper ileum increased the incidence and severity of exudative diathesis, indicating lowered Se status, and reduced protein binding of ^{75}Se in the duodenum. Species that infect the posterior ileum had no effect on manifestation of exudative diathesis or on absorption of Se.

B. Uptake and Release of Selenium by Erythrocytes

Lee *et al.*[20] showed that human erythrocytes rapidly take up selenite. Within 1 min after *in vitro* addition of ^{75}Se-selenite to whole blood, 50-70% of the radiolabel could be recovered with the cells. Within the next 10-15 min, most of the radioactivity was released from the cells, leaving only 5% of the original added amount. This rapid uptake and extrusion has been demonstrated in erythrocytes of other species,[21-23] although Jenkins and Hidiroglou[21] maintain that the processes are not as rapid with bovine, chick, and ovine erythrocytes as with human erythrocytes.

Jenkins and Hidiroglou[21] showed that, during a 3-hr incubation of bovine blood, ^{75}Se from selenite was taken up by red cells to a much greater extent than ^{75}Se from selenate or Se-methionine. (Note the contrast with intestinal cell uptake.) This was indicated by a greater amount of ^{75}Se in the red cells and a greater amount of ^{75}Se associated with plasma proteins when selenite was the Se source. The accumulation of ^{75}Se in the erythrocytes was greatly increased and the occurrence of ^{75}Se in plasma proteins was greatly reduced when certain inhibitors, namely arsenate, chromate, *p*-chloromercuribenzoate, or iodoacetate, were included in the incubation medium with selenite. The same inhibitors had no effect when the ^{75}Se source was Se-methionine or selenate. The inhibitors were shown to affect ^{75}Se release and not cell permeability or binding. Lee *et al.*[20] had earlier shown that *p*-chloromercuriobenzoate and iodoacetate prevented or reduced release of ^{75}Se by human erythrocytes but did not influence uptake. Jenkins and Hidiroglou[21] showed further that red cells dialyzed against a saline buffer accumulated more ^{75}Se from selenite than did undialyzed cells unless glucose was included in the incubation medium. Dialysis did not affect accumulation from Se-methionine or selenate. The increased accumulation with selenite in dialyzed cells was attributed to an interference with Se release resulting from loss of energy sources. The authors concluded that Se uptake by erythrocytes is by diffusion for all three forms tested, but that with selenite, compounds are formed within the cell that are actively extruded. The stimulatory effect of glucose on Se release, however, may have resulted from facilitation of NADPH production and consequent further reduction of the Se rather than from provision of energy for an energy-dependent transport system.

Lee et al.[20] demonstrated that erythrocytes alter the chemical form of selenite. Plasma was separated from whole blood that had been incubated with ^{75}Se-selenite and was then added to washed erythrocytes. There was no uptake of radioactivity by the fresh cells, in contrast to cells incubated with ordinary plasma and selenite. Jenkins and Hidiriglou[21] proposed that the form of Se released from the cells is the selenotrisulfide, selenodiglutathione (GSSeSG). This proposal was based on migration of ^{75}Se into the same area as that of glutathione disulfide (GSSG) during electrophoresis of cell exudates and on appearance of radiolabel in elemental Se and in the cystinylbisglycine (one hydrolysis product of GSSG) area after paper chromatography of hydrolyzed cell exudates.

Gasiewicz and Smith[24] suggested that the protein-bound form of Se produced by erythrocytes was H_2Se, since plasma that had been bubbled with H_2Se in the presence of $CdCl_2$ produced the same gel chromatographic peaks as plasma incubated with erythrocytes and selenite and $CdCl_2$. Other forms of Se incubated with plasma and $CdCl_2$ (selenite, selenate, GSSeSG) did not produce the Cd-Se complex to give the same chromatogram.

Thus, the form or forms of Se released by erythrocytes have not yet been definitively established. The significance of red cell uptake, metabolism, and release by erythrocytes in living animals is itself uncertain. Though the red cell apparently has the capacity to absorb and alter selenite, it may never have the opportunity except under experimental conditions. Dietary Se in whatever form will, if absorbed, first be altered by intestinal cells before ⸗ ,g presented to erythrocytes.

C. Plasma Transfer of Selenium

After dosing chickens with $H_2{}^{75}SeO_3$ by crop intubation, Jenkins et al.[25] separated serum proteins by electrophoresis and examined the distribution of [75]Se. Two hours after dosing, 33-44% of the plasma ^{75}Se was contained in the alpha$_2$-globulin and 20-24% in alpha$_3$-globulin. Over the next 24 hrs, the amount in gamma-globulin rose to 30% or more, and in the period of 24-173 hrs, 50-70% of the label was carried by the alpha$_2$- and gamma-globulin fractions. Because selenite added to chick serum did not complex with proteins,[25] the authors concluded that protein synthesis is required for Se transport by plasma.

Burk[26] also reported no detection of protein-bound ^{75}Se using gel filtration of rat plasma samples incubated with ^{75}Se-selenite with or without erythrocytes, although he found a single Se-containing protein peak (perhaps representing more than one protein) from plasma of Se-deficient rats that had been injected with a tracer dose of $H_2^{75}SeO_3$. A second peak appeared from plasma of Se-adequate rats. That peak, however, disappeared and the radioactivity was transferred to the other peak when NaCl was added to the eluting buffer.

Gasiewicz and Smith[27] also found that incubation of ^{75}Se-selenite with rat plasma yielded no protein-bound ^{75}Se. However, in contrast to Burk's finding,[26] Gasiewicz and Smith found ^{75}Se-containing proteins in plasma when erythrocytes had been included in the incubation medium. Others have reported the same effect of erythrocytes on Se-binding by plasma proteins in cow[21,23] and human[20,28] blood. Gasiewicz and Smith,[27] using a gel filtration technique nearly the same as that of Burk,[26] found ^{75}Se bound to plasma components in a wide range of apparent molecular weights 5 hrs after ^{75}Se-selenite was injected into rats. The differing results may be due to the timing of blood sampling after administration of the ^{75}Se. Burk's samples were taken much later (72 hrs after injection). Sandholm[28] and Jenkins et al.[25] have shown that the relative distribution of ^{75}Se among plasma proteins changes over time.

Motsenbocker and Tappel[29] have proposed that a particular selenocysteine-containing protein, selenoprotein P, found in rat plasma, serves primarily as a Se transport protein. After denaturing plasma with sodium dodecyl sulfate, the selenoprotein P and Se-containing glutathione peroxidase (SeGSHpx) polypeptides were easily distinguishable by gel electrophoresis. ^{75}Se from injected $H_2^{75}SeO_3$ reached a peak in plasma selenoprotein P by 3 hrs and then began to decline. More than twice as much ^{75}Se was found in the selenoprotein P of Se-deficient rats than in that of Se-adequate rats. In SeGSHpx, on the other hand, uptake of ^{75}Se was similar for Se-deficient and Se-adequate rats and rose very slowly from the start. Within 1 hr of administration, half of the ^{75}Se dose was found in liver, and by 9 hrs, the liver concentration had dropped to about one-third its peak value. Liver slices incubated with ^{75}Se-selenite produced both labeled selenoprotein P and SeGSHpx. The rapid incorporation of ^{75}Se into liver, the ability of liver to synthesize selenoprotein P, and the subsequent rapid appearance of high levels of selenoprotein P in plasma are supportive but not conclusive evidence that selenoprotein P functions as a transport protein for Se in plasma. Motsenbocker and Tappel[29] added further support to their hypothesis by showing that ^{75}Se from selenoprotein P, injected intracardially, was taken up by nonhepatic tissues as well as by liver of Se-deficient rats. By 5 hrs, testes and kidney had accumulated more ^{75}Se per unit weight than had liver. Thus, it appears that selenoprotein P can carry Se from liver to tissues where it is needed. The manner in which the Se is freed from the protein is not yet known.

D. Tissue Uptake of ^{75}Se

Studies of tissue uptake of ^{75}Se can give an idea of affinity of particular tissues for Se, of the route followed by Se as it enters and is transported about the body, and of the degree and time course of retention in the body. However, all of these factors are dependent on such things as the Se status of the animal at the time of administration, the mode of administration of the tracer, and the amount of carrier given with the ^{75}Se dose. Interpretation of results of such studies must take into account the composition of the diet, the length of time it is fed prior to the administration of the Se isotope, and the time elapsed between administration of the isotope and collection of tissues.

Brown and Burk[30] carried out a very complete ^{75}Se uptake study with rats, first depleting the rats' Se stores by feeding them a low-Se *Torula* yeast diet for 30 days. Following intraperitoneal injection of tracer quantities of $H_2^{75}SeO_3$, rats were killed over an interval of 10 weeks. Whole body retention and retention in various tissues were determined. The pattern of retention in blood, heart, liver, kidney, spleen, lung, stomach, and small intestine was a biphasic elimination curve, with rather steep drops in activity during the first week or two and much slower rates of decline subsequently. Notably different, however, were the patterns for brain and thymus. Both began at very low levels and rose to peaks at about 2 weeks. Thymus then lost ^{75}Se fairly rapidly, presumably due to incorporation of ^{75}Se into lymphocytes, which then left the thymus. Brain, on the other hand, lost ^{75}Se very slowly. This finding in brain was verified and elaborated by Trapp and Millam,[31] who found the same pattern in distinct regions of the rat brain and in other nervous tissue, such as spinal cord. The authors suggested that the long retention time in brain may be due to limited access of the tissue to the general circulation. The pineal gland, though anatomically close to brain, is not separated from the general circulation by the blood-brain barrier and showed a biphasic disappearance curve for ^{75}Se.

Another interesting finding of Brown and Burk[30] was that rat testis showed a steady uptake of ^{75}Se to a peak at about 2 weeks, accumulating a relatively large quantity, second only to kidney in its amount per gram of tissue. At 3 weeks, testis and epididymis contained nearly 42% of the total body ^{75}Se. Earlier work with mice[32] showed a similarly shaped curve for ^{75}Se uptake by testis but with a shorter period before the peak (1 week) and a much smaller percentage accumulation of the dose per gram of tissue. This difference may be a species-related phenomenon or could be due to a difference in Se status at the time of administration. No mention was made of the pre-treatment diet in the mouse study.

Developing teeth and bone, not surprisingly, take up Se to a much greater extent than do mature teeth and bone.[33,34] Shearer and Hadjimarkos[33] injected pregnant rats with microgram quantities of $H_2^{75}SeO_3$ and found that, 13 days post partum, the concentrations of ^{75}Se (% of dose/100 g tissue) were lower in soft tissues and higher in teeth and bone of pups compared to dams. Higher Se intakes during the period of tooth development have been associated with a greater incidence of dental caries in humans[35,36] and in monkeys.[37] It is hypothesized that high levels of Se, which becomes incorporated into the protein fraction of enamel and dentine,[33,34] interfere with normal crystal nucleation.

Transfer of Se across the placenta was investigated in sheep by dosing either the ewe or fetus with $Na_2^{75}SeO_3$ through indwelling venous catheters and collecting blood over a 6-hr period for plasma analysis for ^{75}Se.[38] The study showed that transfer is bidirectional but very inefficient. The report of effficiencies of transfer (2% from ewe to fetus and 1% from fetus to ewe) requires verification in further experiments, as no evaluation was made of Se status of the ewes or of Se content of their diet. Those factors may influence uptake of ^{75}Se by the placenta. The application of this information to the prevention of nutritional muscular dystrophy in lambs also is uncertain, as selenite is not the form of Se that will circulate in blood if Se is provided through diet or oral dosing.

Hopkins et al.[39] investigated the effects of different types of diets and varied dietary Se levels on the distribution and excretion of ^{75}Se by rats injected with microgram quantities of Se as selenite. Using four levels of Se supplementation (0, 0.1, 1.0, 5.0 ppm) to three diets made from Torula yeast, casein, or a commercially available practical diet, the authors found that the amount of ^{75}Se retained in carcass and tissues at 48 hrs was inversely related to the Se content of the diet. Reduction in carcass ^{75}Se was accounted for largely by increased urine content of ^{75}Se. The general relationship of dietary Se level to carcass retention was the same for all three diets, but less ^{75}Se was retained by those rats eating the practical diet. No explanation was offered for this last observation, but perhaps the practical diet contained more Se before supplementation than did the semipurified diets.

In a study with chickens, Jensen et al.[40] reported that, 7 days after an oral dose (several micrograms) of $H_2^{75}SeO_3$, chicks fed a Torula yeast diet without added Se retained one-half of the original dose, whereas chicks fed the same diet supplemented with 1 ppm Se retained only one-fifth of the dose. Burk et al.,[41] following 10 days of excretion of ^{75}Se from an intraperitoneal injection of $H_2^{75}SeO_3$ in rats, verified that total body retention is inversely related to the dietary Se level. Furthermore, they showed the same type of relationship between whole body retention and the amount of carrier Se delivered with the tracer dose. Some tissues, such as kidney, small intestine, testis, and thymus, took up less ^{75}Se as the level of dietary Se increased, but this relationship did not hold for all tissues. In particular, heart, skeletal muscle, stomach, and blood at 10 weeks all showed ^{75}Se concentrations directly related to dietary Se level.

Hansen and Kristensen,[42] in a study with mice, made the point that the disappearance of ^{75}Se from the whole body or liver, kidney, or lung tissue, expressed as a percentage of the dose administered, was biphasic if the ^{75}Se was delivered as a single dose, either orally or intraperitoneally. In the first phase, within about the first 100 hrs, the elimination of ^{75}Se was rapid and proportional to the dose. However, in the later phase, the rate of elimination was much slower and was independent of the carrier dose. When ^{75}Se was administered in drinking water for 10 days or longer, the elimination curve had a single phase independent of dose. Reports of biological half-life of ^{75}Se in the body can, therefore, be very disparate, depending on dose and mode of administration, unless only the second phase of the elimination curve from a single dose administration is used for calculation. Half-excretion times should not be considered equivalent to biological half-life.

II. EXCRETION OF SELENIUM

Se can be excreted from the body by all three major elimination routes: the lungs, the urinary tract, and the intestinal tract. The amount and distribution of Se eliminated by these routes depend on the level of Se intake,[39,40] the form of Se administered,[9-11,43,44] the composition of the diet,[39] and certain other variables, such as arsenic exposure.[45-47]

Burk et al.,[41] using an injected tracer dose of $H_2{}^{75}SeO_3$, investigated the effect of dietary Se level on the route of Se excretion. Fecal excretion over 10 days remained nearly constant at about 10% of the dose as the dietary Se concentration varied from near zero to 1.0 ppm. Urinary excretion, however, was directly related to the dietary Se level, varying from 6% with the low Se basal diet to 67% with the 1.0 ppm Se-supplemented diet. Their calculation of the respiratory elimination as the percentage of the dose not retained by the body and not eliminated in urine or feces showed a small amount (a few percent), fairly constant over the range of dietary Se levels. Thus, it is through alteration of urinary excretion that the rat adjusts to variations in Se intake over this range of dietary levels.

However, Burk et al.[48] showed that when dietary Se was very low, there was a threshold below which urinary excretion of Se from a $^{75}SeO_3{}^{-2}$ injected dose remained constant (as percentage of dose). Only when the dietary Se, provided as selenite, exceeded 0.054-0.084 ppm did the percentage of the dose excreted in urine increase.

Burk et al.[41] also showed that the amount of carrier added to an injected tracer has a great influence on the amount and route of excretion. As the amount of carrier increased from zero to 50 μg Se, fecal elimination remained fairly constant, but urinary excretion increased from 6 to 50%. With a 200 μg Se carrier, urinary excretion dropped to 42% of the injected dose and respiratory excretion rose to 35%.

To evaluate the significance of these and other studies, it is important to recognize whether a dose is within the range of normal intakes or is toxic, as the dominating metabolic pathways differ in the two situations.[49] The dietary requirement for Se for the rat is estimated to be 0.10 mg/ kg diet.[50] Thus, daily Se intake for a 100 g rat consuming approximately 15 g of feed/day of an Se-adequate diet is approximately 1.5 μg Se, or 15 μg Se/kg body weight. A dietary level of 1 ppm Se corresponds to a 15 μg daily intake of Se or 150 μg Se per kg body weight. Therefore, even a 20 μg carrier dose exceeds the daily intake of Se of a rat consuming a diet containing 10 times its requirement of Se. In the study of Burk et al.,[41] respiratory excretion (expressed as percent of injected dose) remained small throughout the range of dietary levels tested (0.1-1.0 ppm Se) and for carrier doses of 20 and 50 μg Se. The great increase observed in the proportion of the dose excreted by the lungs when a 200 μg dose (1.4 mg/kg body weight) was given suggests that the capacity of normally used pathways for metabolism, distribution, and excretion of the Se load had been exceeded.

McConnell and Roth[43] administered very high doses of selenite to rats, even exceeding the reported minimum lethal dose of 3.5 mg Se/kg body weight for the rat.[51] They found that, as the dose increased, the percentage of Se exhaled increased to levels as high as 60% of the injected dose within 24 hrs, but that the percentage of Se eliminated in urine decreased concomitantly. Of the amount of Se exhaled within 24 hrs, 70% was lost in the first 6 hrs. Thus, volatile Se compounds can be formed rapidly and in large quantity when the Se load is high.

The effect of the form of Se on excretion was reported in a series of studies with rats from the University of Otago, New Zealand.[9-11,18] When oral doses of ^{75}Se were given to rats as selenite, Se-methionine, or Se-cystine, urinary excretion during the first week was 4-5% of the dose for Se-methionine and more than twice that amount for selenite and Se-cystine.[9,18] The difference cannot be accounted for by differences in absorption. When ^{75}Se-methionine was fed to a rabbit and the resulting radiolabeled kidney was fed to rats, the urinary excretion was nearly 12%.[10] This suggests that the form of Se in the rabbit kidney had been changed and was more available to be converted to urinary metabolites. ^{75}Se-methionine or ^{75}Se-selenite mixed with fish muscle homogenate and administered to rats resulted in urinary excretion values similar to those for Se-methionine. Fish muscle labeled *in vivo* with ^{75}Se-methionine or ^{75}Se-selenite gave similar results. The unexpectedly low results from administering selenite mixed with fish muscle homogenate could have been due to binding of the selenite by fish muscle proteins or to some other in vitro reaction which made the Se less available for conversion to urinary metabolites.

Nahapetian *et al.*[49] compared two oral doses of each of three forms of Se and also found that, at a dose of 16 μg Se/kg body weight, urinary excretion of the rat was similar for selenite and Se-cystine but significantly lower for Se-methionine. With a dose of 1.5 mg Se/kg body weight, however, urinary excretion from selenite was reduced to the same percentage of dose as that from Se-methionine, while excretion from Se-cystine remained unchanged. The lowered urinary excretion from selenite was probably compensated for by an increase in respiratory excretion.

Hirooka and Galambos[44] injected rats with 1.4 mg Se as $Na_2^{75}SeO_3$ or $Na_2^{75}SeO_4$ per kg body weight and found that a significantly greater portion of the selenite dose was exhaled compared to the selenate, and significantly more of the selenate than of the selenite was excreted in urine. The authors suggested that selenate is more slowly reduced than selenite in the rat, thereby accounting for the slower appearance and lesser amount of volatile Se from selenate. However, the oxidation state of the Se in dimethylselenide, the main volatile metabolite,[52] is the same as that of the Se in trimethylselenonium, the primary urinary metabolite.[47,49,53,54] Unless the large quantity of urinary Se (ca. 50% of the administered dose) excreted after the selenate injection was in a different form (see below) and in a higher oxidation state, it is unlikely that reduction of selenate was the limiting factor.

Ganther *et al.*[55] were able to manipulate the amount of volatilization of a subacute dose of $Na_2^{75}SeO_3$ (2 mg Se/kg body weight) by varying the composition of the diet. Rats fed a commercially prepared stock diet volatilized about 30% of the dose within 10 hrs, whereas rats eating a casein-based purified diet exhaled about 10%. Testing of various fractions of the stock diet associated organic substances with the higher volatilization. Addition of methionine or more protein (as casein) to the purified diet increased volatilization, but to no more than 70% of the level with the stock diet. Addition of more vitamins was not effective. Pre-feeding rats with the purified diet supplemented with 3 ppm Se resulted in volatilization similar to that due to the stock diet, but the Se content of the diets alone could not explain the degree of volatilization, as the Se content of the stock diet was only 0.5 ppm. The increased volatilization with the addition of methionine might have been due to greater availability of methyl groups for the formation of dimethylselenide. However, Hirooka and Galambos[44] found no impairment in respiratory excretion in rats that had been fed a choline-deficient diet and had developed fatty liver.

Ganther and Baumann[45] verified earlier work[56,57] showing that, in rats injected with subacute doses of Se, arsenite increased blood Se, reduced liver Se, and greatly decreased Se content of expired air. They were able to show further that fecal excretion of Se was increased and body retention was decreased, in accord with the many reports that ιs reduces toxicity of Se.[58-60] Levander and Baumann[46] expanded this work, showing that, without significantly changing bile volume, arsenite caused a ten-fold increase in excretion of Se into bile when rats had been injected with a moderately high dose of selenite (0.5 mg Se/kg body weight). A stimulatory effect of arsenite was seen over the entire range of Se doses tested (0.02-1.0 mg/kg body weight), but the stimulation was greater for higher dosages. The As effect was not altered by whether the diet was purified or a practical type. Because the primary metabolites of respiratory and urinary excretion are methylated forms, one might postulate that urinary excretion would also be reduced by arsenite; however, this was not the case.[45] Ganther[61] has proposed that trimethylselenonium (primary urinary Se metabolite) may be derived from a carbon chain rather than by transfer of a methyl group, obviating the need for dimethylselenide as an intermediate. This is consistent with the finding of Obermeyer et al.[62] that very small amounts of ^{75}Se were excreted in urine of rats given very large doses of ^{75}Se-dimethylselenide.

There are many Se-containing compounds that appear in urine, but, according to Palmer et al.,[47] 75% of urinary Se is contained in two compounds. One has been identified as trimethylselenonium [$(Ch_3)_2Se^+$],[47] and the other, designated U-2, has not been identified. When Palmer et al.[47] gave rats large doses of Se, the organic urinary Se-containing metabolite occurring in the greatest amount was trimethylselenonium, regardless of the form of Se administered. Kiker and Burk[54] were able to identify the same two metabolites in urine from rats injected with tracer doses of $Na_2^{75}SeO_3$, even when the rats had been raised using an Se-deficient (0.006 ppm) diet. However, a very small percentage of the initial Se dose was excreted in the urine by the Se-deficient rats, and more than half of the excreted Se was in a form designated as inorganic, though unidentified. The rats eating a diet containing 0.5 ppm Se excreted 10 times as much ^{75}Se, most of which was trimethylselenonium and U-2. The low excretion of Se by the deficient group and the low concentration of organic forms probably reflects uptake and retention of Se by depleted tissues.

Nahapetian et al.[49] reported results showing similar disparate proportionation between two groups of rats maintained using a practical-type diet containing 0.25 ppm Se and injected with two different levels of Se (either 16 μg Se/kg body weight or 1500 μg Se/kg body weight).

The low percentage excretion (3-4%) in the urine and the relatively low concentration of urinary trimethylselenonium reported for the group receiving the smaller dosage are somewhat surprising, because the dietary level of Se is more than adequate, and 16 μg Se/kg body weight is not a small dose. Therefore, tissues should not have been depleted. Ganther[61] measured trimethylselenonium in urine of men consuming a normal diet based on processed meat and found that it accounted for about one-tenth of the total urinary Se. These reports demonstrate that it is incorrect to assume that trimethylselenonium is the predominant urinary metabolite under all conditions.

At least two volatile Se compounds have been identified in exhaled air — dimethylselenide[52] and dimethyldiselenide[63] — and there may be others as yet unidentified. The relative proportion of dimethylselenide and dimethyldiselenide depends on the form of Se administered, according to Jiang et al.[63] They showed that when mice were given selenite or Se-cystine in their drinking water, dimethylselenide was the predominant volatile species, but when Se-methionine was given, dimethyldiselenide and an unidentified compound were the main species.

Methylation of Se has been regarded as a detoxification mechanism, since, as Se intake increases, the excretion of methylated metabolites increases, as discussed above. Obermeyer et al.[62] lent support to this hypothesis when they determined the acute intraperitoneal LD_{50} for trimethylselenonium to be 49.4 mg Se/kg body weight in the rat. Franke and Moxon[51] had found that 3.25-3.5 mg Se as selenite injected per kilogram body weight killed 75% of their rats in 48 hrs. Thus, trimethylselenonium is very much less toxic than selenite. Tsay et al.[64] also showed that injected trimethylselenonium was excreted very rapidly (70% in the first 6 hrs), whereas the Se from an injected dose of selenite was excreted much more slowly and the amount excreted was less. McConnell and Portman[52] showed that when dimethylselenide was injected into rats, nearly 80% of it appeared in the exhaled air within 6 hrs. The low toxicity and the rapid elimination of these methylated forms makes it reasonable to conclude that methylation is a protective detoxification process.

III. METABOLISM OF SELENIUM

Several excretory end products and intermediates of Se metabolism have been identified and some of the pathways of Se metabolism have been described. Although many reactions have been observed in the test tube, their occurrence *in vivo* has not been firmly established.

Ganther[6] has shown that selenious acid (H_2SeO_3) can react spontaneously with a variety of thiols to form compounds with a S to Se ratio of 4 to 1. Stoichiometry and product analysis conformed to the reaction proposed by Painter in 1941[65]:

$$4\ RSH + H_2SeO_3 \longrightarrow RSSeSR + RSSR + 3\ H_2O$$

The family of compounds of the form RSSeSR has been designated "selenotrisulfides," as Se has been substituted for S in a trisulfide. Selenotrisulfides are unstable and readily decompose to the disulfide and elemental Se at alkaline pH. Ganther,[6] however, was able to verify by thin-layer and column chromatography, elemental analysis and amino acid analysis, that selenodicysteine and a non-Se-containing compound (probably cystine) were the products of reaction of 4 moles cysteine per mole of H_2SeO_3.

To obtain a 4 : 1 stoichiometry in the reaction of glutathione (GSH) and H_2SeO_3, it was necessary that the pH be lowered to 1.3 and that concentrations of reactants be increased ten-fold over the levels used with other thiols.[6] As these conditions do not occur in living animals, the significance of this reaction *in vivo* must be questioned. However, Ganther[66] also showed that, under conditions approximating those *in vivo* (i.e., neutral pH, GSH : Se ratio greatly in excess of 4 : 1), the major product formed from the chemical reaction of selenite and GSH was a selenopersulfide, GSSeH. This selenopersulfide can also be formed by the reaction of glutathione reductase on selenodiglutathione, GSSeSG, in the presence of NADPH. Therefore, if selenodiglutathione is formed *in vivo*, there may be two pathways by which the persulfide can be formed in the body:

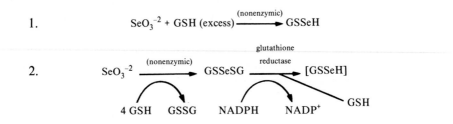

1.
$$SeO_3^{-2} + GSH\ (excess) \xrightarrow{\text{(nonenzymic)}} GSSeH$$

2.
$$SeO_3^{-2} \xrightarrow{\text{(nonenzymic)}} GSSeSG \xrightarrow[\text{reductase}]{\text{glutathione}} [GSSeH]$$

Selenopersulfide, with Se at the zero oxidation state, is unstable and can decompose to GSH and elemental Se. However, under anaerobic conditions, selenopersulfide can be converted to an acid-volatile selenide, presumably H_2Se, either by glutathione reductase in the presence of NADPH or by nonenzymic reduction by excess GSH.[67] Diplock *et al.*[68] showed that acid-volatile Se, which behaved the same as H_2Se and unlike $(CH_3)_3Se^+$, was formed in rat liver homogenate and by a microsomal fraction of liver. Thus, H_2Se apparently can be formed *in vivo* from selenite.

Hsieh and Ganther[69] added further support to the proposal that there are two pathways *in vivo* leading to H_2Se, a presumed intermediate of further metabolism, when they studied formation of dimethylselenide from selenite by cell-free systems derived from rat liver and kidney. Fractionation of the soluble fraction of liver by gel filtration resulted in only one fraction (Fraction C) with activity to form dimethylselenide by itself when incubated with GSH, an NADPH generating system, *S*-adenosylmethionine, and coenzyme A. However, the addition of one other fraction (Fraction A) stimulated dimethylselenide synthesis by Fraction C. Fraction A was found to contain glutathione reductase and another NADPH-linked reductase, which stimulated H_2Se formation. Fraction C contained no glutathione reductase, but apparently contained a methyltransferase that could methylate the selenide produced by nonenzymic reduction of selenite by GSH. Addition of Fraction A provided the glutathione reductase to make more substrate for methylation and, thereby, increased the production of dimethyl selenide.

The production of dimethylselenide has been shown to occur[70] in the 9000 × *g* supernatant fraction of mouse liver, kidney, and lung and to some extent in muscle, spleen, and heart when these fractions are incubated with $Na_2{}^{75}SeO_3$, GSH, an NADPH-generating system, *S*-adenosylmethionine, and ATP. This suggests the presence in these tissues of a methyltransferase and probably glutathione reductase (although selenite can be reduced nonenzymically) but does not indicate whether these tissues are significant sites of dimethylselenide production *in vivo*. The enzymes are not specific for the metabolites of Se.

As discussed previously (see Section II), there is evidence to suggest that trimethylselenonium, which is excreted in the urine, is not formed merely by the methylation of dimethylselenide. Foster and Ganther[71] have developed a technique for the synthesis of ^{75}Se-trimethylselenonium iodide. It and an intermnediate, dimethylselenocysteine selenonium iodide, which can spontaneously degrade to alanine and dimethylselenide, may serve as useful compounds for the study of the formation and metabolism of methylated Se derivatives *in vivo*.

There have been many reports of the substitution of Se from selenite for S in amino acids, producing Se-methionine and Se-cysteine. Rosenfeld[72] fed sheep ^{75}Se- selenite and, after 60 days, was able to identify ^{75}Se-methionine and ^{75}Se-cystine in extracts of wool. In a ruminant, however, one cannot be sure if such compounds result from the mammal's own metabolism or that of its rumen microflora. This study is also subject to the criticism that co-chromatography of the Se compounds with their S- analogues cannot be regarded as definite identification. Schwartz and Sweeney[73] showed that when ^{75}Se-selenite was mixed with various amino acids and immediately spotted on paper, ^{75}Se traveled with cystine in subsequent elution. The same was true with other disulfides, such as homocystine and oxidized glutathione, but not with —SH compounds, such as methionine, cysteine, and GSH.

Olson and Palmer[74] used ion-exchange chromatography to search for Se-containing amino acids in acetone powders from hydrolysates of liver and kidney of rats fed Se as selenite. Identification was based on co-chromatography with standards made from Se-containing amino acids rather than their S-analog. In both liver and kidney, peaks appeared at the position of the selenodisulfide, cysteine-selenocysteine. A small amount appeared at the position of selenocysteine-selenocysteine (i.e., selenocystine). These two peaks, incidentally, were different from the position of cystine. Selenomethionine did not appear. The possibility of Se-binding to amino acids was tested by chromatographing a mixture of the standard amino acid solution and [75]Se- selenite. None of the radioactivity appeared with the amino acids.

When chromatography of samples prepared from liver of a rabbit fed and injected with large amounts of $Na_2{}^{75}SeO_3$ showed no peaks in the elution positions of the Se-containing amino acids, Cummins and Martin[75] concluded that the rabbit does not have the ability to synthesize Se-containing amino acids. However, all their samples were prepared under strongly alkaline conditions, which may have destroyed Se-containing amino acids. Imposing the same treatment conditions on known Se-containing amino acids produced no selenite, an observation which the authors interpreted as verification of efficacy of their technique. However, the Se may have been released from the amino acids and been present in a form other than selenite and, therefore, not detected in their colorimetric assay. Godwin and Fuss,[76] using the same species, were able to detect radioactivity in the selenocystine peak from chromatography of a kidney hydrolysate 48 hrs after the rabbit had been given oral and intravenous ^{75}Se-selenite.

Forstrom et al.[77] used several types of chromatography to show quite convincingly that the Se in GSHpx is in selenocysteine, and Hawkes et al.[78] reported that selenocysteine in protein is the predominant form of Se in the rat, accounting for over 80% of the whole body ^{75}Se in rats that had consumed ^{75}Se-selenite as their main dietary source of Se for 5 months. It is apparent, then, that selenite is reduced in the body and in some manner is incorporated into selenocysteine. There is uncertainty as to whether Se replaces the S in cysteine before or after the amino acid is incorporated into protein. Hawkes et al.[79] have reported success in isolating from rat liver an aminoacyl tRNA that is specific for selenocysteine. The data show that the tRNA has the characteristics necessary to be an intermediate of a pathway of incorporation of intact selenocysteine, but, as pointed out by the authors, they do not show the existence of such a pathway *in vivo*. If such a pathway exists, it may utilize preformed selenocysteine of dietary origin and does not necessarily imply *de novo* synthesis of selenocysteine. Chung and Spallholz[99] reported the *in vivo* incorporation of ^{14}C- radioactivity from uniformly labeled methionine into the Se-cysteinyl moiety of mouse SeGSHpx; they found no incorporation of ^{14}C-label from either serine or alanine. However, Sunde and Everson[100] found specific labeling of Se-cysteine in rat SeGSHpx (using an isolated perfused liver system) with ^{14}C or ^3H from serine, suggesting that serine may be the primary source of carbon for Se-cysteine in the enzyme.

The finding by Sunde and Everson[100] of nearly equal specific activities of label in serine and in carboxymethyl-selenocysteine suggests that the Se-cysteinyl moiety of SeGSHpx is formed subsequent to the incorporation of the serinyl residue into the protein. Further evidence of post-translational modification of SeGSHpx-serinyl residues was provided by the results of Yasumoto *et al.*,[101] who found that the incorporation of Se from selenomethionine is depressed in nutritional pyridoxine deficiency. They proposed that the need for pyridoxine for the utilization of Se from selenomethionine involves a pyridoxine-dependent modification of enzyme cysteinyl residues. Sunde and Hoekstra,[102] using an isotope dilution technique in isolated perfused rat livers, found that selenite and selenide are metabolically closer than selenocysteine to the immediate precursor used for SeGSHpx. They suggested that post-translational modification of enzyme cysteinyl residues may be the mechanism whereby Se is inserted into the active site of the enzyme.

Esaki *et al.*[80] has acquired evidence of the potential for synthesis of selenocysteine in mammalian tissues. They purified cystathionine beta-synthase and cystathionine gamma-lyase from rat liver. The two enzymes, when incubated with selenohomocysteine and serine, catalyzed the formation of selenocystathionine, alpha-ketobutyrate, and NH_3. Cystathionine beta-synthase did not form selenocysteine from serine and H_2Se. Thus, the pathway for selenocysteine synthesis from selenohomocysteine is like that of its sulfur counterparts: homocysteine to cysteine. When rat liver homogenate was substituted for the two purified enzymes, the same products were identified.[80] Selenohomocysteine may be formed *in vivo* by metabolism of selenomethionine, one of the primary forms of Se found in plants. Or, possibly, it is formed by reaction of methionine with selenoalkyl or selenaryl groups with catalysis by L-methionine gamma-lyase.[81] In further studies, the same group[82,83] discovered and purified an enzyme in pig liver that specifically degrades selenocysteine to yield alanine and elemental Se, which then, in the presence of certain reductants, is reduced to H_2Se. Named by these authors selenocysteine lyase, this pyridoxal-phosphate enzyme is the first enzyme known to act specifically on Se compounds. It has been found in many tissues of the rat and of several diverse species.[82] The presence of this enzyme in rat liver explains the apparently lower efficiency of conversion of selenohomocysteine in liver homogenate,[80] compared to that with the purified enzyme system. The wide distribution of this lyase may interfere with observation of selenocysteine formation and incorporation into protein.

Wilhelmsen et al.[103] showed that Se-cysteine can be incorporated directly into proteins in lieu of cysteine. They found that, at relatively high concentrations, Se-cysteine competed with cysteine for incorporation into protein in the mRNA-dependent rabbit reticulocyte lysate protein synthesis system. They suggested that misincorporation of Se-cysteine into protein may be physiologically important in conditions of high tissue levels of Se.

IV. TISSUE CONCENTRATIONS OF SELENIUM

The concentration of Se in organs and tissues depends on the particular tissue considered, the amount and form of Se in the diet, the length of time the diet is consumed, and the species of animal. In young animals, it can also depend on the level of dietary Se consumed by the mother. Table 5.1 lists tissue concentrations for the more commonly analyzed tissues of various species.[89-96]

In general, the greater the animal's Se intake, the greater is the concentration in a particular tissue. This is not a linear relationship, for the tissue concentration approaches a plateau as the diet concentration rises.

The form of dietary Se can make a great difference in certain tissues. For example, Latshaw[87] showed that the Se concentration of chicken liver was doubled by feeding Se in natural feedstuffs instead of feeding the same level mostly as Na_2SeO_3. This was also true for muscle but not for blood (Table 5.1). Osman and Latshaw[84] reported a great increase in pancreas when a supplement of Se-methionine was compared to an equivalent supplement as selenite. This did not affect liver. In turkeys, Cantor et al.[89] showed that Se-methionine had very little effect on liver but, compared to selenite, greatly increased concentrations in pancreas, muscle, and gizzard.

Tissues ranked by Se concentration, on a dry matter basis, generally follow the order kidney > liver > pancreas, heart > skeletal muscle. This is remarkably similar across species. The kidney may be high because of being the primary organ of excretion.

Table 5.1

Selenium Concentrations of Animal Tissues

Animal	Feeding period	Dietary Se (ppm)	Blood (µg/ml)	Liver	Kidney	Pancreas	Muscle	Heart	Other	Reference
Chicken	4 wks	Basal (0.03 ppm)		0.15	0.18	0.19	0.05	0.11		(84)
		Basal + 0.06 as Na_2SeO_3		0.78	1.33	0.43	0.14	0.47		
		Basal + 0.06 as Se-met		0.68	1.18	0.71	0.19	0.38		
		Basal + 0.06 as Se-cys		0.77	1.45	0.53	0.13	0.46		
	4 wks	Basal (0.07 ppm)	0.08	0.74	1.31		0.23			(85)
		Basal + 0.1 as Na_2SeO_3	0.13	1.48	1.85		0.29			
		Basal + 0.2 as Na_2SeO_3	0.19	1.58	2.50		0.40			
		Basal + 0.4 as Na_2SeO_3	0.20	1.82	2.75		0.45			
		Basal + 0.6 as Na_2SeO_3	0.23	2.28	2.81		0.50			
		Basal + 0.8 as Na_2SeO_3	0.24	2.34	3.41		0.58			
		High Se basal (0.67 ppm)	0.33	2.37	3.83		1.20			
		+ 0.2 as Na_2SeO_3	0.39	2.88	4.27		1.63			
	4 wks	(Plasma)								(86)
		Basal (0.012 ppm)	0.002			0.05				
		Basal + 0.02 as Na_2SeO_3	0.005			0.07				
		Basal + 0.04 as Na_2SeO_3				0.13				
		Basal + 0.01 as Se-met				0.14				
		Basal + 0.02 as Se-met	0.006			0.24				
		Basal + 0.02 as Se-cys	0.006			0.09				
		Basal + 0.04 as Se-cys				0.13				
	180 days	(Plasma)								(87)
		Basal (0.10 ppm)	0.09	0.43			0.33			
		Basal + 0.32 as Na_2SeO_3	0.22	0.82			0.42			
		High basal (0.42)	0.26	1.92			1.18			
	24 wks	Basal (0.27)	0.33	2.94[a]	3.72[a]				Cerebellum 1.26[a]	(88)
	1 yr	Basal (0.27)	0.18	1.90[a]	2.59[a]	1.40[a]			3.50[a]	

(continues)

Table 5.1 (*Continued*)

| | | | | Tissue (ppm dry matter basis) | | | | | | |
Animal	Feeding period	Dietary Se (ppm)	Blood ($\mu g/ml$)	Liver	Kidney	Pancreas	Muscle	Heart	Other	Reference
Turkey	4 wks	Basal (0.047 ppm)		0.26		0.34	0.16	0.17	Gizzard 0.20	(89)
		Basal + 0.04 as Na_2SeO_3		0.58		0.43	0.20	0.48	0.30	
		Basal + 0.08 as Na_2SeO_3		1.03		0.49	0.20	0.76	0.44	
		Basal + 0.12 as Na_2SeO_3		1.14		0.52	0.23	0.73	0.45	
		Basal + 0.04 as Se-met		0.60		0.62	0.33	0.51	0.41	
		Basal + 0.08 as Se-met		0.89		0.91	0.49	0.74	0.58	
		Basal + 0.12 as Se-met		1.28		1.21	0.68	0.95	0.73	
	14 wks	Basal (0.2 ppm)	(Blood) 0.20	2.48[a]			0.95[a]			(90)
		Basal + 0.1 as Na_2SeO_3	0.18	2.60[a]			0.87[a]			
		Basal + 0.2 as Na_2SeO_3	0.19	2.56[a]			0.86[a]			
Coturnix	1 yr	Basal (0.35 ppm)	0.17	3.19[a]	4.30[a]	1.91[a]				(88)
	1 yr	Basal (0.35 ppm)	0.46	3.5[a]	6.0[a]	4.8[a]				(88)
Pig (sow)	120 days or more	Basal (0.03–0.05 ppm)	0.06	0.38	5.85					(91)
		Basal + 0.1 as inorganic Se	0.20	1.78	11.07					
		Basal + 0.5 as inorganic Se	0.22	2.57	11.76					
Pig (young)	56 days	Basal (? Se)		0.08	12.5		0.07			(92)
		Basal + 0.5 as $SeO3^{-2}$		1.38	7.50		0.31			
Calf	28 days	Basal (0.3 ppm)		0.91	2.70	1.30	0.50	0.77		(93)
		Basal + 0.1 as Na_2SeO_3		0.89	2.78	1.48	0.46	0.82		
		Basal + 1.0 as Na_2SeO_3		2.66	3.76	1.84	0.84	1.45		
Rat	21 days	0.1 ppm	(Plasma) 0.27	0.42	0.59					(94)
	43 days	0.3 ppm	0.42	4.09	6.01	1.44	0.63	1.57	Testis 6.72	(95)
	70 days	Basal	0.09	0.20[a]	2.03[a]		0.25[a]		6.46	(96)
		Basal + 0.25 ppm	0.42	2.18[a]	5.82[a]		0.50[a]		6.77	

[a]Original data converted to dry matter basis.

Other tissues that are notably high in Se, exceeding the concentration of kidney, are the testis,[95,96] the pineal gland,[88,97] and the pituitary gland.[88,97] Rat testis[95,96] has been reported to have a Se concentration of 6.5-6.7 μg/g dry weight, whether the diet was low in Se (*Torula* yeast diet) or was supplemented to be greater than 0.25 ppm. In this organ of highest Se concentration, less than 1% of the Se is bound to GSHpx.[95] Brown and Burk[30] showed in radiographs that ^{75}Se is concentrated in the midpiece of the sperm.

Although the Se concentration of muscle is low, because of its relatively large mass, muscle contains nearly 40% of total body Se.[95] Liver contains about 30% and all other organs and tissues less than 10% each.

REFERENCES

1. McConnell, K. P., and Cho, G. J., Transmucosal movement of selenium, Am. J. Physiol., 208, 1191, 1965.
2. Spencer, R. P., and Blau, M., Intestinal transport of selenium-75 selenomethionine, Science, 136, 155, 1961.
3. Anundi, I., Hogberg, J., and Stahl, A., Absorption of selenite in the rat small intestine: interactions with glutathione, Acta Pharmacol. Toxicol., 54, 273, 1984.
4. Abbott, W. A., and Meister, A., Biliary glutathione: hepatic and pancreatic contributions, Fed. Proc., 41, 1430, 1982.
5. Eberle, D., Clarke, R., and Kaplowitz, N., Rapid oxidation *in vitro* of endogenous and exogenous glutathione in bile of rats, J. Biol. Chem., 256, 2115,1981.
6. Ganther, H. E., Selenotrisulfides. Formation by the reaction of thiols with selenious acid, Biochemistry, 7, 2898, 1968.
7. Reasbeck, P. G., Barbezat, G. O., Robinson, M.F., and Thomson, C.D., Direct measurement of selenium absorption *in vivo*: triple-lumen gut perfusion in the conscious dog, *Proc. New Zealand Workshop on Trace Elements*, 1981, Univ. Otago, Dunedin, N.Z., p. 107 (abstr.).
8. Thomson, C. D., and Stewart, R. D. H., Metabolic studies of (^{75}Se) selenomethionine and (^{75}Se) selenite in the rat, Br. J. Nutr., 30, 139, 1973.
9. Thomson, C. D., Robinson, B. A., Stewart, R. D. H., and Robinson, M. F., Metabolic studies of (^{75}Se) selenocystine and (^{75}Se) selenomethionine in the rat, Br. J. Nutr., 43, 501, 1975.
10. Thomson, C. D., Stewart, R. D. H., and Robinson, M. F., Metabolic studies in rats of (^{75}Se) selenomethionine and of ^{75}Se incorporated *in vivo* into rabbit kidney, Br. J. Nutr., 33, 45, 1975.
11. Richold, M., Robinson, M. F., and Stewart, R. D. H., Metabolic studies in rats of ^{75}Se incorporated *in vivo* into fish muscle, Br. J. Nutr., 38, 19, 1977.
12. Thomson, C. D., and Stewart, R. D. H., The metabolism of (^{75}Se) selenite in young men, Br. J. Nutr., 32, 47, 1974.
13. Janghorbani, M., Christensen, M. J., Nahapetian, A., and Young, V. R., Selenium metabolism in healthy adults: quantitative aspects using the stable isotope [74]SeO_3^{2-}, Am. J. Clin. Nutr., 35, 647, 1982.

14. Brown, D. G., Burk, R. F., Seely, R. J., and Kiker, K. W., Effect of dietary selenium on the gastrointestinal absorption of $^{75}SeO_3^{-2}$ in the rat, Internat. J. Vit. Nutr. Res., 42, 588, 1972.

15. Mykkanen, H., and Humaloja, T., Effect of lead on the intestinal absorption of sodium selenite and selenomethionine (^{75}Se) in chicks, Biol. Trace Element Res., 6, 11, 1984.

16. Mutanen, M. L., and Mykkanen, H.M., Effect of dietary fat on plasma glutathione peroxidase levels and intestinal absorption of ^{75}Se-labeled sodium selenite in chicks, J. Nutr., 114, 829, 1984.

17. Whanger, P. D., Pedersen, N. D., Hatfield, J., and Weswig, P. H., Absorption of selenite and selenomethionine from ligated digestive tract segments in rats, Proc. Soc. Exper. Biol. Med., 153, 295, 1976.

18. Wright, P. L., and Bell, M. C., Comparative metabolism of selenium and tellurium in sheep and swine, Am. J. Physiol., 211, 6, 1966.

19. Pesti, G. M., and Combs, G. F., Jr., Studies on the enteric absorption of selenium in the chick using localized coccidial infections, Poultry Sci., 55, 2265, 1976.

20. Lee, M., Dong, A., and Yano, J., Metabolism of ^{75}Se-selenite by human whole blood in vitro, Can. J. Biochem., 47, 791, 1969.

21. Jenkins, K. J., and Hidiroglou, M., Comparative metabolism of ^{75}Se-selenite, ^{75}Se-selenate, and ^{75}Se-selenomethionine in bovine erythrocytes, Can. J. Physiol. Pharmacol., 50, 927, 1972.

22. Sandholm, M., The initial fate of a trace amount of intravenously administered selenite, Acta Pharmacol. Toxicol., 33, 1, 1973.

23. Sandholm, M., The metabolism of selenite in cow blood *in vitro*, Acta Pharmacol. Toxicol., 33, 6, 1973.

24. Gasiewicz, T. A. and Smith, J. C., Similar properties of the cadmium (Cd) and selenium (Se) complex formed in rat plasma *in vivo* and *in vitro*, Fed. Proc., 36, 1152, 1977.

25. Jenkins, K. J., Hidiroglou, M., and Ryan, J. F., Intravascular transport of selenium by chick serum proteins, Can. J. Physiol. Pharmacol., 47, 459, 1969.

26. Burk, R. F., Effect of dietary selenium level on ^{75}Se binding to rat plasma proteins, Proc. Soc. Exper. Biol. Med., 143, 719, 1973.

27. Gasiewicz, T. A., and Smith, J. C., Interactions of cadmium and selenium in rat plasma *in vivo* and *in vitro*, Biochim. Biophys. Acta, 428, 113, 1976.

28. Sandholm, M., Function of erythrocytes in attaching selenite-Se onto specific plasma proteins, Acta Pharmacol. Toxicol., 36, 321, 1975.

29. Motsenbocker, M. A., and Tappel, A. L., Selenocysteine-containing selenium-transport protein in rat plasma, Biochim. Biophys. Acta, 719, 147, 1982.

30. Brown, D. G., and Burk, R. F., Selenium retention in tissues and sperm of rats fed a *Torula* yeast diet, J. Nutr., 102, 102, 1972.

31. Trapp, G. A., and Millam, J., The distribution of ^{75}Se in brains of selenium-deficient rats, J. Neurochem., 24, 593, 1975.

32. Gunn, S. A., Gould, C., and Anderson, W. A. D., Incorporation of selenium into spermatogenic pathway of mice, Proc. Soc. Exper. Biol. Med., 124, 1260, 1967.

33. Shearer, T. R., and Hadjimarkos, D. M., Comparative distribution of ^{75}Se in the hard and soft tissue of mother rats and their pups, J. Nutr., 103, 553, 1973.

34. Shearer, T. R., Developmental and postdevelopmental uptake of dietary organic and inorganic selenium into the molar teeth of rats, J. Nutr., 105, 338, 1975.

35. Hadjimarkos, D. M., Effect of selenium on dental caries, Arch. Environ. Health, 10, 893, 1965.

36. Ludwig, T. G., and Bibby, B. G., Geographic variations in the prevalence of dental caries in the United States of America, Caries Res., 3, 32, 1969.

37. Bowen, W. H., The effect of selenium and vanadium on caries activities in monkeys (*Macaca irus*), J. Irish Dent. Ass., 18, 83, 1972.

38. Shariff, M. A., Krishnamurti, C. R., Schaefer, A. L., and Heindze, A. M., Bidirectional transfer of selenium across the sheep placenta in utero, Can. J. Anim. Sci., 64 (Suppl.), 252, 1984.

39. Hopkins, L. L., Jr., Pope, A. L., and Baumann, C. A., Distribution of microgram quantities of selenium in the tissues of the rat, and effects of previous selenium intake, J. Nutr., 88, 61, 1966.

40. Jensen, L. S., Walter, E. D., and Dunlap, J. S., Influence of dietary vitamin E and selenium on distribution of Se^{75} in the chick, Proc. Soc. Exper. Biol. Med., 112, 899, 1963.

41. Burk, R. F., Brown, D. G., Seely, R. J., and Scaief, C. C., III, Influence of dietary and injected selenium on whole body retention, route of excretion, and tissue retention of $^{75}SeO_3^{2-}$ in the rat, J. Nutr., 102, 1049, 1972.

42. Hansen, J. C., and Kristensen, P., The kinetics of ^{75}Se-selenium in relation to dose and mode of administration to mice, J. Nutr., 109, 1223, 1979.

43. McConnell, K. P., and Roth, D. M., Respiratory excretion of selenium, Proc. Soc. Exper. Biol. Med., 123, 919, 1966.

44. Hirooka, T. and Galambos, J. T., Selenium metabolism. I. Respiratory excretion, Biochim. Biophys. Acta, 130, 313, 1966.

45. Ganther, H. E., and Baumann, C. A., Selenium metabolism. I. Effects of diet, arsenic and cadmium, J. Nutr., 77, 210, 1962.

46. Levander, O. A., and Baumann, C. A., Selenium metabolism. VI. Effect of arsenic on the excretion of selenium in the bile, Toxicol. Appl. Pharmacol., 9, 106, 1966.

47. Palmer, I. S., Gunsalus, R. P., Halverson, A. W., and Olson, O. E., Trimethyl selenonium ion as a general excretory product from selenium metabolism in the rat, Biochim. Biophys. Acta, 208, 260, 1970.

48. Burk, R. F., Seely, R. J., and Kiker, K. W., Selenium: dietary threshold for urinary excretion in the rat, Proc. Soc. Exper. Biol. Med., 142, 214, 1973.

49. Nahapetian, A. T., Janghorbani, M., and Young, V.R., Urinary trimethylselenonium excretion by the rat: effect of level and source of selenium-75, J. Nutr., 113, 401, 1983.

50. Committee on Animal Nutrition, National Research Council, *Nutrient Requirements of Domestic Animals,* Number 10, Third ed., Nat'l. Acad. Sci., Washington, D.C., 1978, 19.

51. Franke, K. W., and Moxon, A. L., A comparison of the minimum fatal doses of selenium, tellurium, arsenic and vanadium, J. Pharmacol. Exp. Ther., 58, 454, 1936.

52. McConnell, K. P., and Portman, O. W., Excretion of dimethyl selenide by the rat, J. Biol. Chem., 195, 277, 1952.

53. Byard, J. L., Triinethyl selenide, a urinary metabolite of selenite, Arch. Biochem. Biophys., 130, 556, 1969.

54. Kiker, K. W., and Burk, R. F., Production of urinary selenium metabolites in the rat following $^{75}SeO_3^{2-}$ administration, Am. J. Physiol., 227, 643, 1974.

55. Ganther, H. E., Levander, O. A., and Baumann, C. A., Dietary control of selenium volatilization in the rat, J. Nutr., 88, 55, 1966.

56. Palmer I. S., and Bonhorst C. W., Modification of selenite metabolism by arsenite, J. Agric. Food Chem., 5, 928, 1957.

57. Kamstra, L. S., and Bonhorst, C. W., Effect of arsenic on the expiration of volatile selenium compounds by rats, Proc. S. Dakota Acad. Sci., 32, 72, 1953.

58. Dubois, K. P., Moxon, A. L., and Olson, O. E., Further studies on the effectiveness of arsenic in preventing selenium poisoning, J. Nutr., 19, 477, 1940.

59. Moxon, A. L., The effect of arsenic on the toxicity of seleniferous grains, Science, 88, 81, 1938.

60. Moxon, A. L., Rhian, M. A., Anderson, H. D., and Olson, O. E., Growth of steers on seleniferous range, J. Animal Sci., 3, 299, 1944.

61. Ganther, H. E., Chemistry and metabolism of selenium, in *Proceedings of the Third International Symposium on Selenium in Biology and Medicine*, Combs, G. F., Jr., Spallholz, J. E., Levander, O. A., and Oldfield, J. E., eds., Avi Publ. Co., Westport, Conn., 1986.

62. Obermeyer, B. D., Palmer, I. S., Olson, O. E., and Halverson, A. W., Toxicity of trimethylselenonium chloride in the rat with and without arsenite, Toxicol. Appl. Pharmacol., 20, 135, 1971.

63. Jiang, S., Robberecht, H., and Van den Berghe, D., Elimination of selenium compounds by mice through formation of different volatile selenides, Experientia, 39, 293, 1983.

64. Tsay, D. T., Halverson, A. W., and Palmer, I. S., Inactivity of dietary trimethyl selenonium chloride against the necrogenic syndrome of the rat, Nutr. Report Internat., 2, 203, 1970.

65. Painter, E. P., The chemistry and toxicity of selenium compounds with special reference to the selenium problem, Chem. Rev., 28, 179, 1941.

66. Ganther, H. E., Reduction of the selenotrisulfide derivative of glutathione to a persulfide analog by glutathione reductase, Biochemistry, 10, 4089, 1971.

67. Hsieh, H., and Ganther, H. E., Acid-volatile selenium formation catalyzed by glutathione reductase, Biochemistry, 14, 1632, 1975.

68. Diplock, A. T., Caygill, C. P. J., Jeffrey, E. H., and Thomas, C., The nature of acid-volatile selenium in the liver of the male rat, Biochemistry, 134, 283, 1973.

69. Hsieh, H. S., and Ganther, H. E., Biosynthesis of dimethyl selenide from sodium selenite in rat liver and kidney cell-free systems, Biochim. Biophys. Acta, 497, 205, 1977.

70. Ganther, H. E., Enzymic synthesis of dimethyl selenide from sodium selenite in mouse liver extracts, Biochem., 5, 1089, 1966.

71. Foster, S. J., and Ganther, H. E., Synthesis of (^{75}Se) trimethyl selenoniumiodide from (^{75}Se) selenocystine, Anal. Biochem., 137, 205, 1984.

72. Rosenfeld, I., Biosynthesis of seleno-compounds from inorganic selenium by sheep, Proc. Soc. Exper. Biol. Med., 111, 670, 1962.

73. Schwartz, K., and Sweeney, E., Selenite binding to sulfur amino acids, Fed. Proc., 23, 421, 1964.

74. Olson, O. E., and Palmer, I. S., Selenoamino acids in tissues of rats administered inorganic selenium, Metabolism, 25, 299, 1976.

75. Cummins, L. M., and Martin, J. L., Are selenocystine and selenomethionine synthesized *in vivo* from sodium selenite in mammals? Biochemistry, 6, 3162, 1967.

76. Godwin, D. O., and Fuss, C. N., The entry of selenium into rabbit protein following the administration of $Na_2{}^{75}SeO_3$, Aust. J. Biol. Sci., 25, 865, 1972.

77. Forstrom, J. W., Zakowski, J. J., and Tappel, A. L., Identification of the catalytic site of rat liver glutathione peroxidase as selenocysteine, Biochemistry, 17, 2639, 1978.

78. Hawkes, W. C., Wilhelmsen, E. C., and Tappel, A. L., The biochemical forms and tissue and subcellular distribution of selenium in the rat, Fed. Proc., 42, 928 (abstr. #3723), 1983.

79. Hawkes, W. C., Lyons, D. E., and Tappel, A. L., Identification of a selenocysteine-specific aminoacyl transfer RNA from rat liver, Biochim. Biophys. Acta, 699, 183, 1982.

80. Esaki, N., Nakamura, T., Tanaka, H., Suzuki, T., Morino, Y., and Soda, K., Enzymatic synthesis of selenocysteine in rat liver, Biochem., 20, 4492, 1981.

81. Esaki, N., Tanaka, H., Uemura, S., Suzuki, T., and Soda, K., Catalytic action of L-methionine γ-lyase on selenomethionine in selenols, Biochem., 18, 407, 1979.

82. Esaki, N., Nakamura, T., Tanaka, H., and Soda, K., Selenocysteine lyase, a novel enzyme that specifically acts on selenocysteine, J. Biol. Chem., 257, 4386, 1982.

83. Soda, K., Esaki, N., Nakamura, T., and Tanaka, H., Selenocysteine B-lyase: an enzymological aspect of mammalian selenocysteine metabolism, in *Proceedings of the Third International Symposium on Selenium in Biology and* Medicine, Combs, G. F., Jr., Spallholz, J. E., Levander, O. A., and Oldfield, J. E., eds., Avi Publ. Co., Westport, Conn., 1986.

84. Osman, M., and Latshaw, J. D., Biological potency of selenium from sodium selenite, selenomethionine, selenocystine in the chick, Poultry Sci., 55, 987, 1976.

85. Scott, M. L., and Thompson, J. N., Selenium content of feedstuffs and effects of dietary selenium levels upon tissue selenium in chicks and poults, Poultry Sci., 50, 1742, 1971.

86. Cantor, A. H., Langevin, M. L., Noguchi, T., and Scott, M. L., Efficacy of selenium in selenium compounds and feedstuffs for prevention of pancreatic fibrosis in chicks, J. Nutr., 105, 106, 1975.

87. Latshaw, J. D., Natural and selenite selenium in the hen and eggs, J. Nutr., 105, 32, 1975.

88. McFarland, L. Z., Winget, C. M., Wilson, W. O., and Johnson, C. M., Role of selenium in neural physiology of avian species. I. The distribution of selenium in tissues of chickens, turkeys and coturnix, Poultry Sci., 49, 216, 1970.

89. Cantor, A. H., Moorhead, P. D., and Musser, M. A., Comparative effects of sodium selenite and selenomethionine upon nutritional muscular dystrophy, selenium-dependent glutathione peroxidase, and tissue selenium concentrations of turkey poults, Poultry Sci., 61, 478, 1982.

90. Cantor, A. H., and Scott, M. L., Influence of dietary selenium on tissue selenium levels in turkeys, Poultry Sci., 54, 262, 1975.

91. Mahan, D. C., Moxon, A. L., and Hubbard, M., Efficacy of inorganic selenium supplementation to sow diets on resulting carry-over to their progeny, J. Animal Sci., 46, 738, 1977.

92. Ewan, R. C., Effect of vitamin E and selenium on tissue composition of young pigs, J. Animal Sci., 32, 883, 1971.

93. Kincaid, R. L., Miller, W. J., Neathery, M. W., Gentry, R. P., and Hampton, D. L., Effect of added dietary selenium on metabolism and tissue distribution of radioactive and stable selenium in calves, J. Animal Sci., 44, 147, 1977.

94. Motsenbocker, M. A., and Tappel, A. L., Effect of dietary selenium on plasma selenoprotein P, selenoprotein P1 and glutathione peroxidase in the rat, J. Nutr., 114, 279, 1984.

95. Behne, D. and Wolters, W., Distribution of selenium and glutathione peroxidase in the rat, J. Nutr., 113, 456, 1983.

96. Behne, D., Hofer, T., von Berswordt-Wallrabe, R., and Elger, W., Selenium in the testis of the rat: studies on its regulation and its importance for the organism, J. Nutr., 112, 1682, 1982.

97. Vohra, P., Johnson, C. M., McFarland, L. Z., Siopes, T. D., Wilson, W. O., and Winget, C. M., Role of selenium in neural physiology of avian species. 2. The distribution of ^{75}Se from injected selenomethionine-^{75}Se in the tissues and its fate in livers of chickens, Poultry Sci., 52, 644, 1973.

98. Wolffram, S., Arduser, F., and Scharrer, E., *In vivo* intestinal absorption of selenate and selenite in rats, J. Nutr., 115, 454, 1985.

99. Chung, C. K., and Spallholz, J. E., Methionine: possible precursor to selenocysteine of glutathione peroxidase, Federation Proc., 44, 1670 (abst. #7363), 1985.

100. Sunde, R. A., and Evenson, J. K., Serine incorporation into the selenocysteine moiety of glutathione peroxidase, Federation Proc., 44, 1669 (abst. #7360), 1985.

101. Yasumoto, K., Iwami, K., and Yoshida, M., Vitamin B_6 dependence of selenomethionine and selenite utilization for glutathione peroxidase in the rat, J. Nutr., 109, 760, 1979.
102. Sunde, R. A., and Hoekstra, W. G., Incorporation of selenium from selenite and selenocysteine into glutathione peroxidase in the isolated perfused rat liver, Biochem. Biophys. Res. Commun., 93, 1181, 1980.
103. Wilhelmsen, E. C., Hawkes, W. C., and Tappel, A. L., Substitution of selenocysteine for cysteine in a retiulocyte lysate protein synthesis system, Biol. Trace Elem. Res., 7, 141, 1985.

6

BIOCHEMICAL
FUNCTIONS OF
SELENIUM

Historically, the nutritional role of Se has always been associated with that of vitamin E and, hence, with antioxidant activity. In 1951, Schwarz[1] recognized a factor in certain yeasts that would prevent the liver necrosis in rats caused by the combined deficiency of vitamin E and cysteine. He designated this "Factor 3." In 1957, Schwarz[2] showed that Se salts were effective in preventing liver necrosis and that the activity of Factor 3 preparations preventing liver necrosis was proportional to their Se contents. Simultaneously and independently, Schwarz et al.[3] and Patterson et al.[4] reported that Se was effective in preventing exudative diathesis, a condition characterized by leakage of plasma through the capillaries into subcutaneous spaces and observed in chicks consuming vitamin E-deficient diets. Thus, by 1957, Se was recognized as having nutritional significance and as possibly being an essential nutrient.[3]

During the same period (in the 1950s), Mills[5] and Mills and Randall[6] discovered that the glutathione peroxidase system (Fig. 6.1) of intact erythrocytes protected hemoglobin from ascorbic acid-induced oxidation but only in the presence of glucose. In 1963, Cohen and Hochstein[7] showed that glucose protected against peroxide-induced oxidation of hemoglobin and theorized that the role of glucose was to maintain the reduced glutathione (GSH) concentration by generating NADPH for the reduction of oxidized glutathione (GSSG) by glutathione reductase.

In 1972, Rotruck et al.[8] observed that, although including vitamin E in the diet of rats was known to protect their erythrocytes from oxidative

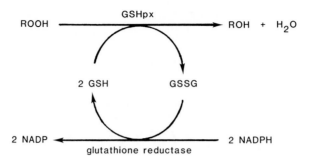

Fig. 6.1 The glutathione redox cycle with glutathione peroxidase (GSHpx) and glutathione reductase.

hemolysis *in vitro*, dietary Se could also fulfill that function but only when glucose was included in the incubation. Furthermore, dietary Se, but not dietary vitamin E, could protect against ascorbate-induced oxidation of hemoglobin to methemoglobin in erythrocytes incubated in the presence of glucose. This report gave the first strong evidence that the function of Se was specific and distinct from that of vitamin E.

The effect of glucose on protection of hemoglobin from oxidation had been attributed to the maintenance of GSH levels in the cell,[7] but GSH in erythrocytes of Se-deficient rats was found to be higher than GSH in erythrocytes of Se-supplemented rats.[8] This suggested that the problem in Se-deficiency was related to the utilization of GSH rather than to its maintenance. Since GSH, along with a peroxide, is a substrate for glutathione peroxidase (GSHpx), Rotruck *et al.*[9] studied this enzyme from rat erythrocytes and found that it contained Se. Subsequently, Se was found to be a part of of the enzyme (hence, SeGSHpx) of other species (Table 6.1).[10-24,94] This discovery explained for the first time a nutritional function of Se in animals.

I. PHYSICAL PROPERTIES OF SELENIUM-DEPENDENT GLUTATHIONE PEROXIDASE

Selenium-dependent glutathione peroxidase from several tissues of several animal species has been purified (Table 6.1). Estimates of molecular weight are remarkably uniform, ranging from 76,000 to 100,000 for the intact enzyme. It is generally agreed that the enzyme is composed of four subunits, apparently identical, with molecular weights ranging from 18,000 to 23,000. Most authors report a stoichiometry of about 4 g-atoms Se/mole of enzyme, although notably, Sunde[25] reported lower values for sheep erythrocytes and

Table 6.1

Physical Properties Reported for Glutathione Peroxidase Purified from Several Species

Species	Tissue	Native enzyme molecular weight	Subunit molecular weight	Se (g-atoms/mole of enzyme)	Reference
Rat	Liver	76,000	19,000	4.09	(10)
		—	19,000	—	(11)
	Lung	84,000	20,000	—	(12)
Hamster	Liver cytosol	23,000	—	—	(13)
Cow	Erythrocytes	85,000	—	—	(14)
		83,800	21,000	—	(15)
		—	—	4.04	(16)
		—	21,900	—	(17)
	Lens	96,600	—	—	(18)
Sheep	Erythrocytes	88,000	22,000	3.8	(19)
		89,000	22,000	2.2	(20)
	Liver	77,000–80,000	18,000	1.6	(20)
Pig	Aorta	84,000	—	—	(21)
Human	Erythrocytes	100,000	—	—	(22)
		95,000	23,000	3.5	(23)
	Placenta	85,500	22,000	ca. 4	(24)
Trout	Liver	95,000	24,800	3.8	(94)

liver. He proposed that his lower values were probably artifactual, being due either to the lability of Se and its resulting release from GSHpx, or to contamination of his GSHpx preparation by other proteins.

The enzyme does not contain heme or, in fact, any metal other than Se.[16] Wendel et al.[26] found by X-ray photoelectron spectroscopy that the active site of GSHpx includes bound Se. Subsequently, Forstrom et al.,[27] by derivatizing the ^{75}Se-labeled enzyme, hydrolyzing it with acid, and isolating the ^{75}Se-labeled products, was able to show that the catalytic site of rat liver GSHpx includes selenocysteine.

The amino acid sequence of SeGSHpx from bovine erythrocytes has been elegantly determined by Gunzler et al.[17] using three different cleavage methods. Their results showed that the monomeric form of the enzyme consists of 198 amino acids with a molecular mass of about 21,900 daltons. The active site selenocysteine was situated at position 45 (from the N-terminal). The amino acid sequence was found to differ at some positions from that predicted by X-ray crystallographic analysis[28] and was found to include some residues at both terminals that were not detected by the X-ray method. The partial N-terminal sequence reported by Condell and Tappel[29] for the rat liver enzyme matches the bovine erythrocyte enzyme sequence in 38 of 46 positions. Gunzler et al.[17] found three cysteine residues in addition to the Se-cysteine residue; however, in the crystal structure, they are located too far from one another and from the Se-cysteine to form disulfide or selenodisulfide bridges in the monomer.

The active sites of SeGSHpx have been shown by X-ray crystallography to lie in flat depressions on the molecular surface, with each active center built up by segments from two subunits.[28,30] Binding studies in solution and in the crystalline state indicate half-site reactivity of SeGSHpx, suggesting that the dimer rather than the monomer is the functional subunit. Under oxidizing conditions, Kraus and Ganther[31] reported that GSH bound covalently to the Se of GSHpx in a 1 : 1 ratio. However, the crystalline enzyme binds only 0.5 mole GSH/mole subunits.[28]

Studies of the incorporation of Se into the active site of SeGSHpx are discussed in Chapter 5, Section III.

II. MECHANISM OF SELENIUM-DEPENDENT GLUTATHIONE PEROXIDASE

The catalytic mechanism of SeGSHpx appears to be complex; hypotheses for its description are still being modified to comply with new findings. In 1975, Ganther[32] proposed the mechanism of action for GSHpx shown in Fig. 6.2. Even before it was discovered that Se is a constituent of SeGSHpx, Flohe et al.[33] published kinetic studies that suggested that the SeGSHpx reaction occurs as a sequence of three bimolecular steps. Plots of the

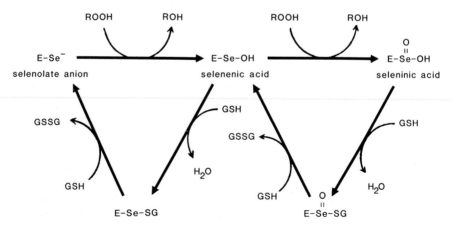

Fig. 6.2 Mechanism of action of selenium-containing glutathione peroxidase as proposed by Ganther.,[32] showing redox changes of selenium at the active site of the enzyme (E).

reciprocals of velocity and substrate concentration, with peroxide as the variable substrate and at several different concentrations of GSH, gave a pattern of parallel lines characteristic of such a ping-pong mechanism, in which a product is released from one enzyme-substrate interaction before a second substrate interacts with the enzyme. This led Flohé[34] to propose a reaction scheme much like Ganther's except that the active site of the enzyme was presumed to contain sulfhydryl groups rather than selenol groups.

Various experimental findings which led to or have supported Ganther's proposed mechanism are shown in Table 6.2.[35-40] There seems to be general agreement that the mechanism is of the "ping-pong" type, that the enzyme cannot be saturated with GSH, and that the enzyme-bound Se occurs in different oxidation states at different steps of the reaction. In its most reduced form, when affinity for GSH is relatively low and affinity for peroxide is high, the enzyme-bound Se is thought to occur as the selenolate anion (enzyme-Se–) at physiological pH.[28] The reduced form is recognized in chemical assay by being inhibitable by iodoacetate (iodoacetate sensitive).[35] Although Kraus et al.[39] demonstrated the existence of at least three oxidized forms of SeGSHpx, it is not known which, if any, of these is involved in the catalytic function of the enzyme. The proposed selenenic acid intermediate (enzyme-SeOH) remains hypothetical, not having been isolated or otherwise identified. Although a seleninic acid form (enzyme-SeOOH) was identified by Epp et al.[28] with X-ray crystallography, it has not been established whether this form occurs in the catalytic reaction.

Chaudiere et al.[41] have proposed two possible mechanisms (Fig. 6.3) that are consistent with their data from inhibition studies and that differ from Ganther's proposed mechanism. As correctly pointed out by Chaudiere et al.,[41] steady state kinetics cannot distinguish the rate constants of the two consecutive steps for which the substrate is GSH unless one of the steps can be manipulated by a specific effector. In search of a suitable effector, they examined various mercaptans and sulfhydryl compounds and selected mercaptosuccinate because it inhibited SeGSHpx quickly and at low concentrations without inhibiting glutathione reductase, to which the SeGSHpx reaction is coupled for assay of activity. Eleven models of enzyme inhibition, considering possible interactions of the inhibitor with the enzyme in either of the steps utilizing GSH, were examined. A rate equation was generated for each model and evaluated by the goodness of fit of experimental data, using nonlinear least squares fitting. The only model to pass the evaluation criteria is shown in Fig. 6.4. According to this model, the inhibitor can interact with either of the forms of the enzyme (F or G) that can react with GSH to yield the inhibited form, H. Because the

Table 6.2

Timetable of Findings Leading to and Supporting Ganther's Proposed Mechanism of Action of GSHpx

Year published	Finding	Implication	Reference
1957	GSHpx discovered, stoichiometry determined.	$H_2O_2 \xrightarrow{\text{GSHpx}} 2\,H_2O$ $2\,GSH \qquad GSSG$	(5)
1968-69	Hydroperoxides, including those of unsaturated fatty acids, can serve as substrates.	$ROOH \xrightarrow{\text{GSHpx}} ROH + H_2O$ $2\,GSH \qquad GSSG$	(35) (36,37)
1972	In kinetic studies, reciprocal plots (1/velocity vs. 1/[peroxide]) show parallel lines for different GSH concentration.	"Ping-pong" mechanism ROOH ROH $_{GSSG\ GSH}$ GSH	(33)
	Apparent K_m and Vmax for peroxide increases with GSH.	Consistent with "ping-pong" mechanism	
1973	Se is constituent of GSHpx.	Se may be part of active site	(8)
1974	After incubation of GSHpx with GSH, enzyme is easily separated by immediate gel chromatography showing that affinity of reduced enzyme for GSH is low, although GSH is highly specific and required substrate for GSHpx reaction.	There must be at least two forms of the enzyme (supports "ping-pong").	(34)
	Rate constants with different hydroperoxides vary, but apparent V_{max} of reaction is constant.	Reaction with peroxide is independent of reaction with GSH (supports ping-pong).	
	GSHpx pre-incubated with GSH is irreversibly and completely inhibited by iodoacetate, whereas if iodoacetate is added first, inhibition is very slow. Adding a hydroperoxide to the enzyme prevents inhibition.	There are at least two forms of the enzyme.	
1975	X-Ray photoelectron spectroscopy shows that GSHpx-bound Se undergoes substrate-induced redox change.	Bound Se may shuttle between R—SeH and a seleninyl (R—SeO—OH) or selenenyl (R—Se—OH) compound.	(26)
1977	Incubation of GSHpx with KCN at alkaline pH releases Se from enzyme and inhibits enzyme activity. GSHpx is protected from KCN inactivation by preincubation with GSH or other reducing agents.	Se is part of active site; there are at least two oxidation states of enzyme; oxidized form may be related to selenenic acid, since CN⁻ reacts with sulfenic acid derivatives of certain enzymes.	(38)

(continues)

Table 6.2 *(Continued)*

Year published	Finding	Implication	Reference
1978	[75]Se is removed from labeled GSHpx by derivatization with iodoacetate (by forming carboxymethyl derivative) and subsequent acid hydrolysis. [75]Se co-elutes with ^{3}H-Se-cysteine from anion exchange, cation exchange, and gel permeation columns.	Se in GSHpx is contained in Se-cysteine.	(27)
	[75]Se GSHpx derivatized with ^{14}C-iodoacetate results in 0.92 and 0.88 iodoacetates bound per Se in the intact protein and hydrolyzed sample, respectively.	The only iodoacetate-reactive site associated with enzyme activity is the Se moiety of the intact enzyme, i.e., Se—Cys is the active site.	
1979	X-Ray crystallography gives tentative amino acid sequence; shows that change from oxidized to reduced form is due to loss of one or more Se-bound oxygens.	Mechanism of action involves changes in binding of oxygen by Se.	(30)
1980	Three different oxidized forms of GSHpx are prepared and show different stabilities and sensitivities to CN⁻. "Form A," formed by autooxidation after separation of GSH from reduced form by gel filtration, rapidly loses activity at 25°C but not at 4°C. Reduced enzyme oxidized with H_2O_2 is stable and not sensitive to CN⁻. "Form C," incubated with GSH and then dialyzed under oxidizing conditions, has GSH tightly bound in equal ratio with Se and is rapidly inactivated by CN⁻.	The enzyme catalytic reaction may involve more than one oxidized form. An enzyme-GSH complex, such as E—SeSG or E—SeOSG may be an intermediate of the catalytic reaction.	(39) (40)
1980	CN⁻ removes GSH from Form C, forming GSCN but causing no loss of enzyme activity. The resulting enzyme form is then inhibitable by iodoacetate. Treatment of Form C with CN⁻ gives change in UV spectrum.	GSH is bound to Se at the active site. Form C underdoes reduction when treated with KCN and probably forms E—Se⁻.	(31)
1983	X-Ray crystallography gives evidence of a selenolate anion (E—Se⁻) rather than a free selenol (E—SeH) in the reduced enzyme at physiological pH and also of a seleninic (E—SeOOH) acid existing in the peroxide-oxidized enzyme.	Reduced form of enzyme is probably E—Se⁻.	(28)

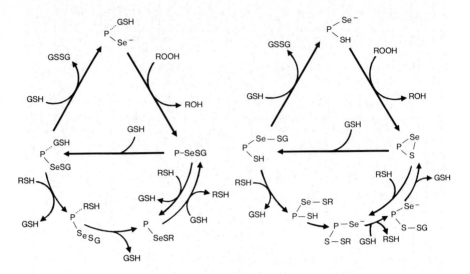

Fig. 6.3 Two possible mechanisms of action of selenium-containing glutathione peroxidase as proposed by Chaudiere *et al.*[41] P represents glutathione peroxidase, with selenium at the active site.

model requires that, in order to return to form F, the inhibited form H must incorporate GSH, form F must contain one bound molecule of GSH or be obtained from the decomposition of an intermediate that contained GSH. Therefore, form F cannot be a selenenic acid, as proposed in Ganther's model.

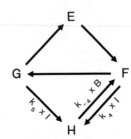

Fig. 6.4 The model of enzyme inhibition that best matched experimental data obtained using an inhibitor of glutathione peroxidase, according to Chaudiere *et al.*[41] E is the form of the enzyme that reacts with a peroxide; F and G are the two forms of the enzyme that react with glutathione. I represents an inhibitor and H, the inhibited form of the enzyme. B is glutathione. The k_4, k_{-4} and k_5 are rate constants.

III. BIOLOGICAL FUNCTION OF SELENIUM-DEPENDENT GLUTATHIONE PEROXIDASE

A. Cellular Oxidant Protection

Selenium-dependent glutathione peroxidase functions in the cell as part of a defense system against oxygen-induced damage. (For reviews of cellular oxidation and antioxidant defense systems, see references 42-45.) Sequential addition of electrons to oxygen can lead to a number of intermediates, some of which can interact with cell constituents, particularly membrane lipids, altering their structures and thereby affecting their roles.

$$O_2 \longrightarrow \underset{\text{(superoxide)}}{O_2^{\cdot-}} \longrightarrow O_2^{-2} \longrightarrow \underset{\text{(peroxide)}}{HO_2^{-}} \longrightarrow H_2O_2$$

The two intermediates, superoxide and peroxide, are particularly important, judging by the fact that animals have evolved several enzyme systems for their removal. Superoxide and peroxide can also be formed by endogenous enzyme systems, such as NADPH oxidase[46] and xanthine oxidase,[46,47] and by exogenous agents, such as carbon tetrachloride.[48] Although superoxide itself is relatively unreactive with unsaturated fatty acids,[46] in the presence of iron (Fe^{+3}), it can interact with peroxide to form the very reactive hydroxyl radical according to the Haber-Weiss reaction[46]:

$$O_2^{\cdot-} + Fe^{+3} \longrightarrow O_2 + Fe^{+2}$$

$$H_2O_2 + Fe^{+2} \longrightarrow \cdot OH + OH^- + Fe^{+3}$$

Whether hydroxyl radical is generated *in vivo* is controversial,[43,49] but it would be expected to be a very active initiator of lipid peroxidation. Singlet oxygen $^1O_2$ is also an initiator of lipid peroxidation, reacting very rapidly with unsaturated compounds[50]; it is thought to be produced in reactions secondary to superoxide generation[44] and also by several peroxidases.[51]

Whatever their source, free radicals are known to be produced in biological systems, and one consequence of free radical production is lipid peroxidation. A free radical initiator can interact with an unsaturated fatty acid to form a lipid free radical ($R\cdot$). This is followed by rearrangement of the double bonds and acceptance of molecular oxygen to form a fatty acid peroxyl radical ($ROO\cdot$). The peroxyl radical can then abstract a hydrogen from another unsaturated fatty acid, forming a fatty acid hydroperoxide ($ROOH$) and another fatty acid free radical, thus establishing a chain reaction. Furthermore, fatty acid peroxides may homolyze and lead to chain branching,[52] further increasing the production of lipid peroxides from a single initiator. Peroxidation of unsaturated fatty acid residues of phospholipids causes changes in bonding within the molecule as well as chain cleavage.[53] This alters its three-dimensional conformation and can alter the structural integrity of membranes in which they are found. The various free radical intermediates in the formation of lipid peroxides can also alter certain amino acids,[54] affecting proteins, including enzymes.[55] Formation of peroxides and free licals can be essential and beneficial, e.g., in polymorphonuclear leukocytes and macrophages for their bactericidal activity[56] or as intermediates in prostaglandin synthesis.[57] However, uncontrolled lipid peroxidation can be very detrimental to the cell.

The defense system against cellular damage due to free radical chain reactions attacks the process at several different stages. The enzyme superoxide dismutase can "dismute" superoxide to hydrogen peroxide:

$$O_2^- + O_2^- + 2\,H^+ \longrightarrow H_2O_2 + O_2$$

Hydrogen peroxide can be converted to water by SeGSHpx:

$$H_2O_2 + 2\,H^+ \longrightarrow 2\,H_2O$$

or to water and oxygen by the heme-containing enzyme, catalase:

$$H_2O_2 \longrightarrow H_2O + \tfrac{1}{2}\,O_2$$

Diminishing the amounts of these two components (O_2^- and H_2O_2) reduces the likelihood of free radical chain reactions. When free radicals are formed, however, they can be scavenged by alpha-tocopherol. This explains the long-observed relationship of vitamin E and Se, and why either one is sufficient to prevent certain disorders, such as exudative diathesis in chicks,[3] liver necrosis in rats,[2] and muscular dystrophy in lambs.[58]

Christophersen[37] showed that peroxides of free fatty acids, as well as hydrogen peroxide, could serve as substrates for SeGSHpx. It was, therefore, suggested that SeGSHpx could serve in the antioxidant defense system by reducing lipid hydroperoxides. McCay et al.[59] reported that when microsomes were incubated in a peroxidizing medium, there was loss of unsaturated fatty acids and accumulation of malonaldehyde, a product of chain cleavage. When a SeGSHpx system was added, however, both malonaldehyde (also called malondialdehyde) accumulation and fatty acid loss were inhibited. If SeGSHpx were reducing the fatty acid peroxides, the authors would have expected to find changes in the composition of fatty acids and appearance of hydroxy fatty acids. Neither were found.

The authors, therefore, concluded that SeGSHpx cannot reduce lipid peroxides when they are acylated, as in phospholipids of biological membranes, and that, therefore, SeGSHpx must act at the stage of reducing hydrogen peroxide and preventing initiation of lipid peroxidation. Grossman and Wendel[60] recently showed in a more direct manner that SeGSHpx did not act on linoleoyl hydroperoxide in phosphatidyl choline. When the peroxidized fatty acid was cleaved from the phospholipid by pancreatic phospholipase A_2, the SeGSHpx reaction proceeded. This supports McCay's contention that esterified fatty acids cannot be substrates for SeGSHpx.

Selenium-dependent glutathione peroxidase is found in the cytosol and the mitochondrial matrix of rat liver.[15,61] Presumably, the compartmentation is the same in other tissues and other species. This would support the hypothesis of McCay et al.[59] that SeGSHpx reduces hydrogen peroxide rather than lipid peroxides, as the lipid peroxides would be situated in the hydrophobic region of the membrane and would not be accessible to SeGSHpx.

B. Prostaglandin Metabolism

However, SeGSHpx is found in very high concentration in platelets[62] and its function there involves the reduction of lipid peroxides. Bryant et al.[63] showed that conversion of L-12-hydroperoxy-5,8,11,14-eicosatetraenoic acid (12-HPETE) in platelets is catalyzed by SeGSHpx. The metabolic pathways of arachidonic acid presented in Fig. 6.5 show that HPETE and other hydroxy acids inhibit prostacyclin synthase.[64] Bryant et al.[65] showed that platelets from Se-deficient rats accumulated seven times more HPETE than did platelets from Se-adequate rats. Therefore, if SeGSHpx activity were low, as in Se deficiency, the resulting accumulation of HPETE would result in an imbalance of prostacyclin and thromboxanes, leading to increased platelet aggregation and vasoconstriction. The recently reported work of Schiavon et al.,[66] using cultured endothelial cells from pig thoracic aorta, is consistent with this scheme. They found that addition of Se (form not specified) to their cell culture medium caused a dose-dependent rise in SeGSHpx activity and an increase in prostacyclin production from arachidonate. These same authors also found a significant increase in bleeding times in human subjects supplemented daily with 10 μg Se (as Na_2SeO_3)/kg bodyweight over a 6-week period. Also in support of this scheme, Guidi et al.[62] showed a reduction of thromboxane B_2 production from arachidonate-stimulated human platelet lysates when SeGSHpx was added to the incubation medium; however, they found no relationship between SeGSHpx activity and platelet aggregation. The absence of an inverse correlation between SeGSHpx activity and

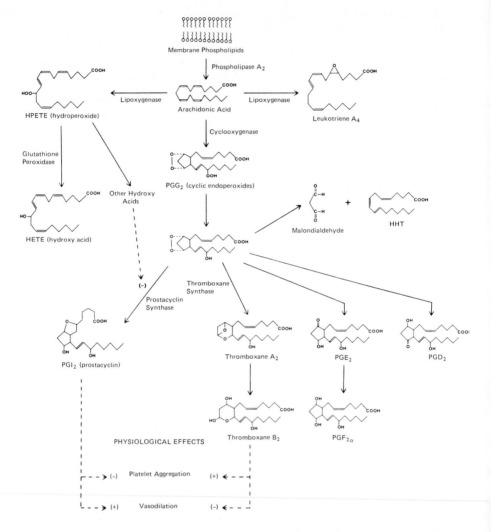

Fig. 6.5 Metabolic pathways of arachidonic acid. SeGSHpx catalyzes conversion of HPETE to HETE. In Se deficiency, accumulation of HPETE causes inhibition of prostacyclin synthase. PG is Prostagliandin.

aggregation, as would be expected by the proposed scheme, is likely due to SeGSHpx never being low in this experiment. Manipulations of SeGSHpx were done by addition of purified enzyme to lysates of normal platelets.

Levander et al.[270] found that the production of prostacyclin-like activity by rat aortas was depressed by 22% due to nutritional Se deficiency and the resultant decrease of SeGSHpx in that tissue. This was thought to relate to increases in plasma lipoperoxides in Se deficiency, which caused an imbalance of the ratio of thromboxane : prostacyclin.

Another possible role of SeGSHpx in prostaglandin metabolism is in the protection of prostaglandin dehydrogenase, a key enzyme in the degradation pathway of prostaglandins. This enzyme has been shown to be depressed under conditions of normobaric hyperoxia,[67] resulting in a rise in vasoconstrictors due to inactivation of the breakdown of prostaglandins. While this may not be the cause of the signs of pulmonary toxicity (edema, congestion, capillary endothelial necrosis), due to excess oxygen, the decline in prostaglandin dehydrogenase activity coincides with onset of signs. North et al.[68] reported that supplementing rats' diets with 600 IU vitamin E/kg maintained nearly 50% of the prostaglandin dehydrogenase activity of lung tissue when the rats were exposed to hyperoxia. Those rats consuming the unsupplemented basal diet (15 IU vitamin E/kg) and exposed to hyperoxia maintained only about 5% of the activity measured in air. Likewise, supplementation of the diet with 0.1 ppm Se (the basal diet contained 0.05 ppm of inherent Se) resulted in significant protection of prostaglandin dehydrogenase. It is presumed that the protective effect on the enzyme occurs through antioxidant activity and that, therefore, Se must in this case function through its role in SeGSHpx. However, in the above-mentioned study, SeGSHpx was not measured.

C. Selenium-Dependent Glutathione Peroxidase in Plasma

The fact that SeGSHpx also occurs in plasma raises the question: What are the source and function of GSHpx in plasma? According to Meister and Anderson,[69] GSH concentrations in plasma are very low (micromolar concentrations, compared to millimolar concentrations in mammalian cells). Flohé et al.[33] reported that the apparent K_m of SeGSHpx for GSH ranges from 10^{-7} to $10^{-4} M$ when the steady-state concentration of peroxide ranges from nanomolar to micromolar amounts. Thus, the concentration of GSH in plasma may be sufficient to allow SeGSHpx to reduce peroxide and hydroperoxides. However, GSH reductase activity in plasma is very low[70] and probably cannot regenerate reduced GSH at a rate sufficient to support significant SeGSHpx activity.

More likely than having a significant protective role against oxidation, plasma SeGSHpx may have no particular function; rather, it may merely spill over from other tissues in which it is abundant. In a study with chicks that had been severely depleted of Se and then re-fed very low levels (0.01-0.04 ppm) of Se for 5 days, Combs et al.[71] found that 12 hrs after a single injection of 2 μg Se (as Na_2SeO_3) per 100 g body weight, plasma SeGSHpx correlated well with the dietary supplemental Se level, and not with the dose of Se injected (Table 6.3). At 0.02 ppm dietary Se, plasma SeGSHpx before injection of selenite was not different from that of the unsupplemented group, but the subsequent increase due to the injected selenite was much greater. This suggests that only when the amount of Se (and, therefore, SeGSHpx) in tissues reached a certain minimum was there a spilling of SeGSHpx into plasma.

Plasma SeGSHpx activity is well correlated with dietary Se intake when the latter is suboptimal, and with tissue levels of SeGSHpx in general.[70,72] It is, therefore, frequently used as a convenient measure of nutritional status with respect to Se. It seems likely, however, that when there is tissue damage (e.g., liver or kidney), SeGSHpx from damaged cells may be introduced into the plasma. In such cases, plasma SeGSHpx measurements may give erroneously elevated indications of nutritional Se status.

D. Other Glutathione Peroxidase Activities Not Dependent on Selenium

Selenium-dependent glutathione peroxidase is not the only enzyme with peroxidase activity that uses glutathione. There is a non-Se-dependent GSHpx that was discovered when considerable GSHpx activity (assayed with lipid hydroperoxides as substrates) was found in livers of Se-depleted rats.[73] This enzyme, subsequently shown to be identical with GSH S-transferase B,[74,75] differs from SeGSHpx in its kinetics, physical properties, substrate specificities, and susceptibility to inhibition by cyanide or iodoacetate.[74,75]

Cumene hydroperoxide and various other hydroperoxides can serve as substrate for both SeGSHpx and non-Se-dependent GSHpx,[75] but the non-Se-dependent enzyme shows very little affinity for H_2O_2.[73] Thus, measuring GSHpx activity using H_2O_2 as substrate will indicate only the Se-dependent enzyme. However, assessment of Se status by measuring GSHpx activity with a lipid hydroperoxide substrate in tissues with both enzymes can give erroneously high results.

In attempting to determine the relative amounts of Se-dependent and non-Se-dependent GSHpx in a tissue preparation, it is not legitimate to subtract the activity measured using H_2O_2 from that measured using a lipid hydroperoxide (e.g., cumene hydroperoxide, t-butyl hydroperoxide) unless the concentrations of the two different substrates are selected so as to give equal rates of activity with the Se-dependent enzyme. The proper concentrations may be determined empirically after physical separation of the two enzymes (e.g., by gel filtration). Of course, relative amounts of the two enzymes can also be determined by physically separating the enzymes for each sample and measuring activity for each with a lipid hydroperoxide.

Table 6.3

Effect of Low Dietary Supplements of Sodium Selenite and Injected Sodium Selenite on Plasma Glutathione Peroxidase in Severely Depleted Chicks[a]

Dietary Se (ppm)	Time after Se injection[b] (hrs)	Plasma SeGSHpx (nmoles NADPH/min/mg protein)[c]
0	0	.31 ± .05
	12	.57 ± .06
.01	0	.35 ± .01
	12	.54 ± .03
.02	0	.29 ± .03
	12	.70 ± .05
.03	0	.47 ± .06
	12	1.07 ± .05

[a]Chicks were fed a low-Se diet (0.007 ppm) for 19 days after hatching and then were fed diets supplemented with Se at the indicated levels for 5 days.
[b]With 2 μg Se/100 g body weight, subcutaneous.
[c]Each value is the mean of three composite samples of six chicks each.

The proportions of total GSHpx activity that are attributable to the Se-dependent and the non-Se-dependent forms vary among tissues. A study by Lawrence and Burk[73] showed that in the rat, adrenal gland and liver had considerable non-Se-dependent GSHpx activity, amounting to about 35% of total GSHpx activity, whereas in the heart and lung, non-Se-dependent GSHpx was not detectable. Most of the total GSHpx activity in testis was from the non-Se enzyme, but total activity per milligram protein was quite small compared to that of liver. Livers of some other species were reported by the same authors to contain a comparatively greater percentage of the GSHpx activity as the non-Se-dependent enzyme: guinea pig, 100%; human, 84%; chicken, 70%; pig, 67%; sheep, 81%.[76] However, the nutritional backgrounds of these animals were not known. In nutritional Se deficiency, SeGSHpx activity is reduced and, in some species, glutathione S-transferase activity is elevated.[74] Therefore, the reported differences among species in the relative amounts of the two enzymes may have been due to differences in nutritional Se status. Another factor that adds uncertainty to reports of relative proportions of Se-dependent and non-Se-dependent GSHpx in tissue is the diurnal variation in activity exhibited by those enzymes. Davies et al.[77] showed that mouse hepatic GSH S-transferase activity reached a high plateau during hours of darkness, while hepatic SeGSHpx reached its low point during that time. Cupp[78] also observed a circadian rhythm of SeGSHpx activity in chick duodenum in organ culture.

Lee et al.[79] reported that nearly half of the total GSHpx activity in rabbit liver is due to the non-Se-dependent form and that total activity is nearly twice that of rat liver. If the dietary Se intakes of the compared animals were equivalent, this might explain why rats show liver necrosis in combined Se- and vitamin E-deficiency but similarly nourished rabbits do not.[79] However, both chickens and pigs would appear to have low total GSHpx activity in liver, a large proportion of which is the non-Se-dependent form, according to the results of Lawrence and Burk[76]; yet pigs develop liver necrosis in Se-deficiency, and Se-deficient chickens do not.

Another enzyme, different from SeGSHpx and GSH S-transferase B but also having GSHpx activity, has been reported in pig liver,[80] heart,[81] and brain.[82] This enzyme, called by Ursini et al.[82] "peroxidation inhibiting protein," or PIP, can reduce phosphatidyl choline hydroperoxides. Rabbit liver microsomes incubated with PIP and glutathione in a peroxidation-promoting system showed 90% inhibition of malonaldehyde formation, but only if the rabbits were fed adequate amounts of vitamin E.[82] The dependence of PIP on vitamin E has not yet been explained. Further studies by Ursini et al.[287] indicate that PIP is an Se-containing enzyme with many of the characteristics (e.g., kinetic properties, inhibitor sensitivity, amino acid content, substrate specificity) of SeGSHpx, but with a molecular weight of only ca. 23,000. It is possible that PIP, renamed by Ursini et al.[287] as "phospolipid hydroperoxide glutathione peroxidase" may prove to be a distinct selenoenzyme with a function similar to that of SeGSHpx. Its many apparent similarities to SeGSHpx suggest that it may actually be a catalytically active monomeric form of the latter enzyme.

E. Organic Selenium Compound with Peroxidase-Catalyzing Activity

A nonprotein, organic Se-compound, 1-phenyl-1,2-benzoisoselenazol-3 (PZ51)*, has been shown to have GSHpx activity with hydrogen peroxide and lipid hydroperoxides as substrates.[83-85] This synthetic Se compound has anti-inflammatory properties[84] and also behaves as an antioxidant, as shown by its ability to increase the lag time before the onset of lipid peroxidation in isolated hepatocytes.[85] The Se in PZ51 was found not to be available to mice for synthesis of SeGSHpx.[83,84] Because of its innate GSHpx activity and its inability to serve as a Se source, PZ51 may prove to be very valuable for investigating nutritional roles of Se that may not involve SeGSHpx.

*Ebselen, A. Nattermann & Cie. GmbH, Cologne, West Germany.

IV. EFFECTS OF DRUGS ON SELENIUM-DEPENDENT GLUTATHIONE PEROXIDASE

Chaudiere *et al.*[41,271] found that two classes of drugs commonly used in the treatment of arthritis, mercaptocarboxylic acids (e.g., penicillamine) and gold compounds (e.g., aurothioglucose), are potent inhibitors of SeGSHpx purified from hamster liver. Each type of drug inhibits SeGSHpx at a different point in its reaction sequence. The mercaptocarboxylic acids are competitive inhibitors of GSH binding to the enzyme; the gold compounds competitively inhibit the peroxide-binding step. Mercurio and Combs[272] showed that these drugs also inhibit crude hepatic SeGSHpx from the chick by the same mechanisms. They also potentiated the manifestation of signs (i.e., exudative diathesis) when given parenterally to vitamin E-deficient chicks fed marginal levels of Se, indicating their inhibitory activities *in vivo*. While both classes of drugs have been used as antiarthritic agents, these effects on SeGSHpx are the only common mechanisms reported to date. Baker *et al.*[273] found that aurothioglucose interacted with Se status to affect the responses of rats to adjuvant. The effects of the drugs may not be specific for SeGSHpx, as Mercurio and Combs[272] found each to inhibit chick liver catalase.

Other drugs (i.e., xenobiotic agents) have been shown to produce decreases in SeGSHpx activities in animal models. These include tri-*o*-cresylphosphate,[274] doxorubicin,[275,276] and polychlorinated biphenyls.[277] High levels of dietary silver (e.g., 750 ppm Ag as silver acetate) also reduce tissue SeGSHpx activities.[278] In the latter case, Ag may remove Se from the metabolically available pool by co-precipitation as selenides; however, the possible mechanisms for these other effects are largely unstudied. Swanson[274] found that tri-*o*-cresylphosphate (at 0.2% of the diet) reduced tissue Se residues apparently by increasing Se excretion (particularly via fecal elimination), but direct effects on SeGSHpx were not investigated. Doxorubicin does not affect SeGSHpx *in vitro*,[275] yet it reduces cardiac activities transiently after drug treatment. These effects are likely to be the results of the cardiotoxicity of the drug (hepatic SeGSHpx activities may be increased within the same time period) rather than those relating to specific antagonisms of Se or SeGSHpx.

V. OTHER FUNCTIONS OF SELENIUM

A. Modification of Drug Metabolism and Toxicity by Selenium

In addition to lowered SeGSHpx levels, nutritional Se-deficiency is accompanied by changes in hepatic enzymes and substrates involved in the metabolism and detoxification of drugs and other foreign compounds.

Some of these enzymes, including the cytochrome P_{450}-dependent mixed function oxidases, transform xenobiotics by such reactions as hydroxylation, dealkylation, deamination, and desulfuration. The transformations, which occur mainly in endoplasmic reticulum of liver and are referred to as Phase I reactions of drug metabolism, may activate a drug, inactivate a previously active form, or create a toxic intermediate. Most of these reactions result in a product that is more water-soluble than the parent compound, thus promoting its renal clearance. The enzymes catalyzing Phase I reactions are versatile and nonspecific. The so-called Phase II reactions are conjugations catalyzed by transferases. The conjugating moieties are generally common intermediates of large molecular size, such as GSH or UDP* glucuronide, and with strong hydrophilic properties, which make the conjugates readily excretable. The conjugates are devoid of pharmacologic activity and are nontoxic.

The changes brought about in the drug metabolizing and detoxifying enzymes by Se-deficiency are not in the same direction for all enzymes; they are not necessarily of the same magnitude or even in the same direction in different species. Reiter and Wendel[86] showed in vitamin E-adequate mice that activities of certain cytosolic enzymes, such as some GSH S-transferases and GSSG reductase, were elevated in long-term (4-month) Se deprivation, while others, such as GSH thioltransferase and sulfotransferase, were simultaneously decreased. These changes did not occur until GSHpx had fallen to 5% or less of the control (Se-fed) level. Of the microsomal enzyme activities examined, cytochrome P_{450}-dependent hydroperoxidase, heme oxygenase, and UDP-glucuronyl transferase were raised; NADPH-cytochrome P_{450} reductase and flavin-containing monooxygenase were lowered; NADH-cytochrome b_5 reductase, analine hydroxylase, and aminopyrine N-demethylase were largely unchanged.[86] Shull et al.[87] reported a significant decrease in aminopyrine N-demethylase activity and in monocrotaline metabolism in liver microsomes of male rats maintained with a low-Se, *Torula* yeast-based diet for 11 months. No changes occurred in those mixed function oxidase activities of females treated similarly. They also found a decrease in aniline hydroxylase in Se-deficient males. (It was not measured in females.) Pilch and Combs[88] did not detect any change due to alteration of Se status in aminopyrine N-demethylation or aniline hydroxylation in vitamin E-adequate chicks, whether male or female, but the chicks were only 13 days old at the termination of the experiment. Perhaps that was insufficient time to bring about changes in the mixed function oxidases. In their studies with Se-deficient mice, Reiter and Wendel[86] observed no changes in enzymes other than GSHpx until the 17th day, with plateaus of change not reached for another 30-40 days.

*Uridine diphosphate.

Glutathione *S*-transferase and UDP-glucuronyl transferase have been shown to be elevated in uncomplicated Se deficiency (i.e., Se deficiency produced using a diet adequate in other nutrients, including vitamin E) in liver of the rat[89-91] and the mouse.[86,92] Masukawa *et al.*[90] showed a 75% increase in GSH *S*-transferase activity (assayed with 1-chloro-2,4-dinitrobenzene as substrate) in rat liver, a smaller change in kidney (20%), and no significant changes in brain, heart, lung, and testis. The activity in testis was high, equaling that in Se-deficient liver, regardless of Se status. Burk and Lane[89] reported an increase in rat liver GSH *S*-transferase, due to Se deficiency, of similar magnitude. Reiter and Wendel[86] found that GSH *S*-transferase in the mouse was about doubled after 60 days of Se depletion. In the chick, no change in GSH *S*-transferase was noted after 2 weeks of consuming a Se-deficient diet.[91] The GSH *S*-transferase levels of Se-adequate chicks were lower (one-half or less) than those of rats or mice. Increases in UDP-glucuronyl transferase were similarly large in rats[91] and mice[92] in Se-deficiency, while in chicks, a small amount was detected in the Se-deficient group and none in the Se-adequate group.[91]

The activities of drug metabolizing enzymes, particularly of the cytochromes P_{450}, can also be modulated by various inducers and inhibitors. Of special interest in relation to Se is phenobarbital, which induces cytochromes P_{450} and b_5 and NADPH-cytochrome *c* reductase in rat liver.[93] Burk and Masters[93] showed that the induction of cytochrome P_{450} is impaired by nutritional Se deficiency, with induction in rat liver being 1.7-fold in Se-deficiency and 2.5-fold in Se-adequacy. The induction of cytochrome b_5 and NADPH-cytochrome *c* reductase was independent of nutritional Se status, however. Stimulation of the same parameters by 3-methylcholanthrene, another inducer, was not altered by Se-deficiency. The dampening of phenobarbital induction by Se-deficiency was evident on the activity of ethylmorphine demethylase but not on that of biphenyl hydroxylase. Whether this could be explained by the presence of Se in certain cytochromes and not in others is not known. It is unlikely that it is explainable by oxidative destruction of certain cytochromes due to the absence of SeGSHpx in Se-deficiency, since, when microsomal preparations from Se-deficient or Se-adequate livers were stored, there was virtually no destruction of cytochrome P_{450} between 2 and 24 hrs. Also, inclusion of alpha-tocopherol in the homogenizing medium was without effect, suggesting that oxidative processes were not responsible for this response.[94]

Pilch and Combs[88] detected no inhibition of phenobarbital induction of cytochrome P_{450} in Se-deficient chicks. Aminopyrine N-demethylation and aniline hydroxylation were less induced by phenobarbital only in male chicks that were deficient in both vitamin E and Se. Females were not thus affected. Siami et al.[95] reported that Se-deficient female rats were not subject to inhibition of induction of mixed function oxidase activity by phenobarbital; however, rats did respond to dietary Se. Apparently, then, there are not only species differences in the effect of Se status on the response to phenobarbital but also sex differences.

Because different xenobiotics are metabolized in different ways, the changes in drug metabolizing enzymes brought about by nutritional Se-deficiency can cause certain toxic compounds to be made more toxic and others to be made less toxic. In order to interpret experimental findings about the effects of changes in Se status on the toxicity of drugs and other xenobiotics, it is necessary to be aware of the types of intermediates of drug metabolism and of the processes which manifest toxicity. According to Mitchell et al.,[96] reactive intermediates responsible for toxic effects can be divided into four categories:

i. Electrophilic alkylators: (e.g., acetaminophen)	Form conjugates with GSH Deplete GSH concentration Bind covalently to macromolecules Show sulfhydryl protective effect
ii. Electrophilic alkylators: (e.g., furosemide)	Do not affect GSH concentration Bind covalently to macromolecules Have no sulfhydryl protective effect
iii. Radical alkylators (e.g., carbon tetrachloride)	Alkylate proteins and lipids Do not affect GSH concentration
iv. Generators of active oxygen (e.g., paraquat, nitrofurantoin)	Nonalkylating Usually do not affect GSH concentration, but more toxic with prior GSH depletion More toxic with vitamin E deficiency

Manifestations of toxicity result from inactivation of critical cellular molecules or loss of integrity of membranes due to structural changes in constituent molecules. Alkylating or arylating intermediates of xenobiotic metabolism can covalently bind to cell macromolecules, such as DNA, RNA, and proteins (including enzymes), thus incapacitating them for their normal functions. Free radical intermediates and various forms of reactive oxygen can cause lipid peroxidation. Peroxidation of fatty acids contained in membranes can lead to changes in three-dimensional structure of the lipid molecules, thus interrupting order in the membrane. Also, products of lipid peroxidation (or of the breakdown of peroxides), such as malonaldehyde, can bind to cell macromolecules.

Toxicity can be manifested as cell damage, recognizable upon histological examination or by appearance in the plasma of enzymes or other metabolites that are usually contained only within cells (e.g., plasma GOT).* In some cases, however, animals may die from xenobiotic toxicity with no apparent cell damage. Lipid peroxidation is another process understood to be a manifestation of toxicity and that is often accompanied by cell damage.

Lipid peroxidation has been determined in biological systems by several methods, including measurement of diene conjugates, malonaldehyde, fluorescent products resulting from reaction of malonaldehyde with amino groups of amino acids and proteins, and volatile hydrocarbons (especially pentane and ethane). Malonaldehyde, often reported as thiobarbituric acid (TBA)-reactive substances, is a nonvolatile breakdown product of lipid peroxides. It must be measured in incubations of tissue preparations (i.e., *in vitro*). Its accuracy in estimating lipid peroxidation that has occurred *in vivo* is questionable, since it can bind to sulfhydryl and amino groups of proteins,[97] and it can be metabolized *in vivo* and *in vitro*.[98] However, alteration of its production by the presence or absence of antioxidants shows that it is an indicator of lipid peroxidation and can, therefore, be useful. Measurements in exhaled air of pentane, a product of breakdown of peroxides of ω-6 fatty acids[99,100] and ethane, from peroxides of ω-3 fatty acids[100,101] have been reported to correlate well with malonaldehyde measurements[102] and with mortality resulting from carbon tetrachloride toxicity.[101] Other volatile hydrocarbons, such as hexanal and acetone, are not as reliable indicators of lipid peroxidation, since they can arise from other sources as well.[103] Although there is little doubt that tissue metabolism can produce pentane and ethane,[104] there is uncertainty as to how great a contribution is made by gut microorganisms to the measured volatile hydrocarbons excreted by a living animal. Hafeman and Hoekstra[101] reported that if rats were not fasted, ethane values were high, especially if a diet containing cod liver oil (high in ω-3 fatty acids) was fed. In their studies with carbon tetrachloride-induced lipid peroxidation, however, those authors[101] were satisfied that, when rats were fasted, ethane evolving from peroxidation of external lipids was insignificant in comparison to that resulting from tissue metabolism. They found that carbon tetrachloride caused lipid peroxidation only in tissues where it was being metabolized, and treatments that inhibit its metabolism also reduced lipid peroxidation. Although standard errors of measured ethane production among similarly treated animals can be large, sometimes greatly exceeding the mean, ethane or pentane production remains useful as a noninvasive index of lipid peroxidation *in vivo* as well as being applicable *in vitro*.

*Glutamic-oxalacetic transaminase.

While lipid peroxidation is sometimes accompanied by liver necrosis, the two are not always correlated, as shown by Burk and Lane[89] with a number of different xenobiotics. As a toxic effect of xenobiotics, lipid peroxidation is likely to be significant only for those compounds that are metabolized to free radicals, those that generate active oxygen, or those that deplete tissue GSH concentrations.

As mentioned before, because of the different ways in which xenobiotics can be metabolized, the changes in drug metabolism occurring during Se-deficiency can cause certain compounds to be more toxic and others to be less toxic. In the first class are such compounds as nitrofurantoin,[105,106] an antibacterial agent used for treatment of urinary tract infections, and paraquat, an herbicide. Both are metabolized to form free radicals and, subsequently, active oxygen (superoxide, singlet oxygen).[107-109] The increased oxygen uptake by mouse lung microsomes treated with nitrofurantoin can be partially inhibited by superoxide dismutase, partially by catalase, and with an additive effect when the two enzymes are added together,[108] verifying that superoxide and hydrogen peroxide have been formed. It is attractive to reason that the protective effect of Se against this form of toxicity is due to removal of H_2O_2 by SeGSHpx and consequent retardation of lipid peroxidation. In accord with this thinking is the finding by Burk and Lane[110] of acute tubular necrosis in kidneys of Se-deficient rats that had been treated with nitrofurantoin but no lesions in similarly treated Se-adequate rats. Although the necrosis in the kidney was associated with elevated ethane production and could, therefore, be attributed to peroxidation, it was not evident that the necrosis was the cause of death. Similarly, in rats given lethal doses of paraquat or diquat (another herbicide), liver necrosis and elevated ethane production were evident in those rats deficient in Se but not in the Se-adequate controls.[110] The absence of increased ethane production or liver lesions suggests that the cause of death in the controls was not lipid peroxidation and raises questions concerning the cause of death in the Se-deficient animals.

Nitrofurantoin is thought to undergo redox cycling, catalyzed by NADPH-cytochrome c reductase, and producing superoxide anion.[108] Because the reductase reaction consumes NADPH, death from nitrofurantoin may be due to NADPH depletion. However, the protective role of Se, if Se is functioning through SeGSHpx, appears inconsistent with that hypothesis, since the SeGSHpx system also uses NADPH. Another observation is that GSH is depleted by nitrofurantoin in erythrocytes.[111,112] However, GSH concentrations are elevated in Se deficiency in the rat[110] and chick,[113] and should reduce rather than increase the toxicity of the drug if GSH depletion is the cause of toxicity and death.

Nitrofurantoin has been shown to cause formation of methemoglobin and superoxide from oxyhemoglobin.[111,112] The degree of loss of oxygen-carrying capacity has not been quantitated but should be considered as a possible cause of death. At the present time, the metabolic basis of the protective role of Se in the toxicities of nitrofurantoin and other oxidant drugs remains unexplained.

Certain other compounds, such as iodipamide, acetaminophen, and aflatoxin B_1, have been reported by Burk and Lane[89] to be rendered less toxic to rats by nutritional Se-deficiency. The protection from toxicity is thought not to be associated with a function of Se per se, but instead with the increases in GSH S-transferase and in GSH that accompany Se-deficiency.[89] In addition to at least one of the family of GSH S-transferases having peroxidase activity,[114] the GSH S-transferases also can bind (and thereby inactivate) hydrophobic compounds.[115] Through their transferase activities, these conjugate foreign compounds with GSH, thereby promoting their excretion.

The reduction in toxicity afforded by nutritional Se deficiency is not consistent among species, however. When Chen et al.[91] administered aflatoxin B_1 to Se-deficient, vitamin E-adequate rats, the animals showed less binding of aflatoxin to hepatic DNA, RNA, and protein than did the Se- and vitamin E-adequate rats, presumably because more of the aflatoxin had been conjugated. This is consistent with the observed elevations of conjugating enzymes observed in the Se-deficient rat liver. In chicks, however, Chen et al.[116] found no changes in binding of aflatoxin to liver macromolecules in Se-deficiency when vitamin E was adequate. This difference between rats and chicks may be due to the lack of enzyme induction and to the relatively low normal activities of the conjugating enzymes in the chick compared to those in the rat.[91] Activity of glutathione S-transferase, with 1-chloro-2,4-dinitrobenzene as substrate, has been found in Se-deficient rat liver to be 1.4 μmoles substrate conjugated/min/mg protein[89] and that in Se-deficient chick liver to be 0.11 μmoles/min/mg protein.[117] The activity of UDP-glucuronide transferase has been reported in rat liver as 38.4 nmoles p-nitrophenol conjugated/min/mg protein and in Se-deficient chick liver as 1.8 nmoles/min/mg protein.[91] The low activities of these conjugating enzymes could explain the absence of a decline in binding of macromolecules by aflatoxin in Se-deficient chick liver. When vitamin E, as well as Se, was inadequate, there was an increase in binding of aflatoxin to cell macromolecules.[116] Although the explanation of this is not known, it is possible that the combined deficiency resulted in some loss of cell integrity, leaving cell constituents less available to conjugating processes and more vulnerable to binding by aflatoxin.

In even more contrast to rats, turkey poults were found to be protected against aflatoxin toxicity by dietary supplements of Se. Gregory and Edds[118] reported that beginning with 0.1 ppm dietary Se, increasing the level of Se resulted in increasing ratios of conjugated to free aflatoxin but with no accompanying changes in activities of conjugating enzymes or in the amount of cytochrome P_{450}. However, activities of certain cytochrome P_{450} isozymes can change without a significant change in the amounts of total cytochrome P_{450} being evident.[119] Since the different P_{450} isozymes differ in activity with respect to particular substrates and also in the products formed from those substrates, it is possible that a change in proportion or distribution of those isozymes could be induced by a change in Se status and thereby affect the rate of activation of aflatoxin or the products formed and the subsequent rates of conjugation or binding.

Acetaminophen, another drug that is rendered less toxic to rats by Se deficiency,[89] is metabolized to a toxic intermediate by the cytochrome P_{450} system [120,121] and then de-toxified by conjugation to glutathione. However, only a relatively small fraction is transformed to the toxic intermediate; most is conjugated with glucuronide or sulfate and excreted as those conjugates.[122-125] Thus, the increase in activity of UDP-glucuronyl transferase that accompanies Se deficiency in the rat[91] probably results in a greater degree of conjugation of the parent compound and a lesser degree of transformation to the toxic intermediate. Glutathione concentration, also increased in rat liver during Se deficiency, probably contributes to an increased rate of conjugation of the toxic intermediate. The elevated activity of GSH S-transferase may contribute to a greater rate of conjugation of the toxic intermediate, but there is evidence that the conjugation occurs by spontaneous adduct formation rather than by enzyme catalysis.[123-125]

In spite of a reported increase in GSH S-transferase in mouse liver during long-term Se deficiency,[86] Peterson[126] found that Se-deficient mice did not respond the same as rats to acetaminophen. In mice fed a low-Se *Torula* yeast-based diet for 9 weeks, the LD_{50} was 167 mg acetaminophen/kg body weight compared to 374 mg/kg in the Se-adequate mice, i.e., Se-deficiency made the mice more susceptible to acetaminophen toxicity. In perfused mouse liver, Thelen and Wendel[127] found that elevated ethane release preceded release by the liver of lactate dehydrogenase, an enzyme whose appearance in plasma indicates cell damage. This led the authors to suggest that lipid peroxidation was not a consequence of cell destruction but may have been the cause. If lipid peroxidation is responsible for toxicity of acetaminophen in mice, it is easy to see how nutritional Se-deficiency would exacerbate that toxicity. By chemically inducing and inhibiting the monoxygenase systems of GSH-depleted mice, Wendel and Feuerstein[128] were able to manipulate *in vivo* ethane production caused by treatment with acetaminophen, suggesting that a metabolic intermediate of acetaminophen was causing lipid peroxidation. Acetaminophen caused little ethane production in uninduced, Se-adequate mice that had been pretreated with diethylmaleate to deplete liver GSH. In similarly treated Se-deficient mice, however, ethane production was very high. These observations led the authors to propose that acetaminophen must be metabolized to a free radical, which causes lipid peroxidation in the absence of GSHpx. Still, it is not clear that lipid peroxidation is the cause of toxicity of acetaminophen. In fact, noninduced mice given 500 mg acetaminophen/kg had less lipid peroxidation and greater mortality than did induced mice given 300 mg/kg. This suggests that lipid peroxidation is not the cause of death in acetaminophen toxicity.

As can be seen from the preceding discussion, the nature of the relationship between Se and drug metabolism is not clear. Although nutritional Se deficiency may result in the increased toxicity of a foreign compound, lipid peroxidation may or may not be increased in the presence of that compound, and cause of death cannot be attributed to lipid peroxidation. Hence, the role of Se in protection against drug toxicity may have nothing to do with its antioxidant function via SeGSHpx. Indeed, the alterations in drug metabolizing enzymes induced in mice by Se deficiency appear not to be mediated by SeGSHpx. Reiter and Wendel[86] showed that after mice had been fed an Se-deficient diet long enough for activities of drug metabolizing enzymes to reach new steady state levels, a single dose of 7 μg Se (as Na_2SeO_3) per kilogram body weight was sufficient to reduce the changes in enzyme activity by 50%, i.e., returning them toward their control levels. At that dose, SeGSHpx was still undetectable; to attain 50% repletion of SeGSHpx required a dose more than 10 times greater.

B. Effects of Selenium on the Metabolism of Glutathione

As mentioned previously, the plasma concentration of GSH increases in Se deficiency.[110] Rotruck et al.[8] also reported that the concentration of GSH in red blood cells was elevated in Se deficiency. However, Hill and Burk[282] found no increase in intracellular concentration of GSH in liver, heart, kidney, brain, or testis of Se-deficient rats. Using isolated rat hepatocytes, Hill and Burk[282] showed that, although initial intracellular GSH concentrations were the same in control and Se-deficient cells, the amount of GSH released to the medium by Se-deficient cells during a 5-hr incubation was nearly twice that of control cells, and the intracellular GSH concentration of the Se-deficient cells was 1.4 times that of the control cells. A conclusion that hepatic GSH synthesis is accelerated by Se-deficiency is supported by the finding of increased (nearly doubled) activity of gamma-glutamylcysteine synthetase activity in Se-deficient liver.

Glutathione has been shown to be released by the hepatocyte into blood and bile.[283] Se-deficiency affects only the release into blood.[282] The renal clearance of glutathione (including oxidized and nonoxidized forms) is elevated in Se-deficiency. Using ^{35}S-GSH, Hill and Burk[284] showed that kidneys of normal rats removed 69% of the GSH presented, while those of Se-deficient rats removed 76%. Renal clearance was 1.6 times greater in Se-deficient rats than in controls.[284]

Hill and Burk[285] also showed that addition of sulfur-containing amino acids to the incubation medium of hepatocytes increased the intracellular concentration of GSH. Addition of propargylglycine, a noncompetitive inhibitor of cystathionase, to the medium prevented the increase in GSH accumulation, although the amount of GSH released to the medium was unaffected. This suggests that the synthesis of GSH during Se deficiency is substrate limited. Combs et al.[286] observed that addition of cysteine to a Se-deficient diet partially overcame growth depression of chicks, whereas an equimolar addition of methionine did not. Perhaps the addition of cysteine provided enough of the amino acid to accommodate the increased capacity for GSH production while still allowing enough for more protein synthesis. Methionine, on the other hand, may not be converted sufficiently fast to cysteine to provide for normal protein synthesis as well as increased GSH production.

C. Modification of Heme Metabolism by Selenium

Another phenomenon that suggests a metabolic role for Se other than as a constituent of SeGSHpx is the net loss of heme observed in rat liver and intestinal mucosal cells in nutritional Se-deficiency. Burk and Correia[129] reported that the activity of microsomal heme oxygenase, the rate-limiting enzyme in heme catabolism, was higher in rats fed a Se-deficient diet for 6 months than in Se-adequate controls. Homogenate cytochrome P_{450}, which is composed of heme-containing proteins, was lower. Since heme oxygenase can be induced by increased heme concentration, these authors subsequently used various agents to elevate heme levels and found that in Se deficiency, heme synthesis was similar to and sometimes less than that of controls.[130] The induction of heme oxygenase, then, was not from increased synthesis of heme. They showed further that activity of tryptophan pyrrolase, a heme-containing enzyme, was impaired in Se deficiency and concluded that induction of heme oxygenase in Se-deficient rats is caused by an increase in heme concentration resulting from impairments in its utilization.[130] Injection of a small dose of heme, insufficient to induce heme oxygenase in control rats, caused a significant induction of the enzyme in the Se-deficient rats, supporting the hypothesis that the heme-binding capacity of Se-deficient rat liver is impaired. The role of Se in heme utilization is apparently not related to SeGSHpx. In Se-depleted rats, an injection of Na_2SeO_3 restored microsomal heme oxygenase to normal by 12 hrs, but during that period there was no significant increase in SeGSHpx.[129]

The case for the effect of Se on heme metabolism being through a mechanism other than SeGSHpx function is even more clear in the intestinal mucosa. Pascoe et al.[131] showed that feeding rats a Se-deficient diet for a single day resulted in a significant drop in villous tip cell cytochrome P_{450} content and activity [measured as activities of arylhydrocarbon hydroxylase and ethoxyresorufin O-deethylase activities (EROD)]. Selenium-dependent glutathione peroxidase activity remained unaltered to that time. After the rats had been fed the Se-deficient for sufficient time to reduce villous tip SeGSHpx (about 3 days), refeeding of Se resulted in recovery of EROD activity before a change in SeGSHpx was evident. Pascoe et al.[131] then showed that nutritional Se deficiency had no effect on cytochrome b_5 or NADPH-cytochrome c-reductase, indicating that the impaired activity of the intestinal mixed function oxidase system was due primarily to decreased cytochrome P_{450} level. Nutritional Se deficiency was also shown to reduce activity of ferrochelatase,[131] the enzyme that inserts iron into the porphyrin moiety. Delta-aminolevulinic acid synthetase and dehydratase, two critical enzymes in porphyrin synthesis, were not affected by Se deficiency. The response of ferrochelatase can perhaps explain the net reduction in heme and in cytochrome P_{450} content observed in villous tip cells in Se deficiency. The mechanism by which Se regulates ferrochelatase remains to be established.

D. Role of Selenium in Spermatogenesis

Normal spermatogenesis in the rat,[132,133] mouse,[134] boar,[135] and bull[136] requires Se. Burk and Brown[137] showed that ^{75}Se injected into male rats appeared in the midpiece of the sperm tail. Others subsequently showed that Se in rodent[138] and bull[136] sperm is associated with a single cysteine-rich[139] keratinous protein found in the mitochondrial capsule (i.e., outer membrane) of the midpiece sheath. Severe dietary Se deficiency results in reduced sperm production and in impaired morphology, motility, and viability of generated sperm. In the mouse, motility is less affected than in the rat and, therefore, fertility is not completely lost, as it is in the second generation Se-deficient rat.[140] Combs and Whitacre[141] maintained young cockerels on Se-deficient diets with very high vitamin E supplementation (500 IU/kg diet). The high levels of vitamin E prevented the pancreatic atrophy that usually develops in severe Se deficiency in chicks, but at 20 weeks of age, five of the seven cockerels failed to show testicular maturation, which is normally expected at 16-18 weeks. This suggests that Se may be required also for the chicken for normal testicular development and spermatogenesis.

E. Other Selenium-Containing Proteins

Several Se-containing proteins other than SeGSHpx have been discovered in rat liver,[142] rat kidney,[143] and rat,[142,144,145] and monkey[145] plasma, and ovine heart and muscle.[280] Whether these proteins have enzymic activity or any other function is not known, but one is thought to be a transport protein for Se. Burk and Gregory[142] isolated proteins of molecular weight 79,000 and 83,000 from plasma and liver, respectively, of rats treated with $^{75}SeO_3^{-2}$. These proteins, both devoid of SeGSHpx activity, eluted from a gel filtration column in the same volume for both tissues and, thus, were both designated ^{75}Se-P. In livers of severely Se-deficient rats, ^{75}Se was preferentially incorporated into ^{75}Se-P, while in livers of Se-adequate rats, more was incorporated into SeGSHpx. This and the presence of ^{75}Se-P in plasma could suggest that ^{75}Se-P serves as a Se-transport protein. However, since drug and heme metabolism in Se-deficient animals can respond to Se before SeGSHpx activity increases, it is possible that ^{75}Se-P may be related to one of those functions. Motsenbocker and Tappel[145] found Se-containing proteins of molecular weight 80,000 in rat and monkey plasma. These may be the same as ^{75}Se-P reported by Burk and Gregory.[142] The rat and monkey proteins had a half-life of Se-binding of only a few hours; this characteristic would be consistent with a transport protein. In a subsequent publication, Motsenbocker and Tappel[144] provided further evidence that the plasma protein, called by those authors selenoprotein P, serves as a transport protein for Se (see discussion of Se transport in Chapter 5).

Motsenbocker and Tappel[143] also reported finding three selenoproteins without SeGSHpx activity in rat kidney: two with molecular weight of 40,000 and one of 75,000. These, like selenoprotein P, contained Se as Se-cysteine. The Se concentration of rat kidney is greater than that of liver, spleen, heart, and lung[146]; however, the specific activity of SeGSHpx is less in kidney than in those other tissues.[76] Furthermore, kidney maintains a higher Se concentration than do liver or plasma during Se-deprivation, at least in the short-term (4 weeks).[279] Whether or to what extent the enduring Se can be accounted for by the above three proteins is not known; neither are the function(s) of the proteins known.

An Se-containing protein with molecular weight of 10,000 has been found in ovine heart and muscle.[280] Designated "G protein," this protein contains Se-cysteine.[281] Its function is not known.

A protein that transiently but specifically binds Se after injections of Na_2SeO_3 has been identified in rat liver mitochondria.[267] The protein is released from mitochondria by freezing and thawing; it is smaller than the mitochondrial SeGSHpx (i.e., 77,000 daltons vs. 100,000 daltons) and contains Se in an inorganic form. Brian et al.[267] speculated that this protein may be involved in Se metabolism.

Mammalian hemoglobin (Hb) has been found to contain Se, which is noteworthy inasmuch as it also possesses glutathione peroxidase activity.[268] Its Se, however, is contained in the globin moiety; the heme moiety, which has the glutathione peroxidase activity, contains no Se. Beilstein and Whanger[268] have found that rats injected with $Na_2{}^{75}SeO_3$ show the predominant radiolabeling of erythrocyte protein as SeGSHpx, whereas rats given ^{75}Se-methionine show labeling predominantly as Hb. Because Hb-bound Se is subsequently made available for SeGSHpx, these findings suggest that protein, such as Hb in which Se is not functional, may serve as Se reserves in the body.[268,269]

Although several Se-containing proteins have been identified in mammalian tissues, the only one known for certain to have enzymic activity is SeGSHpx. Several selenoenzymes, however, have been identified in microorganisms. One, formate dehydrogenase, has been found to be Se-dependent in Escherichia coli[147,148] and in several strictly anaerobic bacteria including Clostridium thermoaceticum,[149] C. formicoaceticum,[150] C. stricklandii,[151] C. cylindrosporum,[152] C. acidiurici,[152] and Methanococcus vannielli.[153] The bacterial formate dehydrogenases catalyze the oxidation of formate to CO_2 with the concomitant reduction of nitrate, fumarate, pyridine nucleotides, cytochromes, or iron-sulfur centers, as well as covalently bound Se. The complex contains four gram-atoms of Se, which appear to be located as single selenocysteinyl residues in each of the 110,000-dalton subunits.[153] The selenocysteinyl residues are thought to participate in catalysis by undergoing reversible oxidation and reduction.[154]

The second bacterial enzyme known to be Se-dependent is glycine reductase. This enzyme catalyzes the reductive deamination of glycine with the concomitant esterification of orthophosphate and ADP to form ATP. This reductive deamination serves as a terminal electron acceptor process for several amino acid-fermenting anaerobes (e.g., Clostridium sporogenes) which are dependent upon normal activities of this selenoenzyme for normal growth.[155] Other bacteria (e.g., C. stricklandii and C. malenominatum) have alternative electron acceptors under normal conditions of cultivation in complex media and, thus, show decreased glycine reductase activity without impaired growth when Se is absent from the medium. It contains one gram-atom of Se per mole of the protein present as a selenocysteinyl residue. The protein also contains two cysteinyl residues which are extremely labile to oxygen, imparting unusually high oxygen sensitivity to this enzyme.

Selenium has been found to be required for the formation of nicotinic acid hydroxylase in *Clostridium barkeri*[156] and xanthine dehydrogenase in *C. acidiurici* and *C. cylindrosporum.*[266] Nicotinic acid hydroxylase catalyzes the hydration of a double bond of nicotinic acid, followed by dehydrogenation of the 6-oxo derivative with reduction of NADP+. Studies cited by Stadtman[154] indicate that the enzyme can incorporate stoichiometric amounts of Se in a form yet to be identified. Xanthine dehydrogenase, like its mammalian counterpart xanthine oxidase, is known to contain molybdenum, FAD, and nonheme iron. It functions *in vivo* to catalyze the reduction of uric acid to xanthine; however, *in vitro* it will oxidize a number of purines and aldehydes using as electron acceptors oxygen, ferricyanide, or tetrazolium salts. It is not known whether xanthine dehydrogenase is a selenoenzyme; however, its function in reduction-oxidation reactions, like that of nicotinic acid hydroxylase, resembles those of enzymes presently known to contain Se.

VI. INTERRELATIONSHIPS OF SELENIUM AND OTHER NUTRIENTS

A. Vitamin E

When both Se and vitamin E are deficient in the diets of animals, particular deficiency syndromes develop, some of which are responsive to either Se or vitamin E supplementation. Such syndromes include liver necrosis in the rat,[2] exudative diathesis in the chick,[3] and white muscle disease in lambs[58] and calves.[157] The lesions in these conditions are thought to result from unchecked oxidative processes that lead to lipid peroxidation and membrane damage.

As discussed earlier in this chapter, Se plays a role in curtailing lipid peroxidation through the enzyme SeGSHpx, which converts hydrogen peroxide to water. Hydrogen peroxide, if not removed, is thought to be capable of interacting with other cell constituents to form free radicals, which can proliferate through chain reactions and chain branching and which can cause structural changes in and cross-linking of lipids and proteins. It is these changes that lead to membrane damage and the lesions characteristic of the deficiency syndromes.

Vitamin E, a lipophilic molecule, is a scavenger of free radicals. On reaction with a free radical, vitamin E (alpha-tocopherol) is oxidized to a tocopherol semiquinone radical, which is rapidly degraded,[158] and the original free radical receives a hydrogen atom, thereby resolving its unpaired electron. Vitamin E is located in cell membranes in close proximity to phospholipids and their unsaturated fatty acid moieties and can, therefore, terminate chain reactions involving fatty acid peroxyl radicals.

Thus, both Se and vitamin E, though functioning at different points in the sequence of reactions, reduce the rate of lipid peroxidation and its resulting membrane damage. Therefore, for some vitamin E-Se deficiency conditions, one of the nutrients can spare the other or each can individually prevent appearance of the deficiency syndrome.

Not all vitamin E-deficiency conditions are responsive to Se. Encephalomalacia in the chick, for instance, can be prevented by vitamin E and synthetic lipid soluble antioxidants (e.g., ethoxyquin, diphenyl-*p*-phenylene diamine) but not by Se.[159] The same is true for muscular dystrophy in the rabbit.[160,161] The responsiveness of these conditions to synthetic antioxidants with structures dissimilar to that of vitamin E suggests that it is the antioxidant properties of vitamin E that make it effective. The ineffectiveness of Se further suggests that the oxidative events are not occurring in the cystosol, where SeGSHpx is located, but in the lipid environment of the membrane.

B. Vitamin C and Other Antioxidants

Most animals (except humans, other primates, guinea pigs, and a few exotic species) can synthesize ascorbic acid (vitamin C), and it is, therefore, not considered for them an essential nutrient. However, supplementation of an Se- and vitamin E-deficient diet with ascorbic acid has been shown to reduce the incidence of exudative diathesis in chicks[78, 162-164] and ducks.[165] Combs and Scott[163] and Combs and Pesti[164] showed that 200 ppm dietary ascorbic acid raised plasma SeGSHpx activities of chicks fed a vitamin E-deficient diet marginal in Se. To determine if ascorbic acid was influencing intestinal absorption of Se, Combs and Pesti[164] measured disappearance of ^{75}Se (from $Na_2{}^{75}SeO_3$) from ligated duodenal loops of chicks fed diets with or without added ascorbic acid and found that immediate disappearance (within the first 5 min) was increased from loops of chicks fed ascorbic acid. By 15 min, there was no significant difference between treatment groups. In the intact chick administered $Na_2{}^{75}SeO_3$, increased absorption was greater at 1 hr in chicks fed ascorbic acid than in those receiving no supplemental ascorbic acid. No differences were detectable by 3 hrs.[164] The authors concluded that ascorbic acid reduced exudative diathesis by promoting intestinal absorption of Se and increasing the incorporation of Se into SeGSHpx.

Using chick duodenum in culture, Cupp[78] was able to show that ascorbic acid increases the post-absorptive utilization of Se. Duodena were incubated with Se (as Na_2SeO_3) and ascorbic acid together or with each nutrient individually in sequence, with washing in between. Simultaneous exposure to both nutrients resulted in an increase of SeGSHpx activity by about 40% compared to exposure to Se alone. When exposure to Se alone was followed by ascorbic acid alone, SeGHSpx activity was increased to the same extent as with simultaneous exposure. This indicated that the interaction of Se and ascorbic acid occurred primarily following absorption. The increased uptake by chicks of ^{75}Se reported by Combs and Pesti[164] must have been secondary to the increased utilization of Se: passive absorption was promoted by post-absorptive removal.

Of the enzymes of the oxidant defense system, GSHpx in erythrocytes (assayed with cumene hydroperoxide as substrate) was the only one found by Chen and Thacker[166] to be affected by ascorbic acid. The authors proposed that ascorbic acid increased lipid peroxidation and thereby stimulated GSHpx activity. Although ascorbic acid in the presence of Fe^{+2} is often used as a pro-oxidant in *in vitro* systems, there is no strong evidence that ascorbic acid is a pro-oxidant *in vivo*. Furthermore, work by Fidler *et al.*[167] showed that lipid hydroperoxides or *t*-butyl peroxide, administered to chicks by crop intubation, reduced, rather than increased, GSHpx activities in liver and plasma. The mechanism by which SeGSHpx is increased by ascorbic acid treatment is unclear, but it does not appear to be by induction due to lipid peroxidation.

Although ascorbic acid affects Se status, Combs and Pesti[164] showed that neither dietary Se nor vitamin E affected ascorbic acid status of chicks. This and a similar finding in ducks by Dean and Combs[168] contradict a report by Brown *et al.*,[169] which reported a decline in ascorbic acid concentration of plasma in Se-deficient ducks. The contention that Se does not affect ascorbic acid status is supported by a study of Chow *et al.*,[170] in which ascorbic acid in rat plasma and lungs was elevated by administration of PCBs (polychlorinated biphenyls), regardless of the Se status.

Ascorbic acid is a scavenger of superoxide radical[171] and may serve directly as part of the biological oxidant defense system. At physiological pH, the rate constant for the reaction of superoxide dismutase (SOD) with superoxide radical is about 3000 times that for the ascorbic acid reaction with superoxide radical.[171,172] However, the level of SOD in most tissues is about one-thousandth of that of ascorbic acid,[171] making the SOD-catalyzed reaction rate only about three times that of the ascorbate-catalyzed reaction. Hence, ascorbic acid could conceivably play a significant role in removal of superoxide radical *in vivo*. Furthermore, GSH is capable of reducing dehydroascorbic acid to ascorbic acid,[173,174] possibly establishing cycling of ascorbic acid.

Ascorbic acid may be most effective in the oxidant defense system in extracellular fluids, where SOD and SeGSHpx are not found. A pool of extracellular ascorbic acid has been shown to be maintained in the lung of the scorbutic guinea pig.[175] Ascorbic acid has also been found to protect rats from lung damage during exposure to hyperbaric oxygen.[176]

Many nonbiological antioxidants produce biological results similar to those of ascorbic acid, vitamin E, and Se. Ethoxyquin, a synthetic antioxidant widely used in feeds, reduced the occurrence of exudative diathesis and raised plasma SeGHSpx in chicks fed vitamin E-deficient diets that were marginal in Se.[163,177] N,N'-Diphenyl-p-phenylene diamine (DPPD) prevents exudative diathesis in chicks[178] and also such other vitamin E-/Se-deficiency syndromes as resorption-gestation in rats[179] and muscular dystrophy in the guinea pig.[180] Downey *et al.*[181] showed that DPPD reduced pentane production by rats when added to a vitamin E-deficient diet. Tappel *et al.*[182] tested mixtures of several antioxidants and antioxygenic nutrients added to mouse diets for their effects on indices of aging. Fluorescent pigments in testes were greatly reduced in mice consuming a diet containing large supplements of vitamin E, butylated hydroxytoluene, ascorbic acid, DL-methionine and a moderate supplement of selenite (0.11 ppm). Since fluorescent pigments are thought to be products of lipid peroxidation, this study suggests that large doses of antioxidants can reduce lipid peroxidation *in vivo*. Other measured parameters, including kidney function, uptake of calcium by muscle microsomes (an indicator of membrane damage), and longevity, were not affected by the antioxidant content of the diet.

It appears that many antioxidants and antioxygenic nutrients reduce the need for Se by terminating or preventing initiation of free radical chain reactions. Ascorbic acid apparently functions in an additional, as yet uncharacterized, way when it causes increased incorporation of Se into SeGSHpx.

C. Sulfur

Belonging to the same family in the periodic table and having similar electronic configurations in their valence shells, Se and S might be expected to substitute for one another in molecules and to compete for transport and binding sites in biological systems. In fact, Se-containing analogs of S compounds, such as selenomethionine and selenocysteine, are found in plants and animals, and some S compounds and their Se-containing analogs do compete for transport (e.g., methionine and selenomethionine compete for transport across the intestinal mucosa of the hamster).[183] However, S compounds tend to follow oxidative pathways, while Se compounds tend to undergo reduction in biological systems. Consequently, the two elements can interact by the oxidation of S being coupled to the reduction of Se. Nuttall and Allen[184] have shown in an *in vitro* system that, as Se^0 is reduced to HSe^-, thiols, such as GSH, are oxidized. In the presence of molecular oxygen, HSe^- is rapidly oxidized to Se^0, resulting in a cycle that catalytically oxidizes thiols.[184] Whether concentrations of HSe^- and molecular oxygen in body fluids are sufficient to make this reaction significant *in vivo* is not known. A reaction that does occur *in vivo* and is thought, at least at one step, to involve a coupled reduction of Se and oxidation of GSH, is the SeGSHpx reaction (see Section II, mechanism of selenium-dependent glutathione peroxidase, this chapter).

An interaction of S and Se has been seen in studies of Se toxicity, where supplemental S has been shown to reduce toxicity signs. Ganther and Baumann[185] found that growth depression and splenomegaly in rats fed excesses of sodium selenate were partially overcome by feeding sulfate. Halverson and Monty[186] had reported similar findings in rats with respect to growth depression and liver damage. Ganther and Baumann[185] noted that sulfate greatly increased the urinary excretion of Se, but that it had no effect on the total amount of Se in the gastrointestinal contents and feces. Following a pulse dose of $Na_2{}^{75}SeO_4$ by stomach tube to rats, Acuff and Smith[187] found exhaled ^{75}Se, as well as urinary ^{75}Se, to be increased by those rats consuming a high level of sulfate. The mechanism by which S increases excretion of Se is not known, but increased excretion undoubtedly accounts, at least partially, for the alleviation of toxicity signs.

Acuff and Smith,[187] after dosing rats with $Na_2{}^{75}SeO_4$ by stomach tube, noticed that the percentage absorption of Se, measured 90 minutes after dosing, was lowest when the diet contained a suboptimal level of sulfate. Thus, although Se status does not appear to affect Se absorption,[188] S status may affect it. It is possible that, when S is limiting, more Se is incorporated into amino acids or other molecules by intestinal microflora and absorption is thereby prevented or delayed. This hypothesis must be tested using a time-course experimental design for following Se absorption, as the use of a single time period for measurement of disposition of the ^{75}Se does not allow recognition of such delays.

White and Somers[189] and White[190] reported that a suboptimal level of S in diets of sheep fed Se as selenomethionine resulted in higher levels of Se in plasma and wool than when the S level was adequate or higher. Urinary and fecal excretion of Se were not significantly affected by the S content of the diet. It seems likely that synthesis of methionine by rumen microflora would have been reduced due to the low level of S in the diet and that, as a consequence, selenomethionine was substituted for methionine in some proteins. Ganther *et al.*[191] found that volatilization of Se was increased by rats given increased dietary protein or increased methionine, suggesting that adequate or excess methionine frees Se for other metabolic routes. Scott[192] showed that 0.1 ppm Se added to a chick diet deficient in vitamin E and sulfur amino acids prevented exudative diathesis but not muscular dystrophy. Cystine, methionine, or 1.0 ppm Se could all prevent muscular dystrophy. This suggests that Se can substitute for S, probably by being incorporated into cysteine, which is thought to be the active agent in prevention of muscular dystrophy.[193] Whether and how animals incorporate Se into methionine or cysteine is still a debated issue (see Chapter 5, Section III, metabolism of selenium).

Vernie et al.[194] reported that, in a cell-free system, various thiols in combination with Na_2SeO_3 inhibited incorporation of ^{14}C-leucine into protein. Reaction products of Se with thiols inhibited protein synthesis also in cultured cells. The blocking agents were shown to be selenotrisulfides (e.g., selenodiglutathione, GSSeSG).[194] Disulfides were not inhibitory. The degree of inhibition of protein synthesis depends on the particular selenotrisulfide and on the type of cell.[194] This could conceivably be useful in the treatment of certain cancers. Whether this interaction of Se and S compounds is significant in animals not being treated with foreign agents is not known.

Smith et al.[195] supplemented grazing steers by monthly injection of Se as Na_2SeO_3 or by a dietary supplement of elemental S or by a combination of the two. The Se treatment improved weight gain but the S treatment did not. Se treatment lowered plasma amino acid levels, suggesting that protein synthesis had been enhanced. Such an increase in protein synthesis would be consistent with the observed improvement in weight gain. Sulfur treatment alone did not reduce plasma amino acids. The combined treatments resulted in plasma amino acid values intermediate between the two individual treatments. The apparent decline in protein synthesis when S was added to the Se treatment may have been caused by a reduction of the Se effect due to increased excretion of Se in the presence of S. Alternatively, it is possible that this effect may have been due to an inhibition of protein synthesis caused by an interaction of Se and thiols as presented by Vernie et al.,[194] if such an interaction occurs in vivo.

Broderius et al.[196] investigated tissue distribution and quantity of sulfhydryl groups in Se-deficient lambs and rats. Lambs with white muscle disease were found to have elevated nonprotein sulfhydryl compounds (including elevated GSH) and decreased protein sulfhydryl groups in skeletal muscle, but not in heart, kidney, or liver. Also, total sulfhydryl content of muscle was decreased. The authors anticipated finding an increase in disulfide concentrations to account for the decline in total sulfhydryl groups, but instead found a decrease in disulfides. A similar pattern was reported in muscle in vitamin E-deficient chicks with nutritional muscular dystrophy.[197] In Se-deficient rats, nonprotein sulfhydryl groups in liver and kidney were greatly increased. However, unlike in lambs and chicks, total sulfhydryls in the target organ (liver, in the case of the rat) were increased. No satisfactory explanation for this effect of Se-deficiency has yet been given.

D. Zinc

There is evidence for interaction between Se and Zn in biological systems, but its nature is not understood. Chmielnicka et al.[198] found that a series of injections of $ZnCl_2$ resulted in a total body retention of about 20% of the amount of Zn administered. However, when Na_2SeO_3 was concurrently given (by mouth), retention of Zn was nearly doubled, with the concentration of Zn in most tissues being doubled. Zinc by itself caused a four-fold increase in the amount of metallothionein in liver.[198] Co-administration of Se greatly reduced that increase. Metallothionein content of kidney was independent of Zn and Se. However, administration of Se with Zn caused a total shift of Zn from low molecular weight to high molecular weight proteins in the soluble fraction of kidney.[198] Alexander and Aaseth[199] reported that oral treatment of rats with a near-toxic dose (ca. 4 ppm) of Se as selenite for 7 days lowered liver Zn and raised kidney Zn. The differing results of these two studies may be explainable by the absence of co-administration of an excess of Zn in the latter study. Alexander and Aaseth[199] found selenite to be without effect on excretion of Zn into bile.

Zinc also affects distribution of Se. When equimolar quantities of $Na_2{}^{75}SeO_3$ and $ZnCl_2$ were injected simultaneously into mice, ^{75}Se uptake by heart and liver was less than when $Na_2{}^{75}SeO_3$ was injected alone.[200] Co-administration of Zn caused no change in ^{75}Se content of plasma, erythrocytes, lung, brain, kidney, spleen, and testis. Sinisalo and Combs,[201] using 0.1 ppm dietary Se and high levels of dietary Zn (100- 2000 ppm), found that SeGSHpx activity of the chick pancreas increased as dietary Zn increased, while plasma SeGSHpx activity was unaffected. Chvapil et al.[202] found that, compared to 40 ppm dietary Zn, 1000 ppm lowered malonaldehyde production by rat liver. This decrease in lipid peroxidation may be due to a Zn-induced increase in SeGSHpx activity.

E. Copper

The effects of Cu administration on apparent Se status of an animal and the effects of Se on Cu status suggest a competition between the two elements. Amer et al.[203] found that supplementation of a calf diet that was marginal in Se content (0.08 ppm) with 0.7 ppm Se as Na_2SeO_3 resulted in a sudden drop in plasma Cu and in plasma ceruloplasmin activity in the presence of 6.5 ppm Cu in the basal diet or when the basal diet was supplemented with 100 or 200 ppm Cu. Thomson and Lawson[204] observed that Se supplementation of lambs born to ewes pastured on Cu-deficient lands resulted in increased plasma and liver Cu levels. Supplementation with both Cu and Se gave lower liver Cu concentrations than supplementation with Cu alone. These observations with calves and lambs of marginal Se or Cu status are consistent with a hypothesis that the two minerals have similar affinities for binding to carrier and/or storage proteins and that providing an excess of one will cause displacement and freeing of the other. Jenkinson et al.[205] found that rats consuming a Cu-deficient diet had low activities of liver superoxide dismutase (SOD), a copper-containing enzyme, and of liver SeGSHpx compared to Cu-adequate controls. Selenium supplementation partly overcame the reduction of SeGSHpx but had no effect on SOD. When Se distribution was traced by injecting ^{75}Se, the authors found an elevation of ^{75}Se in livers of Cu-deficient rats.[205] The pattern of retention of ^{75}Se by organs resembled that of Se deficiency. A possible explanation of these data is that certain binding sites will be filled by one or the other of these (or other) metals, and the more unfilled binding sites there are, the less will be the availability for either of the metals to serve other functions. Dougherty and Hoekstra[206] showed that acute Cu toxicity in rats as a result of injection of $CuSO_4$ caused greater production of ethane than did a comparable injection of Na_2SO_4. Dietary vitamin E (200 IU/kg diet) totally prevented the rise in ethane production after Cu injection. Dietary Se at 0.5 ppm was only slightly less effective. It is likely that the increase in lipid peroxidation, as indicated by the rise in ethane production, was due to decreased SeGSHpx resulting from an interaction of Se and Cu.

When Cu or Se is in excess, administration of the opposing element can alleviate toxicity signs. Jensen[207] reported a decrease in mortality of Se-intoxicated chicks treated with 1000 ppm Cu as $CuSO_4$. Hill[208] also showed that 500 ppm dietary Cu greatly reduced mortality of chicks fed 40 ppm Se. Interestingly, Cu treatment improved growth only slightly compared to treatment with Hg but was much more effective than Hg in reducing mortality. Single oral pretreatment with $CuSO_4$ prevented selenosis in ponies given toxic doses of Se.[209] In Se-intoxicated ponies not pretreated with Cu, serum Se was high and remained elevated throughout the 50-hr study. In those ponies pre-treated with Cu, initial serum Se was high but it dropped rapidly. Chen et al.[210] reported significant increases in Cu content of blood, heart, liver, and kidney of rats given toxic doses of Se in their drinking water compared to those not given excess Se. Jensen[207] also reported that, as dietary Se was increased in chick diets, the Cu level of liver increased. The elevations in tissue Cu in Se toxicity and the decreased mortality when Se toxicity is treated with Cu together suggest that when one or both elements are present in excess, they become metabolically less available, perhaps through formation of a Cu-Se adduct.

Jensen[211] found that when chicks were fed a diet normally regarded as adequate in Se (0.2 ppm Se), added Cu (800 to 4000 ppm) caused a high incidence of exudative diathesis, muscular dystrophy and mortality. When the diet was further supplemented with 0.5 ppm Se, exudative diathesis and muscular dystrophy did not develop and there was no increase in mortality. This too suggests the formation of a nontoxic Se-Cu complex. That Se and Cu interact biologically is evident. The hypothesis of competitive binding to proteins and the formation of a metabolically unavailable form of Cu and Se when the two metals are in excess offers a plausible explanation for the data presented.

VII. INTERRELATIONSHIPS OF SELENIUM AND OTHER ELEMENTS

A. Mercury

In 1967, Parizek and Ostadalova[212] published a report showing that sodium selenite afforded protection to rats from renal necrosis and mortality caused by mercuric chloride. Similar protection against neural signs of toxicity and mortality due to methylmercury have been shown in the Japanese quail[213-216] and in the chick.[215]

The interaction of Se and Hg is complicated and is not well understood. Se administered with Hg changes the tissue distribution of Hg compared to that when Hg is administered alone. Sell and Horani[215] fed chicks and quail diets containing 20 ppm Hg as methylmercury with and without 8 ppm Se as sodium selenite (1:1 molar ratio of Hg and Se) and found that when Se was fed, the concentration of Hg in chick liver was about half of that in livers of chicks not supplemented with Se. Quail, on the other hand, showed the opposite pattern, with a doubling in the livers of the Se-supplemented group compared to the group receiving Hg only.[215] In a subsequent study, using the same concentrations and forms of Hg and Se, Sell[217] showed that Se supplementation increased liver Hg in laying hens of both chickens and quail. In the rat, Se increased liver Hg concentration[218] but in the guinea pig, it decreased liver Hg.[219] Almost uniformly, whether Hg (as methylmercury) was administered chronically through the diet or by single injections or oral doses, co-administration of Se caused an increase in Hg concentration of the brain.[216-221] Although, with the passage of days, Hg concentrations of most tissues, including brain, of Se-treated animals tend to approach those of the non-Se-treated animals,[219,220] the combined facts that brain Hg levels are initially higher in Se-treated animals and that Se confers protection against Hg toxicity suggest that the Hg in brain has been transformed to a less toxic form. Kidney, another target site of Hg toxicity,[212,222] showed reduced Hg levels when Se was co-administered with methyl mercury.[218,219,221] Further, Komsta-Szumska et al.[219] showed in the guinea pig that Se reduced the proportion of inorganic Hg (known to be a more potent renal toxicant than organic Hg[223]) in the kidney.

Various mechanisms have been proposed to explain the protective effect of Se in Hg toxicity. It is generally agreed that Se does not increase fecal or urinary excretion of Hg,[217,219] although one report showed an increase in excretion when chicks were fed Se with methylmercurey but not with mercuric chloride.[224] Komsta-Szumska et al.[219] have proposed that, since Se reduced fecal excretion of Hg in the guinea pig and reduced the concentration of Hg in skin and in all major organs, another route of elimination, namely exhalation, must be involved. Another possible mechanism for the protective effect of Se is the formation of a nontoxic Se-Hg complex. Naganuma and Imura[225] showed that a low molecular weight, short-lived complex, bis(methylmercuric)selenide (BMS), could be formed in vitro from methylmercury and selenite in the presence of GSH. Masukawa et al.[226] found BMS in blood and tissues of methylmercury-treated rats after selenite injection and suggested that short-term formation of BMS is related to the selenite-induced changes in tissue distribution of Hg. Pretreatment of rats with diethylmaleate to deplete tissue GSH resulted in a profound inhibition of BMS formation in blood but a significant increase in total blood mercury.[221] Furthermore, GSH depletion reduced the increase in brain Hg concentration normally observed when Se is co-administered with methylmercury. The authors proposed that the erythrocytes are the primary site of BMS formation and that BMS may be a transport form of Hg. Naganuma et al.[227] showed that Hg levels were higher in brains of mice administered BMS than in those administered Se with Hg as either methylmercury or mercuric chloride. Thus, formation of BMS may be one means by which tissue distribution of Hg is altered.

Ionic Hg, but not methylmercury, has a high affinity for metallothionein-like proteins,[228] and Hg stimulates synthesis of these proteins.[229] Synthesis of thionein may be a protective mechanism at low chronic exposure, providing binding sites for ionic Hg. Selenium eliminates the binding of Hg to metallothionein and increases binding to high molecular weight proteins.[219,229] In kidney, this is likely to be related to the shift of the form of Hg from inorganic to organic, as reported by Komsta-Szumska et al.[219]

Komsta-Szumska et al.[219] reported that Hg is found in the same fraction of high molecular weight proteins as Se in kidney tissue preparations subjected to gel filtration. Affinity of seleno-sulfhydryl groups for methylmercury is higher than that of sulfhydryl groups.[230] Thus, it seems likely that Se combines with a high molecular weight protein, producing a complex that shows greater affinity to Hg than does thionein.

It has also been suggested that methylmercury can be cleaved to form free radicals,[231] which could be responsible for the toxic effects of Hg. This could explain why vitamin E, in addition to Se, confers protection against Hg toxicity, as shown by Welsh and Soares[214] in Japanese quail, but the evidence supporting this hypothesis is not strong.

Methylmercury also has an influence on distribution of Se. Komsta-Szumska[232] showed that a single dose of $Na_2^{75}SeO_3$ (50 μmole Se/kg) to a guinea pig resulted in the largest concentrations of radiolabel in liver and kidney. Pretreatment of animals with methylmercury eliminated the initial accumulation of Se in kidney. Uptake of Se by brain was also higher with methylmercury treatment, with increases in the mitochondrial and nuclear fractions and a decrease in the soluble fraction.

B. Cadmium

In experimental animals, acute exposure to Cd can result in testicular necrosis, placental hemorrhage, hemorrhagic necrosis of nonovulating ovaries, teratogenicity, or death.[229] Chronic exposure can cause kidney damage, depression of pancreatic function, and elevation of hepatic gluconeogenic enzymes.[229] Selenium has been shown to afford protection against many of the signs of acute toxicity due to Cd.

Testicular damage due to Cd^{+2} can be prevented by administration of Zn,[233,234] cysteine and certain other thiols,[235] or Se.[236] Mason and Young[236] showed that Se as SeO_2 in a concentration one-half the equimolar concentration of Cd was sufficient to protect the rat testis from injury when the two compounds were injected simultaneously, but that Zn^{+2} in 160 times the equimolar concentration of Cd had no effect when administered with Cd. To be effective, Zn could be administered hours or days prior to Cd administration. Selenium, on the other hand, when administered up to one day prior to Cd administration, was ineffective. Zinc stimulates synthesis of thionein, at least in liver,[237] and thionein can bind Cd^{+2} as well as Zn^{+2}. It is possible that it is through stimulation of metallothionein formation that Zn gives protection against Cd-induced testis injury.

The mechanism by which Se protects against Cd toxicity probably involves a direct interaction of the two elements. Gasiewicz and Smith[238] showed that when SeO_3^{-2} and Cd^{+2} were incubated in plasma containing erythrocytes, a protein of 130,000 molecular weight, with Cd and Se bound in a 1 : 1 ratio, was formed. The same protein peak was found in gel filtration of plasma that had been incubated with H_2Se and Cd^{+2} without erythrocytes, although erythrocytes were necessary to form the Cd-Se complex when Se was present as SeO_3^{-2}. The authors hypothesized that erythrocytes must absorb and metabolize SeO_3^{-2} and release H_2Se, which then interacts with Cd^{+2}. After SeO_3^{-2} and $CdCl_2$ were injected simultaneously into rats, two peaks representing 330,000 and 130,000 daltons with a Cd:Se stoichiometry of 1 : 1 were found in the gel filtrates of plasma, showing that a Cd-Se complex can also be formed *in vivo*.[238] Chen *et al*.[239] showed that, in kidney and testes, SeO_3^{-2} stimulated the uptake of Cd^{+2} into soluble, high molecular weight proteins and almost completely eliminated the binding of Cd^{+2} to metallothionein.

Coadministration of Se and Cd causes significantly increased uptake of Cd by rat testis, compared to administration of Cd alone.[240] However, studies with the radioactive isotope $^{109}Cd^{+2}$ indicate that Cd is localized in the capillaries and that very little penetrates the tissue.[241] It is possible, then, that an interaction of Se and Cd in the blood, as suggested by Gasiewicz and Smith,[238] renders the Cd harmless to the vascular tissue.

As mentioned previously, cysteine and certain other thiols protect the testis from acute Cd-induced necrosis, but, unlike Se, cysteine causes almost no change in uptake of Cd by testis.[240] However, cysteine causes greatly increased uptake of Cd by kidney, resulting in severe renal damage. Selenium causes very little change in Cd uptake by kidney, and kidney damage is minimal, whether or not Se treatment is given. It is not clear how cysteine protects the testis from damage and simultaneously causes harm to the kidney.

Early and Schnell[242] showed that the administration of Cd^{+2} to rats caused inhibition of certain hepatic monooxygenasses, but that when SeO_3^{-2} was administered simultaneously the inhibition was prevented. However, application of one agent (Se or Cd) *in vitro* to a microsomal preparation made from livers of rats treated with the other agent *in vivo*, or application of both agents *in vitro* to microsomes, resulted in inhibition of the monooxygenases; i.e., Se did not change the effect of Cd. The authors concluded that the protective effect of Se could not be due to the formation of a Cd-Se complex or protection would have been evident also *in vitro*. However, as the authors acknowledged, SeO_3^{+2} may not be the form of Se necessary to form a Cd-Se complex, and, thus, their findings do not contradict the hypothesis of Gasiewicz and Smith.[238]

A study of the effects of Se on the teratogenicity of Cd in the golden hamster[243] showed that co-administration of Se and Cd almost totally overcame the teratogenic effects caused by Cd alone. However, when the injection of the two minerals was separated by 0.5-4 hrs, Se was less effective. When Se was administered 2 hrs or more before Cd, it was less effective than when done in the opposite order. Results of Gasiewicz and Smith[238] suggest that endogenous Se is not available to interact with Cd in plasma. Furthermore, injected SeO_3^{-2} is rapidly taken up by erythrocytes,[238,244] which then metabolize the Se to a form that becomes bound to plasma proteins.[244,245] Thus, the diminished effectiveness of early administered Se in counteracting the teratogenicity of Cd is probably due to binding of much of the Se to proteins, making it unavailable to interact with Cd.

C. Arsenic

In 1938 Moxon[246] discovered that As could protect rats from Se toxicity resulting from consumption of seleniferous grains. Moxon and Wilson[247] later showed that As could counteract reduced hatchability of eggs laid by hens fed 10 ppm Se. Depressed growth in chicks due to excessive dietary Se can also be overcome by As.[248,249]

The interaction of Se and As also gives protective properties to Se when As is in excess. Holmberg and Ferm[243] showed that the teratogenic effects of As injected into golden hamsters on day 8 of gestation were greatly reduced by co-administration of Se. Se alone showed no teratogenicity. The means by which As affords protection against Se toxicity was elucidated by studies of Levander and Baumann[250,251] that showed a great (up to ten-fold) increase in output of Se into bile when selenite-treated rats were injected with sodium arsenite. (Se also increased the biliary excretion of As in arsenite-treated rats.) A concomitant and equivalent decline in liver Se was also observed. Arsenic treatment caused a rise in blood Se levels when selenite was used, and the authors suggested that this might have resulted in increased filtration of Se into bile. They pointed out, however, that when selenate instead of selenite was used, As caused an increase in biliary excretion but there was no accompanying rise in blood Se. Thus, the chemical or biochemical mechanism by which the two minerals interact is not yet clear.

D. Lead

Lead, tin, and tellurium all have valence shell electron structure similar to that of Se, all have high affinity for sulfur-containing compounds, and all interact biologically with Se.

Lead affects the heme synthesis pathway: in particular, the enzymes δ-aminolevulinic acid dehydratase (ALAD) and heme synthetase.[252,253] Manifestations of these effects in the rat include splenomegaly, reduced hematocrit, and increased mechanical fragility of erythrocytes.[254] Vitamin E-deficient rats are especially susceptible to Pb poisoning.[254] Cerklewski and Forbes[252] showed that with 200 ppm dietary Pb and adequate vitamin E, increasing levels of dietary Se from 0.15 to 0.50 ppm reduced urinary excretion of δ-aminolevulinic acid (ALA), suggesting a protective effect of Se. However, 1.0 ppm Se caused an increase in ALA excretion. Also, Pb content of liver and tibia, but not kidney, was reduced with 0.5 ppm dietary Se (200 ppm Pb), but the Pb concentrations of all three tissues were increased at 1.0 ppm Se. The results of Levander et al.[255] differed from those of Cerklewski and Forbes[252] but also displayed an irregular pattern. With 250 ppm Pb in drinking water, supplementation of a vitamin E-adequate, Torula yeast diet with 0.5 ppm Se resulted in splenomegaly and reduced hematocrit, whereas those parameters were normal without Se supplementation. Removal of vitamin E worsened all parameters, including filterability of erythrocytes, which has been shown to be negatively correlated with the degree of lipid peroxidation in erythrocytes incubated in vitro.[256] Addition of excess Se to the vitamin E-deficient diet improved filterability of erythrocytes, reduced splenomegaly, and improved hematocrit.[256] Levander et al.[255] concluded that Se can give some protection against Pb poisoning but that vitamin E status plays a more significant role.

The protective effect of vitamin E and of Se under some conditions suggests that lipid peroxidation may play a role in Pb toxicity. Sifri and Hoekstra[257] and Ramstoeck et al.[258] showed that Pb-poisoned rats produced greater amounts of ethane than did vitamin E- and Se-deficient controls receiving no Pb. Dietary vitamin E and, to a lesser extent, Se provided protection against this sign of Pb-induced lipid peroxidation. Donaldson and Leeming[259] have shown that increasing levels of dietary Pb in chicks cause a decrease in the ratio of linoleic:arachidonic acids in the liver through an apparent stimulation of elongation and desaturation of linoleic acid to form arachidonic acid. The mechanism of this shift is not known, but the greater concentration of polyunsaturated fatty acids could make the liver more susceptible to lipid peroxidation.

Howell and Hill[260] tested the effect of Pb on Se toxicity in chicks. With dietary Se at 20 ppm, addition of 400 ppm improved weight gain but did not restore it to control levels. Thus, Pb may offer some protection against Se toxicity, but its effect is not dramatic.

E. Tin

The interaction of Sn and Se has not been widely studied. Howell and Hill[260] showed that 200 ppm Sn reduced the growth-retarding effects of a toxic level of Se (25 ppm) in chicks. Chiba et al.[261] also found injections of equimolar amounts of Sn or Pb to greatly reduce mortality of mice that had been injected with 100 μmoles Se/kg body weight.

Chiba et al.[261] showed that injection of 10 μmoles Sn/kg body weight into mice dramatically inhibited ALAD activity and that simultaneous injection of an equimolar injection of Se completely restored activity. The mechanism of the interaction of Sn and Se is not known. A study by Dwivedi et al.[262] showed that Sn reduced GSH and increased malonaldehyde production in liver. However, whether the increased lipid peroxidation is a primary or secondary effect of Sn intoxication and, hence, whether Se protects through SeGSHpx is not clear.

F. Tellurium

Because of the similarity of atomic structures of Se and Te, attempts have been made to substitute Te for Se in diets. Whanger et al.[263] found that Te had no effect on white muscle disease in lambs fed a diet low in Se. Krishnamurty and Bieri[178] also found no protection in Se-deficient chicks from exudative diathesis when Te was added to a diet low in vitamin E. However, they did find that Te reduced apparent lipid peroxidation in tissues (as indicated by thiobarbituric acid reactive compounds), although not as effectively as did Se or vitamin E.

Tellurium, when added to a diet adequate in both Se and vitamin E, can induce some signs suggestive of Se-vitamin E deficiency. Van Vleet et al.[264] observed depressed SeGSHpx activity in blood of Te-treated pigs, despite normal levels of Se in liver. Tellurium treatment resulted in histopathological lesions normally associated with Se-vitamin E deficiency. Weight gain of Te-treated pigs was less than 50% of that of control animals, but whether this was associated with depressed feed intake was not indicated. A lowered feed intake and, hence depressed intakes of Se and vitamin E could account for the depressed GSHpx and other deficiency signs.

Tellurium has been shown in other ways to interact with Se. Howell and Hill[260] found that inclusion of Te in a chick diet containing excess Se lead to increased deposition of Se in liver, while reducing both mortality and depression of growth. Any protective effect of Te in Se toxicity, then, must not be through interference with absorption of Se or through reducing its retention. Se can also counter toxicity due to large amounts of Te. Sodium selenide (5 ppm) or 200 IU vitamin E/kg of diet afforded complete protection to ducklings fed 500 ppm Te as $TeCl_4$.[265]

REFERENCES

1. Schwarz, K., Production of dietary necrotic liver degeneration using American *Torula* yeast, Proc. Soc. Exper. Biol. Med., 77, 818, 1951.
2. Schwarz, K., and Foltz, C. M., Selenium as an integral part of Factor 3 against dietary necrotic liver generation, J. Amer. Chem. Soc., 79, 3292, 1957.
3. Schwarz, K., Bieri, J. G., Briggs, G. M., and Scott, M. L., Prevention of exudative diathesis in chicks by Factor 3 and selenium, Proc. Soc. Exper. Biol. Med., 95, 621, 1957.
4. Patterson, E. L., Milstrey, R., and Stokstad, E. L. R., Effect of selenium in preventing exudative diathesis in chicks, Proc. Soc. Exper. Biol. Med., 95, 617, 1957.
5. Mills, G. C., Hemoglobin catabolism, 1. Glutathione peroxidase, an erythrocyte enzyme which protects hemoglobin from oxidative breakdown, J. Biol. Chem., 229, 189, 1957.
6. Mills, G. C., and Randall, H. P., Hemoglobin catabolism. II. The protection of hemoglobin from oxidative breakdown of the intact erythrocyte, J. Biol. Chem., 232, 589, 1958.
7. Cohen, G., and Hochstein, P., Glutathione peroxidase: the primary agent for the elimination of hydrogen peroxide in erythrocytes, Biochemistry, 2, 1420, 1963.
8. Rotruck, J. T., Pope, A. L., Ganther, H. E., and Hoekstra, W. G., Prevention of oxidative damage to rat erythrocytes by dietary selenium, J. Nutr., 102, 689, 1972.
9. Rotruck, J. T., Pope, A. L., Ganther, H. E., Swanson, A. B., Hafeman, D. G., and Hoekstra, W. G., Selenium: Biochemical role as a component of glutathione peroxidase, Science, 179, 588, 1973.
10. Nakamura, W., Hosoda, S., and Hayashi, K., Purification and properties of rat liver glutathione peroxidase, Biochim. Biophys. Acta, 358, 251, 1974.
11. Stults, F. H., Forstrom, J. W., Chiu, D. T., and Tappel, A. L., Rat liver glutathione peroxidase: purification and study of multiple forms, Arch. Biochem. Biophys, 183, 490, 1977.
12. Chiu, D. T., Stults, F. H., and Tappel, A. L., Purification and properties of rat lung soluble glutathione peroxidase, Biochim. Biophys. Acta, 445, 558, 1976.
13. Chaudiere, J., and Tappel, A. L., Purification and characterization of selenium-glutathione peroxidase from hamster liver, Arch. Biochem. Biophys., 226, 448, 1983.
14. Schneider, F., and Flohé, L., Untersuchungen uber die glutathion: H_2O_2-oxydoreductase (glutathion-peroxydase), Hoppe-Seyler's Z. Physiol. Chem., 348, 540, 1967.
15. Flohé, L., and Schlegel, W., Glutathion-peroxidase. IV. Hoppe-Seyler's Z. Physiol. Chem., 352, 1401, 1971.
16. Flohé, L., Gunzler, W. A., and Shock, H. W., Glutathione peroxidase: a selenoenzyme, FEBS Letts., 32, 132, 1973.
17. Gunzler, W. A., Steffens, G. J., Grossman, A., Kim, S. M. A., Otting, F., Wendel, A., and Flohé, L., The amino-acid sequence of bovine glutathione peroxidase, Hoppe-Seyler's Z. Physiol. Chem., 365, 195, 1984.
18. Holmberg, N. J., Purification and properties of glutathione peroxidase from bovine lens, Exp. Eye Res., 7, 570, 1968.
19. Oh, S. H., Ganther, H. E., and Hoekstra, W. G., Selenium as a component of glutathione peroxidase isolated from ovine erythrocytes, Biochemistry, 13, 1825, 1974.
20. Sunde, R. A., Ganther, H. E., and Hoekstra, W. G., A comparison of ovine liver and erythrocyte glutathione peroxidase, Fed. Proc., 37, 757, 1978 (abstr.).
21. Smith, A. G., Harland, W. A., and Brooks, C. J. W., Glutathione peroxidase in human and animal aortas, Steroids Lipids Res., 4, 122, 1973.

22. Paglia, D. E., and Valentine, W. N., Studies on the quantitative and qualitative characterization of erythrocyte glutathione peroxidase, J. Lab. Clin. Med., 70,158,1967.

23. Awasthi, Y. C., Beutler, E., and Srivastava, S. K., Purification and properties of human erythrocyte glutathione peroxidase, J. Biol. Chem., 250, 5144, 1975.

24. Awasthi, Y. C., Dao, D., Lal, K. K., and Srivastava, S. K., Purification and properties of glutathione peroxidase from human placenta, Biochem. J., 177, 471, 1979.

25. Sunde, R. A., The metabolism of selenium in relation to glutathione peroxidase, PhD thesis, University of Wisconsin, Madison, 1980.

26. Wendel, A., Pilz, W., Ladenstein, G., Sawatzki, G., and Weser, V., Substrate-induced redox change of selenium in glutathione peroxidase as studied by x-ray photoelectron spectroscopy, Biochim. Biophys. Acta, 377, 211,1975.

27. Forstrom, J. W., Zakowski, J. J., and Tappel, A. L., Identification of the catalytic site of rat liver glutathione peroxidase as selenocysteine, Biochemistry, 17, 2639, 1978.

28. Epp, O., Ladenstein, R., and Wendel, A., The refined structure of the selenoenzyme glutathione peroxidase at 0.2-nm resolution, Eur. J. Biochem., 133, 51, 1983.

29. Condell, R. A., and Tappel, A. L., Amino acid sequence around the active-site selenocysteine of rat liver glutathione peroxidase, Biochim. Biophys. Acta, 709, 304, 1982.

30. Ladenstein, R., Epp, O., Bartels, K., Jones, A., Huber, R., and Wendel, A., Structure analysis and molecular model of the selenoenzyme glutathione peroxidase at 2.8 Å resolution, J. Mol. Biol., 134, 199, 1979.

31. Kraus, R. J., and Ganther, H. E., Reaction of cyanide with glutathione peroxidase, Biochem. Biophys. Res. Comm., 96, 1116, 1980.

32. Ganther, H. E., Selenoproteins, Chemica Scripta, 8A, 79, 1975.

33. Flohé, L., Loschen, G., Gunzler, W. A., and Eichele, E., Glutathione peroxidase. V. Hoppe-Seyler's Z. Physiol. Chem., 353, 987, 1972.

34. Flohé, L. and Gunzler, W. A., Glutathione peroxidase, in *Glutathione, Proceedings of the 16th Conference of the German Society of Biological Chemistry*, Flohé, L., Benohr, H.Ch., Sies, H., Waller, H. D., and Wendel, A., eds., Georg Thieme Publishers, Stuttgart, Germany, 1974.

35. Little, C., and O'Brien, P. J., An intracellular GSH-peroxidase with a lipid peroxide substrate, Biochem. Biophys. Res. Comm., 31, 145, 1968.

36. Christophersen, B. O., Reduction of linolenic acid hydroperoxide by a glutathione peroxidase, Biochim. Biophys. Acta, 176, 463, 1969.

37. Christophersen, B. O., Formation of monohydroxy-polyenic fatty acids from lipid peroxides by a glutathione peroxidase, Biochim. Biophys. Acta, 164, 35, 1968.

38. Prohaska, J. R., Oh, S. H., Hoekstra, W. G., and Ganther, H. E., Glutathione peroxidase: inhibition by cyanide of release of selenium, Biochem. Biophys. Res. Comm., 74, 64, 1977.

39. Kraus, R. J., Prohaska, J. R., and Ganther, H. E., Oxidized forms of ovine erythrocyte glutathione peroxidase, Biochim. Biophys. Acta, 615, 19, 1980.

40. Ganther, H. E. and Kraus, R. J., Oxidation states of erythrocyte glutathione peroxidase: isolation of an enzyme-glutathione complex, in *Selenium in Biology and Medicine*, Spallholz, J. E., Martin, J. L., and Ganther, H. E., eds., Avi Pub. Co., Westport, Conn., 1981, 865.

41. Chaudiere, G., Wilhelmsen, E. C., and Tappel, A. L., Mechanism of selenium-glutathione peroxidase and its inhibition by mercaptocarboxylic acids and other mercaptans, J. Biol. Chem., 259, 1043, 1984.

42. Chow, C. K., Nutritional influence on ceHular antioxidant systems, Am. J. Clin. Nutr., 32, 1066, 1979.

43. Diplock, A. T., The role of vitamin E and selenium in the prevention of oxygen-induced tissue damage, in *Selenium in Biology and Medicine*, Spallholz, J. E., Martin, J. L., and Ganther, H. E., eds., Avi Pub. Co., Westport, Conn., 1981, 303.

44. Witting, L. A., The role of nutritional factors in free-radical reactions, in *Advances in Nutritional Research*, Draper, H. H., ed., Plenum Press, New York, 1977, Chap. 8.

45. McCay, P. B., and King, M. M., Vitamin E: its role as a biologic free radical scavenger and its relationship to the microsomal mixed-function oxidase system, in *Vitamin E: A Comprehensive Treatise*, Machlin, L. J., ed., Marcel Dekker, New York, 1980, 289.

46. Fong, K. L., McCay, P. B., Poyer, J. L., Keele, B. B., and Misra, H., Evidence that peroxidation of lysosomal membranes is initiated by hydroxyl free radicals produced during flavin enzyme activity, J. Biol. Chem., 248, 7792, 1973.

47. Fridovich, I., Quantitative aspects of the production of superoxide anion radical by milk xanthine oxidase, J. Biol. Chem., 245, 4053, 1970.

48. Recknagel, R. O., and Glende, E. A., Carbon tetrachloride hepatotoxicity: an example of lethal cleavage, CRC Critical Reviews in Toxicology, 2, 263, 1973.

49. Cohen, G., and Cederbaum, A. I., Chemical evidence for production of hydroxyl radicals during microsomal electron transfer, Science, 204, 66, 1979.

50. Foote, C., Photosensitized oxygenations and the role of singlet oxygen, Accounts Chem. Res., 1, 104, 1968.

51. Beuge, J. A., and Aust, S. D., Lactoperoxidase-catalyzed lipid peroxidation of microsomal and artificial membranes, Biochim. Biophys. Acta, 444, 192, 1976.

52. Tappel, A. L., Lipid peroxidation damage to cell components, Fed. Proc., 32, 1870, 1973.

53. Tarn, B. K., and McKay, P. B., Reduced triphosphopyridine nucleotide oxidase-catalyzed alterations of membrane phospholipids, J. Biol. Chem., 245, 2295, 1970.

54. Roubal, W. T., Free radicals, malonaldehyde and protein damage in lipid-protein systems, Lipids, 6, 62, 1971.

55. Roubal, W. T., and Tappel, A. L., Damage to proteins, enzymes, and amino acids by peroxidizing lipids, Arch. Biochem. Biophys., 113, 5, 1966.

56. Babior, B. M., Kipnes, R. S., and Curnutte, J. T., The production by leukocytes of superoxide, a potential bactericidal agent, J. Clin. Invest., 52, 741, 1973.

57. Hamberg, M., and Samuelsson, B., Oxygenation of unsaturated fatty acids by the vesicular gland of sheep, J. Biol. Chem., 242, 5344, 1967.

58. Proctor, J. F., Hogue, D. E., and Warn, R. G., Selenium, vitamin E and linseed oil meal as preventatives of muscular dystrophy in lambs, J. Anim. Sci., 17, 1183, 1958.

59. McKay, P. B., Gibson, D. D., Fong, K. L., and Hornbrook, K. R., Effect of glutathione peroxidase activity on lipid peroxidation in biological membranes, Biochim. Biophys. Acta, 431, 459, 1976.

60. Grossman, A., and Wendel, A., Phospholipid hydroperoxides are not substrates for selenium-dependent glutathione peroxidase, in *Oxygen Radicals in Chemistry and Biology*, Bors, W., Saran, M., and Tait, D., eds., Walter de Gruyter and Co., Berlin, 1984, 719.

61. Green, R. C., and O'Brien, P. J., The cellular localisation of glutathione peroxidase and its release from mitochondria during swelling, Biochim. Biophys. Acta, 197, 31, 1970.

62. Guidi, G., Schiavon, R., Biasioli, A., and Perona, G., The enzyme glutathione peroxidase in arachidonic acid metabolism of human platelets, J. Lab. Clin. Med., 104, 574, 1984.

63. Bryant, R. W., Simon, T. C., and Bailey, J. M., Role of glutathione peroxidase and hexose monophosphate shunt in the platelet lipoxygenase pathway, J. Biol. Chem., 257, 4937, 1982.

64. Ham, E. A., Egan, R. W., Soderman, D. D., Gale, P. H., and Kuehl, F. A., Jr., Peroxidase-dependent deactivation of prostacyclin synthetase, J. Biol. Chem., 254, 2191, 1979.

65. Bryant, R. W., Simon, T. C., and Bailey, J. M., Hydroperoxy fatty acid formation in selenium deficient rat platelets: coupling of glutathione peroxidase to the lipoxygenase pathway, Biochem. Biophys. Res. Comm., 117, 183,1983.

66. Schiavon, R., Freeman, G. E., Guidi, G. C., Perona, G., Zatti, M., and Kakkar, V. V., Selenium enhances prostacyclin production by cultured endothelial cells: possible explanation for increased bleeding times in volunteers taking selenium as a dietary supplement, Thrombosis Res., 34, 389, 1984.

67. Vader, C. R., Mathias, M. M., and Schatte, C. L., Pulmonary prostaglandin metabolism during normobaric hyperoxia, Prostagland. Med., 6, 101, 1981.

68. North, L. N., Mathias, M. M., and Schatte, C. L., Effect of dietary vitamin E or selenium on prostaglandin dehydrogenase in hyperoxic rat lung, Aviation, Space, Environ. Med., July, 1984.

69. Meister, A., and Anderson, M. E., Glutathione, Ann. Rev. Biochem., 52, 711, 1983.

70. Omaye, S. T., and Tappel, A. L., Effect of dietary selenium on glutathione peroxidase in the chick, J. Nutr., 104, 747, 1974.

71. Combs, G. F.,Jr., Liu, C. H., and Su, Q., unpublished results, 1982.

72. Smith, P. J., Tappel, A. L., and Chow, C. K., Glutathione peroxidase activity as a function of dietary selenomethionine, Nature, 247, 392, 1974.

73. Lawrence, R. A., and Burk, R. F., Glutathione peroxidase activity in selenium-deficient rat liver, Biochem. Biophys. Res. Comm., 71, 952, 1976.

74. Lawrence, R. A., Parkhill, L. K., and Burk, R. F., Hepatic cytosolic non Se-dependent glutathione peroxidase activity: its nature and the effect of selenium deficiency, J. Nutr., 108, 981, 1978.

75. Pierce, S., and Tappel, A. L., Glutathione peroxidase activities from rat liver, Biochim. Biophys. Acta, 523, 27, 1978.

76. Lawrence, R. A., and Burk, R. F., Species, tissue, and subcellular distribution of non Se-dependent glutathione peroxidase activity, J. Nutr., 108, 211, 1978.

77. Davies, M. H., Bozigian, H. P., Merrick, B. A., Birt, D. F., and Schnell, R. C., Circadian variations in glutathione-S-transferase and glutathione peroxidase activities in the mouse, Toxicol. Letts., 19, 23, 1983.

78. Cupp, M. S., Studies of the nutritional-biochemical interactions of selenium and ascorbic acid in the chick, PhD thesis, Cornell University, Ithaca, New York, 1984.

79. Lee, V. H., Layman, D. K., and Bell, R. R., Selenium-dependent and non selenium-dependent glutathione peroxidase activity in rabbit tissue, Nutr. Rep. Int., 20, 573, 1979.

80. Ursini, F., Maiorino, M., Valente, M., Ferri, L., and Gregolin, C., Purification from pig liver of a protein which protects liposomes and biomembranes from peroxidative degradation and exhibits glutathione peroxidase activity on phosphatidylcholine hydroperoxides, Biochim. Biophys Acta, 710, 197, 1982.

81. Maiorino, M., Ursini, F., Leonelli, M., Finato, N., and Gregolin, C., A pig heart peroxidation inhibiting protein with glutathione peroxidase activity on phospholipid hydroperoxides, Biochem. Int., 5, 575, 1982.

82. Ursini, F., Maiorino, M., Bonaldo, L., and Gregolin, C., The glutathione peroxidase active on phospholipid hydroperoxides: studies on the enzyme from pig brain, in *Oxygen Radicals in Chemistry and Biology*, Bors, W., Saran, M., and Tait, D., eds., Walter de Gruyter and Co., Berlin, 1984.

83. Wendel, A., Fausel, M., Safayhi, H., Tiegs, G., and Otter, R., A novel biologically active seleno-organic compound. II. Activity of PZ51 in relation to glutathione peroxidase, Biochem. Pharm., 33, 3241, 1984.

84. Wendel, A., Fausel, M., Safayhi, H., Tiegs, G., and Otter, R., Ebselen[+] (PZ51), a seleno organic compound endowed with glutathione peroxidase activity, in Proceedings of the Third International Symposium on Selenium in Biology and Medicine, Combs, G. F., Jr., Spallholz, J. E., Levander, O. A., and Oldfield, J. E., eds., Avi Publ. Co., Westport, Conn., 1986.

85. Sies, H., Akerboom, T., Ishikawa, T., Cadenas, E., Graf, P., Gabriel, H., and Muller, A., Hepatic and cardiac hydroperoxide metabolism: role of selenium, in Proceedings of the Third International Symposium on Selenium in Biology and Medicine, Combs, G. F., Jr., Spallholz, J. E., Levander, O. A., and Oldfield, J. E., eds., Avi Publ. Co., Westport, Conn., 1986.

86. Reiter, R., and Wendel, A., Selenium and drug metabolism-II. Independence of glutathione peroxidase and reversibility of hepatic enzyme modulations in deficient mice, Biochem. Pharm., 33, 1923, 1984.

87. Shull, L. R., Buckmaster, G. W., and Cheeke, P. R., Effect of dietary selenium status on in vitro hepatic mixed-function oxidase enzymes of rats, J. Environ. Path. Toxicol., 2, 1127, 1979.

88. Pilch, S. M. and Combs, G. F., Jr., Effects of dietary vitamin E and selenium on the mixed-function oxygenase system of male and female chicks, Comp. Biochem. Physiol., 69C, 331, 1981.

89. Burk, R. F., and Lane, J. M., Ethane production and liver necrosis in rats after administration of drugs and other chemicals, Tox. Appl. Pharm., 50, 467, 1979.

90. Masukawa, T., Nishimura, T., and Iwata, H., Differential changes of glutathione S-transferase activity by dietary selenium, Biochem. Pharm. 33, 2635, 1984.

91. Chen, J. S., Goetchius, M. P., Campbell, T. C., and Combs, G. F., Jr., Effects of dietary selenium and vitamin E on hepatic mixed-function oxidase activities and in vivo covalent binding of aflatoxin B_1 in rats, J. Nutr., 112, 324, 1982.

92. Reiter, R., and Wendel, A., Selenium and drug metabolism-I. Multiple modulations of mouse liver enzymes, Biochem. Pharm., 32, 3063, 1983.

93. Burk, R. F., and Masters, B. S. S., Some effects of selenium deficiency on the hepatic microsomal cytochrome P-450 system in the rat, Arch. Biochem. Biophys., 170, 124, 1975.

94. Bell, J. G., Cowley, C. B., and Youngson, A., Rainbow trout liver microsomal lipid peroxidation: The effect of purified glutathione peroxidase, glutathione S-transferase and other factors, Biochim. Biophys. Acta, 795, 91, 1984.

95. Siami, G., Schulert, A. R., and Neal, R. A., A possible role for the mixed function oxidase enzyme system in the requirement for selenium in the rat, J. Nutr., 102, 857, 1972.

96. Mitchell, J. R., Hughes, H., Lauterberg, B. H., and Smith, C. V., Chemical nature of reactive intermediates as determinant of toxicologic responses, Drug Metab. Rev., 13, 539, 1982.

97. Shin, B. C., Huggins, J. W., and Karraway, K. L., Effects of pH, concentration and aging on the malonaldehyde reaction with proteins, Lipids, 7, 229, 1972.

98. Siu, G. M., and Draper, H. H., Metabolism of malonaldehyde in vivo and vitro, Lipids, 17, 349, 1982.

99. Donovan, D. H., and Menzel, D. B., Mechanisms of lipid peroxidation: iron catalyzed decomposition of fatty acid hydroperoxides as the basis of hydrocarbon evolution in vivo, Experientia, 34, 775, 1978.

100. Dumelin, E. E., and Tappel, A. L., Hydrocarbon gases produced during *in vitro* peroxidation of polyunsaturated fatty acids and decomposition of preformed hydroperoxides, Lipids, 12, 894, 1977.

101. Hafeman, D. G. and Hoekstra, W. G., Protection against carbon tetrachloride-induced lipid peroxidation in the rat by dietary vitamin E, selenium, and methionine as measured by ethane evolution, J. Nutr., 107, 656, 1977.

102. Riely, C. A., and Cohen, G., Ethane evolution: a new index of lipid peroxidation, Science, 183, 208, 1974.

103. Dillard, C. J., and Tappel, A. L., Volatile hydrocarbon and carbonyl products of lipid peroxidation: a comparison of pentane, ethane, hexanal, and acetone as *in vivo* indices, Lipids, 14, 989, 1979.

104. Gavino, V. C., Dillard, C. J., and Tappel, A. L., Release of ethane and pentane from rat tissue slices: effect of vitamin E, halogenated hydrocarbons, and iron overload, Arch. Biochem. Biophys., 233, 741, 1984.

105. Peterson, F. J., Combs, G. F., Jr., Holtzman, J. L., and Mason, R. L., Effect of Se and vitamin E deficiency on nitrofurantoin toxicity in the chick, J. Nutr., 112, 1741, 1982.

106. Peterson, F. J., Combs, G. F.,Jr., Holtzman, J. L., and Mason, R. P., Metabolic activation of oxygen by nitrofurantoin in the young chick, Toxicol. Appl. Pharm., 65, 162, 1982.

107. Bus, J. S., Aust, S. D., and Gibson, J. E., Superoxide- and oxygen-catalyzed lipid peroxidation as a possible mechanism for paraquat (methyl viologen) toxicity, Biochem. Biophys. Res. Comm., 58, 749, 1974.

108. Mason, R. P., and Holtzman, J. L., The role of catalytic superoxide formation in the O_2 inhibition of nitroreductase, Biochem. Biophys. Res. Comm., 67, 1267, 1975.

109. Sasame, H. A., and Boyd, M. R., Superoxide and hydrogen peroxide production and NADPH oxidation stimulated by nitrofurantoin in lung microsomes: possible implications for toxicity, Life Sci., 24, 1091, 1979.

110. Burk, R. F., and Lane, J. M., Modification of chemical toxicity by selenium deficiency, Fund. Appl. Tox., 3, 218, 1983.

111. Dershwitz, M. and Novak, R. F., Generation of superoxide via the interaction of nitrofurantoin with oxyhemoglobin, J. Biol. Chem., 257, 75, 1982.

112. Dershwitz, M., and Novak, R. F., Studies on the mechanism of nitrofurantoin-mediated red cell toxicity, J. Pharmacol. Exper. Therapeutics, 222, 430, 1982.

113. Combs, G. F., Jr., Influences of dietary vitamin E and selenium on the oxidant defense system of the chick, Poultry Sci., 60, 2098, 1981.

114. Prohaska, J. R., and Ganther, H. E., Glutathione peroxidase activity of glutathione-*S*-transferases purified from rat liver, Biochem. Biophys. Res. Comm., 76, 437, 1977.

115. Jakoby, W. B., Glutathione-*S*-transferases: a group of multifunctional detoxification proteins, Adv. Enzymology, 46, 383, 1977.

116. Chen, J., Goetchius, M. P., Combs, G. F.,Jr., and Campbell, T. C., Effects of dietary selenium and vitamin E on covalent binding of aflatoxin to chick liver cell macromolecules, J. Nutr., 112, 350, 1982.

117. Peterson, F. J., and Combs, G. F., Jr., unpublished results, 1983.

118. Gregory, J. F. III, and Edds, G. T., Effect of dietary selenium on the metabolism of aflatoxin B_1 in turkeys, Fd. Chem. Toxic., 22, 637, 1984.

119. Mercurio, S. D., Lichtblau, L., and Sparber, S. B., Separation of hepatic N-demethylase-inducing and opioid dependence-producing doses of levo-alpha-acetylmethadol in the pregnant rat, Life Sciences, 33, 1127, 1983.

120. Dahlin, D. C., Miwa, G. T., Lu, A. Y.H., and Nelson, S. D., N-Acetyl-p-benzoquinone imine: a cytochrome P-450-mediated oxidation product of acetaminophen, Proc. Natl. Acad. Sci., USA, 81, 1327, 1984.

121. Dahlin, D. C., and Nelson, S. D., Synthesis, decomposition kinetics, and preliminary toxicological studies of pure N-acetyl-p-benzoquinone imine, a proposed toxic metabolite of acetaminophen, J. Med. Chem., 25, 885, 1982.

122. Cummings, A. J., King, M. L., and Martin, B. K., The excretion of paracetamol and its metabolites in man, Br. J. Pharmacol. Chemother., 29, 150, 1967.

123. Mitchell, J. R., Thorgeirsson, S. S., Potter, W. Z., Jollow, D. J., and Keiser, H., Acetaminophen-induced hepatic injury: protective role of glutathione in man and rationale for therapy, Clin. Pharmacol. Ther., 16, 676, 1974.

124. Davis, M., Labadarios, D., and Williams, R. S., Metabolism of paracetamol after therapeutic hepatotoxic doses in man, J. Int. Med. Res., 4, 40, 1976.

125. Davis, M., Simmons, C. J., Harrison, N. G., and Williams, R., Paracetamol overdose in man: relationship between pattern of urinary metabolites and severity of liver damage, Q. J. Med., 178, 181, 1976.

126. Peterson, F. J., personal communication.

127. Thelen, M., and Wendel, A., Drug-induced lipid peroxidation in mice—V: Ethane production and glutathione release in the isolated liver upon perfusion with acetaminophen, Biochem. Pharm., 32, 1701, 1983.

128. Wendel, A., and Feuerstein, S., Drug-induced lipid peroxidation in mice—I: Modulation by monoxygenase activity, glutathione and selenium status, Biochem. Pharm., 30, 2513, 1981.

129. Burk, R. F., and Correia, M. A., Selenium and hepatic heme metabolism, in *Selenium in Biology and Medicine*, Spallholz, J. E., Martin, J. L., and Ganther, H. E., eds., Avi Pub. Co., Westport, Conn., 1981, 86.

130. Correia, M. A., and Burk, R. F., Defective utilization of haem in selenium-deficient rat liver, Biochem. J., 214, 53, 1983.

131. Pascoe, G. A., Sakai-Wong, J., Soliven, E., and Correia, M. A., Regulation of intestinal cytochrome P-450 and heme by dietary nutrients: Critical role of selenium, Biochem. Pharm., 32, 3027, 1983.

132. McCoy, K. E. M., and Weswig, P. H., Some selenium responses in the rat related to vitamin E, J. Nutr., 98, 383, 1969.

133. Wu, S. H., Oldfield, J. E., and Whanger, P. D., Effects of selenium, vitamin E, and antioxidants on testicular function in rats. Biol. Reprod., 8, 625, 1973.

134. Wallace, E., Calvin, H. I., and Cooper, G. W., Progressive defects observed in mouse sperm during the course of three generations of selenium deficiency, Gamete Res., 4, 377, 1981.

135. Liu, C. H., Chen, Y. M., Zhang, J. Z., Huang, M. Y., Su, Q., Lu, Z. H., Yin, R. X., Shao, G. Z., Feng, D., and Zheng, P. L., Preliminary studies on influence of selenium deficiency to the developments of genital organs and spermatogenesis of infant boars, Acta Veterinaria Zootechnica Sinica, 13, 73,1982.

136. Palleni, V., and Bacci, E., Bull sperm selenium is bound to a structural protein of mitochondria, J. Submicr. Cytol., 11, 165, 1979.

137. Brown, D. B., and Burk, R. F., Selenium retention in tissues and sperm of rats fed *Torula* yeast diet, J. Nutr., 102, 102, 1972.

138. Calvin, H. I. and Cooper, G. W., A specific selenopolypeptide associated with the outer membrane of rat sperm mitochondria, in *The Spermatozoan*, Fawcett, D. W., and Bedford, J. M., eds., Urban and Schwarzenberg, Baltimore, 1979, 135.

139. Calvin, H. I., Cooper, G. W., and Wallace, E. W., Evidence that selenium in rat sperm is associated with a cysteine-rich structural protein of the mitochondrial capsule, Gamete Res., 4, 139, 1981.

140. Wallace, E., Calvin, H. I., and Cooper, G. W., Progressive defects observed in mouse sperm during the course of three generations of selenium deficiency, Gamete Res., 4, 377, 1983.

141. Combs, G. F., Jr. and Whitacre, M., unpublished results.

142. Burk, R. F., and Gregory, P. E., Some characteristics of ^{75}Se-P, a selenoprotein found in rat liver and plasma, and comparison of it with seleno-glutathione peroxidase, Arch. Biochem. Biophys., 213, 73, 1982.

143. Motsenbocker, M. A. and Tappel, A. L., Selenium and selenoproteins in the rat kidney, Biochim. Biophys. Acta, 709, 160, 1982.

144. Motsenbocker, M. A. and Tappel, A. L., Selenocysteine-containing selenium transport protein in rat plasma, Biochim. Biophys. Acta, 719, 147, 1982.

145. Motsenbocker, M. A., and Tappel, A. L., Selenocysteine-containing proteins from rat and monkey plasma, Biochim. Biophys. Acta, 704, 253, 1982.

146. Chow, C. K., and Jeng, J., Dietary selenium and distribution of selenium in the tissues of young and mature rats, in *Selenium in Biology and Medicine*, Spallholz, J. E., Martin, J. L., and Ganther, H. E., eds., Avi Pub. Co., Westport, Conn., 1981, 477.

147. Pinsent, J., The need for selenite and molybdate in the formation of formic dehydrogenase by members of the *coli-aerogenes* group of bacteria, Biochem. J., 57, 10, 1954.

148. Enoch, H. G., and Lester, R. L., The purification and properties of formate dehydrogenase and nitrate reductase from *Escherichia coli*, J. Biol. Chem., 250, 6693, 1975.

149. Andreesen, J. R., and Ljungdahl, L. G., Formate dehydrogenase of *Clostridium thermoaceticum*: incorporation of ^{75}Se and the effects of selenite, molybdate and tungstate on the enzyme, J. Bacteriol., 116, 867, 1973.

150. Andreesen, J. R., El Ghazzawi, E., and Gottschalk, G., The effect of ferrous ions, tungstate and selenite on the level of formate dehydrogenase in *Clostridium formicoaceticum* and formate synthesis from CO_2 during pyruvate fermentation. Arch. Microbiol. 96, 103, 1973.

151. Stadtman, T. C., Biochemical function of selenium, Nutr. Rev., 35, 161, 1977.

152. Wagner, R. and Andreesen, J. R., Differentiation between *Clostridium acidiurici* and *Clostridium cylindrosporum*, on the basis of specific metal requirements for formate dehydrogenase formation, Arch. Microbiol., 114, 219, 1977.

153. Jones, J. B., Dilworth, G. L., and Stadtman, T. C., Occurrence of selenocysteine in the selenium-dependent formate dehydrogenase of *Methanococcus vannielli*, Arch. Biochem. Biophys., 195, 255, 1979.

154. Stadtman, T. C., Selenium dependent enzymes, Ann. Rev. Biochem., 49, 93, 1980.

155. Costilow, R. N., Selenium requirement for the growth of *Clostridium sporogenes* with glycine as the oxidant in Strickland reaction systems, J. Bacteriol., 131, 366, 1977.

156. Imhoff, D., and Andreesen, J. R., Nicotinic acid hydroxglase from *Clostridium barker*: selenium dependent formation of active enzyme, FEMS Microbiol. Letts., 5, 155, 1979.

157. McMurray, C. H., and McEldowney, P. K., A possible prophylaxis and model for degenerative myopathy in young cattle, Br. Vet. J., 133, 535, 1977.

158. Michaelis, L., and Wollman, S. H., The semiquinone radical of tocopherol, Science, 109, 313, 1949.

159. Yoshida, M., and Hoshii, H., Preventive effect of selenium, methionine and antioxidants against encephalomalacia of chicks induced by dilauryl succinate, J. Nutr., 107, 35, 1977.

160. Draper, H. H., Ineffectiveness of selenium in the treatment of nutritional muscular dystrophy in the rabbit, Nature, 180, 1419, 1957.

161. Hove, E. L., Fry, G. S., and Schwarz, K., Ineffectiveness of Factor 3-active selenium compounds in muscular dystrophy of rabbits on vitamin E-free diets, Proc. Soc. Exp. Biol. Med., 98, 27, 1958.

162. Dam, H., Kruse, I., Prange, I., and Sondergaard, E., Influence of dietary ascorbic acid, nordihydroguaiaretic acid and cystine on vitamin E deficiency symptoms in chickens, Biochim. Biophys. Acta, 2, 501, 1958.

163. Combs, G. F., Jr., and Scott, M. L., Antioxidant effects on selenium and vitamin E function in the chick, J. Nutr., 104, 1297, 1974.

164. Combs, G. F., Jr., and Pesti, G. M., Influence of ascorbic acid on selenium nutrition in the chick, J. Nutr., 106, 958, 1976.

165. Moran, E. T., Jr., Carlson, H. C., Brown, R. G., Sweeny, P. R., George, J. C., and Stanley, D. W., Alleviating mortality associated with a vitamin E-selenium deficiency by dietary ascorbic acid, Poultry Sci., 54, 266, 1975.

166. Chen, L. H., and Thacker, R. R., An increase in glutathione peroxidase activity induced by high supplementation of vitamin C in rats, Nutr. Res., 4, 657, 1984.

167. Fidler, J. W., Naber, E. C., and Latshaw, J. D., Effect of peroxide administration on selenium utilization, growth, deficiency symptoms, and glutathione peroxidase activity in chicks fed controlled selenium diets, Poultry Sci., 59, 141, 1980.

168. Dean, W. F., and Combs, G. F., Jr., Influence of dietary selenium on performance, tissue selenium content, and plasma concentrations of selenium-dependent glutathione peroxidase, vitamin E, and ascorbic acid in ducklings, Poultry Sci., 60, 2655, 1981.

169. Brown, R. G., Sweeny, P. R., George, J. C., Stanley, D. W., and Moran, E. T., Jr., Selenium deficiency in the duck: serum ascorbic acid levels in developing muscular dystrophy, Poultry Sci., 53, 1235, 1974.

170. Chow, C. K., Thacker, R., and Gairola, C., Dietary selenium and levels of L-ascorbic acid in the plasma, livers, and lungs of polychlorinated biphenyls-treated rats, Internat. J. Vit. Nutr. Res., 51, 279, 1981.

171. Nishikimi, M., Oxidation of ascorbic acid with superoxide anion generated by the xanthine-xanthine oxidase system, Biochem. Biophys. Res. Comm., 63, 463, 1975.

172. Fridovich, I., The biology of oxygen radicals, Science, 201, 875, 1978.

173. Basu, S., Som, S., Deb, S., Mukherjee, D., and Chatterjee, I. B., Dehydroascorbic acid reduction in human erythrocytes, Biochem. Biophys. Res. Comm., 90, 1335, 1979.

174. Som, S., Basu, S., Mukherjee, D., and Chatterjee, I. B., Dehydroascorbic acid reduction in guinea pig tissues Curr. Sci., 49 195, 1980.

175. Willis, P. J., and Kratzing, C. C., Extracellular ascorbic acid in lung, Biochim. Biophys. Acta, 444, 108, 1976.

176. Jamieson, D., and Brenk, H. A.S., The effects of antioxidants on high pressure oxygen toxicity, Biochem. Pharm., 13, 159, 1964.

177. Combs, G. F., Jr., Influence of ethoxyquin on the utilization of selenium by the chick, Poultry Sci., 57, 210, 1978.

178. Krishnamurthy, S., and Bieri, J. G., Dietary antioxidants as related to vitamin E function, J. Nutr., 77, 245, 1962.

179. Draper, H. H., Goodyear, S., Barbee, K. D., and Johnson, B. C., A study of the nutritional role of anti-oxidants in the diet of the rat, Br. J. Nutr., 12, 89, 1958.

180. Shull, R., Alfin-Slater, R. B., Deuel, H. J., Jr., and Ershoff, B. H., Comparative effects of alpha-tocopherol, DPPD and other antioxidants on muscular dystrophy in guinea pig, Proc. Soc. Exper. Biol. Med., 95, 263, 1957.

181. Downey, J. D., Irving, D. H., and Tappel, A. L., Effects of dietary antioxidants on *in vivo* lipid peroxidation in the rat as measured by pentane production, Lipids, 13, 403, 1978.

182. Tappel, A., Fletcher, B., and Deamer, D., Effect of antioxidants and nutrients on lipid peroxidation fluorescent products and aging parameters in the mouse, J. Gerontol., 28, 415, 1973.

183. Whanger, P. D., Sulphur-selenium relationships in animal nutrition, Sulphur Inst. J., 6, 6, 1970.

184. Nuttall, K. L.,and Allen, F. S., Hydrogen selenide ion and colloidal selenium in the catalytic oxidation of thiols, Inorg. Chim. Acta, 93, 85, 1984.

185. Ganther, H. E., and Baumann, C. A., Selenium metabolism II. Modifying effects of sulfate, J. Nutr., 77, 408, 1962.

186. Halverson, A. W., and Monty, K. J., An effect of dietary sulfate on selenium poisoning in the rat, J. Nutr., 70, 100, 1960.

187. Acuff, R. V., and Smith, J. T., Dietary inorganic sulfate status in the rat and its effect on selenium absorption, Radiochem. Radioanal. Lett., 53, 25, 1982.

188. Brown, D. G., Burk, R. F., Seely, R. J., and Kiker, K. W., Effect of dietary selenium on the gastrointestinal absorption of $^{75}SeO_3^{-2}$ in the rat, Internat. J. Vit. Nutr. Res., 42, 588, 1972.

189. White, C. L. and Somers, M., Sulphur-selenium studied in sheep. I. The effects of varying dietary sulphate and selenomethionine on sulphur, nitrogen and selenium metabolism in sheep, Aust. J. Biol. Sci., 30, 47, 1977.

190. White, C. L., Sulfur-selenium studies in sheep. II. Effect of a dietary sulfur deficiency on selenium and sulfur metabolism in sheep fed varying levels of selenomethionine, Aust. J. Biol. Sci., 33, 699, 1980.

191. Ganther, H. E., Levander, O. A. and Baumann, C. A., Dietary control of selenium volatilization in the rat, J. Nutr., 88, 55, 1966.

192. Scott, M. L., Studies on the interrelationship of selenium, vitamin E and sulfur amino acids in a nutritional myopathy of the chick, Ann. N. Y. Acad. Sci., 138, 82, 1966.

193. Hathcock, J. N., Hull, S. J., and Scott, M. L., Derivations and analogs of cysteine and selected sulfhydryl compounds in nutritional muscular dystrophy in chicks, J. Nutr., 94, 147, 1968.

194. Vernie, L. N., deVries, M., Karreman, L., Topp, R. J., and Bont, W. S., Inhibition of amino acid incorporation in a cell-free system and inhibition of protein synthesis in cultured cells by reaction products of selenite and thiols, Biochim. Biophys. Acta, 739, 1, 1983.

195. Smith, S. I., Boling, J. A., Gay, N., and Cantor, A. H., Selenium and sulfur supplementation to steers grazing tall fescue, Biol. Trace Element Res., 6, 347, 1984.

196. Broderius, M. A., Whanger, P. D., and Weswig, P. H., Tissue sulfhydryl groups in selenium-deficient rats and lambs, J. Nutr., 103, 336, 1973.

197. Hull, S. J., and Scott, M. L., Changes in muscle and liver sulfhydryl compounds in chicks with nutritional muscular dystrophy, Fed. Proc., 29, 694 (abstr.), 1970.

198. Chmielnicka, J., Komsta-Szumska, E., and Zareba, G., Effect of interaction between ^{65}Zn, mercury and selenium in rats (retention, metallothionein, endogenous copper), Arch. Toxicol., 53, 165, 1983.

199. Alexander, J., and Aaseth, J., Biliary excretion of copper and zinc in the rat as influenced by diethylmaleate, selenite, and diethyldithiocarbamate, Biochem. Pharmacol., 29, 2129, 1980.

200. Naganuma, A., Tanaka, T., Kyoko, M., Matsuda, R., Tabata-Hanyu, J., and Imura, N., The interaction of selenium with various metals *in vitro* and *in vivo*, Toxicol., 29, 77, 1983.

201. Sinisalo, M., and Combs, G. F., Jr., unpublished results, 1984.
202. Chvapil, M., Peng, Y. M., Aronson, A. L., and Zukoski, C., Effect of zinc on lipid peroxidation and metal content in some tissues of rats, J. Nutr., 104, 434, 1974.
203. Amer, M. A., St-Laurent, G. J., and Brisson, G. J., Supplemental copper and selenium for calves: effects upon ceruloplasmin activity and liver copper concentration, Can. J. Physiol. Pharmacol., 51, 649, 1973.
204. Thomson, G. G., and Lawson, B. M., Copper and selenium interaction in sheep, New Zealand Vet. J., 18, 79, 1970.
205. Jenkinson, S. G., Lawrence, R. A., Burk, R. F., and Williams, D. M., Effects of copper deficiency on the activity of the selenoenzyme glutathione peroxidase and on excretion and tissue retention of $^{75}SeO_3{}^{2-}$, J. Nutr., 112, 197, 1982.
206. Dougherty, J. J., and Hoekstra, W. G., Effects of vitamin E and selenium on copper-induced lipid peroxidation in vivo and on acute copper toxicity, Proc. Soc. Exper. Biol. Med., 169, 201, 1982.
207. Jensen, L. S., Modification of a selenium toxicity in chicks by dietary silver and copper, J. Nutr., 105, 769, 1975.
208. Hill, C. H., Reversal of selenium toxicity by mercury, copper, and cadmium, J. Nutr., 104, 593, 1974.
209. Stowe, H. D., Effects of copper pretreatment upon the toxicity of selenium in ponies, Am. J. Vet. Res., 41, 1925, 1980.
210. Chen, S. Y., Collipp, P. J., and Hsu, J. M., The effect of selenium toxicity on tissue distribution of zinc, iron and copper in rats, in Proceedings of the Third International Symposium on Selenium in Biology and Medicine, Combs, G. F., Jr., Spallholz, J. E., Levander, O. A., and Oldfield, J. E., eds., Avi Publ. Co., Westport, Conn., 1986.
211. Jensen, L. S., Precipitation of a selenium deficiency by high dietary levels of copper and zinc, Proc. Soc. Exper. Biol. Med., 149, 113, 1975.
212. Parizek, J., and Ostadalova, I., The protective effect of small amounts of selenite in sublimate intoxication, Separatum Experientia, 23, 142, 1967.
213. Ganther, H. E., Goudie, C., Sunde, M. L., Kopecky, M. J., Wagner, P., Oh, S. H., and Hoekstra, W. G., Selenium: relation to decreased toxicity of methylmercury added to diets containing tuna, Science, 175, 1122, 1972.
214. Welsh, S. O., and Soares, J. H., Jr., The protective effect of vitamin E and selenium against methyl mercury toxicity in the Japanese quail, Nutr. Reports Int., 13, 43, 1976.
215. Sell, J. L., and Horani, F. G., Influence of selenium on toxicity and metabolism of methylmercury in chicks and quail, Nutr. Reports Int., 14, 439, 1976.
216. El-Begearmi, M. M., Sunde, M. L., and Ganther, H. E., A mutual protective effect of mercury and selenium in Japanese quail, Poultry Sci., 56, 313, 1977.
217. Sell, J. L., Comparative effects of selenium on metabolism of methylmercury by chickens and quail: tissue distribution and transfer into eggs, Poultry Sci., 56, 939, 1977.
218. Thomas, D. J., and Smith, J. C., Effects of coadministered sodium selenite on short-term distribution of methyl mercury in the rat, Environ. Res., 34, 287, 1984.
219. Komsta-Szumska, E., Reuhl, K. R., and Miller, D. R., Effect of selenium on distribution, demethylation, and excretion of methylmercury by the guinea pig, J. Toxicol. Environ. Health, 12, 775, 1983.
220. Ijima, S., Tohyama, C., Lu, C. C., and Matsumoto, N., Placental transfer and body distribution of methylmercury and selenium in pregnant mice, Toxicol. Appl. Pharm., 44, 143, 1978.
221. Masukawa, T., Nishimura, T., Kito, H., and Iwata, H., Influence of diethylmaleate on the formation of bis (methylmercuric) selenide and methylmercury distribution in rats, J. Pharm. Dyn., 6, 950, 1983.

222. Sener, S., Braun, J. P., Rico, A. G., Benard, P., and Burgat-Sacaze, V., Urine gamma-glutamyl transferase in rat kidney toxicology: nephropathy by repeated injections of mercuric chloride. Effects of sodium selenite, Toxicol., 12, 299, 1979.

223. Chang, L. W., Pathological effect of mercury poisoning, in *The Biochemistry of Mercury in the Environment*, Nraigu, J. O., ed., Elsevier North-Holland Biomed. Press, New York, 1979, 51.

224. Rubenstein, D. A., and Soares, J. H., Jr., The effect of selenium on the biliary excretion and tissue deposition of two forms of mercury in the broiler chick, Poultry Sci., 58, 289, 1979.

225. Naganuma, A., and Imura, N., Bis (methylmercuric) selenide as a reaction product from methylmercury and selenite in rabbit blood, Res. Comm. Chem. Pathol. Pharmacol., 27, 163, 1980.

226. Masukawa, T., Kito, H., Hayashi, M., and Iwata, H., Formation and possible role of bis (methylmercuric) selenide in rats treated with methylmercury and selenite, Biochem. Pharmacol., 31, 75, 1982.

227. Naganuma, A., Kojima, Y., and Imura, N., Interaction of methylmercury and selenium compound: formation and behavior of bis(methylmercuric) selenide in animals, 7th Symposium on Environmental Pollutants and Toxicology, Pharmaceutical Society of Japan, Kobe, 1980, 121.

228. Chen, R. W., Ganther, H. E. and Hoekstra, W. G., Studies on the binding of methylmercury by thionein, Biochem. Biophys. Res. Comm., 51, 383, 1973.

229. Magos, L., and Webb, M., The interactions of selenium with cadmium and mercury, CRC Crit. Rev. Toxicol., 8, 1, 1980.

230. Sugiura, Y., Tamai, Y., and Tanaka, H., Selenium protection against mercury toxicity: high binding affinity of methylmercury by selenium-containing ligands in comparison with sulfur-containing ligands, Bioinorg. Chem., 9, 167, 1978.

231. Ganther, H. E., Modification of methylmercury toxicity and metabolism by selenium and vitamin E: possible mechanisms, Environ. Health Perspectives, 25, 71, 1978.

232. Komsta-Szumska, E., Reuhl, K. R., and Miller, D. R., The effect of methylmercury on the distribution and excretion of selenium by the guinea pig, Arch. Toxicol., 54, 303, 1983.

233. Parizek, J., The destructive effect of cadmium ion on testicular tissue and its prevention by zinc, J. Endocrinol., 15, 56, 1957.

234. Gunn, S. A., Gould, T. C., and Anderson, W. A.D., Zinc protection against cadmium injury to rat testis, Arch. Pathol., 71, 274, 1961.

235. Gunn, S. A., Gould, T. C., and Anderson, W. A.D., Protective effect of thiol compounds against cadmium-induced vascular damage to testis, Proc. Soc. Exper. Biol., 122, 1036, 1966.

236. Mason, K. E., and Young, J. O., Effectiveness of selenium and zinc in protecting against cadmium-induced injury of the rat testis, in *Selenium in Biomedicine*, Avi Publ. Co., Westport, Conn., 1967, 383.

237. Bremner, I., and Davies, N. T., The induction of metallothionein in rat liver by zinc injection and restriction of food intake, Biochem. J., 149, 733, 1975.

238. Gasiewicz, T. A., and Smith, J. C., Interactions of cadmium and selenium in rat plasma *in vivo* and *in vitro*, Biochim. Biophys. Acta, 428, 113, 1976.

239. Chen, R. W., Whanger, P. D., and Fang, S. C., Diversion of mercury binding in rat tissues by selenium: a possible mechanism of protection, Pharmacol. Res. Comm., 6, 571, 1974.

240. Gunn, S. A., and Gould, T. C., Specificity of response in relation to cadmium, zinc, and selenium, in *Selenium in Biomedicine*, Avi Publ. Co., Westport, Conn., 1967, 395.

241. Nordberg, G. F., Cadmium metabolism and toxicity. Experimental studies on mice with special reference to the use of biological materials as indices of retention and the possible role of metallothionein in transport and detoxification of cadmium, Environ. Physiol. Biochem., 2, 7, 1972.

242. Early, J. L., Jr., and Schnell, R. C., Selenium antagonism of cadmium-induced inhibition of hepatic drug metabolism in the male rat, Toxicol. Appl. Pharmacol., 58, 57, 1981.

243. Holmberg, R. E., and Ferm, V. H., Interrelationships of selenium, cadmium, and arsenic in mammalian teratogenesis, Arch. Environ. Health, 18, 873, 1969.

244. Sandholm, M., The metabolism of selenite in cow blood *in vitro*, Acta Pharmacol. Toxicol., 33, 6, 1973.

245. Jenkins, K. J., Hidiriglou, M., and Ryan, J. F., Intravascular transport of selenium by chick serum proteins, Can. J. Physiol. Pharmacol., 47, 459, 1969.

246. Moxon, A. L., The effect of arsenic on the toxicity of seleniferous grains, Science, 88, 81, 1938.

247. Moxon, A. L., and Wilson, W. O., Selenium-arsenic antagonism in poultry, Poultry Sci., 23, 149, 1944.

248. Carlson, C. W., Guenther, E., Kohlmeyer, W., and Olson, O. E., Some effects of selenium, arsenicals, and vitamin B_{12} on chick growth, Poultry Sci., 33, 768, 1954.

249. Hill, C. H., Interrelationships of selenium with other trace elements, Fed. Proc., 34, 2096, 1975.

250. Levander, O. A., and Baumann, C. A., Selenium metabolism. V. Studies on the distribution of selenium in rats given arsenic, Toxicol. Appl. Pharm., 9, 98, 1966.

251. Levander, O. A., and Baumann, C. A., Selenium metabolism. VI. Effect of arsenic on the excretion of selenium in the bile, Toxicol. Appl. Pharm., 9, 106, 1966.

252. Cerklewski, F. L., and Forbes, R. M., Influence of dietary selenium on lead toxicity in the rat, J. Nutr., 106, 778, 1976.

253. Chisolm, J. J., Disturbances in the biosynthesis of heme in lead intoxication, J. Pediatr., 64, 174, 1972.

254. Levander, O. A., Morris, V. C., Higgs, D. J., and Ferretti, R. J., Lead poisoning in vitamin E-deficient rat, J. Nutr., 105, 1481, 1975.

255. Levander, O. A., Morris, V. C., and Ferretti, R. J., Comparative effects of selenium and vitamin E in lead-poisoned rats, J. Nutr., 107, 378, 1977.

256. Levander, O. A., Morris, V. C., and Ferretti, R. J., Filterability of erythrocytes from vitamin E-deficient lead-poisoned rats, J. Nutr., 107, 363, 1977.

257. Sifri, M., and Hoekstra, W. G., Effect of lead on lipid peroxidation in rats deficient or adequate in selenium and vitamin E, Fed. Proc., 37, 757 (abstr.), 1978.

258. Ramstoeck, E. R., Hoekstra, W. G., and Ganther, H. E., Triaklyllead metabolism and lipid peroxidation *in vivo* in vitamin E- and Se-deficient rats, as measured by ethane production, Toxicol. Appl. Pharmacol., 54, 251, 1980.

259. Donaldson, W. E., and Leeming, T. K., Dietary lead: effects on hepatic fatty acid composition in chicks, Toxicol. Appl. Pharm., 73, 119, 1984.

260. Howell, G. O., and Hill, C. H., Biological interactions of selenium with other trace elements in chicks, Environ. Health Perspectives, 25, 147, 1978.

261. Chiba, M., Fujimoto, N., and Kikuchi, M., Selenium: its antagonistic effect on the toxicity of tin-injected mice, in *Proceedings of the Third International Symposium on Selenium in Biology and Medicine*, Combs, G. F., Jr., Spallholz, J. E., Levander, O. A., and Oldfield, J. E., eds., Avi Publ. Co., Westport, Conn., 1986.

262. Dwivedi, R. S., Kaur, G., Srivastava, R. C., and Krishna Murti, C. R., Lipid peroxidation in tin-intoxicated partially hepatectomized rats, Bull. Environ. Contam. Toxicol., 33, 200, 1984.

263. Whanger, P. D., Weswig, P. H., Schmitz, J. A., and Oldfield, J. E., Effects of selenium, cadmium, mercury, tellurium, arsenic, silver and cobalt on white muscle disease in lambs and effect of dietary forms of arsenic on its accumulation in tissues, Nutr. Reports Int., 14, 63, 1976.

264. Van Vleet, J. F., Boon, G. D., and Ferrans, V. J., Induction of lesions of selenium-vitamin E deficiency in weanling swine fed silver, cobalt, tellurium, zinc, cadmium and vanadium, Am. J. Vet. Res., 42, 789, 1981.

265. Van Vleet, J. F., Protection by various nutritional supplements against lesions of selenium-vitamin E deficiency induced in ducklings fed tellurium or silver, Am. J. Vet. Res., 38, 1393, 1977.

266. Wagner, R., and Andreesen, J. R., Selenium requirement for active xanthine dehydrogenase from *Clostridium acidiurici* and *Clostridium cylindrosporum*, Arch. Microbiol., 121, 255, 1979.

267. Brian, W. R., Sunde, R. A., and Hoekstra, W. G., A previously unreported [75]Se- binding protein in rat liver mitochondria, Federation Proc., 44, 1669 (abstr. #7361), 1985.

268. Beilstein, M. A. and Whanger, P. D., A comparison of selenium distribution in blood fractions of humans and animals, in *Proceedings of the Third International Symosium on Selenium in Biology and Medicine*, Combs, G. F., Jr., Spallholz, J. E., Levander, O. A., and Oldfield, J. E., eds., Avi Publ. Co., Westport, Conn., 1986.

269. Butler, J. A., Beilstein, M. A., and Whanger, P. D., Incorporation of selenium from selenite and selenomethionine in rat tissues, Federation Proc., 44, 1510 (abstr. #6430), 1985.

270. Levander, O. A., Morris, V. C., and Mutanen, M., Effect of selenium (Se) deficiency on rat aortic glutathione peroxidase activity and on the ability of rat aorta to produce prostacyclin-like activity, Federation Proc., 44, 1670 (abstr. #7364), 1985.

271. Chaudiere, J., and Tappel, A. L., Interaction of gold (I) with the active site of selenium-glutathione peroxidase, J. Inorg. Biochem., 20, 313, 1984.

272. Mercurio, S. D. and Combs, G. F., Jr., Drug-induced changes in selenium- dependent glutathione peroxidase activity in the chick, J. Nutr., 115, 1459, 1985.

273. Baker, M. A., Dillard, C. J., and Tappel, A. L., Interactions of the antiarthritic drug, gold thioglucose, with selenium and glutathione peroxidase: investigations in the adjuvant-treated rat, Federation Proc., 44, 1509 (abstr. #6425), 1985.

274. Swanson, A. B., Effects of tri-*o*-cresylphosphate in selenium metabolism in the rat, PhD thesis, University of Wisconsin, Madison, 1975.

275. Revis, N. W., and Marusic, N., Glutathione peroxidase and selenium concentration in the hearts of doxorubicin-treated rabbits, J. Mol. Cell Cardiol., 10, 945, 1978.

276. Doroshaw, J. H., Locker, G. Y., and Myers, C. E., Doxorubicin toxicity: the interactions of drugs and endogenous defenses against free radical attack, Clin. Res., 26, 434A (abstr.), 1978.

277. Combs, G. F., Jr., and Scott, M. L., Polychlorinated biphenyl-stimulated selenium deficiency in the chick, Poultry Sci., 54, 1152, 1975.

278. Wagner, P. A., Hoekstra, W. G., and Ganther, H. E., Alleviation of silver toxicity by selenite in the rat in relation to tissue glutathione peroxidase, Proc. Soc. Exp. Biol. Med., 148, 1106, 1975.

279. Burk, R. F., Jr., Whitney, H. F., and Pearson, W. N., Tissue selenium levels during the development of dietary liver necrosis in rats fed *Torula* yeast diets, J. Nutr., 95, 420, 1968.

280. Whanger, P. D., Evidence for non-glutathione peroxidase selenium containing proteins in mammalian tissues, in *Proceedings of the Third International Symposium on Selenium in Biology and Medicine*, Combs, G. F., Jr., Spallholz, J. E., Levander, O. A., and Oldfield, J. E., eds., Avi Publ. Co., Westport, Conn., 1986.

281. Beilstein, M. A., Tripp, M. J., and Whanger, P. D., Evidence for selenocysteine in ovine tissue organelles, J. Inorg. Biochem., 15, 339, 1981.
282. Hill, K. E., and Burk, R. R., Glutathione metabolism in selenium deficiency, in *Proceedings of the Third International Symosium on Selenium in Biology and Medicine*, Combs, G. F., Jr., Spallholz, J. E., Levander, O. A., and Oldfield, J. E., eds., Avi Publ. Co., Westport, Conn., 1986.
283. Bartoli, G. M., and Sies, H., Reduced and oxidized glutathione efflux from liver, FEBS Lett., 86, 80, 1978.
284. Hill, K. E., and Burk, R. F., Disposition of plasma glutathione in selenium-deficient rats, Federation Proc., 44 (abstr. #6426), 1985.
285. Hill, K. E., and Burk, R. F., Effect of methionine and cysteine on glutathione synthesis by selenium-deficient isolated rat hepatocytes, in *Functions of Glutathione*, Larsson, A., Orrenius, S., Holmgren, A., and Mannervik, B., Eds., Raven Press, New York, 1983.
286. Combs, G. F., Jr., Bunk, M. J., and LaVorgna, M. W., Vitamin E and selenium in the metabolism of the sulfur-containing amino acids, Proc. Cornell Nutr. Conf., 1980, 109.
287. Usini, F., Maiorini, M., and Gregolin, C., The selenoenzyme phospholipid hydroperoxide glutathione peroxidase, Biochim. Biophys. Acta, 839, 62, 1985.

7

SELENIUM DEFICIENCY DISEASES OF ANIMALS

Selenium was first recognized to have a nutritional role in 1957 when Schwarz *et al.*[1,2] and Patterson *et al.*[3] found that it could replace vitamin E in the diets of rats and chicks, thus preventing dietary hepatic necrosis in the former species and exudative diathesis in the latter species. During the decade following this discovery, many investigators reported the activity of Se in preventing or ameliorating vitamin E-deficiency disorders in several other species. These included nutritional myopathies in lambs, calves, goats, rabbits, mink, chickens, turkeys, and ducks; testicular degeneration in rats, rabbits, hamsters, dogs, pigs, monkeys, and chickens; failures of gestation in cows and sheep; hepatic degeneration in rats, mice, and pigs; exudative diathesis in chickens; and growth retardation in immature animals of most species. Because vitamin E had come, by that time, to be regarded in function as a biologically specific lipid antioxidant,[4] the nutritional interactions of Se and vitamin E were interpreted by many researchers as evidence of an antioxidant function of Se. As the mode of action of Se remained unclear, controversy developed concerning its nutritional role. One school of thought held that Se was nothing more than a factor that spared the function of vitamin E; another held that it must be a nutrient in its own right.

This controversy was settled in the early 1970s upon the finding of a specific deficiency syndrome resulting from uncomplicated Se-deficiency (e.g., nutritional pancreatic atrophy) in the vitamin E-fed chick,[5] and the finding of a specific biochemical function of Se as an essential constituent of the enzyme glutathione peroxidase.[6] These findings and the great body of subsequent research indicate that Se is, indeed, an essential nutrient, the function of which is intimately related to that of vitamin E in normal metabolism. Therefore, the physiological impact of nutritional Se-deficiency must be considered in the context of combined Se-vitamin E status.

The Se- and vitamin E-related diseases of laboratory animals and livestock species have been reviewed.[7,8] It is the purpose of this chapter to describe, as much as possible from a diagnostic point of view, these disorders. Summaries of the Se-related deficiency diseases of animals are presented in Tables 7.1 and 7.2.

I. SELENIUM DEFICIENCY DISEASES OF LABORATORY AND DOMESTIC ANIMALS

A. Rats

1. Dietary Necrotic Liver Degeneration

The combined deficiency of Se and vitamin E in the rat results in the disease described in 1948 by Schwarz[9] as dietary necrotic liver degeneration. This disease had been produced by several investigators by feeding semi-purified low-fat diets that were low in cystine,[10-16] were high in cod liver oil,[9] or were based on European yeasts as major sources of protein.[14-20] While the disease was initially regarded as the result of dietary cystine deficiency, Schwarz[21] showed that a second factor, vitamin E, could also prevent it. His further studies[22] showed that some American yeasts contained a third factor (i.e., "Factor 3") that could also prevent dietary liver necrosis in the vitamin E-deficient rat. Factor 3 was identified in American brewer's yeasts,[22] casein,[23] and pork kidney powder hydrolysates[1]; it was concentrated from the latter source and was found to contain as much as 7% Se by weight.[1] Schwarz and Foltz[1] demonstrated that it was Se in preparations with Factor 3 activity that effected prevention of dietary necrotic liver degeneration in the rat,* and subsequent investigation[24] showed that the apparent activity of dietary cystine in preventing this disease owed to its incidental contamination with trace amounts of Se. Hence, dietary liver necrosis in the rat was recognized to be the result of the combined deficiency of Se and vitamin E.

Dietary necrotic liver degeneration in the Se- and vitamin E-deficient rat can be produced readily in weanling animals and is usually terminal

---

*Although the active principle of Factor 3 was found to be Se, the chemical form of Factor 3-Se has not been determined. Schwarz and colleagues[25-30] conducted extensive studies to compare the efficacy of Factor 3 prepared from pork kidney powder with almost 300 discrete Se compounds; they found none to be as active as the Se in Factor 3, which was more than three times as efficacious in preventing liver necrosis as the Se in sodium selenite (see Table 4.2). The chemical identity of Factor 3 thus remains to be elucidated.

Table 7.1

Selenium-Deficiency Syndromes of Laboratory and Domestic Animals

Species	Syndrome	Specific conditions	System affected	Preventative factors	
				Se	Vitamin E
Rat	Slightly reduced appetite			+	
	Slightly reduced growth			+	
	Poor hair coat	Second generation	Hair follicle	+	
	Sterility		Germinal epithelium: aspermatogenesis	+	
			Spermatozoa: midpiece breakage, decreased motility	+	
	Hepatic necrosis		Liver	+	+
	Cataracts	Second generation	Lens	+	+
Mouse	Reduced growth		Liver, kidney, pancreas, skeletal and cardiac muscle	+	+
	Multi-site necrosis			+	+
	Sterility	Second, third generations	Germinal, epithelium: reduced spermatogenesis	+	
			Spermatozoa: morphological abberration, decreased motility	+	
	Increased susceptibility to coxsacki viral infection		Myocardium	+	
Squirrel monkey	Wasting, lassitude			+	
	Alopecia		Hair follicles	+	
	Multi-site necrosis		Liver, kidney, skeletal and cardiac muscle	+	+
Dog	Muscular weakness		Skeletal muscle, mycardium, diaphragm: degeneration	+[a]	
	Edema		Subcutaneous areas	+	+
	Anorexia, dyspnea			+	+
	Intestinal lipofuscinosis		Intestinal musculature		+

[a]Confer only partial protection.

Table 7.2

Selenium-Deficiency Syndromes of Livestock

Species	Syndrome	Systems affected	Preventative factors	
			Se	Vitamin E
Chicken	Exudative diathesis	Subcutaneous capillaries: edema, hemorrhage	+	+
	Nutritional muscular dystrophy	Skeletal muscles: degeneration	+[a]	+[c]
	Nutritional pancreatic atrophy	Acinar pancreas: atrophy, periacinar fibrosis	+[f]	+[b]
	Encephalomalacia		?[g]	+[f]
	Impaired immunodevelopment	Bursa of fabricius: epithelial vacuolization	+	+
	Reduced egg production	Ovary	+	+
	Increased embryonic mortality	Embryo	+	+
	Reduced growth		+	+[a]
Turkey	Nutritional muscular dystrophy	Gizzard smooth muscle, myocardium, skeletal muscle: degeneration	+	+[a]
	Exudative diathesis	Subcutaneous capillaries: slight edema, hemorrhage	+	+
	Reduced growth		+	+[c]
Duck	Nutritional muscular dystrophy	Smooth muscle of gizzard and duodenum, skeletal muscle: degeneration	+	+
	Altered collagen metabolism	Fibroblasts in tendons: degeneration	+	+
	Exudative diathesis	Subcutaneous capillaries: edema, hemorrhage	+	+
	Reduced growth, survival		+	+
Japanese quail	Reduced growth, feed intake, survival		+	+
	Exudative diathesis	Subcutaneous capillaries	+	+
	Reduced embryonic survival	Embryo	+	+

Species	Disorder	Lesions / affected tissue		
Pig	Hepatosis dietetica	Liver: degeneration	+	+
	Mulberry heart disease	Myocardium: degeneration	+	+
	Nutritional muscular dystrophy	Skeletal muscles: degeneration	+	+
	Edema	Mesenteries, lung, subcutaneous tissues	+	+
	Impaired spermatogenesis	Spermatozoa: malformations	+[e]	?[g]
	Increased susceptibility to swine dysentery	Colonic mucosa: decreased nonspecific immunity (?)	+[e]	+
Sheep	Nutritional muscular dystrophy	Skeletal muscle, diaphragm, myocardium: degeneration	+[f]	+
	Infertility in ewes	Uterine musculature: loss of tone (?)	+[d,e]	+
	Se-responsive "unthriftiness"		+[d,e]	+
Cow	Nutritional muscular dystrophy in calves	Myocardium, skeletal muscle: degeneration	+	+
	Retained placenta in cows	Placenta-uterine attachment	+	+[d]
	Cystic ovarian disease	Ovary	+[d,e]	+[d]
	Se-responsive "unthriftiness"		+	+
	Anemia	Erythrocytes	+	?[g]
Horse	Nutritional muscular dystrophy	Skeletal muscles, myocardium: degeneration	+	+
Fish	Nutritional muscular dystrophy (Atlantic salmon)	Skeletal muscle: degeneration	+	+

[a] Provides only partial protection.

[b] Protects at only very high levels of intake.

[c] At least partial protection is provided by cyst(e)ine.

[d] Etiology of disorder is not well understood, other factors may also protect.

[e] May be related to immune function.

[f] Disorder exacerbated by feeding high levels of polyunsaturated fatty acids.

[g] Role not well understood.

within 20-40 days, depending primarily upon the Se-vitamin E status of the animals at the commencement of nutritional depletion. If a low-methionine diet is used, survival is usually no longer than 4-5 weeks, and pathological signs are restricted to the liver; however, Christensen et al.[31] reported that, if the diet is supplemented with methionine, it may be possible to prolong survival such that animals die showing both hepatic and pulmonary necrosis and hematuria. Ultrastructural changes[32-34] in the hepatocyte precede, by as much as a week, pathological changes observable by light microscopy. The earliest changes observed by electron microscopy are swelling of endoplasmic reticulum and mitochondria with accumulation of Ca by the latter. This so-called latent phase of the deficiency can last up to a week; it is characterized biochemically by decreased respiratory metabolism in liver homogenate or slice preparations,[35] a condition often referred to as the "respiratory decline." After the latent phase, degeneration of the sinusoidal plasma membrane is observed concommitant with increases in lactate dehydrogenase activity in the plasma.[34] Shortly thereafter, focal necrosis of centrilobular hepatocytes is observed by light microscopy; this progresses to massive involvement of the liver, and death due to hepatogenic hypoglycemia[36,37] follows within 48 hrs.

2. Other Effects

Combined Se- and vitamin E-deficiency in rats has been shown to increase deposition of lipids in the retinal pigment epithelium and to decrease photoreceptor outer segment phagocytosis.[38] This is thought to reflect the lack of antioxidant protection of those cells that normally are rich in SeGSHpx.[39] Multifocal coagulation necrosis of the myocardium was reported recently in rats fed a Se- and vitamin E-deficient semi-purified diet.[40]

Rats that are fed Se-deficient diets containing adequate amounts of vitamin E to prevent liver necrosis show slightly impaired appetite and rates of growth and have been shown to experience lens cataracts and sterility (males). Rats, particularly males, reared with Se-deficient diets usually weigh about 10% less than their Se-fed littermates by 6 months of age and thereafter.[41-43] This effect is associated with reductions in food consumption and efficiency of utilization[43]; however, it is usually of such magnitude only in the progeny of Se-deficient dams when the young are also reared with Se-deficient diets. Second-generation Se-depleted rats also routinely show sparse hair coats[44] (see Fig. 7.1) and have been found to show lens cataracts.[45,46]

Sterility due to reduced sperm motility was reported in rats depleted of Se for one[47,48] or two[41,49,50] generations. In these cases, decreased sperm

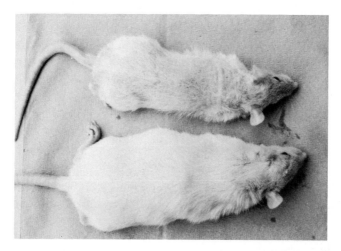

Fig. 7.1 Impaired growth and hair coat development due to two-generational Se-deficiency in the vitamin E-fed rat. Control (i.e., Se-fed) rat is shown at the bottom of the picture. Photograph from the authors' laboratory.

motility was due to a characteristic midpiece breakage.[47] Brown and Burk[51] showed that Se is concentrated in the sperm midpiece. Studies by Calvin *et al.*[52-55] have described a cysteine-rich selenoprotein that is a structural component of the sperm mitochondrial capsule. It appears that the loss of this selenoprotein in nutritional Se-deficiency may be involved with midpiece breakage and consequent loss of sperm motility. Aspermatogenesis due to severe Se-deficiency has also been observed in the rat[46]; the high retention of Se in the testis of the rat,[56] even during conditions of nutritional Se depletion, supports the hypothesis that Se is important in both the germinal epithelium and in the spermatozoa itself.

B. Mice

1. Multi-Site Necrotic Degeneration

A multi-site necrotic degeneration in the Se- and vitamin E-deficient mouse was reported in 1958 by DeWitt and Schwarz.[57] That condition involved necrosis of the liver and kidney, with apparent involvement of the pancreas and the skeletal and cardiac muscles, and with occasional hematuria. It was prevented by feeding either Factor 3 (i.e., Se) or vitamin E. This finding, however, has not been repeated. Bunk[58] studied uncomplicated Se-deficiency (e.g., the purified diet contained 0.01 ppm Se) in the second-generation deficient mouse; his results revealed a slight reduction (i.e., 12% after 180 days) in body weight, marked reductions of SeGSHpx activities in plasma (e.g., decreased by 93% at 120 days) and liver (e.g., decreased by 99% at 120 days), but no gross or histological abnormalities in the major organs. Similar reductions in body weight gains were observed by Lane *et al.*[59] in mice fed a low dietary level of Se (i.e., 0.03 ppm), in comparison to a very high level of Se (i.e., 1.5 ppm), which was significant only during the phases of most rapid growth (e.g., during pregnancy).

2. Infertility in Males

More recently, Wallace *et al.*[60-62] have demonstrated the essentiality of Se for the maintenance of fertility in the male mouse. Nutritional deprivation of Se of these animals results in abnormal development of the mitochondrial capsule of spermatozoa; this effect is observed by transmission electron microscopy as abnormal alignment of sperm tail mitochondria with disorientation of other tail structures.[62] Abnormal sperm morphology is seen with increased incidence through successive generations of Se deprivation[60,61]; however, the predominance of grossly abnormal morphology is associated with only moderately reduced sperm motility,[60] in contrast to findings with the Se-deficient rat.[47] Second-generation Se-deficient males show reduced sperm counts and corresponding decreases in the cross sectional areas of the seminiferous tubules.[60,62] These changes are thought to relate to the absence of a specific selenoprotein, similar to that described in the rat, associated with the mitochondria of developing spermatozoa.[62] Selenium is known to be taken up by the mouse testis[63] and pancreas,[64] but dietary deficiency of the mineral has been shown to affect the physiological activity of only the former organ. Nutritional Se status appears to be unrelated to the etiology of hereditary muscular dystrophy in the mouse, as dystrophic muscle contains elevated activities of SeGSHpx[65] and has a greater capacity for the uptake and retention of Se.[66]

3. Increased Susceptibility to Viral Myocarditis

Uncomplicated Se-deficiency was found to potentiate viral myocarditis in the mouse.[67,68] Both the incidence and severity of heart lesions among mice treated with Coxsackie B_4 virus was high for mice maintained with either a semi-purified or practical type Se-deficient diet, and the incidence of heart lesions was reduced by dietary supplementation with Se.

C. Monkeys

Muth *et al.*[69] studied nutritional Se-deficiency in the squirrel monkey (*Saimiri sciureus*). They maintained a small number of individuals for several months using a semi-purified diet that was deficient in Se but contained an apparently adequate level (i.e., 60 IU/kg) of vitamin E. Reduced body weight, alopecia, and lassitude were observed after 9 months. Biweekly administration of sodium selenite (40 μg Se/monkey) effected recovery. Untreated individuals did not survive; they showed hepatic necrosis, nephrosis, and skeletal and myocardial degeneration at autopsy.

Studies by Butler et al.[70] demonstrated no physiological abnormalities in rhesus monkeys (*Macaca mulatta*) after prolonged periods of nutritional Se deprivation. Adults fed a Se-deficient diet for as long as 18 months or young animals reared using a Se-deficient diet for 14 months showed reduced levels of Se in blood and activities of SeGSHpx in plasma and erythrocytes[70,71] but showed no other differences from Se-supplemented controls with respect to a variety of clinical and biochemical indices.

Certain strains of owl monkeys (*Aotus trivirgatus*) develop spontaneous hemolytic anemias that have been found to respond to intramuscular injections of Se and vitamin E.[72] However, because treatment with Se alone has no therapeutic value against this condition,[72] it must be concluded that it is related to vitamin E per se.

D. Dogs

Van Vleet[73] produced combined Se-vitamin E-deficiency in beagle pups within 40-60 days. At that time, the deficiency was manifest clinically by generalized muscular weakness, subcutaneous edema (limbs, ventral abdomen, ventral neck, and submandibular area), anorexia, depression, dyspnea, and eventual coma. Dogs examined at necropsy after 10-15 days of progressive clinical signs showed the following gross lesions: ventral subcutaneous edema (see Fig. 7.2), generalized pallor and edema of the skeletal muscle with scattered white longitudinal streaking (see Fig. 7.3), brown-yellow discoloration of the intestinal musculature, and white chalky deposits at the renal corticomedullary junction. Microscopic examination showed degeneration and regeneration of the skeletal muscles, focal subendocardial necrosis of the ventral myocardium, intestinal lipofuscinosis, and renal mineralization. Supplementation of the basal diet with 0.5 ppm Se prevented all clinical signs of deficiency; it reduced but did not completely prevent the skeletal myopathy or intestinal lipofuscinosis, both of which responded to vitamin E.

E. Species in Which Selenium-Deficiency Does Not Produce Clinical Signs

Selenium has been shown to be required for the support of normal activities of SeGSHpx in rabbits,[74,75] hamsters,[76] and guinea pigs,[77] although the normal hepatic activity is so low in the latter species as to elude detection

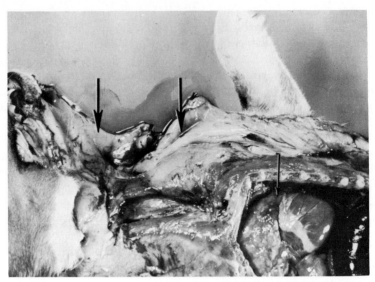

Fig. 7.2 Ventral edema in the Se- and vitamin E-deficient dog. Photograph courtesy of Dr. J. F. Van Vleet, Purdue University, with permission of the Journal of the American Veterinary Medical Association (see reference 73).

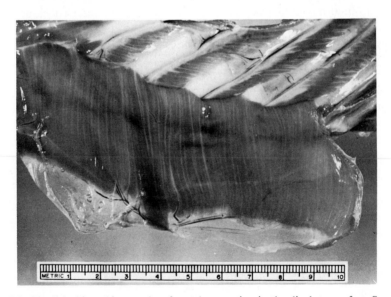

Fig. 7.3 Parallel, thin, white streaks of myodegeneration in the diaphragm of an Se- and vitamin E-deficient dog. Photograph courtesy of Dr. J. F. Van Vleet, Purdue University, with permission of the Journal of the American Veterinary Medical Association (see reference 73).

in an earlier study.[76] Each of these species shows specific deficiency syndromes resultant of vitamin E-deprivation that are not reduced or prevented by Se (e.g., muscular dystrophy in the rabbit[78-80]; sterility, hepatic degeneration, and myopathies in the hamster[81]; myopathies in the guinea pig[82,83]). The rhesus and owl monkeys, already discussed, also have been found to show no disease signs that respond to Se.

II. SELENIUM DEFICIENCY DISEASES OF LIVESTOCK

A. Chickens

The growing chick may show any of three Se-deficiency diseases, depending upon specific dietary circumstances. These diseases include exudative diathesis, nutritional muscular dystrophy, and nutritional pancreatic atrophy. The first two of these diseases are completely prevented by dietary supplements of nutritional levels of vitamin E. The last disease, nutritional pancreatic atrophy, is strictly dependent on dietary Se under such circumstances; only very high dietary concentrations of vitamin E or other antioxidants can protect the chick pancreas in the absence of Se. Therefore, all three of these Se deficiency diseases are related in some manner to dietary antioxidant status. In addition to these known Se-deficiency diseases, several other Se-related disorders have been reported.

1. Exudative Diathesis in Chicks

Exudative diathesis was described by Dam and Glavind[84] as a disorder among vitamin E-deficient chicks. It is characterized by severe subcutaneous edema, particularly in the depending regions of the body (e.g., abdomen, feet, and ventral aspects of the neck and wings).[85] The edema appears to result from abnormally increased permeability of the capillaries; this was indicated by the study of Dam and Glavind,[86] which showed that escape of trypan blue from the capillaries was increased in chicks with exudative diathesis. Affected chicks are also anemic and hypoproteinemic,[87] which state also contributes to the edema. Exudative diathesis in the vitamin E-deficient chick was found to be prevented by a factor in brewer's yeast,[88] which was subsequently identified as Factor 3-Se.[2,3,87,89]

The combined deficiency of Se and vitamin E produces exudative diathesis in young chicks within 2-4 weeks when they are reared with deficient diets from hatching. By that time, hepatic SeGSHpx activities have dropped to less than one-third of control (Se-fed) levels, and significant declines in erythrocyte SeGSHpx are noted.[90] The effect of Se-deprivation is seen much earlier in the plasma, wherein SeGSHpx drops to less than 15% of control levels within 6 days, at which time the initial signs of exudative diathesis are not yet observed.[90] Noguchi *et al.*[90] found that the activity of SeGSHpx in plasma assayed at 7 days was significantly correlated with the subsequent incidence of exudative diathesis among chicks at 13 days. The probable direct involvement of SeGSHpx in the etiology of exudative diathesis is also indicated by the findings of Mercurio and Combs[91] that *in vivo* inhibitors of SeGSHpx (e.g., aurothioglucose, DL-penicillamine hydrochloride) potentiate the manifestation of exudates in chicks fed marginal levels of Se.

Both the incidence and rate of appearance of the disease are dependent upon the Se-vitamin E status of the flock. Chicks produced from Se- and vitamin E-depleted hens will show exudative diathesis within 6-12 days when they are reared using a low-Se (e.g., less than 0.02 ppm), vitamin E-free diet; however, chicks from adequately nourished hens will show exudates much later if fed such a deficient diet, and chicks fed marginal levels of Se and/or vitamin E will show exudates with lower incidence. Exudative diathesis is readily diagnosed by the appearance of the subcutaneous edema (see Fig. 7.4), which soon progresses to a hemorrhagic stage, producing a blue-green discoloration of the skin (see Fig 7.5). Affected

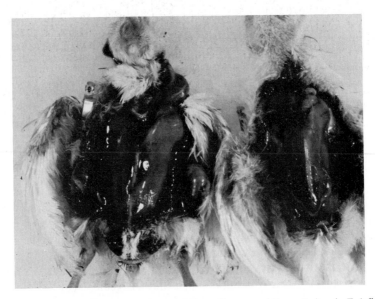

Fig. 7.4 Edema of the subcutaneous tissues of viscerally exposed Se- and vitamin E-deficient chicks with exudative diathesis. Photograph courtesy of Dr. M. L. Scott, Cornell University.

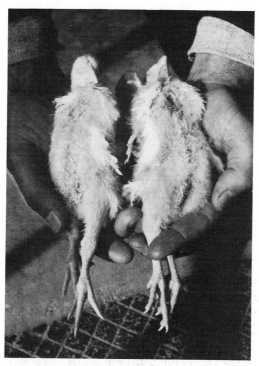

Fig. 7.5 External appearance of exudative diathesis in the Se- and vitamin E-deficient chick. Note blue-green discoloration of the ventral aspect of the body and edema of the feet in the chick of the left-hand side of the picture. Photograph courtesy of Dr. M. L. Scott, Cornell University.

chicks show reduced spontaneous activity and food intake; if not treated with Se or vitamin E, they survive usually no more than 2-6 days. Selenium and vitamin E spare the dietary requirements for one another in the prevention of exudative diathesis. When fed diets severely deficient with respect to Se, chicks require 100-110 IU vitamin E per kilogram of diet to prevent the disorder[92]; when fed diets containing no vitamin E, they require 0.10-0.15 ppm Se.[93-95] The amount of Se required to prevent exudative diathesis in the chick is reduced not only by dietary supplements of vitamin E, but also by supplements of synthetic antioxidants. (The antioxidant effect on the utilization of Se is discussed in Chapter 4.)

2. Nutritional Muscular Dystrophy in Chicks

Nutritional muscular dystrophy was described in the vitamin E-deficient chick by Dam and colleagues.[86,96] Subsequent investigations showed that this disease is produced only when diets are moderately deficient in the sulfur-containing amino acid cystine.[97-102] The disease is characterized by degeneration of the skeletal muscles, which is especially prominent in the pectorals and gastrocnemius. It is seen as longitudinal white striations of the muscle fibers, usually visible through the skin (see Fig. 7.6). Affected chicks show generalized muscular weakness and marked decreases in spontaneous activity. Microscopic examination reveals Zenker's degeneration of muscle fibers, with perivascular infiltration of eosinophils and macrophages[97]; the condition progresses to fibrosis. Hence, dystrophic muscles show elevated levels of lysosomal enzymes[103]; plasma samples from affected individuals show elevated transaminase activities.[104] Lesions are not found in other organs. Myopathy generally is observable grossly within 20-25 days when day-old chicks are reared using a dystrophigenic diet. In general, synthetic antioxidants are without effect in preventing nutritional muscular dystrophy in the chick[85]; however, Machlin and Shalkop[98] found that diphenyl-p-phenylene diamine (DPPD) was effective when added at high levels to low-fat diets (indeed, the addition of 4% lard to the dystrophigenic diet negated the protective effect of DPPD). On the basis of these findings, low levels of synthetic antioxidants are used in vitamin E-deficient dystrophigenic diets to prevent other vitamin E- and antioxidant-related disorders (e.g., encephalomalacia) that would otherwise be produced in the chick.

Dietary supplements of Se are effective in reducing (by some 10-15%) but not fully preventing nutritional muscular dystrophy in the chick.[105-107] Calvert and Scott[99] showed that although supplemental Se markedly reduced the amount of vitamin E required by the chick for preventing myopathy, it did not affect the level of cystine needed for similar protection. This has been interpreted as indicating that nutritional muscular dystrophy in the chick is primarily a disorder of vitamin E and cysteine metabolism, and that the role of Se in this disorder is only to improve the tissue utilization of vitamin E.[85,108] The mode of action of Se in sparing vitamin E in the prevention of this disorder is unclear at the present time. Hull and Scott[104] found that both the activity of SeGSHpx and the concentration of reduced glutathione (GSH) were significantly greater in muscle from dystrophic vs. nondystrophic chicks when each was fed dystrophigenic diets supplemented with 0.10 ppm Se. This suggests that the metabolic conditions leading to muscular dystrophy in vitamin E and cyst(e)ine deficiency may relate to oxidative stresses associated with either reduced utilization of or increased needs for the SeGSHpx system. This hypothesis is supported by the findings of Shih et al.[109] of increases by twofold to threefold in the ratios of protein-bound disulfide : sulfhydryl content, and of appearances of low molecular weight proteins (presumed to be derived from proteolysis) in dystrophic chick muscle. The apparent oxidation of muscle proteins during

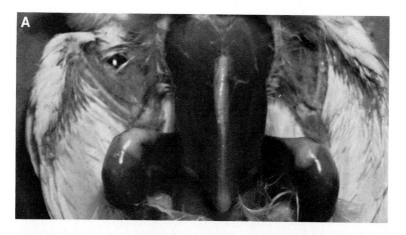

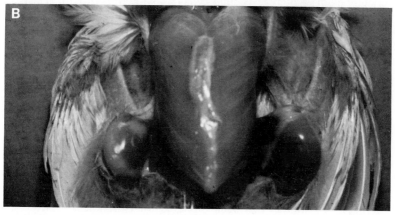

Fig. 7.6 Gross appearance of breast musculature in (B) Se- and vitamin E-deficient chick with nutritional muscular dystrophy compared to (A) Se- and vitamin E-fed chick. Photographs courtesy of Dr. M. L. Scott, Cornell University.

nutritional muscular dystrophy suggests that the need for sulfur-containing amino acids by the vitamin E-deficient chick may relate to an increased need for essential amino acids under these circumstances of rapid turnover of muscle proteins. That cysteine is much more effective in this regard than is methionine[99] was explained by Hathcock,[110] who found evidence that both the transsulfuration of methionine to cysteine and the conversion of cysteine to taurine were depressed in the vitamin E-deficient chick. It is doubtful that Se has even an indirect role in this interrelationship between vitamin E and metabolism of the sulfur-containing amino acids, as Hathcock's diet contained 0.10 ppm Se (added as Na_2SeO_3).[110]

3. Nutritional Pancreatic Atrophy in Chicks

The discovery by Thompson and Scott[111,112] of a specific requirement for Se by the vitamin E-fed chick ended the controversy concerning the nutritional role of the mineral that had developed over the dozen years since the recognition of its interrelationship with vitamin E in rats and chicks. Using low-Se (e.g., ca. 0.01 ppm) purified diets supplemented with what was believed to be an excess of vitamin E (e.g., 100 IU/kg), Thompson and Scott found that the chick required supplemental Se for growth and survival,[111] and that Se-deprivation resulted in impaired utilization of dietary lipids coincident with decreased pancreatic enzyme production.[112] The pathogenesis of this condition was studied by Gries and Scott,[113] who found that this uncomplicated Se-deficiency resulted in degeneration of the acinar pancreas and consequent loss of pancreatic exocrine function. In the severely Se-deficient chick, pancreatic acinar cells first show vacuolation and hyaline body formation; this is followed by loss of zymogen, cytoplasmic shrinkage and dilation of the acinar lumina (see Fig. 7.7). Finally, infiltration with fibroblasts and macrophages occurs; the terminal phase is characterized by severe periacinar fibrosis.* These histological changes are associated with progressive decreases in the activities of lipase and proteases.[113] It is the insufficiency of pancreatic lipase in the intestinal lumen that results in impairment in the digestion of dietary triglycerides and the consequent impairment of intestinal micelle formation. Impaired micellar solubilization of dietary lipids results in their impaired enteric absorption. Thus, nutritional pancreatic atrophy due to severe Se-deficiency in the chick results in steatorrhea and impaired absorption of vitamin E.[112] Typically, therefore, a primary deficiency of Se in the chick will result in a secondary deficiency of vitamin E. This effect has been obviated for experimental purposes to produce Se-deficiency uncomplicated by vitamin E-deficiency through the use of low-fat (e.g., 4%) diets supplemented with high levels (e.g. 100 IU/kg) of vitamin E in microdispersible form, and with sodium taurocholate (0.1%), linoleic acid (0.5%), and mono-olein (0.5%), added to promote lumenal micelle formation.[118] Nutritional pancreatic atrophy in the Se-deficient chick involves only the acinar pancreas and not the islets of Langerhans[112]; therefore, affected chicks show no effects of altered pancreatic endocrine function and have normal plasma concentrations of glucose.[122] The pathogenesis of nutritional pancreatic atrophy in second-generation Se-deficient chicks was described by Combs and Bunk.[121] The first signs

---

*On this basis, Scott and associates[113-116] referred to this disease as "pancreatic fibrosis"; however, Combs and associates[117-120] have renamed this condition "nutritional pancreatic atrophy" in recognition that the effect of Se-deficiency is the atrophy of acinar cells, the consequence of which is fibrotic infiltration.

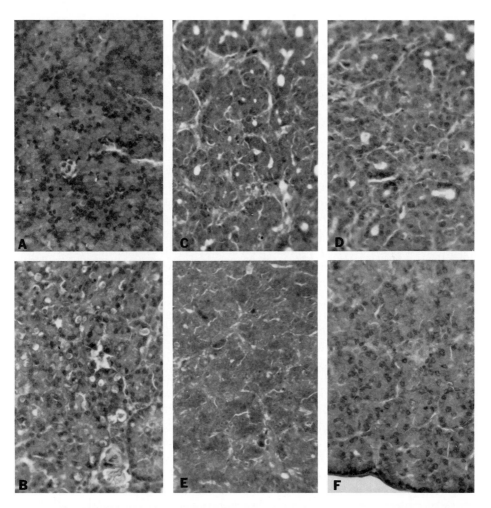

Fig. 7.7 Sections of pancreas from chicks. (A) at 1 day of age (hematoxylin and eosin staining, 250×), (B) After 6 days of feeding a Se-deficient diet (H&E, 250×). (C) After 10 days with the Se-deficient diet (Ladewig's staining showing connective tissue 250×). (D) Same as C, except stained with H&E (250×). (E) After 10 days with the Se-supplemented (0.10 ppm) diet (Ladewig's, 250×). (F) Same as E, except stained with H&E (250×). Photographs from the authors' laboratory, with permission of the Journal of Nutrition (see reference 118).

of abnormal acinar cell appearance are usually seen within 4-6 days after hatching when chicks are reared using a Se-deficient, vitamin E-supplemented diet. By that time, chicks appear normal; however, feed intake starts to decline and a slight (e.g., 5%) depression in rate of gain in body weight is seen. By 6-12 days, as acinar cytoplasm diminishes, feed intake is markedly reduced, chicks may lose body weight, and poor feathering is noted. At 12-15 days some chicks die with pronounced acinar atrophy and mild periacinar fibrosis; mortality increases to ca. 95% by 28 days with all chicks developing severe pancreatic fibrosis. Nutritional pancreatic atrophy can be produced in first-generation Se-deficient chicks, in which the time of onset of the disorder is delayed by 5-7 days.[119] The pancreatic degeneration is reversible upon treatment with Se by as late as 14 days. Selenium-treated chicks show a recovery of appetite within 4 hrs,[117] an appearance of histological signs of acinar regeneration within 1-2 days,[113-119] and a return to normal gross appearance and near normal acinar histological appearance within 2 weeks.

Whitacre and Combs[119] demonstrated that the early (i.e., 6- to 8-day) phase of nutritional pancreatic atrophy is associated with a decrease in the rates of synthesis of RNA and protein (but not DNA), and that this effect is specific for the chick pancreas (i.e., the hepatic synthesis of macromolecules was not affected by Se-deficiency). Upon treatment of deficient chicks with Se, the pancreatic synthesis of RNA and protein returns to normal rates within 12 hrs. Those authors suggested that these lesions in biosynthetic rates may relate to altered function of acinar mitochondria.* Their results confirmed those of Bunk and Combs[118] that respiratory function of mitochondria prepared from chick pancreas was not affected by nutritional Se deficiency. However, Whitacre and Combs[119] found that the recovery of mitochondria from Se-deficient pancreases was only 63% of that from Se-fed controls. This effect probably resulted from the loss of acinar cells in the Se-deficient chick pancreas. Decreases in RNA and protein synthesis appear to result from the disappearance of endoplasmic reticulum from degenerating acinar cells. This hypothesis is consistent with ultrastructural examinations of the atrophic acinar cell, which show marked depletion of endoplasmic reticulum[119,123] (see Fig. 7.8).

The growth depression associated with severe uncomplicated Se-deficiency in the chick is due in part to a depression in appetite. Bunk and Combs[117] found that approximately two-thirds of the growth depression in chicks with nutritional pancreatic atrophy could be overcome by force-feeding to levels of intake comparable to the *ad libitum* levels of Se-adequate chicks.

---

*An effect of Se-deficiency on mitochondrial function had been suggested previously by Shih *et al.*[116]; however, it is probable that the changes in mitochondrial stability they observed were artifactual. Due to the fact that they chose to work with chicks in the advanced stages of pancreatic fibrosis, they found it necessary to subject fibrotic pancreases to mechanical homogenization for as long as 30 min. This severe procedure would, undoubtedly, result in a great amount of mitochondrial disruption and would explain their results. In order to avoid this problem, Combs's group[118,119] conducted their studies of pancreatic mitochondrial function using chicks in the earliest stages of acinar atrophy and without any fibrosis.

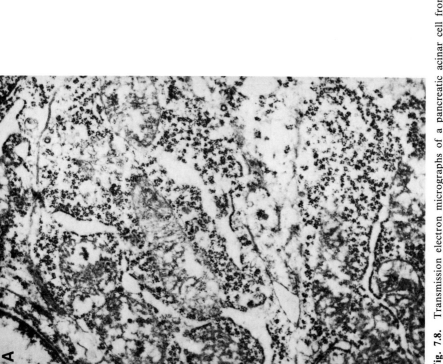

Fig. 7.8. Transmission electron micrographs of a pancreatic acinar cell from (A) an Se-deficient chick (27,750×) and (B) an Se-fed (0.10 ppm dietary Se) chick (28,500×). Note the enlarged and disrupted mitochondria (MIT) and depletion of endoplasmic reticulum (ER) in Se deficiency. Photographs from the authors' laboratory, with permission of the Journal of Nutrition (see reference 119).

Bunk and Combs[124] demonstrated that growth was promoted in Se-deficient chicks by dietary supplements of cystine, whereas supplements of methionine were without such effect. Subsequent studies by Halpin and Baker[126] have confirmed this finding for at least some strains of chickens. Therefore, it appears that the Se-deficient chick with nutritional pancreatic atrophy either has an increased metabolic demand for cysteine that cannot be met by further transsulfuration from methionine or has an impairment in the transsulfuration pathway itself. Findings by Bunk and Combs[124] that Se-deficient chicks had decreased concentrations of homocysteine, cystathionine, and cysteine in the free amino acid pool of plasma, and by LaVorgna and Combs[125] that Se-deficient chicks had increased rates of methionine-methyl group oxidation are consistent with a hypothesis of relative insufficiency in the metabolic conversion of methionine to cysteine in Se-deficiency; however, the metabolic basis of this effect remains to be elucidated. Combs et al.[120] found that nutritional pancreatic atrophy could be produced using a practical-type (i.e., corn-soy based) diet that contained less than 0.01 ppm Se.* In that study, Se deprivation produced only a very slight reduction in growth rate after 30 days, even though it produced clear pancreatic atrophy. That finding suggests the presence of a factor contained in the practical diet, apparently not cystine, that prevents the growth depression associated with severe Se-deficiency in studies using purified diets.

Nutritional pancreatic atrophy has been considered to be the only clearly delineated pathological condition that results from the deficiency of Se uncomplicated by deficiencies of vitamin E, cystine, etc. However, Whitacre and Combs[127] found that the condition could also be prevented by dietary supplements with high levels of vitamin E, butylated hydroxytoluene (BHT), DPPD, ethoxyquin, or ascorbic acid. Although normal pancreatic function is maintained when chicks consume diets containing at least 0.05 ppm Se,[112,115] pancreatic atrophy was also prevented with dietary additions of at least 300 IU vitamin E per kilogram of diet or of 500 ppm of any of these synthetic antioxidants or ascorbic acid.[127] Each of these treatments was fully effective in supporting normal pancreatic histological appearance as well as normal chick growth in the Se-deficient (0.010 ppm) purified diet. That antioxidant supplementation did not act to increase the utilization of the trace amount of Se in the diet was indicated by the lack of increase in either the Se content of pancreas, or the SeGSHpx activities of plasma, pancreas, or liver. Therefore, nutritional pancreatic atrophy, while highly responsive to exceedingly low dietary concentrations of Se, must be

*That study was conducted in the Peoples' Republic of China using, as major ingredients in the basal diet, low-Se corn and soybean meal grown in areas of endemic Se deficiency in that country.

considered as a disorder involving in a more general way the total antioxidant status of the chick.

4. Encephalomalacia in Chicks

Century and Horwitt[128] reported that dietary supplements of Se reduced the incidence of encephalomalacia in chicks. This disorder, characterized by separation of the molecular and granular layers of the cerebellum accompanied by hemorrhages and edema, is manifest as a severe ataxia and is produced by the deficiency of vitamin E in chick diets containing no synthetic antioxidants.[129-131] Studies by Dam[130] and Yoshida and Hoshii[132] have found Se to be without protective effect against encephalomalacia; Century and Horwitt[128] refuted these types of observations by suggesting that the protective effect of Se was weak and, thus, observable only when the diet did not contain overwhelming amounts of oxidant "stressors." However, it is also possible that the diet used by Century and Horwitt[128] may have contained a small amount of vitamin E,* the utilization of which was enhanced by correcting the dietary Se-deficiency. The lack of confirmation of this proposed effect of Se would support the latter hypothesis. It is the opinion of the present authors that encephalomalacia in the chick is a vitamin E/lipid antioxidant-related disorder that does not involve Se.

5. Impaired Development of Immunocompetence in Chicks

Marsh et al.[134] showed that Se was required for normal development of immunocompetence in the chick. Chicks made deficient with respect to either Se or vitamin E within the first 2 weeks after hatching showed impaired humoral responses to ovine erythrocytes; however, Se and vitamin E appeared to be mutually replaceable for this function by 3 weeks of age. Dietary concentrations of Se greater than or equal to 0.20 ppm produced significant immunosuppression, but only in male chicks. Subsequent studies[135] have shown lesions of the epithelial tissue of the bursa of Fabricius in Se- and vitamin E-deficient chicks (see Fig. 7.9); these lesions appear to be associated with depletion of lymphoid cells in that organ and may explain the diminished B cell function observed in chicks with the combined deficiency. These results would suggest that Se- and/or vitamin E-deficiency may affect disease resistance in young chicks; however, that hypothesis has not been tested.

---

*A commercial preparation of "stripped" corn oil was used in those experiments. Although it was assumed to be free of vitamin E activity, no analyses of either the oil or chick tissues were reported. Machlin[133] has indicated that such preparations may contain detectable amounts of vitamin E.

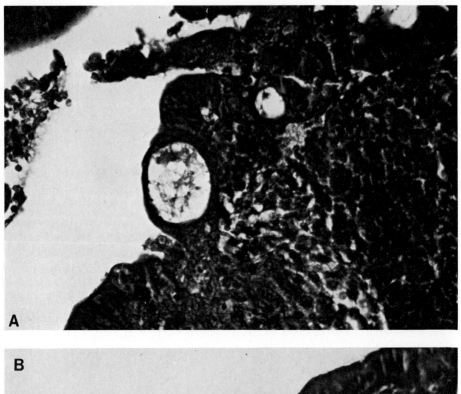

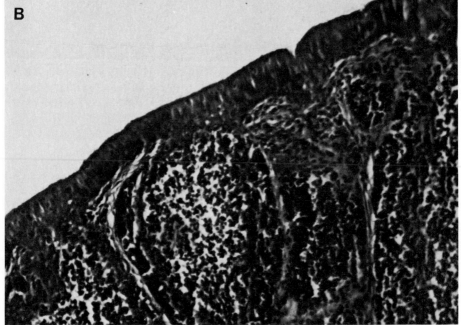

Fig. 7.9. Sections (hematoxylin and eosin, 500×) of bursa of Fabricius from (A) an Se- and vitamin E-deficient chick (panel A) and (B) an Se- (0.10 ppm) and vitamin E- (100 IU/kg) fed chick. Note vacuolation of bursal epithelium in Se and vitamin E deficiency. Photographs courtesy of Dr. J. A. Marsh, Cornell University.

6. Reproductive Failure in Breeding Chickens

Cantor and Scott[136] observed significant reductions in rates of egg production and embryonic survival among single-comb White Leghorn hens fed a corn-soy-based diet containing less than 0.03 ppm total Se without supplemental vitamin E. Both parameters returned to normal by supplementing the diet with 0.10 ppm Se as Na_2SeO_3. That level of added Se resulted in concentrations of Se in eggs averaging 0.121 ppm after 3 weeks of feeding and was associated with a protective effect against exudative diathesis among progeny reared using a diet deficient in both Se and vitamin E. The studies of Latshaw et al.[137] support a requirement of ca. 0.05 ppm for sustaining egg production in the laying hen. Combs and Scott[138] found that dietary levels of ca. 0.05 ppm Se are adequate to sustain egg production in laying pullets, but that levels less than 0.10 ppm Se resulted in deficiencies of SeGSHpx in hens and impaired hatchability and post-hatching performance of progeny. Progeny of Se- and vitamin E-deficient hens show late-stage embryonic mortality, with a high incidence of hemorrhages in the subcutaneous tissue (see Fig 7.10). There is no evidence that Se-deficiency affects reproductive performance in the male chicken, although testicular degeneration has been reported in roosters after chronic vitamin E-deficiency.

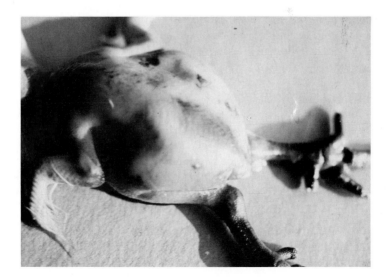

Fig. 7.10 Hemorrhages and edema of 19-day-old embryonic chick from an Se- and vitamin E-deficient dam. Feathers have been removed. Photograph from the authors' laboratory.

B. Turkeys

1. Muscular Dystrophies in Poults

Degeneration of the smooth muscle of the proventriculus (gizzard) is the most characteristic sign of Se-deficiency in the young turkey poult. This condition, orginally reported as a sign of vitamin E-deficiency,[139] was later shown to be prevented by dietary supplements of Se.[140-142] It is characterized by a hyaline degeneration of smooth muscle (see Fig. 7.11), resulting in a pale gross appearance of the organ (see Fig. 7.12). Degenerative lesions are sometimes also observed in the myocardium and skeletal muscle. These myopathies are associated with increased activity of glutamic oxaloacetic transaminase in serum, and slightly decreased hematocrit and blood hemoglobin concentration,[141] and with hypoalbuminemia and decreased activities of SeGSHpx in plasma and other tissues.[143] In marked contrast to the skeletal myopathy of the vitamin E-deficient chick, gizzard myopathy in the Se- and vitamin E-deficient poult is not prevented by dietary sulfur-containing amino acids[140] but is completely prevented by supplements of Se.[140-142] However, the dietary level of vitamin E affects the amount of Se required for the prevention of the disorder. Walter and Jensen[141] reported that it was necessary to use a basal diet low in methionine and vitamin E, as well as Se, in order to produce gizzard myopathy experimentally. Scott et al.[144] found that while a dietary level of ca. 0.18 ppm Se was required to prevent gizzard myopathy in vitamin E-fed poults, a level of ca. 0.28 ppm was required when the diet was not supplemented with vitamin E. In the latter studies, methionine and vitamin E supplementation of the dystrophigenic diet produced improvements in growth but did not affect the incidence of gizzard myopathy. Selenium, vitamin E, and methionine are not effective in amelioration of the hereditary degenerative skeletal myopathy in turkeys.[145]

2. Exudative Diathesis in Poults

The combined deficiency of Se and vitamin E in poults was found to produce a mild type of exudative diathesis.[146,147] This condition was characterized by hemorrhaging on the inner margins of the thighs and caudal breast muscles; in contrast to the exudative diathesis of the Se- and vitamin E-deficient chick, it involved only a mild edema. Affected poults also showed a macrocytic anemia[146] and occasional hydropericardium.[141] The disorder is prevented by dietary supplements of vitamin E or Se.[146,147]

C. Ducks

1. Nutritional Muscular Dystrophy in Ducklings

A nutritional muscular dystrophy was described by Pappenheimer and Goettsch[148] among ducklings fed a vitamin E-deficient diet. Yarrington et al.[149] showed that this disorder was also prevented by dietary supplements

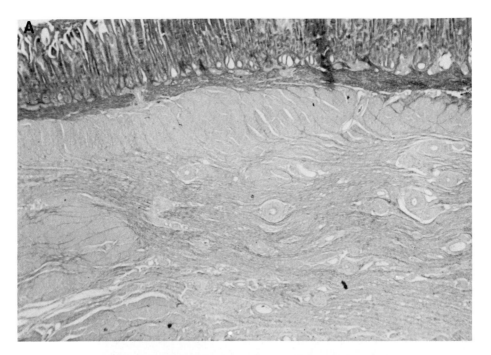

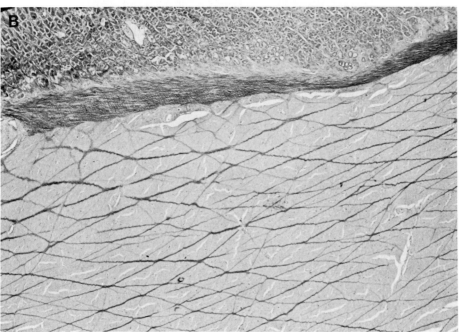

Fig. 7.11 Sections of gizzard from (A) an Se- and vitamin E-deficient turkey poult and (B) an Se- and vitamin E-fed turkey poult. Note extensive fibrosis in gizzard smooth muscle in Se- and vitamin E-deficiency. Photographs courtesy of Dr. M. L. Scott, Cornell University.

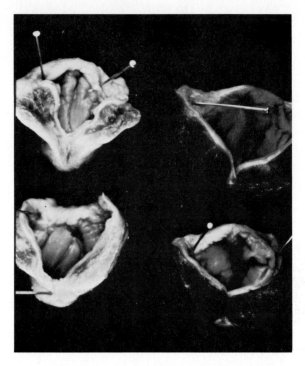

Fig. 7.12   Gross appearance of gizzards from Se- and vitamin E-deficient turkey poults (left) and Se- and vitamin E-fed turkey poults (right). Note pallor and reduction in amount of gizzard smooth muscle due to Se- and vitamin E-deficiency. Photograph courtesy of Dr. M. L. Scott, Cornell University.

of Se. Subsequent studies have been conducted by several investigators[150-155] to provide a description of the pathogenesis of muscular dystrophy in the Se- and vitamin E-deficient duckling. The first ultrastructural lesions observed in the deficient duckling are degeneration of the sarcoplasmic reticulum and mitochondria of the smooth muscle of the duodenum and gizzard.[150,152] The condition is readily detected on gross examination by pale areas of necrosis seen in the dystrophic gizzard (see Fig. 7.13). These changes are accompanied by mineralization of sarcoplasmic debris in necrotic cells and are followed by invasion of macrophages and infiltration of fibroblasts. Abnormalities of capillaries and nonmyelinated nerve fibers are not observed extensively subsequent to the development of extensive necrosis of the muscle.[150] Involvement of the myocardium and skeletal muscles is also seen.[153,156] Skeletal muscle appears hyalinized by light microscopy; extensive myofibrillar lysis is seen, and electron-microscopic examination reveals mitochondrial swelling with disruption of critical

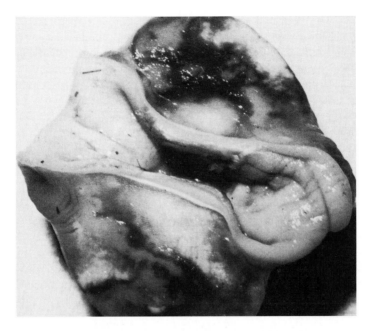

Fig. 7.13 Gizzard myopathy in the Se- and vitamin E-deficient duckling. Note pale areas of necrosis of the gizzard smooth muscle. Photograph courtesy of Dr. J. F. Van Vleet, Purdue University, with permission of the American Journal of Veterinary Research (see reference 154).

membranes. Dean and Combs[157] found that nutritional muscular dystrophy in the duckling was prevented by supplementing a corn-soy-based practical diet (containing 10 IU vitamin E per kilogram and 0.04 ppm inherent Se) with 0.10 ppm Se as Na_2SeO_3; however, higher levels of Se were required to produce maximal activities of SeGSHpx in plasma and liver.

Brown *et al.*[158] proposed that the metabolism of connective tissue may be impaired in the Se- and vitamin E-deficient duckling. They found that the contents of total and soluble collagen were decreased in tendons from ducklings fed a low-Se and low-vitamin E practical type diet vs. ducklings fed the diet supplemented with 0.5 ppm Se (as Na_2SeO_3). Degenerate fibroblasts were observed in tendons from Se-deficient animals. Brown *et al.*[158] interpreted their findings as indicating an impairment of normal collagen maturation and suggested that the functional failure of tendons resulting from such an impairment may lead to the myofibrillar degeneration seen in nutritional muscular dystrophy. This hypothesis is supported by the observations of Bartlett *et al.*,[159] who reported structural alterations in collagen in tendons from Se-deficient ducklings, and of Brown *et al.*,[158,160,161] who reported beneficial effects of supplemental ascorbic acid, a substance known to be involved in collagen metabolism, as a protective factor in Se-deficiency. While supplements of ascorbic acid may have some benefits for Se-deficient ducklings as reported by Moran *et al.*,[161] it is likely that any such response is due to metabolic effects of high-level antioxidant treatment, rather than to the correction of an impairment in the biosynthesis of this compound. Studies by Dean and Combs[157] in the duckling and by Combs and Pesti[94] in the chick provide no support for the latter hypothesis.

2. Exudative Diathesis in Ducklings

Exudative diathesis has been reported in association with nutritional muscular dystrophy in Se- and vitamin E-deficient ducklings.[161,162] The condition would appear to be similar to that of the chick, i.e., green-colored edema of the subcutaneous tissues seen most frequently on the thigh with associated petechial hemorrhages of the thigh musculature. According to Jager,[162] the appearance of exudative diathesis is infrequent and occurs in association with only the more severe cases of nutritional muscular dystrophy in deficient ducklings.

D. Japanese Quail

Severely depressed growth, reduced feed consumption, poor feathering, and poor survival were reported by Scott and Thompson[163] in young Japanese quail (*Coturnix coturnix japonica*) reared using a diet deficient only in Se. The combined deficiency of Se and vitamin E produced exudative diathesis in some animals. Jensen[164] found that while oviposition and fertility were not affected by the combined deficiency of Se and vitamin E, embryonic survival (i.e., egg hatchability) was markedly depressed among females reared to maturity with the deficient diet. Many of the surviving progeny of Se- and vitamin E-deficient females showed extreme generalized muscular weakness and prostration after hatching. Supplementation with either Se or vitamin E returned embryonic survival to normal and reduced quail hen mortality.

E. Pigs

Pigs may show a variety of deficiency diseases that are related to their nutritional status with respect to Se, vitamin E, synthetic antioxidants, and polyunsaturated fats. These diseases include degeneration of liver and heart, visceral edema, and abnormal spermatogenesis. Altered epithelial cell morphology and reduced tolerance to parenterally administered iron have also been reported as consequences of Se/vitamin E-deficiency. These conditions have been reviewed.[165]

1. Hepatosis Dietetica

The combined deficiency of Se and vitamin E in the pig frequently leads to hepatic degeneration referred to as "hepatosis dietetica." This condition was first produced experimentally in vitamin E-deficient swine[166] but was subsequently described in the field.[167] It was recognized to involve the combined deficiency of Se and vitamin E shortly after the discovery[1-3] of a nutritional role of Se.[168,169] Hepatosis dietetica shows two clinical patterns: an acute type with acute liver failure usually in rapidly growing young (e.g., 3-4 months old) pigs and resulting in sudden death, and a subacute type with ascites and jaundice, which generally accompanies edema and/ or cardiomyopathy. The liver lesions of the disease have been described.[167,170-173] The acute lesions are seen as multiple scattered swollen red lobules with hemorrhagic necrosis, and edema of the wall of the gallbladder (see Fig. 7.14). Microscopic examination reveals massive necrosis often with hemorrhage. The subacute lesions appear as scattered collapsed

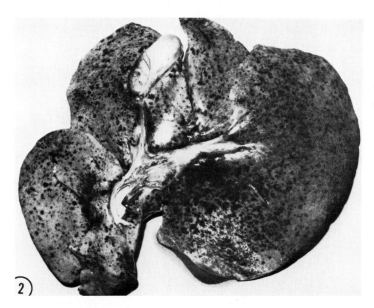

Fig. 7.14 Gross appearance of liver of Se- and vitamin E-deficient pig showing hemorrhagic necrosis. Photograph courtesy of Dr. J. F. Van Vleet, Purdue University, with permission of the American Journal of Veterinary Research (see reference 173).

lobules that yield a rough and granular appearance to the surface of the liver with some lobules remaining unaffected.

Affected pigs show increased plasma activities of aspartate aminotransferase, isocitrate dehydrogenase, and (moderately) alanine aminotransferase.[174] Of these, isocitrate dehydrogenase appears to be the most specific indicator of hepatic damage in the pig.

2. Mulberry Heart Disease

Growing pigs (i.e., 2-4 months old) fed Se- and vitamin E-deficient diets can develop a severe cardiomyopathy characterized by epicardial and myocardial hemorrhages.[170,175] The widespread appearance of hemorrhage in this condition suggested the name "mulberry heart." This condition frequently occurs in pigs with hepatosis dietetica (particularly the subacute form), but may occur without hepatic involvement. The pathology of mulberry heart disease has been described.[170-182] In addition to the signs already indicated, affected animals show scattered pale streaks on the ventricular myocardium (see Figs. 7.15 and 7.16) and abundant serous

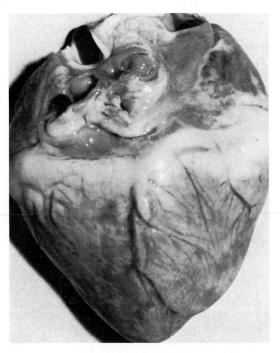

Fig. 7.15   Gross appearance of heart of Se- and vitamin E-deficient pig showing numerous pale white streaks of necrosis. Photograph courtesy of Dr. J. F. Van Vleet, Purdue University, with permission of the American Journal of Veterinary Research (see reference 173).

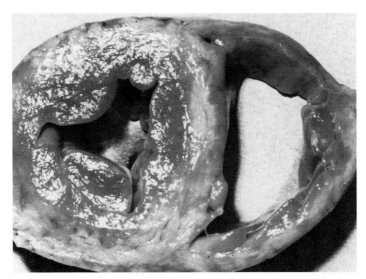

Fig. 7.16 Cross section of heart of Se- and vitamin E-deficient pig showing pale areas of necrosis extensive in the subepicardial myocardium of the left ventricular free wall, and diffusely scattered in the right ventricular free wall and ventricular septum. Photograph courtesy of Dr. J. F. Van Vleet, Purdue University, with permission of the American Journal of Veterinary Research (see reference 173).

exudates in the body cavities with pulmonary congestion and edema. Microscopic examination reveals both vascular and myocytic lesions. The former lesions include fibrinoid necrosis in intramyocardial arteries and arterioles with fibrin microthrombi in the myocardial capillaries. This results in myocardial hemorrhage and edema. The latter lesions involve multifocal hyaline necrosis (see Fig. 7.17) and calcification. Pigs that survive for prolonged periods of time show myocardial fibrosis with macrophage infiltration. Myocyte lesions are observed throughout the heart but are most severe in the atria. The ultrastructural basis for myocyte lesions in Se/vitamin E-deficiency appear to include mitochondrial swelling and mineralization, myofibrillar lysis, and contraction band necrosis.[179,180] Affected vessels show endothelial cell damage and necrosis with fibrin accumulation.[181] Affected animals show increased plasma activities of aspartate aminotransferase and alanine aminotransferase[174]; however, because these enzymes may also be elevated in the plasma due to liver damage, their diagnostic value is low.

3. Nutritional Muscular Dystrophy

Skeletal myopathies are freqently observed in Se- and vitamin E-deficient pigs with hepatosis dietetica and/or mulberry heart disease. Affected pigs show generalized muscular weakness and walk with an unsteady gait. They

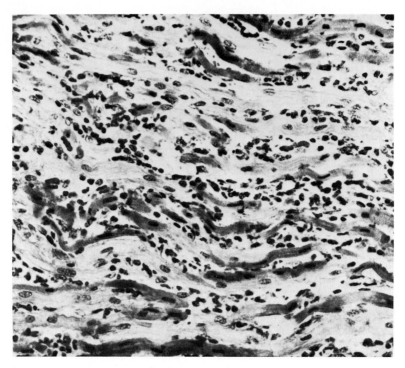

Fig. 7.17   Section (250×) of right atrium of Se- and vitamin E-deficient pig showing extensive
myocardial necrosis and calcification. Photograph courtesy of Dr. J. F. Van Vleet,
Purdue University, with permission of the American Journal of Veterinary Research
(see reference 173).

show a characteristic spread leg posture and are, therefore, referred to as
"splay-legged" or "spraddle-legged." The histopathology of the condition
has been described.[175,176,183] In some cases, lesions may be apparent upon
gross examination as areas of pallor most commonly in the quadriceps
femoris, gracilis, adductor, psoas, and longissimus dorsi muscles.
Microscopic examination reveals Zenker's degeneration with loss of
striations, vacuolization, and disruption of muscle fiber groups. Myofibrillar
lysis and disruption of subcellular membranes systems (i.e., mitchondria,
sarcoplasmic reticulum, plasma membranes) is seen by electron microscopy.
Indicative of muscle degeneration are increases in the activity of creatine
phosphokinase that are observed in plasma or serum from Se- and vitamin
E-deficient pigs affected with nutritional muscular dystrophy.[184] Elevated
activities of aspartate aminotransferase and ornithine carbamyl transferase
have also been reported to be indicative of nutritional muscular dystrophy
in the pig[185]; however, these may be elevated also as the result of hepatic
dysfunction[174] and are, therefore, of less diagnostic value.

4. Edema

Edema has been described in Se- and vitamin E-deficient pigs.[165,175,182] It is most prominent on gross examination in the mesenteries of the gastrointestinal tract and is also seen in the lungs and subcutaneous tissues. This condition has been discussed as a type of exudative diathesis by Van Vleet.[180]

5. Impaired Spermatogenesis

Studies by Liu *et al.*[186] have shown that severe Se-deficiency in boars results in an impairment in spermatogenesis. This finding contradicts earlier studies[187,188]; however, the basis for these apparently discrepant reports is probably the difference in the severity of Se-deficiencies that were produced in these studies. Segerson *et al.*[187] maintained boars with a low-Se (0.025 ppm) semi-purified diet based on cornstarch and *Torula* yeast; Henson *et al.*[188] used a low-Se (0.05 ppm) practical diet based on corn and soybean meal. Neither of these groups observed significant effects due to dietary Se on any parameters of reproductive function. The studies by Liu,[186] however, were conducted using a very low Se practical-type diet based on Se-deficient corn and soybean meal grown in Se-deficient areas of China; their basal diet contained only 0.01 ppm Se. Boars raised with this diet showed significantly reduced (i.e., –46%) sizes of the semeniferous vessicles. Epididymal spermatozoa showed significant reductions in total count (–38%) and viable sperm count (–57%), and significant increases in the incidence of malformations of the head (+73%) or tail (+131%). It appears, therefore, that normal spermatogenesis in the pig, like that in the rat and bull, requires at least low intakes of dietary Se.

6. Susceptibility to Swine Dysentery

Studies by Tiege *et al.*[189-192] have shown that susceptibility to dysentery resulting from exposure to the spirochete, *Troponema hyodysenteriae*, was greatly increased by the combined dietary deficiencies of Se and vitamin E. This organism has been isolated from field cases of "swine dysentery"[193] and is regarded as the primary cause of that disease in practical swine production.[186] Nordstoga[194] suggested that vitamin E status may play a role in the etiology of swine dysentery. This was confirmed by Tiege *et al.*,[189-192] who showed that Se is more important than vitamin E in this respect.[192] Although the mechanism is unclear for the protection by dietary Se against swine dysentery, the effect is seen upon the first exposure of pigs to *T. hyodysenteriae*, and Tiege *et al.*[192] have suggested that Se may act by stimulating the nonspecific immunity of the colonic mucosa.

7. Other Effects

Several reports have indicated that combined Se- and vitamin E-deficiency can reduce the tolerance of baby pigs to parenteral iron supplements.[195-200] Iron-induced myopathy and death among Se- and vitamin E-deficient pigs was shown by Tollerz and Hanneck[196] and Cook.[201]

Adkins and Ewan[202] found that Se-deficiency does not affect pancreatic exocrine function in the baby pig fed vitamin E (100 IU/kg), but that the apparent digestibility of total dry matter and total nitrogen is depressed.

Schanus et al.[203] found that pigs sensitive to chemically induced malignant hyperthermia had a high incidence of SeGSHpx deficiency. Their results showed that those animals in which this condition was induced by exposure to the general anesthetic halothane (2-bromo-2-chloro-1,1,1-trifluoroethane) had erythrocyte SeGSHpx activities at only 20-50% of those of nonreactive individuals. Because the expression of malignant hyperthermia is thought to be under genetic control, these results suggest that the biochemical basis for the syndrome may be the deficiency of SeGSHpx in susceptible genotypes. This hypothesis is supported by observations that the signs of the disorder are consistent with oxidative damage, especially to membranes. It would follow from this that dietary deficiency of Se would also be expected to increase the incidence of halothane sensitivity in pigs.

F. Sheep

The establishment of sheep production in several low-Se parts of the world (e.g., western Oregon, USA; New Zealand) led to the early recognition of the practical consequences of dietary Se-deficiency in this species. The discovery of a nutritional role of Se in the late 1950s[1-3] led to the recognition that deficient intakes of the element were associated with several practical problems in sheep production. These include nutritional muscular dystrophy in lambs, infertility in ewes, and what has been called "selenium-responsive unthriftiness" in lambs.

1. Nutritional Muscular Dystrophy

Nutritional muscular dystrophy in Se- and vitamin E-deficient lambs has been called "stiff lamb disease" and "white muscle disease." It has been enzootic in areas where the Se contents of soils[204] and forages[205,206] are low; its prevention by Se was first shown by Hogue[207] and Muth et al.[208] It is most prevalent in young growing lambs consuming diets that contain less than ca. 0.03 ppm Se (dry matter basis) and are also deficient with respect to vitamin E (usually as the result of poor curing of forages). It occurs with two clinical patterns.[209-212] The first pattern is a congenital type of muscular dystrophy ("congenital white muscle disease") in which lambs are stillborn or die within a few days of birth after sudden physical exertion such as nursing or running. Post-mortem examination reveals straw-colored serous exudates and congestive heart failure. The heart (see Fig. 7.18) can show varying degrees of subendocardial focal or diffuse gray-white discolorations extending into the myocardium; the subepicardial myocardium may also be involved. Such lesions are generally found in one or both ventricles and, less frequently, in the auricles. The initial lesion, as evidenced by microscopic examination, is myofibrillar lysis resulting in noninflammatory coagulative myonecrosis. Involvement of the skeletal muscles is not common.

The second pattern ("delayed white muscle disease") develops after birth; it is observed most frequently in lambs within 3-6 weeks of birth but may occur as late as 4 months after birth. Affected lambs move reluctantly with a stiff, unsteady gait and arched back (see Fig. 7.19). Ultimately, they lose body weight and become prostrate before death. The condition does not appear to be precipitated by physical exertion in most cases; however, some affected lambs with massive heart involvement have suffered sudden death while being driven. Post-mortem examination reveals bilaterally symmetrical, focal or diffuse, yellow-gray discoloration of skeletal muscles

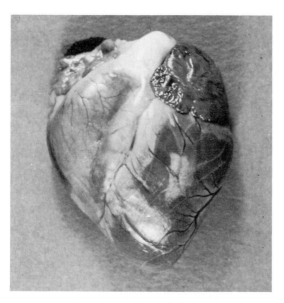

Fig. 7.18 Gross appearance of heart of Se- and vitamin E-deficient lamb showing white areas of myocardial necrosis. Photograph courtesy of Dr. J. E. Oldfield, Oregon State University.

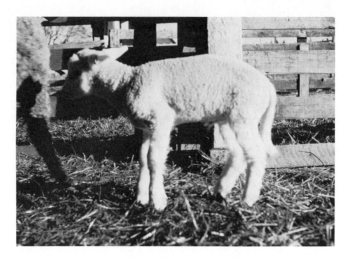

Fig. 7.19 Se- and vitamin E-deficient lamb with "stiff lamb disease." Note characteristic arched back stance. Photograph courtesy of Dr. J. E. Oldfield, Oregon State University.

(see Fig. 7.20) (most frequently diaphragm, intercostals, abductors, longissimus dorsi, triceps femoris). These lesions are seen microscopically as extensive areas of hyaline degeneration and noninflammatory coagulative myonecrosis with myofibrillar lysis or calcification. The incidence of cardiomyopathy is low; however, in some cases heart lesions are seen that resemble those seen in "congenital white muscle disease." Circulatory failure appears to be the ultimate cause of the sudden death that is characteristic of "delayed white muscle disease." Fraser[211] demonstrated progressively abnormal electrocardiograms of Se- and vitamin E-deficient lambs. Just before death, many showed grossly abnormal patterns, with elevated S-T segments. These changes occurred concomitantly with a fall in blood pressure that was most pronounced in the limbs.

Nutritional muscular dystrophy may also be produced by Se-deficiency in yearling sheep.[212,213] In sheep of 9-12 months of age, the disease is frequently observed following driving with the rapid onset of listlessness, stiffness, inability to stand, prostration, and, in the most acute cases, death within 24 hrs.

Sheep affected with nutritional muscular dystrophy show increased activities of several enzymes in the plasma (e.g., lactate dehydrogenase, creatine phosphokinase, glutamic-oxaloacetic transaminase, alpha-hydroxybutyrate dehydrogenase, malic dehydrogenase, fructose diphosphate aldolase).[214-216] Affected tissues show increased activities of collagenase[217] and several lysosomal enzymes (e.g., beta-glucuronidase,

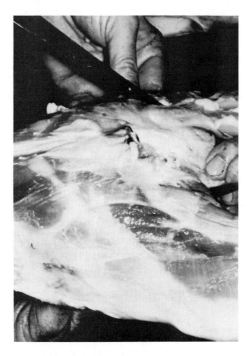

Fig. 7.20   Gross appearance of skeletal muscles of Se- and vitamin E-deficient lamb with "white muscle disease." Note white streaks of muscle degeneration. Photograph courtesy of Dr. J. E. Oldfield, Oregon State University.

alkaline phosphatase, acid phosphatase, proteases).[218] Dystrophic muscles of affected lambs show significant increases in reduced glutathione and nonprotein sulfhydryls but significant decreases in total and protein sulfhydryls.[219]

Nutritional muscular dystrophies in sheep are prevented by adequate intakes of either Se or vitamin E. Despite the early reports of Muth *et al.*[208,220-223] to the contrary, several investigators found that vitamin E could provide effective prophylaxis against this syndrome.[212,224-226] Whanger *et al.*[216] resolved this apparent discrepancy by showing that the form of vitamin E used by Muth *et al.*[208,220-223] had very low biopotency and that forms with good biopotency were fully able to prevent white muscle disease in lambs when administered either orally or parenterally. The occurrence of nutritional muscular dystrophy in the field, therefore, appears to result from the combined deficiency of Se and vitamin E, due to geographic variations in the Se contents of available feedstuffs and to particular conditions of growing, harvesting, and storing that result in vitamin E destruction in those feedstuffs.

2. Infertility in Ewes

Hartley and Grant[212] and Andrews et al.[213] have discussed problems due to a high incidence of barren ewes in flocks with histories of nutritional muscular dystrophy, particularly the congenital type of white muscle disease. Field intervention studies showed that oral administration of Se was effective in reducing the incidence of barren ewes (i.e., 2.5-4% of Se-treated ewes vs. 30% in controls), and in increasing lambing percentages (i.e., 85.7% for Se-treated ewes vs. 52.2% for controls). While the mechanism of action of Se (as well as the extent of involvment, if any, of vitamin E) in this effect has not been elucidated, Segerson and Ganapathy[227] found that Se supplementation increased the strength of uterine contractions. They suggested that this effect increased the number of spermatozoa successfully reaching the ova. However, according to Hartley,[228] a major cause of this apparent infertility is early embryonic mortality (i.e., at 3-4 weeks of gestation). Supplementation with Se thus would appear to increase lamb yield by preventing losses in both ova fertilization rates and embryonic survival.

3. Selenium-Responsive Unthriftiness in Lambs

Andrews et al.[213] described a selenium-responsive condition called "unthriftiness" in sheep. The incidence of this condition is greatest in young and yearling lambs during the autumn and winter months. The syndrome is not characterized by specific clinical signs (e.g., plasma enzymes are not elevated), but rather by a subclinical growth depression, reduction in feed consumption, reduction in wool production, and, in some flocks, increase in rate of mortality. Diarrhea is an occasional feature. Supplemental Se has proven to be effective therapy for this condition.[212,229] Present information does not indicate whether the effect of Se in preventing unthriftiness in sheep is the result of an effect on the immune system (i.e., protection against subclinical disease) or an effect of more direct metabolic nature.

Andrews et al.[213] cited unpublished Se-intervention studies that supported a role of Se in reducing the incidence of peridontal disease in ewes.

G. Cattle

The combined dietary deficiency of Se and vitamin E in cattle can produce several diseases very similar in nature to those observed in Se- and vitamin E-deficient sheep.[212,213] These include nutritional muscular dystrophy, reproductive disorders, and Se-responsive unthriftiness.

1. Nutritional Muscular Dystrophy

Nutritional muscular dystrophy in cattle is generally manifested at 1-4 months of age.[212] This condition is usually called "white muscle disease" and resembles very closely the delayed type of white muscle disease of lambs. Affected individuals become listless and walk reluctantly with a stiff gait; this is followed by prostration and, often, death. Signs show rapid onset frequently after some physical exertion (e.g., being driven). The syndrome is sometimes characterized as sudden death, which may occur within 1 min after a period of excitement.[230] Histological examination of affected calves post mortem reveals peracute myocardial degeneration. This condition can be produced experimentally by feeding a practical diet low in both Se and vitamin E.[231] It is exacerbated by increasing the dietary level of polyunsaturated fats, and is prevented by supplements of either Se or vitamin E.

2. Reproductive Disorders in Cows

Retained placenta is a disorder of dairy cows that involves the combined deficiency of Se and vitamin E. The incidence of the condition has been estimated to be approximately 10% among parturient dairy cows in North America but may be as great as 50% in local areas of endemic Se-deficiency.[232] The disorder involves failure of the placenta to separate from the maternal crypts in the caruncles. This process, which normally occurs over 2-8 hrs post-partum, is called "retained placenta" when the placenta remains attached to the uterus for more than 12 hrs. The major health risk of placental retention is increased incidence of uterine infection from ca. 10% to more than 50%.[233] That Se-deficiency is a factor in the etiology of retained placenta was shown by Trinder *et al.*[234] and has been confirmed[235-238]; these studies demonstrated the efficacy of combined Se-vitamin E treatment in reducing the incidence of the disorder in parturient cows. Some studies[239,240] have not demonstrated such benefits of Se-vitamin E treatments, suggesting that other factors may be involved in the etiology of this syndrome. Harrison *et al.*[241] showed that the incidence of retained placenta was inversely related to nutritional Se status as measured by plasma Se or SeGSHpx at calving (see Figs. 7.21 and 7.22). In most cases, parenteral Se supplements (50 mg of Se as Na_2SeO_3 given 21 days pre-partum) have good prophylactic effects[235,236]; however, Harrison *et al.*[232] have shown that supplements of vitamin E may also be required for preventing the condition in cows fed stored ensiled fodder (of low vitamin E content).

3. Cystic Ovarian Disease

Harrison *et al.*[232,242] reported increases in the incidence of cystic ovarian disease in adult dairy cows of low nutritional Se status (see Fig. 7.23).

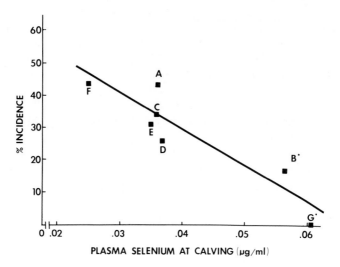

Fig. 7.21   Inverse relationship of the incidence of retained placenta in dairy cows with plasma Se concentration determined at calving. Asterisks denote those injected with Se 21 days before calving.($n = 146$, $r^2 = .83$) Courtesy of Dr. J. H. Harrison and Dr. H. R. Conrad, Ohio Agricultural Research and Development Center.

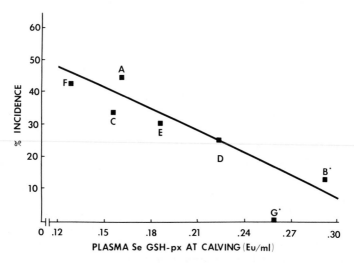

Fig. 7.22   Inverse relationship of the incidence of retained placenta in dairy cows with the activity of SeGSHpx in plasma determined at calving. Eu Enzyme unit. Asterisks denote those injected with Se 21 days before calving ($n = 148$, $r^2 = .69$). Courtesy of Dr. J. H. Harrison and Dr. H. R. Conrad, Ohio Agricultural Research and Development Center.

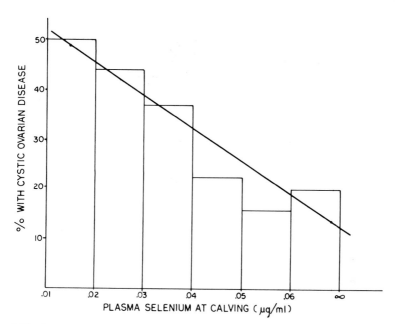

Fig. 7.23   Inverse relationship of the incidence of cystic ovarian disease in dairy cows with nutritional Se state, as indicated by the plasma Se concentration determined at calving. Courtesy of Dr. J. H. Harrison and Dr. H. R. Conrad, Ohio Agricultural Research and Develpment Center.

This condition (see Fig. 7.24) involves the failure of the ovarian follicle to rupture and can result in anestrus or persistent estrus. Parenteral supplementation with Se has been shown to reduce significantly the incidence of this syndrome (see Fig. 7.25).[232]

4. Selenium-Responsive Unthriftiness

Andrews et al.[213] and Hartley and Grant[212] described a subclinical condition usually characterized by slightly reduced growth or loss of body weight but sometimes associated with diarrhea and, in severe cases, death. Like the analogous condition in sheep, this has been referred to a "unthriftiness"; however, the syndrome in cattle is generally not as severe as it is in sheep.

5. Other Disorders

Morris et al.[243] described an anemia of cattle that was associated with the presence of Heinz bodies. This condition occurred in animals grazing on low-Se (0.02-0.055 ppm Se, dry matter basis) St. Augustine grass in peaty muck soils in Florida, USA; it was corrected by dietary supplementation with Se.

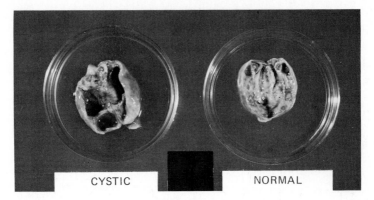

Fig. 7.24 Sectioned ovaries from a cow with cystic ovarian disease and from a normal cow. Photograph courtesy of Dr. J. H. Harrison and H. R. Conrad, Ohio Agricultural Research and Development Center.

Todd and Krook[244] showed that parenteral administration with Se partially prevented the multifocal hepatic necrosis referred to as "sawdust liver." This condition was produced in Hereford steers by feeding a diet rich in polyunsaturated fatty acids, low in protein, and deficient in Se and vitamin E. A protein supplement also reduced the condition, which apparently results primarily from the dietary deficiency of vitamin E.

H. Horses

Horses can experience nutritional muscular dystrophy that appears to involve the combined deficiency of Se and vitamin E. Several investigators

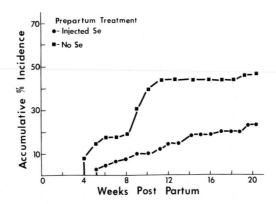

Fig. 7.25 Effect of parenteral Se on the incidence of cystic ovarian disease in dairy cows. Courtesy of Dr. J. H. Harrison and H. R. Conrad, Ohio Agricultural Research and Development Center.

have associated Se/vitamin E-deficiency with generalized muscular dystrophy in foals.[245-248] The condition has been diagnosed with greatest frequency in low-Se areas [209,247-249] including parts of North America, New Zealand, and China. The clinical signs of the disease, as found in one of the most severely Se-deficient areas of the world (i.e., Gansu Province, China), were described by Zhiang et al.[249] as having three clinical patterns. The first is an acute form characterized by sudden death in some cases and, in other cases, by rapid onset of dullness, generalized muscular weakness, sweating, and trembling during movement, which progress to respiratory distress, recumbency, and death. Affected foals show tachycardia (100-120 beats/min) usually with systolic murmurs, and hematuria. Death ensues within 24 hrs. The mortality rate of the condition in Gansu Province, China, is 95%.[249]

The second and most commonly observed form of nutritional muscular dystrophy in foals is a subacute form that is induced by exercise.[249] This form is characterized by initial signs of hindered movement and hematuria. Affected animals show lassitude and generalized muscular weakness. Heart rate is rapid (e.g., 100-120 beats/min) with arrhythmia and systolic murmurs. Foals show increased ventilation rates; swelling of the masseter and lingual muscles causes dysphagia. Within 3-4 days, affected animals become recumbent, salivate excessively, and regurgitate. The mortality rate for animals affected with this condition is estimated to be 30-45%.[249]

The third form of nutritional muscular dystrophy in horses is a chronic form usually seen in older animals.[249] Affected animals show anorexia, emaciation, generalized muscular weakness, tachycardia (80-100 beats/min), and diarrhea. Examination at necropsy reveals bilaterally symmetric necrosis of the masseter, triceps brachii, and quadriceps femoris muscles. These lesions appear at gross examination as gray or gray-yellow streaked or radially striated areas. Enlargement of the liver and kidney is also seen with hemorrhagic areas in each. Lungs are edematous and hyperemic, and the heart shows hypertrophy with gray or gray-yellow necrotic areas on the endocardium of the left ventricle and multiple hemorrhagic areas in the epicardium. Hydropericardium is observed. Affected animals show elevations in serum glutamic-oxaloacetic transaminase activities.[248,249]

The basis of the induction by exercise of myopathy in the horse has been studied.[250,251] Results have showed that exercise produces significant increases in hematocrit, in the blood concentrations of hemoglobin and Se, and in the plasma activities of glutamic-oxaloacetic transaminase. These changes are accompanied by changes in the erythrocyte: decreased concentrations of reduced glutathione and increased concentrations of malondialdehyde (these changes are indicative of sulfhydryl oxidation and lipid peroxidation).

Maylin *et al.*[252] found that effective prevention of nutritional muscular dystrophy in foals could be achieved by oral or parenteral supplementation with Se (1 mg/d). They suggested prevention of the condition by parenteral supplementation of mares during gestation and lactation, or by oral supplementation of foals beginning at birth.

I. Fishes

Poston *et al.*[253] demonstrated that the combined deficiency of Se and vitamin E produced nutritional muscular dystrophy in the Atlantic salmon (*Salmo salar*). Affected individuals showed a Zenker's degeneration of skeletal muscles; supplementation with both Se and vitamin E were required to prevent the condition (see Fig. 7.26). Deficiency of Se alone resulted in reduced SeGSHpx activities in plasma and liver and reduced vitamin E concentrations in liver (but did not affect the vitamin E content of skeletal muscle); however, changes in Se status did not affect the incidence or severity

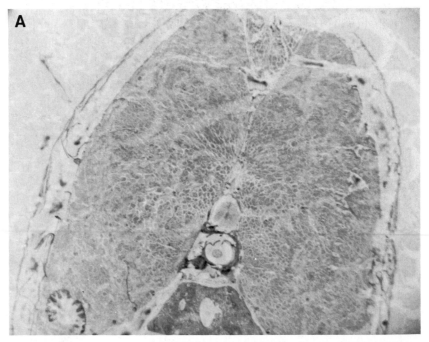

Fig. 7.26 Transverse sections of the dorsal musculature of (A) Se- and vitamin E-deficient and (B) Se- (0.10 ppm) and vitamin E- (100 IU/kg) fed Atlantic salmon (hematoxylin and eosin, 10×). Note the variation in size of and loss of definition of degenerating muscle fibers in Se- and vitamin E- deficiency. Photographs courtesy of Dr. H. A. Poston, Tunison Laboratory of Fish Nutrition, United States Fish and Wildlife Service, with permission of the Journal of Nutrition (see reference 253).

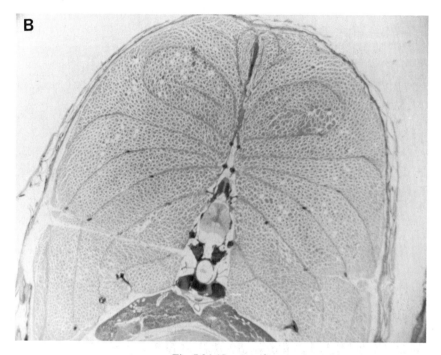

Fig. 7.26 *(Continued)*

of other vitamin E-responsive disorders (e.g., anemia, gall bladder hypertrophy, liver discoloration, edema, dermal depigmentation).

Hilton et al.[254] found that a dietary deficiency of Se alone (i.e., in the presence of an adequate amount of vitamin E) produced no histopathological changes in the rainbow trout (*Salmo gairdneri*). Selenium-deficient animals showed no pathological signs in skeletal muscles or other organs examined (i.e., liver, kidney, spleen). The basal diet used in the studies of Hilton et al.[254] was reported to contain 400 IU vitamin E per kilogram of diet. This level is in the range found by Whitacre and Combs[127] to prevent the otherwise Se-specific syndrome of the chick, nutritional pancreatic atrophy; it is possible that, in like manner, this high level of dietary vitamin E for the rainbow trout may have prevented myopathy of the type reported for the related salmonid fish, the Atlantic salmon.[253] The study of Bell and Cowey[255] supports the hypothesis that the rainbow trout, like the Atlantic salmon, may actually be susceptible to nutritional muscular dystrophy under conditions of combined Se- and vitamin E-deficiency. Those investigators detected elevated activities of pyruvate kinase (indicative of muscle damage) in plasma of Se- and vitamin E-deficient rainbow trout even though no histological evidence of myopathy was observed.

Gatlin and Wilson[256] demonstrated the need for Se by the channel catfish (*Ictalurus punctatus*) for optimal growth and support of SeGSHpx activities. Their study indicated a dietary requirement for Se of ca. 0.25 ppm (dry diet basis) in a diet containing 30 IU vitamin E/kg. Catfish fed lower concentrations of the mineral showed depressed growth rate; however, no organ pathology or dysfunction was reported.

J. Other Species

Muscular dystrophy, often precipitated by exertion, has been reported in the antelope,[257,258] red hartebeeste,[258,259] oryx,[258,260] springbok,[258] eland,[258] kudu,[258] nyala,[258] zebras,[258] buffalo,[258] black rhinoceros,[258] elephant,[258] baboon,[261] mountain goat,[262] tsessebe,[263] oribi,[263] white-tailed deer,[264,265] and flamingo.[266] Many of these conditions have been termed "capture myopathy" or "over-straining disease." The roles, if any, of nutritional Se and vitamin E status in the myopathies of any of these species is not known. However, studies with the white-tailed deer have found that myopathy can occur in does fed diets containing an apparently adequate concentration of Se (i.e., 0.15 ppm) in the presence of a marginal amount (i.e., 5 IU/kg) of vitamin E.[264] Brady et al.[265] showed that supplemental Se (i.e., 0.2 ppm) was effective in reducing blood malondialdehyde concentrations in does and fawns following capture, although this effect was not associated with protection against myopathy or mortality.

Keating and Dagbusan[267] have demonstrated that Se is required in the culture of *Daphnia pulex* and *Daphnia magna*. These crustaceans cannot be maintained in defined media containing less than 1 ppb Se. Under conditions of Se-deficiency, these animals show premature cuticle deterioration, progressive loss of distal segments of the second antennae, and shortened lifespan. Elsey and Lance[268] found SeGSHpx of the alligator to respond to dietary supplementation with Se; however, no adverse effects of feeding a low-Se diet were observed.

III. DIETARY REQUIREMENTS OF SELENIUM FOR LABORATORY AND LIVESTOCK SPECIES

The dietary requirements of various species for Se have been estimated by several expert subcommittees of the Committee on Animal Nutrition, Board on Agriculture, National Research Council. These estimates are presented in Table 7.3.[269-283] It can be seen from the table that the dietary requirements of most species for Se are held to be in the range of 0.10-0.20 ppm (air-dry basis). Also, while it is now apparent that Se is required

Table 7.3

Dietary Requirements for Se of Various Laboratory and Livestock Species

Species	Se requirement (ppm diet)[a]	Criteria	Reference
Laboratory animals			
Rat	0.10	SeGSHpx levels	269
Mouse	+[b]		269
Gerbil	+[b]		269
Guinea pig	0.10	Estimated from adequate diets	269
Hamster	0.10		269
Nonhuman primate	+[b]		270
Dog	0.10	Protection from cardiomyopathy	271
Cat	0.10[b]	Based on needs of other species	272
Rabbit	+[b]		273
Livestock species			
Chicken	0.15	Prevention of exudative diathesis, SeGSHpx levels	274
Turkey	0.20	Prevention of muscular dystrophy	274
Goose	+[b]		274
Duck	0.14	Prevention of muscular dystrophy	274
Pheasant	+[b]		274
Bobwhite quail	+[b]		274
Japanese quail	+[b]		274
Pig	0.15	SeGSHpx level; prevention of lesion of muscles, liver, heart	275
Sheep	0.10	SeGSHpx levels; prevention of white muscle disease	276
Dairy cow	0.10	SeGSHpx levels; prevention of white muscle disease	277
Beef cow	0.20[c]	Prevention of white muscle disease	278
Goat	+[b]		279
Horse	0.10	Prevention of muscular dystrophy	280
Mink	+[b]		281
Fox	+[b]		281
Warm water fish	+[b]		282
Cold water fish	+[b]		283

[a] 10% moisture basis.
[b] Considered to be required, but dietary requirement not estimated due to lack of sufficient quantitative information.
[c] Based on studies in dairy cattle.

in the metabolism of all species, sufficient quantitative information concerning nutritional roles of Se is not available for all. In fact, the greatest amount of available nutritional information has been derived from investigations with only a few species, i.e., the rat, the chick, the pig, and the sheep. For this reason, the estimated Se requirements of several species for which little information is available (e.g., guinea pig, cat, beef cattle)

Table 7.4

Comparison of the Se Needs of the Rat, Chick, Pig, and Lamb

Species	Body weight (kg)	Gain/day (g)	Feed consumed/day (g)
Rat, 21-day-old	.005	5.0	10
Chick, week-old	.070	5.7	8
Pig	5	250	365
Lamb, early weaned	10	250	550

	Dietary Se requirement[a] (ppm)	Se consumed/day		
		μg	μg/kg body weight	μg/kg gain
Rat, 21-day-old	0.10	1.0	16.7	200
Chick, week-old	0.15	1.2	17.1	211
Pig	0.15	54.8	11.0	219
Lamb, early weaned	0.10	55.0	5.5	220
Average				213

[a]Source: Table 7.3.

represent reasonable extrapolations from this body of data. A comparison of the Se needs of rats, chicks, pigs, and lambs (according to the average intakes of Se by these species from diets containing estimated required levels of the mineral) reveals that, although rates of Se intake vary considerably between species when expressed per day or per unit body weight per day, Se intakes are remarkably consistent relative to the rates of daily gain (see Table 7.4). It may be inferred from this consistency that the Se needs of growing animals may be similar, and that adequate Se nutriture is achieved when growing animals consume ca. 210 μg/kg gain/day.

REFERENCES

1. Schwarz, K., and Foltz, C. M., Selenium as an integral part of factor 3 against dietary liver degeneration, J. Am. Chem. Soc., 79, 3292, 1957.
2. Schwarz, K., Bieri, J. G., Briggs, G. M., and Scott, M. L., Prevention of exudative diathesis in chicks by factor 3 and selenium, Proc. Soc. Exp. Biol. Med., 95, 621, 1957.
3. Patterson, E. L., Milstrey, R., and Stokstad, E. L. R., Effect of selenium in preventing exudative diathesis in chicks, Proc. Soc. Exp. Biol. Med., 95, 617, 1957.
4. Tappel, A. L., Vitamin E as the biological lipid antioxidant, Vit. Horm., 20, 493, 1962.
5. Thompson, J. N., and Scott, M. L., Impaired lipid and vitamin E absorption related to atrophy of the pancreas in selenium-deficient chicks, J. Nutr., 100, 797, 1970.
6. Rotruck, J. T., Pope, A. L., Ganther, H. E., Swanson, A. B., Hafeman, D. G., and Hoekstra, W. G., Selenium: biochemical role as a component of glutathione peroxidase, Science, 179, 588, 1973.

7. Anonymous, *Selenium in Nutrition*, Revised Edition, National Academy Press, Washington, D.C., 174 pp., 1983.

8. Shamberger, R. J., *Biochemistry of Selenium*, Plenum Press, New York, 334 pp., 1983.

9. Schwarz, K., Uber die lebertranschadigung der ratte und ihre verhutung durch tocopherol, Z. Physiol. Chem., 283, 106, 1948.

10. Weichselbaum, T. E., Cystine deficiency in the albino rat, Quart. J. Exp. Physiol., 25, 363, 1935.

11. DuVigneaud, V., Hyer, H. M., and Kies, M. W., A relationship between the nature of the vitamin B complex supplement on the ability of homocystine to replace methionine in the diet, J. Biol. Chem., 130, 325, 1939.

12. Glynn, L. E., Himsworth, H. P., and Neuberger, A., Pathological states due to deficiency of the sulfur-containing amino acids, Brit. J. Exp. Pathol., 26, 326, 1945.

13. Daft, F. S., Sebrell, W. H., and Lillie, R. D., Prevention by cystine or methionine of hemorrhage and necrosis of the liver in rats, Proc. Soc. Exp. Biol. Med., 50, 1, 1942.

14. Gyorgy, P. and Goldblatt, H., Hepatic injury on a nutritional basis in rats, J. Exp. Med., 70, 185, 1939.

15. Hove, E. L., and Harris, P. L., Interrelationship between alpha-tocopherol and protein metabolism, J. Nutr., 40, 177, 1950.

16. Schwarz, K., Uber einen ernahrungsbedingten, todlichen leberschaden und seine verhutung durch leberschutzstoffe, Z. Physiol. Chem., 281, 101, 1944.

17. Hock, A., and Fink, H., Uber eine schwere ernahrungsbedingte staffwechselotorung und ihre verhutung durch cystin, Z. Physiol. Chem., 278, 136, 1943.

18. Hock, A., and Fink, H., Uber die Bedentung des Cystins fur den stoffwechsel, zugleich eun Beihrag zur Verbesserung des Hefeeiweibes, Z. Physiol. Chem., 279, 187, 1943.

19. Glynn, L. E., and Himsworth, H. P., Massive crude necrosis of the liver: its significance and experimental production, J. Pathol. Bact., 56, 297, 1944.

20. Schwarz, K., Die ratten-sklampsie, eine ambogene mangelkrankheit, Z. Physiol. Chem., 283, 186, 1948.

21. Schwarz, K., Tocopherol als leberschutzstoff, Z. Physiol. Chem., 281, 109, 1944.

22. Schwarz, K., A hitherto unrecognized factor against dietary necrotic liver degeneration in American yeast (Factor 3), Proc. Soc. Exp. Biol. Med., 78, 852, 1951.

23. Schwarz, K., Casein and Factor 3 in dietary necrotic liver degeneration; concentration of factor 3 from casein, Proc. Soc. Exp. Biol. Med., 80, 319, 1952.

24. Schwarz, K., Stesney, J. A., and Fotz, C. M., Realtionship between selenium traces in L-cystine and protection against dietary liver necrosis, Metab. Clin. Exp., 8, 88, 1959.

25. Schwarz, K., Foltz, C. M., and Bergson, C., Factor 3 and 6-selenoctic acid, Acta Chem. Scand., 12, 1330, 1958.

26. Schwarz, K., and Fredga, A., Biological potency of organic selenium compounds. Aliphatic monoseleno- and diseleno-dicarboxylic acids, J. Biol. Chem., 244, 2103, 1969.

27. Schwarz, K., and Fredga, A., Biological potency of organic selenium compounds. II. Aliphatic selena-carboxylic acids and acid amides, Bioinorg. Chem., 2, 47, 1972.

28. Schwarz, K., and Fredga, A., Biological potency of organic selenium compounds. III. Phenyl-, benzyl-, and phenylethylseleno-carboxylic acids, and related compounds, Bioinorg. Chem., 2, 171, 1972.

29. Schwarz, K., Porter, L. A., and Fredga, A., Biological potency of organic selenium compounds. IV. Straight-chain dialkylmono- and diselenides, Bioinorg. Chem., 3, 145, 1974.

30. Schwarz, K., and Fredga, A., Biological potency of organic selenium compounds. V. Diselenides of alcohols and amines, and some selenium-containing ketones, Bioinorg. Chem., 3, 153, 1974.

31. Christensen, F., Dam, H., Prange, I., and Sondergaard, E., The effect of selenium on vitamin E-deficient rats, Acta Pharmacol. Toxicol., 15, 181, 1958.

32. Piccardo, M. G., and Schwarz, K., The electron microscopy of dietary liver degeneration, in *Liver Function*, Braver, R. W., ed., Am. Inst. Biol. Sci., Washington, D. C., p. 528, 1958.

33. Svboda, D., and Higginson, J., Ultrastructural hepatic changes in rats on a necrogenic diet, Am. J. Pathol., 43, 477, 1963.

34. Porta, E. A., de la Inglesia, F. A., and Hartcroft, W. S., Studies on dietary hepatic necrosis, Lab. Invest., 18, 283, 1968.

35. Schwarz, K., and Corwin, L. M., Prevention of decline of alpha-ketoglutarate and succinate oxidation in vitamin E-deficient rat liver homogenates, J. Biol. Chem., 235, 3387, 1960.

36. Schwarz, K., Dietary necrotic liver degeneration, an approach to the concept of the biochemical lesion, in *Liver Function*, Braver, R. W., ed., Am. Inst. Biol. Sci., Washington, D. C., p. 509, 1958.

37. Schwarz, K., and Mertz, W., Terminal phase of dietary liver necrosis in the rat (hepatogenic hypoglycemia), Metabolism, 8, 79, 1959.

38. Katz, M. L., Parker, K. R., Handelman, G. J., Bramel, J. L., and Dratz, E. A., Effects of antioxidant nutrient deficiency on the retina and retinal pigment epithelium of albino rats: a light and electron microscopic study, Exp. Eye Res., 34, 339, 1982.

39. Stone, W. L., and Dratz, E. A., Selenium-dependent and selenium-independent glutathione peroxidase activities in selected ocular and non-ocular tissues, Exp. Eye Res., 35, 405, 1982.

40. Ren, H. Z., Wei, F. Q., Guan, J. Y., Shu, T. Y., Meng, L. Y., Zhao, Y. H., Li, G. Z., Cheng, B., and Jin, Q., Histopathological and ultrastructural studies on heart muscle of Se-deficient rats, Chin. J. Pathol., 13, 24, 1984.

41. McCoy, K. E. M., and Weswig, P. H., Some selenium responses in the rat not related to vitamin E., J. Nutr., 98, 383, 1969.

42. Siami, G., Schulert, A. R., and Nekel, R. A., A possible role for the mixed function oxidases in the requirement for selenium in the rat, J. Nutr., 102, 857, 1972.

43. Ewan, R. C., Effect of selenium on rat growth, growth hormone and diet utilization, J. Nutr., 106, 702, 1976.

44. Hurt, H. D., Cary, E. E., and Visek, W. J., Growth, reproduction and tissue concentration of selenium in the selenium-depleted rat, J. Nutr., 101, 761, 1971.

45. Whanger, P. D., and Weswig, P. H., Effects of selenium, chromium and antioxidants on growth, eye cataracts, plasma cholesterol and blood glucose in selenium-deficient, vitamin E-supplemented rats, Nutr. Rep. Int., 12, 345, 1975.

46. Sprinker, L. H., Harr, J. R., Newberne, P. M., Whanger, P. D., and Weswig, P. H., Selenium deficiency lesions in rats fed vitamin E-supplemented rations, Nutr. Rep. Int., 4, 335, 1971.

47. Wu, A. S.H., Oldfield, J. E., Whanger, P. D., and Weswig, P. H., Effect of selenium, vitamin E and antioxidants on testicular function in rats, Biol. Reprod., 8, 625, 1973.

48. Wu, A. S.H., Oldfield, J. E., Shull, L. R., and Cheeke, P. R., Specific effect of selenium deficiency on rat sperm., Biol. Reprod., 20, 793, 1979.

49. Wu, A. S.H., Oldfield, J. E., Muth, O. H., Whanger, P. D., and Weswig, P. H., Effect of selenium on reproduction, Proc. West. Soc., Am. Soc. An. Sci., 20, 85, 1969.

50. Wu, A. S.H., Oldfield, J. E., and Whanger, P. D., Effect of selenium, chromium and vitamin E on spermatogenesis, J. An. Sci., 33, 273 (abstract), 1971.

51. Brown, D. G., and Burk, R. F., Selenium retention in tissues and sperm of rats fed a torula yeast diet, J. Nutr., 103, 102, 1973.

52. Calvin, H. I., Selective incorporation of selenium-75 into a polypeptide of the rat sperm tail, J. Exp. Zool., 204, 445, 1978.

53. Calvin, H. I., and Cooper, G. W., A specific selenopolypeptide associated with the outer membrane of rat sperm mitochondria, in *The Spermatozoan: Maturation, Motility, Surface Properties and Comparative Aspects*, Fawcett, D. W., and Bedford, J. M., eds., Urban and Schwarzenberg, Baltimore, p. 135, 1979.

54. Calvin, H. I., Cooper, G. W., and Wallace, E., Evidence that selenium in rat sperm is associated with a cysteine-rich structural protein of the mitochondrial capsules, Gamete Res., 4, 139, 1981.

55. Calvin, H. I., Wallace, E., and Cooper, G. W., Role of selenium in the organization of the mitochondrial sheath in rodent spermatozoa, in *Selenium in Biology and Medicine*, Spallholz, J. E., Martin, J. L., and Ganther, H. E., eds., Avi Publ. Co., Westport, Conn., p. 319, 1981.

56. Behne, D., and Hofer-Bosse, T., Effects of a low selenium status on the distribution and retention of selenium in the rat, J. Nutr., 114, 1289, 1984.

57. DeWitt, W. B., and Schwarz, K., Multiple dietary necrotic degeneration of the mouse, Experientia, 14, 28, 1958.

58. Bunk, M. J., Relationship of appetite, glutathione peroxidase activity, and dietary sulfur-containing amino acids to the onset of nutritional pancreatic atrophy in the selenium-deficient chick and rat, Ph. D. Thesis, Cornell University, Ithaca, New York, 1980.

59. Lane, H. W., Tracy, C. K., and Medina, D., Growth, reproduction rates and mammary gland selenium concentration and glutathione peroxidase activity of BALB/c female mice fed two dietary levels of selenium, J. Nutr., 114, 323, 1984.

60. Wallace, E., Calvin, H. I., and Cooper, G. W., Progressive defects observed in mouse sperm during the course of three generations of selenium deficiency, Gamete Res., 4, 377, 1983.

61. Wallace, E., Cooper, G. W., and Calvin, H.I., Effects of selenium deficiency on the shape and arrangement of rodent sperm mitochondria, Gamete Res., 4, 389, 1983.

62. Wallace, E., Calvin, H. I., Ploetz, K., and Cooper, G. W., Functional and developmental studies on the role of selenium in spermatogenesis, in *Proceedings of the Third International Symposium on Selenium in Biology and Medicine*, Combs, G. F., Jr., Spallholz, J. E., Levander, O. A., and Oldfield, J. E., eds., Avi Publ. Co., Westport, Conn., 1986.

63. Gunn, S. A., Gould, T. C., and Anderson, W. A.D., Incorporation of selenium into spermatogenic pathway in mice, Proc. Soc. Exp. Biol. Med., 124, 1260, 1967.

64. Jones, G. B., and Godwin, K. O., Distribution of radioactive selenium in mice, Nature, 191, 1294, 1962.

65. Bell, R. R., and Draper, H. H., Glutathione peroxidase activity and glutathione concentration in genetically dystrophic mice, Proc. Soc. Exp. Biol. Med., 152, 520, 1976.

66. Revis, N. W., Horton, C. Y., and Curtis, S., Metabolism of selenium in skeletal muscle and liver of mice with genetic muscular dystrophy, Proc. Soc. Exp. Biol. Med., 160, 139, 1979.

67. Bai, J., Ge, K. Y., Deng, X. J., Wu, S. Z., Wang, S. Q., Xue, A. N., and Su, C. Q., Effects of selenium intake on myocardial necrosis induced by coxsackie viral infection in mice, Yingyang Xuebao, 4, 235, 1982.

68. Ge, K. Y., Bai, J., Deng, X. J., Wu, S. Z., Wang, S. Q., Xue, A. N., and Su, C. Q., The protective effect of selenium against viral myocarditis in mice, in *Proceedings of the Third International Symposium on Selenium in Biology and Medicine*, Combs, G. F., Jr., Spallholz, J. E., Levander, O. A., and Oldfield, J. E., eds., Avi Publ. Co., Westport, Conn., 1986.

69. Muth, O. H., Weswig, P. H., Whanger, P. D., and Oldfield, J. E., Effect of feeding selenium-deficient ration to the subhuman primate (*Saimiri sciureus*), Am. J. Vet. Res., 32, 1603, 1971.

70. Butler, J. A., Whanger, P. D., Patton, N. M., and Weswig, P. H., Dietary selenium and pregnancy—a primate study, Fed. Proc., 39, 339, 1980.

71. Butler, J. A., Whanger, P. D., and Tripp, M. J., Blood selenium and glutathione peroxidase activity in pregnant women: comparative assays in primates and other animals, Am. J. Clin. Nutr., 36, 15, 1982.

72. Sehgal, P. K., Bronson, R. T., Brady, P. S., McIntyre, K. W., and Elliott, M. W., Therapeutic efficacy of vitamin E and selenium in treating hemolytic anemia of owl monkeys, Lab. Animal Sci., 30, 92, 1980.

73. Van Vleet, J. F., Experimentally induced vitamin E-selenium deficiency in the growing dog, J. Am. Vet. Med. Assoc., 166, 769, 1975.

74. Cheeke, P. R., and Whanger, P. D., Glutathione peroxidase activity in rabbit tissues, Nutr. Rep. Int., 13, 287, 1976.

75. Lee, Y. H., Layman, D. K., and Bell, R. R., Selenium-dependent and nonselenium-dependent glutathione peroxidase activity in rabbit tissue, Nutr. Rep. Int., 20, 573, 1979.

76. Lawrence, R. A., and Burk, R. F., Species, tissue and subcellular distribution of non-Se-dependent glutathione peroxidase, J. Nutr. 108, 211, 1978.

77. Burk, R. F., Lane, J. M., Lawrence, R. A., and Gregory, P. E., Effect of selenium deficiency in liver and blood glutathione peroxidase activity in guinea pigs, J. Nutr., 111, 690, 1981.

78. Draper, H. H., Ineffectiveness of selenium in the treatment of nutritional muscular dystrophy in the rabbit, Nature, 180, 1419, 1957.

79. Hove, E. L., Fry, G. S., and Schwarz, K., Ineffectiveness of Factor 3-active selenium compounds in muscular dystrophy of rabbits on vitamin E-free diets, Proc. Soc. Exp. Biol. Med., 98, 27, 1958.

80. Jenkins, K. J., Hidiroglou, M., Mackay, R. R., and Proulx, J. G., Influence of selenium and linoleic acid on the development of nutritional muscular dystrophy in beef calves, lambs and rabbits, Can. J. Anim. Sci., 50, 137, 1970.

81. Bieri, J. G., and Evarts, R. P., Vitamin E activity of alpha-tocopherol in the rat, chick and hamster, J. Nutr., 107, 850, 1974.

82. Seidel, J. C., and Harper, A. E., Some observations on vitamin E deficiency in the guinea pig, J. Nutr., 70, 147, 1960.

83. Bonetti, E., and Stirpe, F., Effect of selenium on muscular dystrophy in vitamin E-deficient rats and guinea pigs, Proc. Soc. Exp. Biol. Med., 114, 109, 1963.

84. Dam, H., and Glavind, J., Alimentary exudative diathesis, Nature, 142, 1077, 1938.

85. Scott, M. L., Lesions of vitamin E and selenium deficiencies in poultry and their pathogenesis, Folia Vet. Lat., 4, 113, 1974.

86. Dam, H., and Glavind, J., Vitamin E and kapillarpermeabilitat, Naturwiss., 28, 207, 1940.

87. Reid, B. L., Rahman, M. M., Greech, B. G., and Couch, J. R., Selenium and development of exudative diathesis in chicks, Proc. Soc. Exp. Biol Med., 97, 590, 1958.

88. Scott, M. L., Norris, L. C., Heuser, G. F., and Nelson, T. S., Further chick studies on vitamin E and a vitamin E-like factor in dried brewer's yeast, Poultry Sci., 34, 1220, 1955.

89. Nesheim, M. C., and Scott, M. L., Studies on the nutritional effects of selenium for chicks, J. Nutr., 65, 601, 1958.

90. Noguchi, T., Cantor, A. H., and Scott, M. L., Mode of action of selenium and vitamin E in prevention of exudative diathesis in chicks, J. Nutr., 103, 1502, 1973.

91. Mercurio, S. D., and Combs, G. F., Jr., unpublished research, 1983.

92. Combs, G. F., Jr., Effects of dietary polychlorinated biphenyls on the vitamin E-selenium nutrition of the chick, Ph. D. Thesis, Cornell University, Ithaca, New York, 1974.

93. Combs, G. F., Jr., and Scott, M. L., Antioxidant effects on selenium and vitamin E function in the chick, J. Nutr., 104, 1297, 1974.

94. Combs, G. F., Jr., and Pesti, G. M., Influence of ascorbic acid on selenium nutrition in the chick, J. Nutr., 106, 958, 1976.

95. Pesti, G. M., and Combs, G. F., Jr., Studies on the enteric absorption of selenium in the chick using localized coccidial infections, Poultry Sci., 55, 2265, 1976.

96. Dam, H., Prange, I., and Stodergaard, E., Muscular degeneration (white striation of the muscles) in chicks reared on vitamin E-deficient, low fat diets, Acta Pathol. Microbiol. Scand., 31, 172, 1952.

97. Machlin, L. J., Studies on the growth response in the chicken from the addition of sodium sulfate to a low-sulfur diet, Poultry Sci., 34, 1209, 1955.

98. Machlin, L. J., and Shalkop, W. T., Muscular degeneration in chickens fed diets low in vitamin E and sulfur, J. Nutr., 60, 87, 1956.

99. Calvert, C. C., and Scott, M. L., Effect of selenium on the requirement for vitamin E and cystine for the prevention of nutritional muscular dystrophy in the chick, Fed. Proc., 22, 318, 1963.

100. Jenkins, K. J., Hill, D. C., Hutcheson, L. M., and Branion, H. D., The efficacy of sulfur amino acids and related compounds for protection against development of muscular dystrophy in the chick, Poultry Sci., 41, 672, 1962.

101. Jenkins, K. J., Hill, D. C., Hutcheson, L. M., and Branion, H. D., Relation of arginine and sulfur amino acids to the development of muscular dystrophy in the chick, Poultry Sci., 41, 61, 1962.

102. Hathcock, J., Hull, S. J., and Scott, M. L., Derivatives and analogs of cysteine and selected sulfydryl compounds in nutritional muscular dystrophy in chicks, J. Nutr., 94, 147, 1968.

103. Desai, I. D., Calvert, C. C., and Scott, M. L., A time-sequence study of the relationship of peroxidation, lysosomal activities, and nutritional muscular dystrophy, Arch. Biochem. Biophys., 108, 60, 1964.

104. Hull, S. J., and Scott, M. L., A study of the relationship of plasma glutamic-oxaloacetic transaminase activity to nutritional muscular dystrophy in the chick, J. Nutr., 102, 1367, 1972.

105. Dam, H., and Sondergaard, E., Prophylactic effect of selenium dioxide against degeneration (white striation) of muscle in chicks, Experientia, 13, 494, 1957.

106. Nesheim, M. C., and Scott, M. L., Studies on the nutritive effect of selenium for chicks, J. Nutr., 65, 601, 1958.

107. Ewen, L. M., and Jenkins, K. J., Antidystrophic effect of selenium and other agents on chicks from vitamin E-depleted hens, J. Nutr., 93, 470, 1967.

108. Scott, M. L., Antioxidants, selenium and sulfur-amino acids in the vitamin E nutrition of chicks, Nutr. Abst. Rev., 32, 1, 1962.

109. Shih, J. C.H., Jonas, R. H., and Scott, M. L., Oxidative deterioration of the muscle proteins during nutritional muscular dystrophy in chicks, J. Nutr., 107, 1786, 1977.

110. Hathcock, J., Sulfur metabolism in nutritional muscular dystrophy in the chicken, Ph. D. Thesis, Cornell University, Ithaca, New York, 1967.

111. Thompson, J. N., and Scott, M. L., Role of selenium in the nutrition of the chick, J. Nutr., 97, 335, 1969.

112. Thompson, J. N., and Scott, M. L., Impaired lipid and vitamin E absorption related to atrophy of the pancreas in selenium-deficient chicks, J. Nutr., 100, 797, 1970.

113. Gries, C. L., and Scott, M. L., Pathology of selenium deficiency in the chick, J. Nutr., 102, 1287, 1972.

114. Noguchi, T., Langevin, M. L., Combs, G. F., Jr., and Scott, M. L., Biochemical and histochemical studies of the selenium-deficient pancreas in chicks, J. Nutr., 103, 444, 1973.

115. Cantor, A. H., Langevin, M. L., Noguchi, T. N., and Scott, M. L., Efficacy of selenium in selenium compounds and feedstuffs for prevention of pancreatic fibrosis in chicks, J. Nutr., 105, 106, 1975.

116. Shih, J. C. H., Sandholm, M., and Scott, M. L., Changes of lipoamide dehydrogenase and mitochondrial structure in selenium-deficient chicks, J. Nutr., 107, 1583, 1977.

117. Bunk, M. J., and Combs, G. F., Jr., Effect of selenium on appetite in the selenium-deficient chick, J. Nutr., 110, 743, 1980.

118. Bunk, M. J., and Combs, G. F., Jr., Relationship of selenium-dependent glutathione peroxidase activity and nutritional pancreatic atrophy in selenium-deficient chicks, J. Nutr., 111, 1611, 1981.

119. Whitacre, M. E., and Combs, G. F., Jr., Selenium and mitochondrial integrity in the pancreas of the chick, J. Nutr., 113, 1972, 1983.

120. Combs, G. F., Jr., Liu, C. H., Lu, Z. H., and Su, Q., Uncomplicated selenium deficiency produced in chicks fed a corn-soy-based diet, J. Nutr., 114, 964, 1984.

121. Combs, G. F., Jr., and Bunk, M. J., The role of selenium in pancreatic function, in Selenium in Biology and Medicine, Spallholz, J. E., Martin, J. L., and Ganther, H. E., eds., Avi Publ. Co., Westport, Conn., p. 70, 1981.

122. Cupp, M. S., and Combs, G. F., Jr., unpublished research, 1983.

123. Rebar, A. H., and VanVleet, J. F., Ultrastructural changes in the pancreata of selenium-vitamin E-deficient chicks, Vet. Pathol., 14, 629, 1977.

124. Bunk, M. J., and Combs, G. F., Jr., Evidence for an impairment in the conversion of methionine to cysteine in the selenium-deficient chick, Proc. Soc. Exp. Biol. Med., 167, 87, 1981.

125. LaVorgna, M. W., and Combs, G. F., Jr., Evidence of a hereditary factor affecting the chick's response to uncomplicated selenum deficiency, Poultry Sci., 62, 164, 1983.

126. Halpin, K. M., and Baker, D. H., Selenium deficiency and transsulfuration in the chick, J. Nutr., 114, 606, 1984.

127. Whitacre, M. E., and Combs, G. F., Jr., Peroxidative damage in nutritional pancreatic atrophy due to selenium deficiency in the chick, Federation Proc., 42, 928, 1983.

128. Century, B., and Horwitt, M. K., Effect of dietary selenium on incidence of nutritional encephalomalacia in chicks, Proc. Soc. Exp. Biol. Med., 117, 320, 1964.

129. Dam, H. and Granados, H., Peroxidation of body fat in vitamin E deficiency, Acta Physiol. Scand., 10, 162, 1945.

130. Dam, H., Influence of antioxidants and redox substances on signs of vitamin E deficiency, Pharmacol. Rev., 9, 1, 1957.

131. Bunnell, R. H., Matterson, L. D., Singsen, E. P., Potter, L. M., and Koyeft, A., Studies on encephalomalacia in the chick. 3. The influence of feeding or injecting various tocopherols and other antioxidants on the incidence of encephalomalacia, Poultry Sci., 34, 1068, 1955.

132. Yoshida, M., and Hoshii, H., Preventive effect of selenium, methionine and antioxidants against encephalomalacia of chicks induced by dilauryl succinate, J. Nutr., 107, 35, 1977.

133. Machlin, L. J., personal com munication, 1982.

134. Marsh, J. A., Dietert, R. R., and Combs, G. F., Jr., Influence of dietary selenium and vitamin E on the humoral immune response of the chick, Proc. Soc. Exp. Biol. Med., 166, 228, 1981.

135. Marsh, J. A., Dietert, R. R., and Combs, G. F., Jr., unpublished research, 1983.

136. Cantor, A. H., and Scott, M. L., The effect of selenium in the hen's diet on egg production, hatchability, performance of progeny and selenium concentration in eggs, Poultry Sci., 53, 1870, 1974.

137. Latshaw, J. D., Ort, J. F., and Diesem, C. D., The selenium requirements of the hen and effects of a deficiency, Poultry Sci., 56, 1876, 1977.

138. Combs, G. F., Jr., and Scott, M. L., The selenium needs of laying and breeding hens, Poultry Sci., 58, 871, 1979.

139. Jungherr, E., and Pappenheimer, A. M., Nutritional myopathy of gizzard in turkeys, Proc. Soc. Exp. Biol. Med., 37, 520, 1937.

140. Walter, W. D., and Jensen, L. S., Effectiveness of selenium and noneffectiveness of sulfur amino acids in preventing muscular dystrophy in the turkey poult, J. Nutr., 80, 327, 1963.

141. Walter, E. D., and Jensen, L. S., Serum glutamic-oxaloacetic transaminase levels, muscular dystrophy and certain hematological measurements in chicks and poults as influenced by vitamin E, selenium and methionine, Poultry Sci., 43, 919, 1964.

142. Scott, M. L., Metabolic role of selenium in nutritional myopathies of chicks and poults, Proc. 7th Int. Congr. Nut., p. 265, 1965.

143. Cantor, A. H., Moorhead, P. D., and Musser, M. A., Comparative effects of selenite and selenomethionine upon nutritional muscular dystrophy, selenium-dependent glutathione peroxidase, and tissue selenium concentrations of turkey poults, Poultry Sci., 61, 478, 1982.

144. Scott, M. L., Olson, G., Krook, L., and Brown, W. R., Selenium-responsive myopathies of myocardium of smooth muscle in the young poult, J. Nutr., 91, 573, 1967.

145. Harper, J. A., and Helfer, D. H., The effect of vitamin E, methionine and selenium on degenerative myopathy in turkeys, Poultry Sci., 51, 1757, 1972.

146. Creech, B. G., Feldman, G. L., Ferguson, T. M., Reid, R. L., and Couch, J. R., Exudative diathesis and vitamin E deficiency in turkey poults, J. Nutr., 62, 83, 1957.

147. Rahman, M. M., Davies, R. E., Deyoe, C. W., and Couch, J. R., Selenium and *Torula* yeast in production of exudative diathesis in chicks, Proc. Soc. Exp. Biol. Med., 105, 227, 1960.

148. Pappenheimer, A. M., and Goettsch, M., Nutritional myopathy in ducklings, J. Exp. Med., 59, 35, 1934.

149. Yarington, J. T., Whitehair, C. K., and Corwin, R. M., Vitamin E-selenium deficiency and its influence on avian malarial infection in the duck, J. Nutr., 103, 231, 1973.

150. Yarrington, J. E., and Whitehair, C. K., Ultrastructure of gastrointestinal smooth muscle in ducks with a vitamin E-selenium deficiency, J. Nutr., 105, 782, 1975.

151. Hulstaert, C. E., Molensa, I., deGoeij, J. J. M., Zegers, C., and Van Pijpen, P. L., Selenium and vitamin E-deficient diets and the occurrence of myopathy as a symptom of vitamin E deficiency, Nutr. Metab., 14, 210, 1976.

152. Van Vleet, J. F., and Farrans, V. J., Ultrastructural alterations in gizzard smooth muscle of selenium-vitamin E-deficient ducklings, Avian Dis., 21, 531, 1977.

153. Van Vleet, J. F., and Farrans, V. J., Ultrastructural alteration in skeletal muscle of ducklings fed a selenium-vitamin E-deficient diet, Am. J. Vet. Res., 38, 1399, 1977.

154. Van Vleet, J. F., Amounts of twelve elements required to induce selenium-vitamin E deficiency in ducklings, Am. J. Vet. Res., 43, 851, 1982.

155. Van Vleet, J. F., Amounts of eight combined elements required to induce selenium-vitamin E deficiency in ducklings and protection by supplements of selenium and vitamin E, Am. J. Vet. Res., 43, 1049, 1982.

156. Vos, J., Hulstaert, C. E., and Molenaar, I., Nutritional myopathy in ducklings in a growth-rate-dependent symptom of "tissue peroxidosis" due to a net nutritional shortage of vitamin E plus selenium in skeletal muscle, Nutr. Metab., 25, 299, 1981.

157. Dean, W. F., and Combs, G. F., Jr., Influence of dietary selenium in performance, tissue selenium content, and plasma concentrations of selenium-dependent glutathione peroxidase, vitamin E and ascorbic acid in ducklings, Poultry Sci., 60, 2655, 1980.

158. Brown, R. G., Sweeny, P. R., and Moray, E. T., Jr., Collagen levels in tissues from selenium-deficient ducks, Comp. Biochem. Physiol., 72A, 383, 1982.

159. Bartlett, M. W., Egelstaff, P. A., Holden, T. M., Stinson, R. H., and Sweeny, P. R., Structural changes in tendon collagen resulting from muscular dystrophy, Biochim. Biophys. Acta, 328, 213, 1973.

160. Brown, R. G., Sweeney, P. R., George, J. C., Stanley, D. W., and Moran, E. T., Jr., Selenium deficiency in the duck: serum ascorbic acid levels in developing muscular dystrophy, Poultry Sci., 53, 1235, 1974.

161. Moran, E. T., Jr., Carlson, H. C., Brown, R. G., Sweeney, P. R., George, J. C., and Stanley, D. W., Alleviating mortality associated with a vitamin E-selenium deficiency by dietary ascorbic acid, Poultry Sci., 54, 266, 1975.

162. Jager, F. C., Effect of dietary linoleic acid and selenium on the requirement of vitamin E in ducklings, Nutr. Metabl., 14, 210, 1977.

163. Scott, M. L., and Thompson, J. N., Selenium in nutrition and metabolism, Proc. Maryland Nutr. Conf., 1, 1968.

164. Jensen, L. S., Selenium deficiency and impaired reproduction in Japanese quail, Proc. Soc. Exp. Biol. Med., 128, 970, 1968.

165. Subcommittee on Selenium, Committee on Animal Nutrition, Board on Agriculture, National Research Council, Selenium in Nutrition, Revised Edition, National Academy Press, Washington, D. C., p. 87, 1983.

166. Adamstone, F. B., Krider, J. L., and James, M. F., Response of swine to vitamin E-deficient rations, Ann. N. Y. Acad. Sci., 52, 260, 1949.

167. Obel, A. L., Studies on the morphology and etiology of so-called toxic liver dystrophy (hepatosis dietetica) in swine, Acta Pathol. Microbiol. Scand., Suppl. 94, 1, 1953.

168. Eggert, R. G., Patterson, E., Akers, W. T., and Stokstad, E. L.R., The role of vitamin E and selenium in the nutrition of the pig, J. Anim. Sci. 16, 1032, 1957.

169. Grant, C. A., and Thafrelin, B., Selenium and hepatosis dietetica in pigs, Nord. Veterinaermed., 10, 657, 1958.

170. Harding, J. D.J., Some observations in the histopathology of mulberry heart disease in pigs, Res. Vet. Sci., 1, 129, 1960.

171. Grant, C. A., Morphological and etiological studies of dietetic microangiopathy in pigs ("mulberry heart"), Acta Vet. Scand, 2, Suppl. 3, 1, 1961.

172. Seffner, W., Wittig, W., and Rittenbach, P., Investigations on mulberry heart disease (microangiopathy) of pigs, Dtsch. Tieraerztl. Wochehuschr., 74, 213, 1967.

173. VanVleet, J. F., Comparative efficacy of five supplementation procedures to control selenium-vitamin E deficiency in swine, Am. J. Vet. Res., 43, 1180, 1982.

174. Tollersrud, S., Changes in the enzymatic profile in blood and tissues in preclinical and clinical vitamin E deficiency in pigs, Acta Agric. Scand., Suppl. 19, 124, 1973.

175. Trapp, A. L., Keahey, K. K., Whitenack, D. L., and Whitehair, C. K., Vitamin E-selenium deficiency in swine: differential diagnosis and nature of field problem, J. Am. Vet. Med. Assoc., 157, 289, 1970.

176. Van Vleet, J. F., Carlton, and W. Olander, H. J., Hepatosis dietetica and mulberry heart disease associated with selenium deficiency in Indiana swine, J. Am. Vet. Med. Assoc., 157, 1208, 1970.

177. Nafstad, I., and Tollersrud, S., The vitamin E-deficiency syndrome in pigs. I. Pathological changes, Acta Vet. Scand., 11, 452, 1970.

178. Natstad, I., The vitamin E-deficiency syndrome in pigs. III. Light and electron microscopic studies on myocardial vascular injury, Vet. Pathol., 8, 239, 1971.

179. Sweeney, P. R., and Brown, R. G., Ultrastructural changes in muscular dystrophy. I. Cardiac tissue of piglets deprived of vitamin E and selenium, Am. J. Pathol., 68, 479, 1973.

180. Van Vleet, J. F., Ferrans, V. J., and Ruth, G. R., Ultrastructural alternatives in nutritional cardiomyopathy of selenium-vitamin E deficient swine. I. Fiber lesions, Lab. Invest., 37, 188, 1977.

181. Van Vleet, J. F., Ferrans, V. J., and Ruth, G. R., Ultrastructural alterations in nutritional cardiomyopathy of selenium-vitamin E deficient swine. II. Vascular lesions, Lab. Invest., 37, 201, 1977.

182. Van Vleet, J. F., Pathology of selenium and vitamin E deficiency in animals, in *Proceedings of the Third International Symposium on Selenium in Biology and Medicine*, Combs, G. F., Jr., Spallholz, J. E., Levander, O. A., and Oldfield, J. E., eds., Avi Publ. Co., Westport, Conn., 1986.

183. Van Vleet, J. F., Ruth, G., and Ferraus, V., Ultrasturctural alterations in skeletal muscles of pigs with selenium-vitamin E deficiency Am. J. Vet. Res., 37, 911, 1976.

184. Fontaine, M., Valli, V. E.O., and Young, L. G., Studies on vitamin E and selenium deficiency in young pigs. III. Effect in kinetics of erythrocyte production and destruction, Can. J. Comp. Med., 41, 57, 1977.

185. Orstadius, K., Nutritional muscular dystrophy in pigs. Studies on the aetiology, diagnosis and therapy, Ph. D. Thesis, University of Uppsala, 1961.

186. Liu, C. H., Chen, Y. M., Zhang, J. Z., Huang, M. Y., Su. Q., Lu, Z. H., Yin, R. X., Shao, G. Z., Feng, D., and Zheng, P. L., Preliminary studies on influence of selenium deficiency to the developments of genital organs and spermatogenesis in young boars, Acta Vet. Zootech. Sinica, 13, 73, 1982.

187. Segerson, E. C., Getz, W. R., and Johnson, B. H., Selenium and reproductive function in boars fed a low selenium diet, J. Anim. Sci., 53, 1360, 1981.

188. Henson, H. C., Kattesh, H. G., Hitchcock, J. P., and Kincaid, J. A., The effects of dietary selenium on growth and selected reproductive parameters of young boars, Anim. Prod., 37, 401, 1983.

189. Tiege, J., Jr., Nordstoga, K., and Aursjo, J., Influence of diet on experimental swine dysentery. 1. Effects of a vitamin E and selenium deficient diet supplemented with 6.8% cod liver oil, Acta Vet. Scand., 18, 384, 1977.

190. Tiege, J., Jr., Saxegaard, F., and Froslie, A., Influence of diet on experimental swine dysentery. 2. Effects of a vitamin E and selenium deficient diet supplemented with 3% cod liver oil, vitamin E or selenium, Acta Vet. Scand., 19, 133, 1978.

191. Tiege, J., Jr., Swine dysentery: the influence of dietary vitamin E and selenium on the clinical and pathological effects of *Treponema hyodysenterial* infection in pigs, Res. Vet. Sci., 32, 95, 1982.

192. Tiege, J., Jr., Larsen, H. J., and Tollersrud, J., Swine dysentery: the influence of dietary selenium on clinical and pathological effects of *Treponema hyodysenterial* infection, Acta Vet. Scand., 25, 1, 1984.

193. Harris, D. L., Current status of research on swine dysentery, J. Am. Vet. Med. Assoc., 164, 809, 1974.

194. Nordstoga, K., Fibrinous colitis in swine, a manifestation of Schwartzman reaction?, Vet. Rec., 92, 698, 1973.

195. Lanneck, N., Lindberg, P., and Tollerz, G., Lowered resistance to iron in vitamin E-deficient piglets and mice, Nature, 195, 1006, 1962.

196. Tollerz, A. L., and Hanneck, N., Protection against iron toxicity in vitamin E-deficient piglets and mice by vitamin E and synthetic antioxidants, Nature 201, 846, 1964.

197. Patterson, D. S.P., Allen, V. M., Thurley, D. C., and Done, J. T., The role of tissue peroxidation in iron-induced myodegeneration in piglets, Biochem. J., 104, 2, 1967.

198. Patterson, D. S.P., Allen, W. M., Berrett, S., Sweasy, D., Thurley, D. C., and Done, J. T., A biochemical study of the pathogenesis of iron-induced myodegeneration of piglets, Zentralbl. Veterinaermed., 16, 199, 1969.

199. Patterson, D. S.P., Allen, W. M., Berrett, S., Sweasy, D., and Done, J. T., The toxicity of parenteral iron preparation in the rabbit and the dog with a comparison of the chemical and biochemical responses to iron-dextran in 2 days old and 8 days old piglets, Zentralbl. Veterinaermed., 18, 453, 1971.

200. Patterson, D. S.P., and Allen, W. M., Biochemical aspects of some pig muscle disorders, Br. Vet. J., 128, 101, 1972.

201. Cook, R. W., Iron tolerance in the young pig, M. S. Thesis, Michigan State University, East Lansing, Mich., 1974.

202. Adkins, R. J., and Ewan, R. C., Effect of supplemental selenium on pancreatic function and nutrient digestibility in the pig, J. Anim. Sci., 58, 351, 1984.

203. Schanus, E. G., Schendel, F., Lovrieu, R. E., Rempel, W. E., and McGrath, C., Malignant hyperthermia (MH): Erythrocyte damage from oxidation and glutathione peroxidase deficiency, The Red Cell, Fifth Ann Arbor Conf., p. 323, 1981.

204. Muth, O. H., and Allaway, W. A., The relationship of white muscle disease to the distribution of naturally occurring selenium, J. Am. Vet. Med. Assoc., 142, 1379, 1963.

205. Allaway, W. H., and Hodgson, J. F., Symposium on nutrition, forage and pastures: selenium in forages as related to the geographic distribution of muscular dystrophy in livestock, J. Anim. Sci., 23, 271, 1964.

206. Kubota, J., Allaway, W. H., Carter, D. L., Cary, E. E., and Lazar, V. A., Selenium in crops in the United States in relation to selenium-responsive diseases of animals, Agr. Food Chem., 15, 448, 1967.

207. Hogue, D. E., Vitamin E, selenium and other factors related to nutritional muscular dystrophy in lambs, Proc. Cornell Nutr. Conf., Ithaca, New York, p. 32, 1958.

208. Muth, O. H., Oldfield, J. E., Remment, L. F., and Schubert, J. R., Effects of selenium and vitamin E on white muscle disease, Science, 128, 1090, 1958.

209. Hartley, W. J., and Dodd, D. C., Muscular dystrophy in New Zealand livestock, N. Z. Vet. J., 5, 61, 1957.

210. Grant, A. B., Drake, C., and Hartley, W. J., Further observations on white muscle disease in lambs, N. Z. Vet. J., 8, 1, 1960.

211. Fraser, F. J., Abnormal electrocardiograms, blood pressure changes and some aspects of the histopathology of selenium deficiency in lambs, Quart. J. Expt. Physiol., 51, 94, 1966.

212. Hartley, W. J., and Grant, A. B., A review of selenium responsive diseases in New Zealand livestock, Federation Proc., 20, 679, 1961.

213. Andrews, E. D., Hartley, W. J., and Grant, A. B., Selenium-responsive diseases of animals in New Zealand, N. Z. Vet. J., 16, 3, 1968.

214. Whanger, P. D., Weswig, P. H., Muth, O. H., and Oldfield, J. E., Tissue lactic dehydrogenase, glutamic-oxalacetic transaminase and peroxidase changes of selenium-deficient myopathic lambs, J. Nutr., 99, 331, 1969.

215. Buchanan-Smith, J. G., Nelson, E. C., and Tillman, A. D., Effect of vitamin E and selenium on lysosomal and cytoplasmic enzymes in sheep tissues, J. Nutr., 99, 387, 1969.

216. Whanger, P. D., Weswig, P. H., Oldfield, J. E., Cheeke, P. R., and Schmitz, J. A., Selenium and white muscle disease in lambs: effects of vitamin E and ethoxyquin, Nutr. Rep. Int., 13, 159, 1976.

217. Broderius, M. A., Whanger, P. D., and Weswig, P. H., Collagenase activity in tissues of selenium responsive myopathic lambs, Proc. Soc. Exp. Biol. Med., 143, 297, 1973.

218. Whanger, P. D., Weswig, P. H., Muth, O. H., and Oldfield, J. E., Tissue lysosomal enzyme changes in selenium-deficient myopathic lambs, J. Nutr., 100, 773, 1970.

219. Broderius, M. A., Whanger, P. D., and Weswig, P. H., Tissue sulfhydryl groups in selenium-deficient rats and lambs, J. Nutr., 103, 336, 1973.

220. Muth, O. H., White muscle disease (myopathy) in lambs and calves. I. Occurrence and nature of the disease under Oregon conditions, J. Am. Vet. Med. Assoc., 126, 355, 1955.

221. Muth, O. H., Oldfield, J. E., Schubert, J. R., and Remmert, L. F., White muscle disease (myopathy) in lambs and calves. VI. Effects of selenium and vitamin E on lambs, Am. J. Vet. Res., 20, 231, 1959.

222. Muth, O. H., Schubert, J. R., and Oldfield, J. E., White muscle disease (myopathy) in lambs and calves. VII. Etiology and prophylaxis, Am. J. Vet. Res., 22, 466, 1961.

223. Schubert, J. R., Muth, O. H., Oldfield, J. E., and Remmert, L. F., Experimental results with selenium in white muscle disease of lambs and calves, Federation Proc., 20, 689, 1961.

224. Oldfield, J. E., Muth, O. H., and Schubert, J. R., Selenium and vitamin E as related to growth and white muscle disease in lambs, Proc. Soc. Exp. Biol. Med., 103, 799, 1960.

225. Whiting, F., Willman, J. P., and Loosli, J. R., Tocopherol (vitamin E) deficiency among sheep fed natural feeds, J. Anim. Sci., 8, 234, 1949.

226. Hogue, D. E., Proctor, J. F., Warner, R. G., and Loosli, J. K., Relation of selenium, vitamin E, and an unidentified factor to muscular dystrophy (stiff-lamb or white muscle disease) in the lamb, J. Anim. Sci., 21, 25, 1962.

227. Segerson, E. C., and Ganapathy, S. N., Fertility of ova in ewes receiving selenium and vitamin E supplementation, J. Anim. Sci., 49, Suppl. 1, 335, 1979.

228. Hartley, W. J., Selenium and ewe fertility, Proc. N. Z. Soc. Anim. Prod. 23, 20, 1963.

229. Drake, C., Grant, A. B., and Hartley, W. J., Selenium and animal health. Part 1. The effect of alpha-tocopherol and selenium in the control of field outbreaks of white muscle disease, N. Z. Vet. J., 8, 4, 1960.

230. Cawley, G. D., and Bradley, R., Sudden death in calves associated with acute myocardial degeneration and selenium deficiency, Vet. Rec., 103, 239, 1978.

231. Kennedy, S., Rice, D. A., and McMurray, C. H., Experimental induction of cardiomyopathy in the young bovine, in Proceedings of the Third International Symposium on Selenium in Biology and Medicine, Combs, G. F., Jr., Spallholz, J. E., Levander, O. A., and Oldfield, J. E., eds., Avi Publ. Co., Westport, Conn., 1986.

232. Harrison, J. H., Hancock, D. D., and Conrad, H. R., Vitamin E and selenium for reproduction of the dairy cow, J. Dairy Sci., 67, 132, 1984.

233. Callahan, C. J., Post parturient infection of dairy cattle, J. Am. Vet. Med. Assoc., 155, 1963, 1969.

234. Trinder, N., Woodhouse, C. D., and Renton, C. P., The effect of vitamin E and selenium on the incidence of retained placenta in dairy cows, Vet. Rec., 85, 550, 1969.

235. Julien, W. E., Conrad, H. R., Jones, J. E., and Moxon, A. L., Selenium and vitamin E and incidence of retained placenta in parturient dairy cows, J. Dairy Sci., 59, 1954, 1976.

236. Trinder, N., Hall, R. J., and Renton, C. P., The relationship between intake of selenium and vitamin E on the incidence of retained placenta in dairy cows, Vet. Rec., 93, 641, 1973.

237. Julien, W. E., Conrad, H. R., and Moxon, A. L., Selenium and vitamin E and incidence of retained placenta in parturient dairy cows. II. Prevention in commercial herds in the prepartum treatment, J. Dairy Sci., 59, 1960, 1976.

238. Segerson, E. C., Riviere, G. J., Dalton, H. L., and Whitacre, M. D., Retained placenta of Holstein cows treated with selenium and vitamin E, J. Dairy Sci., 64, 1833, 1981.

239. Gwazdauskas, F. C., Bibb, J. L., McGilliard, M. L., and Lineweaver, J. A., Effect of prepartum selenium-vitamin E injection on time for placenta to pass and on reproductive functions, J. Dairy Sci., 62, 978, 1979.

240. Schingoethe, D. J., Kirkbride, C. A., Olson, O. E., Owens, M. J., Ludens, F. C., and Tucker, W. W., Influence of vitamin E and selenium on retained placentas in parturient dairy cows, J. Dairy Sci., 64, Suppl. 1, 120, 1981.

241. Harrison, J. H., Hancock, D. D., and Conrad, H. R., Selenium deficiency and ovarian function in dairy cattle, Federation Proc., 41, 786, 1982.

242. Harrison, J. H., Hancock, D. D., and Conrad, H. R., Selenium and vitamin E in control of cystic overies and retained placenta, Ohio Agr. Res. Dev. Cent. Dairy Day Rep., 1983.

243. Morris, J. G., Cripe, W. S., Chapman, H. L., Jr., Walker, D. F., Armstrong, J. B., Alexander, J. D., Jr., Miranda, R., Sanchez, A., Jr., Balir-West, J. R., and Denton, D. A., Selenium deficiency in cattle associated with Heinz bodies and anemia, Science, 223, 491, 1984.

244. Todd, G. C., and Krook, L., Nutritional hepatic necrosis in beef cattle, Path. Vet., 3, 379, 1966.

245. Schongaard, H., Basse, A., Gissel-Nielsen, G., and Simesen, M. G., Nutritional muscular dystrophy (NMD) in foals, Nord. Veterinaermed., 24, 67, 1972.

246. Lanneck, N., The importance of vitamin E for domestic animals in sickness and in health, Acta Agric. Scand., Suppl. 19, 13, 1973.

247. Wilson, T. M., Morrison, H. A., Palmer, N. C., Finley, G. F., and Van Dreumel, A. A., Myodegeneration and suspected selenium/vitamin E deficiency in horses, J. Am. Vet. Med. Assoc., 169, 213, 1976.

248. Stowe, H. D., Serum selenium and related parameters of naturally and experimentally fed horses, J. Nutr., 93, 60, 1967.

249. Zhiang, J., Chen, Z., Liu, S., Deng, Y., Zhou, K., and Zhai, X., A study on selenium deficiency of equines, in *Proceedings of the Third International Symposium on Selenium in Biology and Medicine*, Combs, G. F., Jr., Spallholz, J. E., Levander, O. A., and Oldfield, J. E., eds., Avi Publ. Co., Westport, Conn., 1986.

250. Gallagher, K., and Stow, H. D., Influence of exercise on serum selenium and peroxide reduction system of racing standard breds, Am. J. Vet. Res., 41, 1333, 1980.

251. Brady, P. S., Ku, P. K., and Ullrey, D. E., Lack of effect of selenium supplementation in the response of the equine erythrocyte glutathione system and plasma enzymes to exercise, J. Anim. Sci., 47, 492, 1978.

252. Maylin, G. A., Rubin, D. S., and Lein, D. H., Selenium and vitamin E in horses, Cornell Vet., 70, 272, 1980.

253. Poston, H. A., Combs, G. F., Jr., and Leibovitz, L., Vitamin E and selenium interrelations in the diet of Atlantic salmon (*Salmo salar*): gross, histological and biochemical deficiency signs, J. Nutr., 106, 892, 1976.

254. Hilton, J. W., Hodson, P. V., and Slinger, S. J., The requirement and toxicity of selenium in rainbow trout (*Salmo gairdneri*), J. Nutr., 110, 2527, 1980.

255. Bell, J. G., Cowey, C. B., and Youngsen, A., rainbow trout liver microsomal lipid peroxidation. The effect of purified glutathione peroxidase glutathione *S*-transferase and other factors, Biochim. Biophys. Acta 795, 91, 1984.

256. Gatlin, D. M., and Wilson, R. P., Dietary selenium requirement of fingerling channel catfish, J. Nutr., 114, 627, 1984.

257. Jarrett, W. H.F., Jennings, F. W., Murray, M., and Harthoorn, A. M., Muscular dystrophy in a wild Hunter's antelope, E. Afr. Wildl. J., 2, 158, 1964.

258. Basson, P. A., and Hofmeyer, J. M., Mortalities associated with wildlife capture operations, in *The Capture and Care of Wild Animals*, Young, E., ed., Human and Rousseau, Capetown, p. 161, 1973.

259. Young, E., Muscle necrosis in captive red harte beaste (*Alcelaphus buselaphus*), J. S., Afr. Vet. Med. Assoc., 37, 101, 1966.

260. Ebedes, H., Notes on the immobilization of gemsbok (*Oryx gazella gazella*) in South West Africa using etorphine hydrochloride (M99), Madogua, 1, 35, 1969.

261. McConnell, E. E., Basson, P. A., deVos, V., Myers, B. J., and Kuntz, R. F., A survey of diseases among 100 free-ranging baboons (*Papio ursinus*) from the Kruger National Park, Onderstepoort J. Vet. Res., 41, 97, 1974.

262. Herbert, D. M., and Cowan, I. M., White muscle disease in the mountain goat, J. Wildl. Manage., 35, 752, 1971.

263. Young, E., Overstraining disease (*capture myopathy*) in tessebe (*Damaliscus lunatus*) and oribi (*Ourebia ourebi*), Koedoe, 15, 143, 1972.

264. Stuht, J. N., Ullrey, D. E., Trapp, A. L., Youatt, W. G., and Johnson, H. E., White muscle disease in white-tailed deer, Paper presented at the Ann. Conf. Wildl. Dis. Assoc., Ft. Collins, Colo., 1971.

265. Brady, P. S., Brady, L. J., Whetter, P. A., Ullrey, D. E., and Fay, L. D., The effect of dietary selenium and vitamin E on biochemical parameters and survival of young among white-tailed deer (*Odocoileus virginianus*), J. Nutr., 108, 1439, 1978.

266. Young, E., Leg paralysis in the greater flamingo and lesser flamingo *Phoenicopterus ruber roseus* and *Phoeniconaias minor* following capture and transportation, Inter. Zoo. Yearb., 7, 226, 1967.

267. Keating, K. I., and Dagbusan, B. C., Effect of selenium deficiency on cuticle integrity in the *Cladocera* (crustacea), Proc. Nat. Acad. Sci. USA, 81, 3433, 1984.

268. Elsey, R. M., and Lance, V., Effect of diet on blood selenium and glutathione peroxidase activity in the alligator, Comp. Biochem. Physiol., 76B, 831, 1983.

269. Anonymous, *Nutrient Requirements of Laboratory Animals*, Third Revised Edition, National Academy Press, Washington, D. C., 1978.

270. Anonymous, *Nutrition Requirement of Nonhuman Primates*, National Academy Press, Washington, D. C., 1978.

271. Anonymous, *Nutrient Requirements of Dogs*, National Academy Press, Washington, D. C., 1974.

272. Anonymous, *Nutrient Requirements of Cats*, Revised, National Academy Press, Washington, D. C., 1978.

273. Anonymous, *Nutrient Requirements of Rabbits*, Second Revised Edition, National Academy Press, Washington, D. C., 1977.

274. Anonymous, *Nutrient Requirements of Poultry*, Eighth Revised Edition, National Academy Press, Washington, D. C., 1984.

275. Anonymous, *Nutrient Requirements of Swine*, Eighth Revised Edition, National Academy Press, Washington, D. C., 1979.

276. Anonymous, *Nutrient Requirements of Sheep*, Fifth Revised Edition, National Academy Press, Washington, D. C., 1979.

277. Anonymous, *Nutrient Requirements of Dairy Cattle*, Fifth Revised Edition, National Academy Press, Washington, D. C., 1978.
278. Anonymous, *Nutrient Requirements of Beef Cattle*, Sixth Revised Edition, National Academy Press, Washington, D. C., 1984.
279. Anonymous, *Nutrient Requirements of Goats: Angora, Dairy, and Meat Goats in Temperate and Tropical Countries*, National Academy Press, Washington, D. C., 1981.
280. Anonymous, *Nutrient Requirements of Horses*, Fourth Revised Edition, National Academy Press, Washington, D. C., 1978.
281. Anonymous, *Nutrient Requirements of Mink and Foxes*, Second Revised Edition, National Academy Press, Washington, D. C., 1982.
282. Anonymous, *Nutrient Requirements of Warmwater Fishes and Shellfishes*, Revised Edition, National Academy Press, Washington, D. C., 1983.
283. Anonymous, *Nutrient Requirements of Coldwater Fishes*, National Academy Press, Washington, D. C., 1981.

8

SELENIUM IN HUMAN
NUTRITION AND HEALTH

Even after the recognition of the nutritional activities of Se in experimental animals in the late 1950s, the role of Se in human nutrition and health remained unclear until the late 1970s. Although rapid advances were made during that period in the understanding of the nature of and the metabolic bases for the nutritional essentiality of Se for several laboratory and domestic animal species, no ill health effects in humans were attributable to differences in Se intakes, even among populations that differed greatly in Se status. Without signs of some functional impairment associated with changes in Se status, propositions that Se may have an essential role in human health were based largely on considerations of its function in human SeGSHpx and, consequently, were rather academic in nature. This situation changed dramatically in the late 1970s when studies conducted in China received worldwide attention, reporting that severe nutritional Se deficiency in discrete regions of that country was associated with an endemic juvenile cardiomyopathy (i.e., Keshan disease). This finding, as well as further observations implicating Se as a factor in the etiology of a chondrodystrophic disease (Kaschin-Beck disease) of children in severely Se-deficient parts of China, has provided the first firm evidence of an important role of Se in human health.

I. THE NUTRITIONAL SELENIUM STATUS OF HUMAN POPULATIONS

Investigators in several countries have assessed the nutritional Se status of their resident populations on the basis of tissue concentrations of Se and/or activities of SeGSHpx. Table 8.1 summarizes the results of 93 studies

327

Table 8.1

Selenium Contents of Selected Human Tissues as Reported for Various Countries[a]

			Se contents		
Country	Whole blood (ppb)	Plasma/serum (ppb)	Erythrocytes (ppb)	Urine (μg/24hrs)	Hair (ppb)
Australia	110 (1)				
Belgium	130 (2)	73 (2)	200 (2)	20-27 (110)	
	123 (3)	97 (3)	161 (3)	90 (110)	
		82,95,96(4)	343,404,439 (4)[b]		
Canada	182 (5)	144 (5)	236 (5)	125±76 (111)	
China					
Se-deficient area	17 (6)			3.1[c] (6)	98(6)
	15,19,19,19(7)[b]				68,77 94 101(7)[b]
				4.2[c] (9)	184[d] (9)
					61 (10)
	21 (8)			4.2 (10)	44[d] (11)
	17(12)				56,71,107[d] (13)[b]
					72 (14)
					73 (15)
					74 (16)
					74 (17)
					85 (18)
					60,[d] 82 (19)
					66[d] (20)
					73,[d]111 (21)[b]
					119 (22)
					186 (6)
					262 (7)

Moderate-Se area	33 (6)		5.0 (6)	362 (10)
	95 (8)		6.7 (10)	131[d] (11)
	136 (12)		(26 ng/ml) (23)	170 (13)
	95 (24)			203 (14)
	91,125 (25)[b]			634 (15)
				190 (17)
				187 (18)
				410 (22)
				360 (23)
				23,340 (23)
				32,200 (23)
				21,580 (25)
High-Se area	3200 (23)		(2.6 µg/ml) (23)	
	3480 (25)			
Denmark		210 (26)		
England	124 (27)	106 (27)		
Finland	69 (28)	56 (28)		
	56-90 (30)	55 (29)		
	79-103 (32)	46-109 (30)		
		60 (31)		
		74 (33)		
		77(34)		
		54 (35)		
		99 (94)		
France		96 (4)	343 (4)	
		122 (36)	345 (37)	
		98 (37)		

(continues)

329

Table 8.1 (*Continued*)

Country	Whole blood (ppb)	Se contents		Urine (µg/24hrs)	Hair (ppb)
		Plasma/serum (ppb)	Erythrocytes (ppb)		
Germany		32 (38)	140 (40)		
		51 (39)			
		88 (40)			
Guatemala	140 (41)	100 (41)	230 (41)		
Holland	133 (42)	110 (42)	145 (42)		
Italy		61 (43)	39 (44)		
Japan	285 (44)	91 (45)			
		51,[d] 99 (46)[b]			
New Zealand	54 (47)	43 (47)	66 (47)	6-20 (48)	
	57,87 (48)[e]	48 (48)	74 (48)	7 (112)	
	71 (49)	54 (50)	86 (50)	17,24 (113)	
	69 (50)	48 (52)	74 (52)		
	80 (51)				
	59 (52)				
	69 (53)				
	59 (54)				
	60,62,83 (102)				
Norway		153 (55)			
Poland		81 (56)			
Sweden	119 (57)	101 (57)	100 (58)	30 (59)	
		81 (58)		30 (61)	
		65[d] (60)			

330

USA	183 (44)	78,102 (62)[b]	73 (63)	33 (64)	570 (65)
	109 (66)	96 (63)	126 (66)	54 (67)	470 (68)
	166 (68)	135 (64)	158 (73)	39 (74)	440 (91)
	137 (69)	95 (66)	159 (75)	53 (78)	
	70 (71)	116 (69)	200 (77)	115 (114)	
	168,[f] 206,[g] 228[h] (76)	157 (70)	191 (81)		
	229 (79)	122 (72)			
	237 (80)	104 (73)			
	100 (82)	134 (74)			
	89 (83)	94 (75)			
	90 (91)	100 (77)			
		106 (81)			
		100 (86)			
		91 (87)			
		127 (88)			
		137 (89)			
		104 (90)			
USSR	102 (92)			(10 ng/ml) (92)	
Venezuela	355;813 (93)				

[a]References are shown parenthetically; value presented on fresh weight basis.
[b]Individual values are means of different groups of subjects.
[c]Estimated from the authors' reported data.
[d]Value for children (< 15 years of age).
[e]Values for 1973 and 1980, respectively.
[f]Average value for five lowest ranking cities.
[g]Average value for 19 cities sampled.
[h]Average value for five highest ranking cities.

331

in 20 countries in which Se concentrations were measured in human tissues most readily available as biological specimens (i.e., whole blood, plasma/ serum, erythrocytes, urine, hair). These results demonstrate a strong geographic variation in Se status, which correlates with the geographic variation in the Se contents of food supplies (see Table 3.15). Populations with the lowest estimated intakes of Se (i.e., the Se-deficient regions of China, New Zealand, Finland) also have the lowest concentrations of Se in these accessible tissues. Geographic variation within the USA was demonstrated by Allaway et al.,[76] who found that the mean Se concentrations of whole blood from blood banks in 19 cities varied from 157 to 256 ppb (Table 8.2). This variation appears to relate to differences in local intakes of Se, as the cities ranking at the extremes of that range were located in areas known to be either high (e.g., northern Great Plains states) or low (northeastern states) with respect to Se (see Fig. 2.2). Limited data are available for the Se contents of other human tissues (Table 8.3); however, these also indicate a correlation between tissue Se levels and the average Se intakes of populations (i.e., tissue Se levels are substantially higher in the USA than in the low-Se countries Finland and New Zealand).

Nutritional Se status has been assessed on the basis of SeGSHpx activities in blood plasma and cells; however, these data are not extensive (see Table

Table 8.2

Selenium Concentrations of Samples of Whole Blood from 19 Cities in the USA[a]

City, state	Blood Se (ppb)
Rapid City, South Dakota	256
Cheyenne, Wyoming	234
Spokane, Washington	230
Fargo, North Dakota	217
Little Rock, Arkansas	201
Phoenix, Arizona	197
Meridian, Mississippi	195
Missoula, Montana	194
El Paso, Texas	192
Jacksonville, Florida	188
Red Bluff, California	182
Geneva, New York	182
Billings, Montana	180
Montpelier, Vermont	180
Lubbock, Texas	178
Lafayette, Louisiana	176
Canandaigua, New York	176
Munci, Indiana	158
Lima, Ohio	157

[a]From Allaway et al.[76]

Table 8.3

Selenium Contents of Human Tissues as Reported in
North America, Finland, and New Zealand

Tissue	Selenium contents (ppb)[a]					
	North America		Finland		New Zealand	
Liver	365	(5)[b]	175-365[c]	(28)	720	(48)
	280-720	(65)				
	85-825	(85)				
	400-650	(94)				
	480	(95)				
Lung	190	(5)				
	50-240	(65)				
	180	(95)				
Heart	385	(5)	90-200[c]	(28)		
	250-370	(65)				
	25	(95)				
Aorta	270	(5)				
	270	(95)				
Kidney	780	(5)	350-445[c]	(28)		
	610-1840	(65)				
	860	(95)				
Spleen	320	(5)				
	280-470	(65)				
	270	(95)				
Thyroid	1240	(95)				
Pancreas	90	(5)				
	270-340	(65)				
	190[c]	(85)				
Testes	150-380	(65)				
	390	(95)				
Adrenals	360	(95)				
Bone (rib)	420	(65)				
Skeletal muscle	355	(5)				
	110-380	(65)				
Brain	40-210	(65)	140-190[c]	(28)		
Cerebrospinal fluid	19	(96)				
Synovial membrane	190[c]	(85)				
Small intestine	265	(5)				
	120-320	(65)				
	220	(95)				
Colon	220	(95)				
Trachea	190	(5)				
Adipose	105	(5)				
Saliva	3	(97)				

[a]Fresh weight basis.

[b]References indicated in parentheses.

[c]Estimated from authors' original data.

8.4). It is also important to recognize that the quality of this information base is likely to be inferior to that of the tissue Se data. This has to do with the lack of uniforinity of specific assay conditions, acceptor substrate selection (e.g., H_2O_2, t-butyl hydroperoxide, or cumene hydroperoxide, each of which have different apparent Km values for SeGSHpx), and means of expressing results (e.g., as U_{37}; or as nanomoles NADPH oxidized per milliliter, per milligram protein, or per gram hemoglobin). Therefore, while the within-laboratory variation for such measurements may be expected to be acceptably small, the between-laboratory variation may be considerable. The data presented in Table 8.4 have, in several cases, been recalculated from the original reports to provide a consistent basis for their comparison; the limitations of this comparison should be kept in mind in using this table.

The activity of SeGSHpx in blood can be a useful parameter of nutritional Se status in individuals with low to moderate intakes of the element. Numerous measurements of Se and SeGSHpx in whole blood by Thomson et al.[51] have demonstrated that these parameters show a good correlation ($r=0.74$ for 222 subjects, $p < 0.001$) at blood Se concentrations less than 100 ppb, but no significant relationship at greater blood Se levels ($r=0.17$ for 42 subjects) (see Fig. 8.1). In a study of Americans whose whole blood Se concentrations were greater than the range of apparent linearity identified by Thomson et al.,[51] Lane et al.[87] found the correlation between Se and SeGSHpx in whole blood to be relatively weak ($r=0.45$ for 43 subjects, $p < 0.001$). Studies by Rea et al.[52] (Fig. 8.2) and Lane et al.[63] (Fig. 8.3) have demonstrated significant correlations between Se and SeGSHpx activity in erythrocytes from individuals of low to moderate Se status (i.e., erythrocyte Se less than ca. 100-120 ppb, or ca. 1 μg Se/g hemoglobin). Rudolph and Wong[105] also found these factors to be highly correlated ($r=0.86$ for 24 paired samples of erythrocytes from maternal and cord blood, all of which contained less than 70 ppb Se), but this correlation was found by Verlinden et al.[3] to be rather weak ($r=0.31$ for 155 subjects) for Belgians with erythrocyte Se concentrations greater than 90 ppb. Rea et al.[52] demonstrated a good correlation between the Se contents of plasma and erythrocytes for subjects with plasma Se levels up to ca. 120 ppb (see Fig. 8.4); however, the correlation between plasma Se and erythrocyte SeGSHpx activity was found to be weak (Lane et al.[63] reported $r=0.30$ for 65 university students in the United States; Verlinden et al.[2] reported $r=0.33$ for 40 elderly subjects in Belgium) (see Fig. 8.5). Lack of significant correlation was reported by McAdam et al.[90] ($r=0.011$, $p=0.436$) for 291 Americans with plasma Se levels generally above 90 ppb. Such data suggest that Se resides in forms other than active SeGSHpx in increasing amounts in individuals with adequate or greater intakes of Se.

Table 8.4

Glutathione Peroxidase Activities[a] Reported for Residents of Various Countries

Country	Plasma (nmoles NADPH/min/ml)	Plasma (nmoles NADPH/min/mg protein)	Erythrocytes (μmoles NADPH/min/g Hb)	Lymphocytes (nmoles NADPH/min/mg protein)	Granulocytes (nmoles NADPH/min/mg protein)	Platelets (nmoles NADPH/min/mg protein)	Reference
Belgium			15.30 ± 3.30 (40)[bc]				(2)
			13.74 ± 3.20 (159)[c]				(3)
Denmark				38–194[de]	13–61[de]		(26)
England			19.8 ± 4.9 (391)				(69)
Finland	128.5 ± 2.3(56)[c]						(98)
		6.4 ± 6.7[f]				210–235[f]	(34)
France			9.0 ± 2.3 (22)				(37)
Germany	41.1 ± 7.8 (16)[c]						(99)
	37.6 ± 8.4(13)[ce]						(99)
	49.2 ± 8.1 (17)[c]		22.0 ± 9.0 (17)[c]				(40)
Ireland			30.1 ± 4.6(19)[e]				(100)
Israel			24.5 ± 5.6 (25)	139.9 ± 52.3 (22)	36.5 ± 12.1 (21)	174.4 ± 57.1 (16)	(101)
			31.4 ± 8.0 (10)[e]	143.9 ± 29.9 (22)[e]	40.7 ± 12.4 (21)[e]	151.0 ± 88.8 (6)[e]	(101)
Italy			7.78 ± 1.41 (16)[e]		40 ± 9 (16)[e]		(43)
New Zealand			12.5 ± 3.5 (84)				(52)
			15.5 ± 2.6 (7)				(50)
			14.9 ± 1.7 (4)				(50)
			14.8 ± 3.4 (4)				(50)
			12.2 ± 4.8 (23)				(102)
			11.0 ± 2.9 (16)				(102)

(continues)

Table 8.4 (*Continued*)

Country	Plasma		Erythrocytes	Lymphocytes	Granulocytes	Platelets	Reference
	nmoles NADPH/ min/ml	nmoles NADPH/ min/mg protein	(μmoles NADPH/ min/g Hb)	(nmoles NADPH/ min/mg protein)	(nmoles NADPH/ min/mg protein)	(nmoles NADPH/ min/mg protein)	
Sweden	561 ± 26 (16)		45 ± 3 (16)			298 ± 32 (16)	(57)
			21.3 ± 4.8 (9)				(103)
USA			40.5 ± 11.9 (100)[e]				(63)
			26.5 ± 0.5[eg]				(73)
			27.5[hi]				(77)
			25.2 ± 5.4 (6)[e]			271 ± 166[e]	(86)
			26.6(206)[e]				(90)
			35.0 ± 15.3 (174)[ej]				(104)
			28.9 ± 13.7 (86)[ek]				(104)
	195 ± 44 (16)[e]						(105)

[a]Assayed with *t*-butyl hydroperoxide as acceptor substrate unless otherwise noted.
[b]Mean ± SD (*n*) unless otherwise noted.
[c]Recalculated from authors' data.
[d]Range of observations reported by authors.
[e]Assayed with hydrogen peroxide as acceptor substrate.
[f]Range of observations estimated by present authors.
[g]Value of *n* not reported by authors.
[h]Assayed with cumene hydroperoxide as substrate.
[i]Single observation reported by authors.
[j]Nonindustrial workers.
[k]Industrial workers.

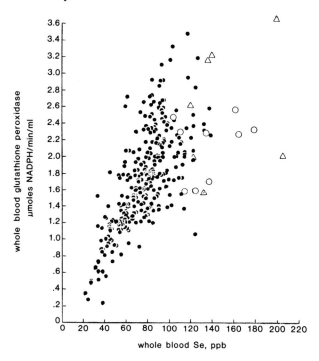

Fig. 8.1   Relationship of Se and glutathione peroxidase activity (measured with *t*-butyl hydroperoxide as the acceptor substrate) in whole blood from 264 New Zealand residents (closed circles), 9 New Zealanders returning home after overseas visits (open circles), and 7 immigrants to New Zealand (triangles). After Thomson *et al.*[51]

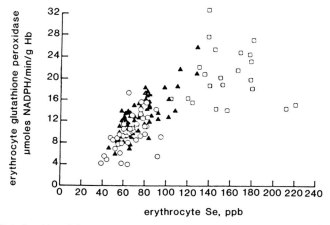

Fig. 8.2   Relationship of Se and glutathione peroxidase activity (measured with H_2O_2 as the acceptor substrate) in erythrocytes from blood donors (closed triangles), hospital patients (open circles) and overseas visitors (open squares) in New Zealand. After Rea *et al.*[52]

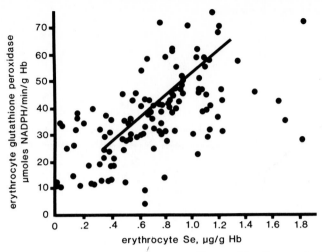

Fig. 8.3 Relationship of Se and glutathione peroxidase activity (measured with H_2O_2 as the acceptor substrate) in erythrocytes of USA residents. After Lane et al.[63]

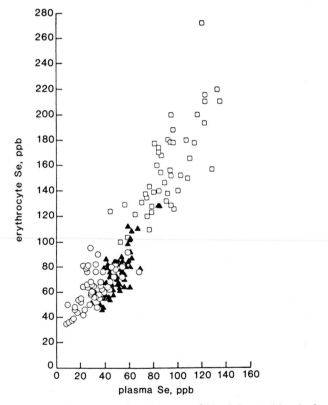

Fig. 8.4 Relationship of Se in plasma and erythrocytes of blood donors (closed triangles), hospital patients (open circles), and overseas visitors (open squares) to New Zealand. After Rea et al.[52]

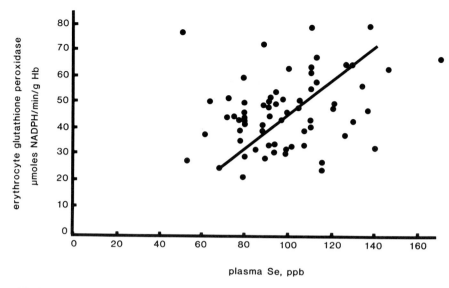

Fig. 8.5 Relationship of plasma Se and erythrocyte glutathione peroxidase activity (measured with H_2O_2 as the acceptor substrate) in USA residents. After Lane *et al.*[63]

A few investigators have measured SeGSHpx activities in other human blood cells including lymphocytes,[26,101] granulocytes,[26,101] and platelets.[34,57,86,101] Of these, platelets would appear to offer the greatest prospects for usefulness in the assessment of nutritional Se status of humans. Platelets show relatively high activities of SeGSHpx (e.g., specific activity ca. 35 times that of plasma[34]), and these activities show rapid responses to changes in Se intake. Levander *et al.*[34] found that platelet SeGSHpx increased by about two-fold due to Se supplementation (200 μg Se per person per day) of low-Se Finnish men (whose pre-experimental plasma Se levels were ca. 70 ppb), and that these increases occurred within 2-4 weeks, by which time plasma SeGSHpx had increased by less than 20%. Levander *et al.*[34] estimated that plasma Se levels of 100-135 ppb (depending upon whether the dietary Se source was inorganic or organic) are associated with maximal platelet SeGSHpx activity.

Isozymes of human SeGSHpx have been identified. Polymorphism with respect to the electrophoretic properties of the human erythrocyte enzyme was discovered by Beutler and colleagues.[106,107] Those investigators found a variant electrophoretic polymorphic form of SeGSHpx, which they called the "Thomas" variant, in Afro-Americans and Ashkenazi Jews. Those populations showed the variant phenotype in 6.4 and 2.2%, respectively; but the variant was not found among a sampling of 300 non-Jewish Euro-Americans. A variant SeGSHpx labeled "GPX1 2-1," but apparently identical with the Thomas variant, was identified by Khan et al.[108] in one Afro-Jamaican (of 72 persons sampled) and three Punjabis (of 116 persons sampled) from the Indian subcontinent. They did not find the variant among samplings of 398 Dutch, 76 Sardinians, 99 mainland Italians, 110 Norwegians, 149 Quecha-speaking Peruvians, 312 Wajana, 504 Trio Amerindians, or 269 non-Punjabi Indians. Khan et al.[108] proposed that the variant forms of erythrocyte SeGSHpx that are found in Africans, Ashkenazi Jews, and Punjabis may be due to a common allele present at frequencies of 0.0111-0.0319 in those populations. Variant forms of SeGSHpx have also been suggested in patients with multiple sclerosis or Down's syndrome (trisomy 21). Multiple sclerosis patients have been found to show moderate reductions in SeGSHpx activities (relative to controls) in erythrocytes but not in other blood cells including lymphocytes, granulocytes and platelets.[101,109] Individuals with Down's syndrome are consistently observed to have markedly increased erythrocyte SeGSHpx activities,[37] which may relate to the increased gene dose.

Within individual locales, there appear to be no significant differences in tissue SeGSHpx activities due to gender.[69,90] McAdam et al.[90] observed no significant differences in erythrocyte SeGSHpx activities between white and black Americans, although they found a significant interactive effect of age, race, and sex on plasma Se concentration. In view of the finding of hereditary differences in SeGSHpx isozymes, it would seem appropriate to investigate more extensively the possiblitity of differences in SeGSHpx levels and/or activities due to such factors as gender and ethnic background. Such information has immediate bearing on the interpretation of SeGSHpx data in the assessment of nutritional Se status.

Several investigators in China[6,7,9-11,13-23,25] and the USA[65,68,91] have assessed nutritional Se status on the basis of the Se content of scalp hair. This method has the obvious advantage of ease of sample availability, storage and preparation; however, standardization of the scalp location and amount of hair is important to maximize reproducibility. It is also important to screen subjects to ascertain which may have had recent use of a Se-containing shampoo, as hair from such subjects will bear Se residues that do not reflect nutritional Se status. Gallagher et al.[91] found that unwashed hair gave the same results as solvent washed and dried hair, indicating that it is not necessary to remove grease and oils for using hair to assess Se status. Studies in China, where the use of hair Se for nutritional assessment has been important in epidemiological studies of Keshan disease and Kaschin-Beck disease, have demonstrated a log-log correlation between the Se contents of hair and whole blood[17] (see Fig. 8.6). Chinese studies have shown good correlations of hair Se content and dietary Se intake[7,8] (see Figs. 8.7 and 8.8) on a log-log basis over a wide range of Se intakes. However, such good correlations may be observed only in populations with relatively

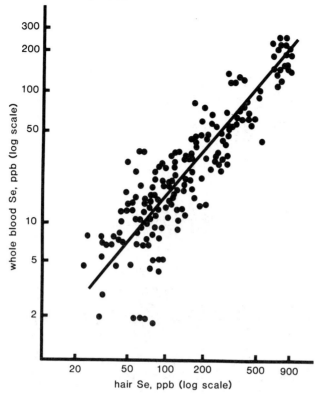

Fig. 8.6 Correlation of hair Se and blood Se in 200 residents of China. After Chen *et al.*[17]

homogeneous hair color, texture, etc. Wahlstrom *et al.*[196] found that Se content of hair was related to hair color in pigs. Animals with black, red, or white hair had different hair concentrations of Se after being raised on normal Se-adequate diets (e.g., hair Se 650, 830, or 740 ppb, respectively) and after being fed a high-Se diet (i.e., 8.13 ppm Se) for 35 days (e.g., final hair Se 980, 1080, or 1150 ppb, respectively), although no differences in other parameters of Se status (i.e., blood Se, plasma SeGSHpx, erythrocyte SeGSHpx) were noted.

The renal clearance of Se is important in the homeostasis of the element; therefore, measurment of urinary Se excretion can provide useful information for the assessment of nutritional Se status in humans. Such use of this parameter has been reviewed.[52,115-118] The urinary excretion of Se is generally greater than the fecal excretion of the element; urine Se content is a function of the level and form of Se intake and the nature of the diet, as well as the Se status of the individual. Because several factors can influence urine volume, measurements of urine Se concentration are generally of only limited usefulness in the assessment of Se status. It is,

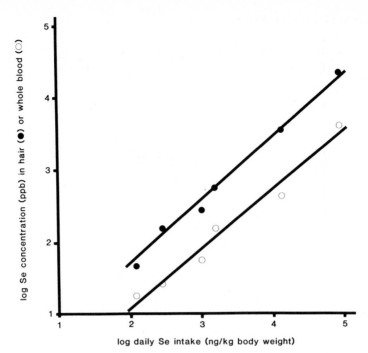

Fig. 8.7 Correlations between daily Se intake and the Se contents of hair and whole blood. Hair Se (●) $y = .8885x - .0496$, $r^2 = .9944$; blood (○) $y = .8275x - .5657$, $r^2 = .9714$. Adapted from the data of Yang.[7]

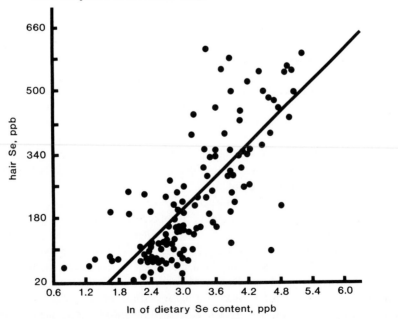

Fig. 8.8 Relationship of hair Se and dietary intake of Se in children in China. $y = 142.8$ ln x - 232.9, $r = 0.83$. After Yang *et al.*[8]

therefore, recommended to make 24-hr urine collections, expressing urinary Se as micrograms per day, or to measure also creatinine in urine specimens and express results as micrograms Se per gram creatinine. The former method is preferred in view of the findings of significant diurnal variation in urinary Se demonstrated by Thomson[112] and Palmquist et al.,[119] showing great variations between individuals. When determined in this manner, urinary Se excretion is closely correlated with the Se concentrations of blood[120,121] or plasma[120,122,123] and can be useful in assessing nutritional Se status of healthy individuals. Table 8.1 presents some values that have been reported for urinary Se excretion in various countries; further references to urinary Se concentrations were reviewed by Robberecht and Deelstra.[115,116]

Morris et al.[124] demonstrated that toenail Se can be used in the assessment of nutritional Se status. They showed that the Se content of toenails reflected the geographic variation in blood Se concentrations: toenail Se was found to be 1.17±0.35 ppm in South Dakota, 0.81±0.14 ppm in Georgia, 0.74±0.13 ppm in Massachusetts, and 0.26±0.09 ppm in New Zealand. Although the authors failed to observe significant correlations between toenail or hair Se and blood Se, the individuals from whom samples were obtained for that experiment had blood Se levels that were relatively high and fell within a narrow range (i.e., 110-200 ppb) and did not constitute, therefore, an adequate sampling to evaluate appropriately the expected correlations. The substantial differences in toenail Se, which were found to be consistent with expectations based on other reports of geographical variations in nutritional Se status, support the uselfulness of toenails as a tissue for assessment of Se status. Morris et al.[124] have pointed out certain advantages offered by the use of this tissue: toenails are easily collected, transported, and stored, and they reflect long-term intake (because clippings from different toes represent different time periods of formation, samples from all toes provide information concerning Se status integrated over an extended period of time).

II. SELENIUM STATUS IN DIFFERENT LIFE CYCLE PHASES

Nutritional Se status is altered in the pregnant woman; however, it is not at all clear whether the changes observed relate to endocrine effects associated with pregnancy or to altered patterns of Se intake during that phase of the life cycle. Several investigators[40,82,102,105,125,126] have found that plasma/serum Se concentrations are significantly lower in pregnant women than in nonpregnant women; these differences can be 10-45% by the last trimester or delivery (see Table 8.5). Butler et al.[82] found the Se content of whole blood to be similarly depressed (i.e., 34%) during the third trimester. These decreases in blood Se concentrations have been suggested as possible

Table 8.5

Changes in Selenium Status During Pregnancy

Country	Nonpregnant women	Pregnant women					Reference
		First trimester	Second trimester	Third trimester	At delivery	Post-partum	
Plasma Se, ppb							
USA	210 ± 30 (16)[c]	110[a]	70[a]	60[a]	—	80[a,b]	(82)
	—				190 ± 30 (25)[c]	—	(105)
Germany	88 ± 11 (17)[c]	89 ± 1 (2)[c]	83 ± 10 (14)[c]	74 ± 12 (21)[c]	—	—	(40)
Finland	72 ± 19 (32)[c]	—	60 ± 6 (9)[c]	52 ± 7 (11)[c]	—	70 ± 7 (6)[c,d]	(125)
				28 ± 10 (10)[c]	—	—	(126)
New Zealand	—				69 ± 18 (23)	—	(102)
	—				61 ± 17 (15)	—	(102)
Plasma glutathione peroxidase, (nmoles NADPH oxidized/min/ml)							
USA	195 ± 44 (16)[c,e]	142[a,e]	162[a,e]	179[a,e]	—	210[a,e]	(82)
	—				140 ± 32 (13)[c,e]	—	(105)
Germany	49.2 ± 8.1 (17)[c,f,g]	41.7 ± 0.6 (2)[c,f,g]	37.6 ± 8.4 (14)[c,f,g]	33.6 ± 10.1 (21)[c,f,g]			(40)
Whole blood Se (ppb)							
USA	—	117[a]	105[a]	77[a]	—	80[a]	(82)
Erythrocyte Se (ppb)							
USA	520 ± 50 (16)[c]	—	—	—	520 ± 70 (34)[c]	—	(105)
Erythrocyte glutathione peroxidase[e] (nmoles NADPH oxidized/min/mg Hb)							
USA	28.7 ± 5.7 (16)[c,e]	13.8[a,e]	18.7[a,e]	28.8[a,e]	—	28.0[a,e]	(82)
	—				34.0 ± 7.1 (24)[c,e,h]	—	(105)

[a] Estimated from the authors' original report.

[b] Ca. 6 weeks after delivery.

[c] Mean ± SD (n).

[d] 3-5 Weeks after delivery.

[e] Assayed with H_2O_2 as acceptor substrate.

[f] Assayed with t-butyl hydroperoxide as acceptor substrate.

[g] Recalculated from authors' data.

[h] Recalculated from authors' data to per milligram Hb basis, assuming average Hb content of samples to be 29 μg/100 ml erythrocytes.

factors in the etiology of pre-eclampsia; however, this suggestion is not supported by the studies of Kauppila et al.,[125] who found no differences in blood Se levels in normal and pre-eclamptic pregnancies. The results of Rudolph and Wong[105] indicate that erythrocyte Se contents are not affected. It is likely that at least a portion of the decrease in plasma and whole blood Se is due to the hemodilution of pregnancy; this is suggested by the rapid recovery of blood Se concentration to nonpregnancy levels after delivery.[82,125] Butler et al.[82] suggested that the effect of hemodilution was insufficient to account for the magnitude of the changes observed. On the basis of studies with rats,[127] they suggested that these changes are related to hormonal factors. The changes in plasma Se concentration during pregnancy appear to be reflected by changes of similar magnitude (i.e., decreases of ca. 30%) in the activity of SeGSHpx in that tissue.[40,105] However, Butler et al.[82] found plasma SeGSHpx to increase by 26% during the course of pregnancy. Substantial increases have also been found in SeGSHpx activities of erythrocytes,[82,105] although the report of Rudolph and Wong[105] would suggest that erythrocyte Se concentrations do not appear to change during pregnancy. These nonuniform changes in the parameters of Se nutrition that occur in pregnancy raise questions concerning whether nutritional Se needs increase during pregnancy, as well as about the validity of these parameters in the assessment of nutritional Se status in pregnant women.

The transfer of Se from mother to fetus appears to be most efficient in women of low Se status. Studies of mothers in New Zealand[102] and Finland[128] found that the concentrations of Se in fetal (umbilical cord) plasma were not significantly different from those of the mother (all were ca. 58-70 ppb) (see Table 8.6). However, similar studies in the USA[102] and Belgium,[2] where maternal plasma Se levels were 190 and 88 ppb, respectively, found that fetal plasma concentrations of the element were only 75% of those of the mothers.

Premature infants are born with low Se status[30,129-133]; however, Se status, as indicated by the concentrations of Se in blood[30,130,131] and other tissues,[134] of these individuals has not been found to be significantly lower than those of full-term infants at the time of delivery. However, because hospitalized premature infants are frequently maintained with low-Se parenteral nutrient solutions or are fed low-Se formula diets (see Chapter 3) for as long as several weeks, it has been common that these low birth weight neonates show progressive declines in blood Se and SeGSHpx activities.[129,132] Because these infants also have lower (than full-term) plasma levels of vitamin E,[135] it may be expected that low Se status and its attendant reduction in antioxidant protection may have significant consequences. Rudolph et al.[132] found no relationship of blood Se concentrations and the early anemia

Table 8.6

Selenium Concentrations of Maternal and Fetal (Umbilical Cord) Plasma at Delivery

Country	Maternal plasma Se (ppb)	Fetal plasma Se (ppb)	Reference
USA	190 ± 30 $(25)^a$	140 ± 30 $(25)^a$	(102)
Belgium	$88 \pm 15(9)^a$	$66 \pm 14(9)^a$	(2)
New Zealand	69 ± 18 $(22)^{a,b}$	70 ± 17 $(22)^{a,c}$	(102)
	$61 \pm 17(15)^a$	$63 \pm 22(15)^a$	(102)
Finland	—	$16 \pm 7(21)^a$	(126)
	$58 \pm 10(17)^a$	$63 \pm 15(17)^a$	(128)

[a] Mean $\pm$ SD (n).

[b] These subjects had erythrocyte glutathione peroxidase activity of 122 ± 4.8 $(21)^a$ μmoles NADPH/min/ g Hb.

[c] These subjects had erythrocyte glutathione peroxidase activity of 9.9 ± 2.5 $(23)^a$ μmoles NADPH/min/ g Hb.

of prematurity, but they did find that Se supplementation was partially effective in protecting against the pro-oxidative effects of dietary iron. They found that the use of a milk-based formula containing 4.8 ppb Se (in comparison to a soy-based formula containing 3.4 ppb Se) was effective in reducing the *in vitro* H_2O_2-induced hemolysis that was stimulated by the use of an iron-supplemented (20 ppm) formula.

Money[136,137] pointed out several apparently common features of the epidemiology and pathology of sudden infant death syndrome (SIDS) and acute fatal Se/vitamin E-responsive diseases of the young of other species, implying that Se and/or vitamin E may have some role(s) in the etiology of SIDS. Victims of SIDS have been found to have low blood levels of Se and vitamin E, but both of these parameters were in the normal range for full-term and premature infants.[138] The hepatic concentrations of each of these nutrients in SIDS cases were also not signifcantly different from those of non-SIDS children.[139] Money[139] found that SIDS livers contained significantly greater concentrations of iron but lower concentrations of retinyl esters than did controls. This finding suggests that the pro-oxidative stress of a tissue iron oversupply in circumstances of low antioxidant protection, by virtue of the low Se and vitamin E status of the neonate, may be a factor in the etiology of SIDS. According to this hypothesis, Se status is not a primary factor in the syndrome. This is consistent with the report of Cowgill,[140] which showed that the neonatal death rate (deaths per 1000 live births) is not significantly different between geographic regions of the USA differing with respect to Se.

The Se status of free-living populations is quite variable within the constraints of the geographic effects on Se intake. In general, the influence of age has minimal effects on nutritional Se status (see Tables 8.7 and 8.8). Studies in Belgium,[2] Finland,[30] and Germany[102] have shown that blood Se levels decline during the first year of life, likely due to the effects of weaning to low-Se foods. By about 1 year, most children show blood Se levels comparable to those found in older children in the general population. Adults tend to have greater levels of tissue Se and blood SeGSHpx than children, and the elderly tend to show slight decreases in these parameters. The causes of these changes in apparent Se status are not clear; however, present information does not suggest that these effects may be due to factors other than age-related changes in food habits with associated changes in dietary Se intake.

III. DISEASES ASSOCIATED WITH NUTRITIONAL DEFICIENCIES OF SELENIUM

The role of Se in human nutrition remained unclear for almost two decades after the recognition of the nutritional essentiality of the element in experimental animals. However, during the latter 1970s, two human diseases were presented to the international community as being associated with severe nutritional Se-deficiency. These include a juvenile cardiomyopathy named for the county in Heilongjiang Province, China, in which it was first described, Keshan disease; and a chondrodystrophy of children called in Mandarin "da gu jie bing" (big joint disease) and referred to in the west as Kaschin-Beck disease (after the physicians who first described it in the USSR). Both diseases occur in rural areas of China that lie in a belt extending from the northeast provinces (Heilongjiang, Jilin, northeastern Inner Mongolia) to the south-central provinces (Sichuan, Yunnan) of the country (see Fig. 8.9). The endemic distributions of Keshan and Kaschin-Beck diseases are similar but not always identical; both correspond to the distribution of endemic Se-deficiency in foods and feeds (see Fig. 2.3).

A. Keshan Disease

Although prevalent in China for more than a century,[141] the disease now called Keshan disease was first studied with respect to its epidemiology, clinical signs, and pathology on the occasion of an outbreak in Keshan County, Heilongjiang Province, China, in 1935.[142] Since then, Keshan disease has been diagnosed in more than a dozen provinces and autonomous regions within the belt of endemic Se-deficiency in that country,[141] almost exclusively among people living in the mountainous and hilly areas of that belt while the alluvial plains are free of the disease.[143] Affected areas are low in soil

Table 8.7

Selenium Status of Various Human Populations According to Subject Age

Country	Age group	Plasma/serum Se (ppb)	Whole blood Se (ppb)	Erythrocyte Se (ppb)	Hair Se (ppb)	Reference
Belgium	Newborn	66 ± 14 (9)[a]	—	—	—	(2)
	2-6 mos	27 (8)[b]	—	—	—	
	7-12 mos	48 (2)[b]	—	—	—	
	1-2 yrs	42 (3)[b]	—	—	—	
	2-6 yrs	59 (10)[b]	—	—	—	
	7-15 yrs	65 ± 13 (15)	—	—	—	
	Adults[c]	85 ± 15 (9)	—	—	—	
	Elderly (82 ± 7 yrs)	73 ± 12 (31)	—	—	—	
Belgium	≤19 yrs	99(1)[b]	112 (1)[b]	130 (1)[b]	—	(3)
	20-24 yrs	96 ± 12 (29)	122 ± 29 (27)	160 ± 30 (27)	—	
	25-29 yrs	97 ± 13 (30)	119 ± 15 (30)	147 ± 22 (29)	—	
	30-34 yrs	98 ± 14 (42)	126 ± 18 (41)	166 ± 33 (41)	—	
	35-39 yrs	93 ± 11 (22)	122 ± 17 (22)	162 ± 32 (22)	—	
	40-44 yrs	95 ± 12 (23)	126 ± 16 (23)	172 ± 31 (23)	—	
	45-49yrs	96 ± 9 (11)	128 ± 13 (11)	173 ± 35 (11)	—	
	50-54 yrs	107 ± 6 (2)	126 ± 17 (4)	164 ± 31 (3)	—	
	55-59 yrs	99 ± 9 (3)	102 ± 6 (3)	106 ± 14 (3)	—	
China	<7 yrs.	—	—	—	57 ± 5 (15)[d.f]	(19)
					50 ± 3 (32)[e.f]	
	7-13 yrs.	—	—	—	77 ± 7 (11)[df]	
					67 ± 4 (32)[ef]	
	Adults	—	—	—	96 ± 15 (11)[df]	
					68 ± 4 (32)[e]f	
England	18-55 yrs	116 ± 16 (338)	138 ± 19 (338)	—	—	(69)
	56-85 yrs	112 ± 13 (53)	130 ± 15 (53)	—	—	

348

Country	Age				
Finland	1 wk	—	49±12 (3)	—	(30)
	1-6 yrs	50±17 (9)	59±11 (14)	—	
	7-12yrs	51±14 (8)	60±14 (13)	—	
Finland	1-6 yrs	50±17 (9)	59±11 (14)	—	(28)
	7-12 yrs.	51±14 (8)	60±14 (13)	—	
	24-81 yrs.	66±11 (21)	87±17 (25)	—	
Germany	Infant	50[g]	—	—	(102)
	6 mos	32[g]	—	—	
	9 mos	68[g]	—	—	
	3 yrs	82[g]	—	—	
	9 yrs	90[g]	—	—	
	22 yrs	98[g]	—	—	
New Zealand					
Aukland	7±3 yrs	—	60±12 (13)	—	(102)
Dunedin	36±4 yrs	—	83±12 (12)	—	(102)
	9±3 yrs	—	59±11 (18)	—	(102)
	33±12 yrs	—	62±12 (59)	—	
Tapansi	11±2 yrs	—	48±10 (52)	—	(102)
	35±3 yrs	—	60±12 (49)	—	
USA	11-20 yrs	98±19 (46)	—	149±27	(90)
	21-30 yrs	108±33 (57)	—	164±33	
	31-45 yrs	103±22 (64)	—	156±29	
	46-60 yrs	102±20 (39)	—	159±38	
USA	>80 yrs	88±8 (6)	—	—	(86)
USA	18-49 yrs	220±30[hi]	—	—	
		235±47[hi]			
	50-80 yrs	224±31[hi]	—	—	
		238±37[hj]			

(continues)

Table 8.7 (*Continued*)

Country	Age group	Plasma/serum Se (ppb)	Whole blood Se (ppb)	Erythrocyte Se (ppb)	Hair Se (ppb)	Reference
USA	20-39 yrs	$99 \pm 3\ (42)^f$	—	—	—	(75)
	40-49 yrs	$92 \pm 4\ (14)^f$	—	—	—	
	50-59 yrs	$91 \pm 5\ (12)^f$	—	—	—	
	60-69 yrs	$90 \pm 7\ (12)^f$	—	—	—	
	70-79 yrs	$89 \pm 8\ (8)^f$	—	—	—	
	80-89 yrs	$87 \pm 8\ (4)^f$	—	—	—	
USSR	Newborn	n.d.^{k}	—	—	—	(92)
	6 mos.-2 yrs	75^b	—	—	—	
	4-6 yrs	85^b	—	—	—	
	7-9 yrs	127^b	—	—	—	
	10-15 yrs.	122^b	—	—	—	

^{a}Mean $\pm$ SD (n), unless otherwise noted.
^{b}No estimate of variance was presented or calculable.
^{c}Women at delivery.
^{d}Mianing, Sichuan Province.
^{e}Xide, Sichuan Province.
^{f}Mean $\pm$ SEM (n).
^{g}Estimated from graph of unpublished data of McKenzie and Ren as cited by Thomson and Robinson.[102]
^{h}Value of n not specified by authors.
^{i}Males.
^{j}Females.
^{k}Authors were unable to detect Se in these samples.

Table 8.8

Glutathione Peroxidase Activities in Various Human Populations According to Subject Age

Country	Age group	Plasma (nmoles NADPH/min/l)	Erythrocytes (μmoles NADPH/min/g Hb)	Reference
Belgium	≤19 yrs		7.0 (1)[abd]	(3)
	20-24 yrs		13.1 ± 3.0 (28)[c]	
	25-29 yrs		12.7 ± 2.7 (29)	
	30-34 yrs		14.6 ± 3.7 (40)	
	35-39 yrs		13.3 ± 2.8 (22)	
	40-44 yrs		15.6 ± 2.8 (22)	
	45-49 yrs		13.6 ± 2.1 (10)	
	50-54 yrs		12.8 ± 5.2 (4)	
	55-59 yrs		13.3 ± 1.4 (3)	
	60-99 yrs		15.3 ± 3.3 (40)[acd]	(2)
England	18-55 yrs		19.6 ± 4.9 (338)[a]c	(69)
	56-85 yrs		20.9 ± 5.0 (53)	
Germany	3-9 yrs	31 ± 3 (12)[acd]		(99)
		30 ± 4 (12)[de]		
	20-46 yrs	41 ± 8 (16)[ad]		
		38 ± 8 (3)[de]		
USA	infant[f]		19.5 ± 1.1[ce]	(132)
	11-20 yrs		24.8 ± 5.7 (46)[ce]	(90)
	21-30 yrs		27.0 ± 7.6 (57)	
	31-45 yrs		26.8 ± 6.6 (64)	
	46-60 yrs		28.0 ± 7.4 (39)	
	>80 yrs		25.2 ± 5.4 (6)[ce]	(86)

[a] Assayed with t-butyl hydroperoxide as acceptor substrate.
[b] Single observation reported by authors.
[c] Mean ± SD (n).
[d] Recalculated from authors' report.
[e] Assayed with hydrogen peroxide as acceptor substrate.
[f] Low-birth weight infants (i.e., 1000-1600 g).

351

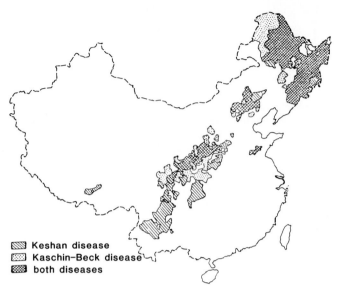

Fig. 8.9 Distribution of Keshan disease and Kaschin-Beck disease in China. After Tan *et al*[144]

Se (i.e., topsoils containing less than 125 ppb Se, of which less than 3 ppb is water-soluble[144]), thereby producing plant foods and feeds of low Se content (e.g., food and feed grains in affected areas generally contain less than 40 ppb Se[143,144]). Selenium-deficiency diseases of livestock (e.g., white muscle disease in lambs) is also endemic in these areas.[144] Therefore, it is not surprising that humans living and consuming locally produced low-Se foods (see Fig. 3.1) in these areas are of low nutritional Se status (see Table 8.9). What is surprising is the severity of the low Se status of residents of Keshan disease areas; studies of Se status have revealed the lowest tissue Se levels of any free-living populations anywhere on earth. Blood Se levels of people in these areas are consistently less than one-half of those of New Zealanders or Finns (see Table 8.1), whose countries also experience endemic Se deficiencies as practical problems in livestock production. Residents of Keshan disease areas tend to have blood Se levels less than ca. 25 ppb and hair Se concentrations less than ca. 100 ppb.[145] The disease has been more prevalent among farming families in rural districts than among residents of urban centers; this difference probably relates to the more monotonous dietary habits of rural residents and to their stronger dependency on food produced in their immediate locales. Studies by Chen *et al*.[17] and Yang *et al*.[22] have shown that urban residents within Keshan disease areas of Heilongjiang and Sichuan provinces have substantially better Se status, as indicated by significantly greater hair Se concentrations, than

Table 8.9

Selenium Status of Children in Keshan Disease-Endemic and Nonendemic Areas of China

Region	Hair Se (ppb)		Whole blood Se (ppb)		Reference
	Endemic area	Nonendemic area	Endemic area	Nonendemic area	
Unspecified	—	—	15 ± 1 (115)[b]	39 ± 7 (134)[b]	(7)
			19 ± 2 (25)[b]		
Sichuan Province[a]	71 ± 3[c]	112 ± 6[c]	—	—	(13)
	88 ± 6[c]	106 ± 7[c]			
	68 ± 4[c]	96 ± 7[c]			
	80 ± 4[c]	113 ± 6[c]			
	47 ± 4[c]	106 ± 7[c]			
	57 ± 5 (15)[b]	—	—	—	(19)
	77 ± 7 (11)[b]				
	50 ± 3 (11)[b]				
	67 ± 4 (11)[b]				
	51 ± 4 (20)[b]				
	50 ± 3 (20)[b]				
Northeast Provinces[d]	69 ± 27[ef]	146 ± 32[e]	—	—	(145)
Northwest Provinces[g]	93 ± 32[ef]	209 ± 108[e]	—	—	(145)
Southwest Provinces[h]	87 ± 32[ef]	170 ± 57[e]	—	—	(145)
Tibet	67 ± 36[i]	343[j]			(145)
	70[i]		21 ± 1[fk]	95 ± 9[k]	(8)
	58 ± 3 (22)[ef]	237 ± 8 (18)[c]	23 (16)[l]	65 (11)[l]	(146)

[a] Results from several different sampling sites shown.
[b] Mean ± SE (n).
[c] Mean ± SE, n nonspecified; statistical analyses not reported.
[d] Primarily Heilongjiang Province.
[e] Mean ± SD, n unspecified.
[f] Significantly different from controls, $p < .05$.
[g] Primarily Shaanxi Province.
[h] Primarily Sichuan Province.
[i] It is not clear whether Keshan disease is endemic in Tibet.
[j] No n or estimate of variance reported.
[k] Mean±SE; n not reported.
[l] Mean (n); no estimate of variance reported.

did residents of neighboring rural districts (see Table 8.10). Ge *et al.*[141] stated that migrants do not suffer from Keshan disease until they have lived in the endemic area for at least 3 months.

Keshan disease is a multifocal myocarditis that occurs primarily in children between the ages of 2 and 10 years,[147] but also to a lesser extent among women of child-bearing age.[141] According to Chen and Yang,[148] infants are rarely affected by Keshan disease. Their intakes of Se from breast milk, even in these deficient areas, is usually ca. 3 μg per infant per day; this level is thought to protect them from the cardiomyopathy, as the first signs of the disease are normally not observed until after children are weaned to solid (and, in these areas, low-Se) foods at which time their intakes drop to ca. 1.5 μg Se per child per day.[148] The incidence shows marked seasonal[141] and annual[149] variations, suggesting that other factors must play roles in the etiology of the disease. The fact that the seasonal patterns of Keshan disease incidence are quite different in northern and southern China[141] (see Fig. 8.10) counterindicate vitamin E as one such factor. The finding that 72% of southern cases are observed between May and August, inclusive, when fresh produce providing vitamin E in the diet is most available, suggests that the incidence of the disease is not related to seasonal changes in vitamin E nutriture. In addition, Chen[146] has stated that the plasma concentrations of vitamin E in Keshan disease patients [0.55 $\pm$ 0.09 (SEM) μg/dl, n=16] were not significantly different from those of healthy children [0.48 $\pm$ 0.06 μg/dl, n=19] in the same villages.* Because the organic forms of Se in the major food sources (e.g., cereals and meats) would be expected to be stable to storage, seasonal variation in Se nutriture is not expected; parameters of Se status of residents of several Keshan disease areas do not indicate that such seasonal variation occurs (see Table 8.11). Therefore, it seems likely that some other presently unidentified environmental factor(s) may be involved in the etiology of Keshan disease.

Keshan disease is diagnosed on the basis of signs of acute or chronic insufficiency of cardiac function, cardiac enlargement, gallop rhythm, cardiac arrhythmias, and electrocardiographic (EKG) and radiographic abnormalities[17,141,146] (see Table 8.12). Subjects may show cardiogenic shock or congestive heart failure; embolic episodes from cardiac thromboses have been reported.[141,146] Four clinical subtypes of Keshan disease have been identified† (see Table 8.12); they have been discussed by Chen *et al.*[17] and Ge *et al.*[141]

---

*The concentrations of Se in whole blood was also not significantly different between these newly diagnosed Keshan disease patients [19 $\pm$ 3 (SEM) ppb, n=16] and healthy children (26 $\pm$ 5, n=19) in the same villages.

†Standard clinical subtyping was delineated at the National Seminar on the Etiology of Keshan Disease, Qiqihar, China, October 1974, as outlined by Chen *et al.*[17]

Table 8.10

Differences in Selenium Status Between Urban and Rural Residents Within Adjacent Areas Within Two Provinces in China

	Hair Se (ppb)		
Province	Urban residents	Rural residents	Reference[d]
Heilongjiang[a]	390 ± 18 (20)[bc]	151 ± 11 (20)[b]	(17)
	295 ± 23 (11)[bc]	151 ± 11 (20)[b]	(22)
	357 ± 21 (22)[bc]	146 ± 13 (21)[b]	
	238 ± 11 (7)[bc]	128 ± 9 (14)[b]	
Sichuan[a]	131 ± 14 (16)[bc]	69 ± 1 (10)[b]	(17)
	161 ± 7 (16)[bc]	58 ± 3 (22)[b]	(22)

[a]Results from different sampling sites are shown.

[b]Mean $\pm$ SE (n).

[c]Significantly different from controls, $p < .001$.

[d]There is some, but apparently not complete, redundancy in these two reports.

The acute type of Keshan disease is observed with sudden onset of signs and symptoms in otherwise apparently healthy children with no history of cardiac disorders. Symptoms include dizziness, malaise, loss of appetite, nausea, vomiting, chills, precardial and substernal discomfort, and dyspnea. The principle physical signs result from cardiogenic shock (e.g., pallor, vasoconstriction in the extremities, arterial blood pressure below 80 mm/ 60 mm Hg); patients show severe arrhythmia and pulmonary edema. Abnormalities noted upon EKG examination include proximal tachycardia, reduced voltage of QRS waves, prolonged atrio-ventricular conduction time

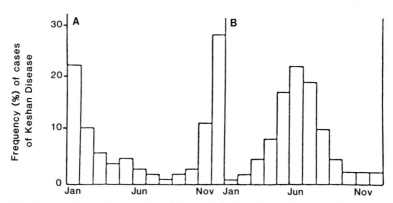

Fig. 8.10 Seasonal variations in the incidence of Keshan disease in (A) northern (primarily Heilongjiang Province) (n = 187 cases) and (B) southern (primarily Sichuan Province) China (n = 315 cases). After Ge et al.[141]

Table 8.11

Seasonal Variations in Se Status of Residents of Several Chinese Provinces

Province	Year - month	Hair Se[a] (ppb)			Reference
		Site 1[b]	Site 2	Site 3	
Sichuan	1974 -Mar	85 ± 17 (21)	—	—	(21)
	-Jun	88 ± 6 (22)	—	—	
	-Oct	69 ± 5 (10)	—	—	
	1975 -Jan	64 ± 6 (18)	48 ± 4 (16)	120 ± 11 (8)	
	-Apr	57 ± 4(20)	69 ± 7 (20)	117 ± 35 (7)	
	-Jul	58 ± 3 (22)	64 ± 4 (19)	126 ± 11 (6)	
	-Oct	53 ± 3 (20)	44 ± 4 (19)	103 ± 6 (7)	
Shandong	1974 -Feb	96 ± 7 (13)	105 ± 6 (24)	—	(21)
	-Apr	121 ± 10 (10)	110 ± 6 (18)	—	
	-Oct	128 ± 9 (14)	105 ± 5 (25)	—	
Heilongjiang	1975 -Apr	54 ± 6 (12)	93 ± 5 (20)	—	
	-Aug	50 ± 8 (22)	86 ± 4 (22)	—	
	-Dec	52 ± 4 (21)	83 ± 5 (20)	—	
Yunan	1975 -Mar	51 ± 6 (13)	59 ± 7 (17)	—	(21)
	-Jun	49 ± 2 (13)	57 ± 3 (17)	—	
	-Sep	58 ± 7 (13)	55 ± 7 (17)	—	
	-Dec	46 ± 15 (7)	54 ± 7 (17)	—	
Sichuan	"Prevalent" season	175 ± 67 (29)	165 ± 10 (20)	141 ± 8 (24)	(19)
		148 ± 5 (28)	136 ± 7 (20)	157 ± 8 (24)	
	"Nonprevalent" season	156 ± 6 (28)	163 ± 10 (20)	142 ± 8 (25)	
		158 ± 7(26)	142 ± 9(20)	151 ± 7(20)	

[a]Mean ± SE (n).

[b]Sites represent different villages within the province.

Table 8.12

Criteria for the Diagnosis and Subtyping of Keshan Disease[a]

History: Living in endemic area in the same conditions as the local people for at least 3 months

Diagnosis: a) Acute or chronic heart function insufficiency
    b) Cardiac enlargement
    c) Gallop rhythm
    d) Arrhythmia
      i. Multiple ventricular extrasystoles
      ii. Atrial fibrilation
      iii. Ventricular or supraventricular tachycardia
    e) EKG changes
      i. A-V block
      ii. Right bundle branch block and/or left bundle branch block
      iii. ST-T changes
      iv. Prolonged Q-T
      v. Multiple ventricular extrasystoles of various origins
    f) Changes noted by X-ray examination
      i. Cardiac enlargement
      ii. Changes in heart shape and cardiac lung
      iii. Left ventricular prominent and pulsation decreased

(People living in areas of prevalent Keshan disease and having one of these symptoms and signs can be diagnosed as suffering from Keshan disease when other diseases can be excluded.)

Clinical subtyping:

a)	Acute type:	acute onset with acute heart function insufficiency (e.g., cardiogenic shock, heart-brain syndrome, pulmonary edema, severe arrhythmia).
b)	Chronic type:	moderate or severe cardiac enlargement, usually with congestive heart failure.
c)	Subacute type:	moderately rapid (but not acute) onset; usually with symptoms and signs of both acute and chronic types; most prevalent in children; most cases have facial edema and gallop rhythm.
d)	Latent type:	mild cardiac enlargement without abnormal heart function.

[a]From the national seminar on the Etiology of Keshan Disease, October, 1974, Quiqihar, China, as presented by Chen et al.[17]

and Q-T intervals, A-V block, right bundle branch block, changes in S-T segments, and inverted T waves. Radiographic examination reveals slight to moderate cardiac enlargment with diminished pulsation.

The chronic type of Keshan disease is characterized by chronic congestive heart failure with varying degrees of heart function insufficiency. Symptoms vary according to the degree of cardiac insufficiency and include palpitation with conciousness of heart beat at rest, shortness of breath, cough with hemoptysis, right upper quadrant pain, edema, and oliguria. Physical signs include cardiac enlargement, reduced intensity of heart sound, soft and changeable systolic murmer, gallop rhythm, rales on the base of the lung, hepatomegaly, and edema. Pronounced EKG changes are observed: ventricular or supraventricular tachycardia, atrial fibrillation, frequent ventricular premature beats, right bundle branch block, A-V block, changes in S-T segment, and inverted T wave. Radiographic examination reveals cardiac enlargement with flask-shaped profile, and weak pulsation. The chronic type of Keshan disease is seen as a late-stage development of patients with the acute or subacute types of the disease.

The most prevalent form of Keshan disease, especially in children, is the subacute type. Its clinical manifestations are similar to those of the chronic type, with signs and symptoms varying with the degree of cardiac insufficiency; however, its course is more accelerated (the insidious period lasting 1-2 weeks), during which time patients appear to be on the verge of collapse. Most patients report malaise and restlessness and show facial edema, gallop rhythm, and slight cardiac dilation.

The latent type of Keshan disease is characterized by normal heart function with mild cardiac dilation and associated EKG changes (right bundle branch block, first or second degree A-V block, occasional ventricular extrasystoles). Cardiac effects are generally so mild that the patient may be unaware of the disease; it may be discovered only as an incidental finding upon autopsy or examination for some other reason. After being informed of their EKG irregularities, some patients have complained of dizziness, fatigue, and palpitation after exercise.

The pathology of Keshan disease has been reviewed by Ge et al.[141] They point out that the primary target organ of the disease is the heart muscle. In addition, several cases show hepatic congestion with fatty metamorphosis and mesenteric lymphadenosis. A few cases show slight degenerative changes in the diaphragm. The gross pathology of the Keshan disease heart involves dilation of the chambers of the organ (primarily the ventricles, but sometimes also the atria) with only moderate myocardial hypertrophy. The gross appearance of the heart in acute cases may be rather normal, but chronic cases usually show a highly expanded ball-shaped heart that is evidenced by a prominent heart shadow upon radiographic examination (see Fig. 8.11). Subacute cases show moderate cardiac enlargement (see Fig. 8.12). Microscopic examination at autopsy reveals multifocal necrosis and fibrous replacement of the myocardium as the main pathological feature of Keshan disease (see Fig. 8.13). Although focal lesions are found throughout the myocardium, they are more frequent in the walls of the ventricles than

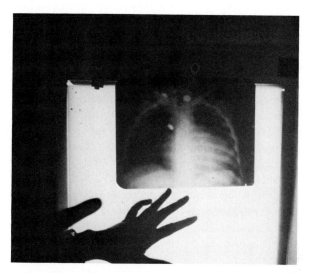

Fig. 8.11 Chest radiograph of a 5-year-old girl with subacute type Keshan disease in Sichang, Sichuan Province, China. Note the severe cardiac enlargement.Photograph made by the senior author a few days before the little girl's death.

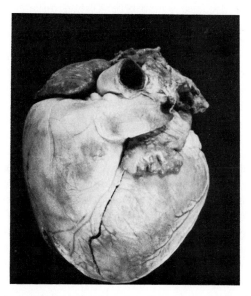

Fig. 8.12 Post-mortem specimen of moderately enlarged heart from a 5-year-old boy with subacute type Keshan disease. Photograph courtesy of Dr. Ge Keyou and Dr. Jin Daxun, China National Center for Preventive Medicine.

of the atria, and on the left side more so than on the right. Ge *et al.*[141] have distinguished two processes of myocardial necrosis in the Keshan disease heart: myocytolysis (see Fig. 8.14), which they regard as the representative lesion particularly in the subacute disease; and contraction band necrosis, which was obvious only in acute cases where it was identified by myofibrillar degeneration. Ultrastructural studies by Ge *et al.*[141] indicate that myocytolysis is initiated by mitochondrial degeneration. Chen *et al.*[150] found, using histochemical procedures, marked losses of succinic dehydrogenase from myocardiocytes of Keshan disease patients. This supported the suggestion of Ge *et al.*[141] that impaired myocardial mitochondrial function may be the initial physiological lesion in Keshan disease. The studies of Ge *et al.*[141] also revealed clusters of small electron-dense particulate cytoplasmic and mitochondrial inclusions; although these bodies were not identified, Ge *et al.*[141] acknowledged the possibility that they may have been cardiophilic virus particles with some role in the etiology of Keshan disease.

Chen[146] has stated that the case-fatality of Keshan disease in China was greater than 80% in the 1940s, but has been ca. 30% in recent years. This improved outcome may result from improvements in both specific medical care procedures and health care in general that have occurred in that country over the last four decades. Acute type Keshan disease cases are treated with massive intravenous doses of ascorbic acid,* which have proven to be effective management of the cardiogenic shock.[146,151] Patients with congestive heart failure are treated with digitalis, diuretics, reduction of sodium intake, and antibiotics. No specific treatments for Keshan disease have been specified.

Hypotheses for the etiology of Keshan disease have proposed that it may be caused by food- and/or water-borne toxins (e.g., mycotoxins, heavy metals, nitrite), certain infectious agents (e.g., cardiophilic viruses), or specific nutrient deficiencies (e.g., Se, Mo, Mg, riboflavin). Available experimental evidence provides support for only the last two of these hypotheses. Su *et al.*[152] isolated several different strains of enterovirus (e.g., echo, Coxsackie) from the tissues of Keshan disease patients. One of these viruses (Coxsackie B_4) was shown by Bai *et al.*[153] and Ge *et al.*[154] to produce Se-responsive myocarditis in mice. Other studies implicate dietary factors in the potentiation of Keshan disease. Wang *et al.*[155] showed that oral treatment with $NaNO_2$ (75 mg per kilogram body weight twice daily for

---

*According to Chen[146] and Ge,[151] this treatment was introduced at Xian Medical College. Treatment for an adult involves an initial dose of 5-10 g ascorbic acid by slow intravenous injection followed by at least another 30 g ascorbic acid within 24 hrs. Half of this dose is used for children under 10 years of age. This treatment is repeated at intervals of 2-3 days; thereafter, the dose is reduced as symptoms subside.

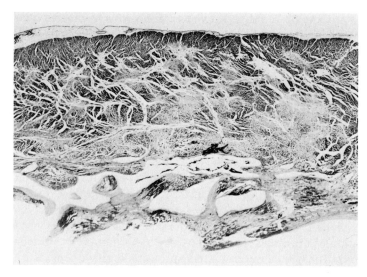

Fig. 8.13 Histology of Keshan disease heart showing multifocal necrosis and fibrous replacement of the myocardium of the left ventricular wall. H & E stain (6×). Photograph courtesy of Dr. Ge Keyou and Dr. Jin Daxun, China National Center for Preventive Medicine.

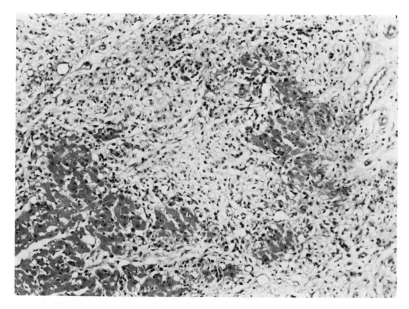

Fig. 8.14 Typical histological appearance of Keshan disease heart showing myocytolysis and fibrosis. H & E stain (130×). Photograph courtesy of Dr. Ge Keyou and Dr. Jin Daxuan, China National Center for Preventive Medicine.

10 days) produced a multifocal myocardial necrosis in rats fed diets based on (low-Se) grains grown in an area of endemic Keshan disease (in Heilongjiang Province, China). Nitrite-induced myocardial lesions reminiscent of Keshan disease and associated with increases in myocardial calcium levels were reduced either by use of similar grains grown in Beijing (and, thus, higher in Se) or by supplementation of the basal diet with either Se (as Na_2SeO_3) or Mo (as ammonium molybdate). Ren et al.[156] reported multifocal coagulation necrosis of the myocardium of rats raised using an Se-deficient semipurified diet. However, the lack of such an observation in the numerous previous studies of Se-deficiency in the rat suggests that the experimental conditions of Ren et al.[156] must have included an unknown and important potentiating factor of the cardiomyopathy.

While the nature and, perhaps, existence of a potentiating factor on Keshan disease may be unclear at present, it is clear that the endemic distribution of the disease is related to the pattern of severe environmental Se-deficiency in China. Several intervention studies have demonstrated that Se can be very effective in the prevention of this disease. Wen et al.[20] evaluated the efficacy of two nutritional supplements of Se for the prevention of Keshan disease in free-living children in Sichuan Province, China: Se-fortified (15 ppm as Na_2SeO_3) table salt made available to the general population within designated study sites, and oral tablets containing 0.5 (for younger children) or 1.0 mg (for older children) Se (as Na_2SeO_3) given once per week. Their results (Table 8.13) show that improvements in the Se status of the juvenile population could be achieved by either means, both of which reduced but did not eliminate the numbers of cases of Keshan disease. A larger intervention study was conducted by the Keshan Disease Research Group[157,158] of the Institute of Health, Chinese Academy of Medical Sciences.* That study evaluated the efficacy of oral tablets containing of Na_2SeO_3 (administered in the same manner as used by Wen et al.[20]) for the prevention of Keshan disease over several years in an endemic area of Sichuan Province. Their results (Table 8.14) also demonstrate that Se treatment was very effective in reducing, but not eliminating, the incidence of Keshan disease. Selenium supplementation was found to reduce the severity of disease manifestations (i.e., it reduced the incidences of cases turning chronic, of cardiac dysfunctions, of EKG abnormalities and of cardiac enlargement). In fact, the results were so encouraging that after 2 years, the control groups were abolished and the entire population was treated with Se for the balance of the study. The results of three other large scale Se-intervention studies are presented in Table 8.15. These also demonstrate that improvements in the Se status of populations otherwise

*This unit was reorganized in 1983 as the China National Center for Preventive Medicine.

Table 8.13

Effects of Selenium-Supplementation on Keshan Disease in Children in Sichuan Province, China[a]

Treatment	Hair Se (ppb)	Normal heart size[b]		Slight dilation[c]		Moderate dilation[d]		EKG
		Normal Total subjects	Abnormal EKG	Normal EKG	Abnormal EKG	Normal EKG	Abnormal EKG	
Pre-treatment	72 ± 2 (20)[e]	183	175	1	2	3	2	0
Control	59 ± 8 (20)	218	204	5	4	3	1	1
Se-supplemented salt[f]	155 ± 7 (16)	211	206	2	3	0	0	0
Oral Se tablets[g]	107 ± 8 (22)	194	190	1	3	0	0	0

[a]From report of Wen et al.[20]

[b]Heart:chest ratio <.50.

[c]Heart:chest ratio =.51 -.55.

[d]Heart:chest ratio =.56 -.60.

[e]Mean ± SE (n).

[f]Normal use of table salt supplemented with 15 ppm Se as Na_2SeO_3.

[g]Orally administered tablets of 0.5 or 1.0 mg Se as Na_2SeO_3 given once per week to each child.

Table 8.14

Effect of Selenium Intervention on the Incidence and Prognosis of Keshan Disease[a]

Parameters	Controls		Se-treated[b]			
	1974	1975[c]	1974	1975	1976	1977
General statistics						
Total subjects	3,985	5,445	4,510	6,767	12,579	12,747
Total cases	54	52	10	7	4	0
Cases turned latent	16	13	9	6	2	0
Cases improved	9	10	0	0	0	0
Cases turned chronic	2	3	1	0	0	0
Deaths	27	26	0	1	2	0
Main signs						
Cases examined	53	52	10	7	4	0
Gallop rhythm	51	48	10	2	2	0
Heart failure	50	47	9	1	3	0
Cardiogenic shock	3	4	0	1	0	0
Arrhythmia	1	3	0	0	0	0
Hemiplegia	2	0	0	0	0	0
Electrocardiographic signs						
Cases examined	54	38	10	7	2	0
Normal	11	5	6	1	1	0
Low voltage	16	12	2	1	0	0
Right bundle branch block	5	9	0	0	0	0
Intraventricular block	0	0	0	0	0	0
ST-T change	16	18	0	6	1	0
Prolonged QT	0	0	0	0	0	0
AV block	1	3	0	0	0	0
Ventricular extra systole	1	2	0	0	0	0
Supraventricular tachycardia	0	1	0	0	0	0
Radiographic signs						
Cases examined	36	35	8	6	2	0
Normal[d]	7	11	2	6	1	0
Slight dilation[e]	0	4	0	0	1	0
Moderate dilation[f]	29	10	6	0	0	0
Severe dilation[g]	0	10	0	0	0	0

[a]From report by the Keshan Disease Research Group of the Chinese Academy of Medical Sciences.[157] The data presented in this table are those for the first year follow-up of new cases within each year. See the original report[158] for results of subsequent years of follow-up.

[b]Oral supplements of Na_2SeO_3 as one tablet per child per week to provide 0.5 or 1.0 mg Se per child per week.

[c]Control groups were abolished after 1975 when all children were given Se.

[d]Heart:chest ratio =.46 -.51.

[e]Heart:chest ratio =.52 -.55.

[f]Heart:chest ratio =.56 -.60.

[g]Heart:chest ratio >.60.

Table 8.15

Effect of Selenium Intervention on the Incidence of Keshan Disease in Selected Regions of China

Region	Year	Controls			Se-treated			Reference
		Total subjects	Cases	Cases/10,000 subjects	Total subjects	Cases	Cases/10,000 subjects	
Mianning County Sichuan Province (selected communes)								(19)
Before intervention								
	1972-1973	3,580	29	81.0	24,225	172	71.0	
Se intervention[a]								
	1976	1,833	33	180.0	12,578	4	3.2	
	1977	1,855	10	53.9	12,747	1	.8	
	1978	1,878	31	165.1	12,465	1	.8	
	1979	1,901	22	115.7	11,146	3	2.7	
	1980	1,915	18	94.0	10,624	1	.9	
	1981	2,013	16	79.5	10,282	0	0	
	1982	2,063	12	58.1	9,801	0	0	
	1983	2,093	4	19.1	8,730	1	1.1	
	Total	15,553	146	93.9	88,373	11	1.2	
Mianning County Sichuan Province (whole county)[a]								(19)
	1977	22,525	83	36.0	32,194	1	.3	
	1978	22,315	104	42.8	29,332	8	2.7	
	1979	24,616	126	51.2	22,582	22	9.7	
	1980	25,051	99	32.5	25,364	17	6.7	
	1981	25,616	77	30.1	24,991	6	2.4	
	1982	25,954	55	21.2	17,027	5	2.9	
	Total	146,071	544	37.2	151,490	59	3.9	

(continues)

Table 8.15 (*Continued*)

Region	Year	Controls			Se-treated			Reference
		Total subjects	Cases	Cases/10,000 subjects	Total subjects	Cases	Cases/10,000 subjects	
Sichuan Province 5 counties[a]								(146)
	1976	243,649	488	20.0	45,515	8	1.7	
	1977	222,944	350	15.7	67,754	15	2.2	
	1978	220,599	373	16.9	65,953	10	1.5	
	1979	223,280	300	13.4	69,910	33	4.7	
	1980	197,096	202	10.7	74,740	22	2.9	
	Total	1,107,568	1,713	15.5	323,872	88	2.7	
Sichuan Province								(19)
Before intervention								
	1974-1976	29,850	33	11.1	19,122	61	31.9	
After intervention[b]								
	1977-1983	87,888	76	8.6	56,440	11	2.0	

[a]Se supplementation was accomplished with orally administered tablets of Na_2SeO_3 given at 0.5 or 1.0 mg Se per child per week, according to body weight.
[b]Se supplementation was accomplished with the use of table salt containing 15 pm Se added as Na_2SeO_3.

of very low Se status is very effective in reducing the incidence of Keshan disease. However, even after several years of supplementation, Se is not able to prevent completely this disease. It is, therefore, most likely that Keshan disease is potentiated in circumstances of nutritional Se deficiency by one or more factors that remain to be identified. The identification of such potentiation factors will provide the missing information necessary to the understanding of the etiology of this disease associated with severe Se-deficiency.

Cardiomyopathies associated with low Se status have been reported in a few cases outside of China[71,159-161,174,176]; however, it cannot be determined at this time the extent to which (if at all) Se deficiency may have been involved in the pathogenesis of those cases. Sartiano et al.[81] have noted that low Se status is not a general feature of cardiomyopathy patients in the USA.

B. Kaschin-Beck Disease

Kaschin-Beck disease is an osteoarthropathy endemic to eastern Siberia, northern Korea, and parts of China. According to Mo,[9] it was first observed in 1849 in the area of the Urow River in the Transbaikal district of what is now the USSR, and was described by Kaschin in 1859 and by Beck and Beck in 1906. In the 1970s, studies in China indicated that the prevalence of Kaschin-Beck disease was greatest in areas of severe Se-deficiency.[9,11,14,15,144] This relationship, identified shortly after that of Se and Keshan disease, prompted Se-intervention studies that have produced promising results.

Kaschin-Beck disease, as reviewed by Mo,[9] affects primarily the epiphyseal cartilage, articular cartilage, and epiphyseal growth plates of growing bones. The long bones are most frequently affected; however, the cartilage tissue associated with any bone in the skeleton may be involved. Affected cartilage shows atrophy and necrosis with repair and disturbance on endochondral ossification. The most striking histological feature of Kaschin-Beck disease is chondronecrosis with proliferation of surviving chondrocytes in clusters. Mo[9] has categorized this process as a coagulation necrosis. The condition results in enlarged joints (especially of the fingers, toes, and knees), shortened fingers, toes and extremities, and, in severe cases, dwarfism. The enlargement of joints characteristic of the disease gives rise to its name in Mandarin "da gu jie bing," i.e., "big joint disease." Radiographic examination of the hands of patients with Kaschin-Beck disease can distinguish four lesion sites.[162] These include the metaphyseal regions (which appear widened with semilunar depressions), the epiphyseal regions (which appear similar to the metaphyseal type, but also include bone sclerosis and epiphyseal early closure), the distal phalanges (which appear as bone edge semilunar depressions), and the joint capsules (which appear uneven and narrow with spur formation).

Like Keshan disease, Kaschin-Beck disease is endemic to the severely Se-deficient regions of China. Residents of Kaschin-Beck disease-endemic areas show very low Se status when compared to residents of neighboring nonendemic areas (see Table 8.16 and Fig. 8.15). The endemic distribution of the disease (see Fig. 8.9) is very similar to that of Keshan disease; both diseases are prevalent only in the long belt of Se-deficiency in that country. However, the fact that the endemic distributions of these two diseases are not identical within this belt indicates that the etiology of one or both involves some other potentiating factor(s). Although vitamin E has not been investigated extensively with regard to its possible role in the etiology of Kaschin-Beck disease, Liang et al.[163] reported that the nutritional vitamin E status of residents of endemic area was within the adequate range but somewhat lower than that of residents of nonendemic areas (i.e., plasma

Table 8.16

Selenium Status of Children in Kaschin-Beck Disease-Endemic and
Non-endemic Areas of China

Hair Se (ppb)		
Endemic areas	Non-endemic areas	Reference
$81 \pm 11 \ (19)^a$	$195 \pm 11 \ (25)^a$	$(7)^b$
$77 \pm 8 \ (25)^a$	$144 \pm 14 \ (20)^a$	
$81 \pm 2 \ (42)^{ac}$	$251 \pm 54 \ (22)^a$	
$165 \pm 7 \ (41)^{ad}$	$357 \pm 19 \ (20)^a$	
49 ± 10^e	93 ± 8^e	(11)
$71 \ (389)^f$	$208 \ (353)^f$	(14)
$72 \ (2)^g$	$231 \pm 118 \ (4)^h$	$(15)^b$
$84 \pm 17 \ (13)^h$	$228 \pm 78 \ (9)^h$	
$59 \pm 21 \ (25)^h$	$212 \pm 67 \ (16)^h$	
$68 \pm 29 \ (9)^h$	$167 \pm 55 \ (15)^h$	
	$392 \pm 171 \ (9)^h$	
	$2965 \pm 1221 \ (8)^h$	
$44 \pm 2 \ (86)^h$	$212 \pm 6 \ (16)^h$	(162)

[a] Mean $\pm$ SEM (n).
[b] Results of different sampling sites reported.
[c] Blood Se was 16 ± 2 ppb (n = 10).
[d] Blood Se was 21 ± 2 ppb (n = 16).
[e] Mean $\pm$ SD, n not reported.
[f] Mean (n); no estimate of variance reported.
[g] No estimate of variance calculable.
[h] Mean $\pm$ SD (n).

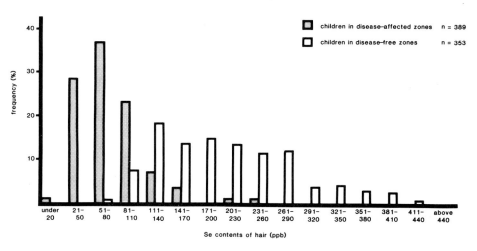

Fig. 8.15 Frequency distributions of hair Se in children in Kaschin-Beck disease-affected areas ($n = 389$) and in nonaffected areas ($n = 353$) of Shaanxi Province, China. Drawn from the data of Li et al.[14]

vitamin E concentrations were 0.85 ± 0.18 mg/dl and 1.02 ± 0.20 mg/dl, respectively). Like Keshan disease, Kaschin-Beck disease is a disease of children; however, unlike the cardiomyopathy, which is most prevalent among children aged 2-7 years, the big joint disease appears to be more prevalent among older children (e.g., 84% of cases in Gansu Province were among children aged 6-15 years[164]; see Table 8.17). Hou et al.,[164] however, have stated that the disease has been diagnosed by radiographic examination as early as 13 weeks of age. Hou et al.[164] stated that Kaschin-Beck disease occurs more frequently in the winter and spring months, during which time changes in food intake patterns result in decreases in nutritional Se status. The limited published information (see Table 8.18) supports this suggestion that some seasonal variation in Se status may occur in Kaschin-Beck disease-endemic areas.

Studies of the effects of Se supplementation in the prevention and therapy of Kaschin-Beck disease have yielded some encouraging results. A study conducted in Gansu Province, China, reported that combined Se (oral administration of an aqueous solution of Na_2SeO_3 weekly according to age: under 5 years., 0.5 mg; 6-10 years., 1.0 mg; above 10 years., 2.0 mg) and vitamin E therapy (either weekly intramuscular injections of 100 IU or oral administration of 65 IU/day) was effective in the recovery of 83% of cases diagnosed radiographically; however, results from control treatment groups were not reported. The results of two controlled Se-intervention studies were summarized by Liang et al.[162] Those studies evaluated the efficacy of Se-supplementation of the susceptible population in Kaschin-

Table 8.17

Age-Distribution of Different Clinical Types of Kaschin-Beck Disease[a]

Age	Metaphyseal type	Epiphyseal type	Distal phalanges	Bone joint type	Total cases
<5 yrs	24	5	0	0	29(13%)[b]
6-10 yrs	60	37	3	0	100 (45%)[b]
11-15 yrs	15	62	8	3	88 (39%)[b]
>16 yrs	1	0	3	3	7 (3%)[b]
Total cases	100 (45%)[b]	104 (46%)[b]	14 (6%)[b]	6 (3%)[b]	224 (100%)[d]
Cases recovered after Se-vitamin E therapy[c]	100 (100%)[d]	87 (84%)[d]	0 (0%)[d]	0 (0%)[d]	187 (83%)[d]

[a]Data from Kaschin-Beck Disease Prevention and Therapy Research Team, Ning County, Gansu Province.[161]

[b]Percentage total cases shown in parentheses.

[c]Details of therapy not reported.

[d]Percentage original cases of respective type shown in parentheses.

Beck disease-endemic areas by the use of weekly oral supplements of Na_2SeO_3 in tablet form (3-10 years., 1 mg Se; 10-13 years., 2 mg Se) or by the routine food use of Na_2SeO_3-supplemented (20 ppm Se) table salt. The results (see Table 8.19) showed that the Se tablets were effective in reducing the severity and in facilitating improvement of Kaschin-Beck disease cases; however, intervention via selenized salt was ineffective. A study reported by Li et al.[165] (Table 8.20) indicates that the use of Na_2SeO_3 tablets for long-term Se intervention in a susceptible population reduced the incidence of Kaschin-Beck disease substantially; however, that conclusion is based only upon the disease incidence in an historic control.

Table 8.18

Seasonal Effects on Selenium Status of Residents of
Kaschin-Beck Disease Areas of Shaanxi Province, China

Month	Hair Se (ppb)		Urine Se ($\mu g/24$ hrs)[a]		Reference
	Site I	Site II	Site I	Site II	
Mar	175 ± 14 (17)	110 ± 7 (20)	4.96 ± 0.49 (16)	2.88 ± 0.22 (21)	(9)
Jan	257 ± 20 (20)	144 ± 10 (26)	4.90 ± 0.41 (24)	3.93 ± 0.40 (29)	
Sep	211 ± 19 (20)	200 ± 17 (25)	5.30 ± 0.55 (18)	3.82 ± 0.37 (2)	
Dec	156 ± 18 (17)	122 ± 10 (23)	4.05 ± 0.30 (17)	3.79 ± 0.28 (21)	
	Site III	Site IV			
Apr	121 ± 16 (6)	32 ± 7 (7)	—	—	(11)
Aug	128 ± 34 (25)	48 ± 26 (21)	—	—	
Feb	134 ± 50 (10)	33 ± 9 (8)	—	—	
Jun	139 ± 41 (10)	63 ± 22 (10)	—	—	

[a]Mean $\pm$ SD (n).

Table 8.19

Effects of Selenium-Supplementation for One Year, by Oral Tablets or Selenized Table Salt, on the Course of Kaschin-Beck Disease in Children in Shaanxi Province, China[a]

Parameter	Se-tablet study		Se-salt study	
	Control	Se-treatment	Control	Se-treatment
Subjects observed	204	220	151	409
Hair Se (ppb)				
Before study	40 ± 2^{b}	40 ± 3^{b}	—	—
After study	47 ± 2^{b}	278 ± 46^{b}	—	—
Radiographic findings				
Total cases detected	174 (85%)[c]	182 (83%)[c]	105 (70%)[c]	266 (65%)[c]
Moderate metaphyseal lesions	159 (78%)	166 (75%)	31 (20%)	110 (27%)
Severe metaphyseal lesions	56 (27%)	15 (7%)	6 (4%)	32 (8%)
Clinical findings				
Cases examined	159	166	52	152
Worsened	30	0	6	6
No changes	66	30	12	45
Marked improvement	4	27	2	31
Moderate improvement	38	86	15	27
Slight improvement	21	23	18	43
Total improved	63 (40%)[d]	136 (82%)[d]	35 (67%)[d]	101 (66%)[d]

[a]From Liang et al.[162]

[b]Mean ± SD for subsample; n not reported.

[c]Percentage subjects observed indicated in parentheses.

[d]Percentage cases examined indicated in parentheses.

The etiology of Kaschin-Beck disease is unclear at the present time. However, the coincidence of its endemic distribution with that of severe environmental Se-deficiency and the apparent effectiveness of supplemental Se in reducing its incidence and/or severity both suggest that Se plays some role in the etiology of Kaschin-Beck disease. While the "big joint disease" cannot be considered a manifestation of Se-deficiency per se, present evidence indicates that it can be considered a Se-responsive disorder in humans.

IV. SELENIUM STATUS OF PATIENTS WITH OTHER NONMALIGNANT DISEASES

Several investigators have assessed the Se status of patients with a variety of diseases to determine whether altered Se nutrition and/or metabolism may be involved in these diseases, either as a contributing agent or a consequence. Those studies for which the Se status of healthy controls

Table 8.20

Incidence of Kaschin-Beck Disease Among Children in Gansu Province, China, after Selenium Intervention[a]

Year	Children examined[b]	Cases diagnosed
Before Se-intervention		
1977	47	20 (43%)[c]
After Se-intervention:[d]		
1978	46	11 (24%)[e]
1979	49	11 (22%)
1980	51	10 (20%)
1981	52	6 (12%)
1982	48	4 (8%)
1983	49	2 (4%)

[a]Data of Li et al.[165]

[b]Radiographic examination of the right hand, children aged 3-10 years.

[c]Percentage total children examined shown in parentheses.

[d]Children aged <6 years given 0.5 mg Se (as Na_2SeO_3) per child per week as oral tablet; children 6-10 years given 1.0 mg Se (as Na_2SeO_3) per child per week as oral tablet; lactating women given 2.0 mg Se (as Na_2SeO_3) per women per week as oral tablets.

[e]All intervention-years incidences significantly different from pre-intervention results, $p < .001$.

was also assessed are summarized in Tables 8.21 and 8.22. Data from patients with malignant diseases have not been included in these tables; those data are included in the discussion on Se and cancer (Chapter 10).

Altered Se status has been found consistently in association with relatively few human diseases. Reduced blood Se levels (by 21-60%) have been measured in patients with alcoholic liver disease[66] and cirrhosis[57,75,84]; however, these effects may be without significant biological consequences inasmuch as they have not been found to be associated with reductions in blood SeGSHpx.[57] Patients with neuronal ceroid lipofuscinosis,[28] acrodermatitis enteropathica,[28] kwashiorkor,[41] and chronic renal failure[75] have been found to show reductions in blood Se by 17-45%, while patients with muscular dystrophy have been found with increased (by ca. 40%) plasma Se levels.[31] Multiple sclerosis patients have had reductions of blood SeGSHpx by as much as 23%[43,101]; yet their plasma Se concentrations appear not to be affected.[43,58,73] Particularly interesting are the consistent reports of decreases in plasma Se concentrations (by ca. 27%) among patients with Down's syndrome (trisomy 21),[4,36,37] even though these individuals also show increased (by ca. 55%) erythrocyte SeGSHpx.[37,103] Many of these apparent differences in Se status between healthy persons and those with particular diseases may relate to differences in diet and, therefore, in Se intake. Such an effect is to be expected in the case of a disorder such as kwashiorkor

Table 8.21

Selenium Status Reported for Patients with Selected Nonmalignant Diseases

Disease	Country	Plasma/serum Se (ppb)		Whole blood Se (ppb)		Reference
		Patients	Controls	Patients	Controls	
Liver diseases						
Alcoholic liver disease	Sweden	78 ± 6 (15)[a]	80 ± 3 (16)	—	—	(57)
	USA	38 ± 7 (16)[c]	95 ± 16 (27)	47 ± 6 (16)[c]	109 ± 14 (27)	(66)
Cirrhosis	Sweden	59 ± 2 (22)	80 ± 3 (16)	69 ± 5 (22)	94 ± 5 (16)	(57)
	USA	90 ± 20 (14)	120 ± 10 (37)	—	—	(84)
	USA	62 ± 4 (18)[df]	94 ± 2 (92)	—	—	(75)
	USA	74 ± 5 (18)[df]	94 ± 2 (92)[d]	—	—	(75)
Chronic active hepatitis	USA	98 ± 14 (4)[d]	94 ± 2 (92)[d]	—	—	(75)
Lung disease						
chronic obstructive pulmonary disease	USA	130 ± 30 (22)	120 ± 10 (37)	—	—	(84)
Pancreatic diseases						
Alcoholic pancreatitis	USA	110 ± 30 (13)	120 ± 10 (37)	—	—	(84)
Diabetes	USA	130 ± 50 (19)	120 ± 10 (37)	—	—	(84)
	Sweden	74 ± 8 (27)[b]	65 ± 8 (13)	—	—	(60)
Cystic fibrosis	France	63 ± 15 (24)[c]	82 ± 13 (20)	—	—	(4)
Gastrointestinal disorders						
Gastric ulcer	USA	120 ± 20 (11)	120 ± 10 (37)	—	—	(84)
Short bowel syndrome	Norway	117 ± 32 (12)	153 ± 25 (30)	—	—	(55)

(continues)

Table 8.21 (Continued)

Disease	Country	Plasma/serum Se (ppb)		Whole blood Se (ppb)		Reference
		Patients	Controls	Patients	Controls	
Neuromuscular disorders						
	USA	76±15 (30)	88±8 (27)	—	—	(165)
Muscular dystrophy, Becker type	Finland	89±18 (2)	60±15 (5)	—	—	(31)
Muscular dystrophy, Duchenne type	Finland	78±21 (5)	60±15 (5)	—	—	(31)
	Finland	—	—	45±10 (6)	60±14 (13)	(28)
Multiple sclerosis	Sweden	77±18 (15)	81±14 (50)	—	—	(58)
	USA	107±4 (27)^d	104±2^{de}	—	—	(73)
	Italy	86±16 (20)^c	61±18 (16)	—	—	(43)
Spinal muscular atrophies	Australia	—	—	70-160 (8)^i	90-150 (9)^i	(1)
Heart diseases						
Arteriosclerosis	USA	120±30 (42)	120±10 (37)	—	—	(84)
	USA	105±4 (33)^d	136±7 (15)^d	—	—	(167)
	Finland	52 (283)^{fj}	55 (283)^j	—	—	(29)
Myocardial infarction	Finland	48±12 (13)	66±11 (21)	64±15 (13)	87±17 (25)	(28)
Cardiomyopathy^k	USA	—	—	35 (1)^l	70±160 (40)^i	(71)
	USA	106±29 (21)	—	—	—	(28)
Neurologic disorder						
Neuronal ceroid lipofuscinosis	Finland	49±7 (10)	60±14 (13)	37±10 (8)	51±14 (8)	(28)
Other diseases						
Arthritis	USA	120±30 (10)	120±10 (37)	—	—	(84)
Acrodermatitis enteropathica	Finland	37±8 (4)	51±14 (8)	59±13 (4)	60±14 (3)	(28)
Hypertension	USA	130±30 (9)	120±10 (37)	—	—	(84)
Fibrocystic disease	Japan	—	—	200±46 (10)	285±32 (25)	(44)
	USA	—	—	142±10 (8)	183±24 (14)	(44)

Down's syndrome (trisomy 21)	France	$71 \pm 14 (27)^c$	$96 \pm 21 (30)$	—	(4)
	France	$69 \pm 12 (13)^c$	$103 \pm 21 (10)$	—	(37)[g]
	France	$72 \pm 11 (10)^f$	$92 \pm 21 (22)$	—	(37)[h]
	France	$90 \pm 18 (28)^c$	$122 \pm 27 (32)$	—	(36)
Pre-eclampsia	Finland	$51 \pm 10 (21)$	$52 \pm 7 (11)$	—	(125)
Kwashiorker	Guatemala	$55 (2)^j$	$100 \pm 20 (6)$	$80 \pm 20 (6)^c$	(41)
Psychoses	USA	$120 \pm 40 (11)$	$120 \pm 10 (37)$	$140 \pm 10 (6)$	(84)
Infection	USA	$120 \pm 30 (14)$	$120 \pm 10 (37)$	—	(84)
Chronic cholecystitis	USA	$89 \pm 14 (9)^d$	$94 \pm 2 (92)^d$	—	(84)
Chronic renal failure	USA	$78 \pm 3 (49)^{df}$	$94 \pm 2 (92)^d$	—	(75)

[a] Mean ± SD (*n*) unless otherwise noted.
[b] Significantly different from control group ($p < .05$).
[c] Significantly different from control group ($p < .001$).
[d] Mean ± SEM.
[e] Value of *n* not reported.
[f] Significantly different from control group ($p < .01$).
[g] Patients less than 15 years of age.
[h] Patients 15 years of age or older.
[i] Range of observations.
[j] No estimate of variance reported or calculable.
[k] Does not include Keshan Disease in China (see Table 8.13).
[l] Measurement of single patient.

Table 8.22

Glutathione Peroxidase Activities[a] Reported for Patients with Selected Nonmalignant Disease

Disease	Country	Plasma (nmoles NADPH/min/ml)		Erythrocytes (μmoles NADPH/min/mg protein)	
		Patients	Controls	Patients	Controls
Alcoholic liver disease	Sweden	508 ± 37 (15)[b,c]	561 ± 26 (16)[b,c]	—	—
Liver cirrhosis	Sweden	595 ± 30 (21)[b,c]	561 ± 26 (16)[b,c]	—	—
Celiac disease	Ireland	—	—	28.5 ± 5.8 (19)[e]	38–194[e,f]
Multiple sclerosis	Denmark	—	—	18.9 ± 4.8 (27)[c,d]	139.9 ± 52.3 (22)[c]
	Israel	—	—	24.2 ± 5.4 (10)[e,g]	143.9 ± 29.9 (22)[e]
	Israel	—	—	6.21 ± 1.56 (20)[d,e]	—
	Italy	—	—	27.8 ± 2.0 (27)[e]	—
	USA	—	—	13.4 ± 2.6 (13)[c,i,j]	—
Down's syndrome (trisomy 21)	France	—	—	14.0 ± 2.6 (10)[c,i,k]	—
	Sweden	—	—	29.9 ± 6.9 (14)[c,d]	—

(continues)

Table 8.22 (Continued)

Disease	Country	Granulocytes (nmoles NADPH/min/mg protein)			Reference
		Patients	Controls		
Alcoholic liver disease	Sweden	—	—		(57)
Liver cirrhosis	Sweden	—	—		(57)
Celiac disease	Ireland	—	—		(100)
Multiple sclerosis	Denmark	4-25[efh]	13-61[efh]		(26)
	Israel	36.7 ± 11.5 (20)[cd]	36.5 ± 12.5 (21)[c]		(101)
		41.2 ± 11.2 (9)[eg]	40.7 ± 12.4 (21)[e]		
	Italy	35 ± 7 (20)[e]	40 ± 9 (16)[e]		(43)
	USA	—	—		(73)
Down's syndrome (trisomy 21)	France	—	—		(37)
	Sweden	—	—		(103)

[a] Mean ± SD (*n*), unless otherwise noted.
[b] Mean ± Se (*n*).
[c] Assayed using *t*-butyl hydroperoxide as acceptor substrate
[d] Significantly different form control group, $p < .01$.
[e] Assayed using H_2O_2 as acceptor substrate.
[f] Range of observations as reported by the authors.
[g] Significantly different from control group, $p < .05$.
[h] Value of *n* not reported by authors.
[i] Significantly different from control group, $p < .001$.
[j] Subjects less than or equal to 15 years of age.
[k] Subjects greater than 15 years of age.

377

wherein inadequate intake of protein, the vehicle for most dietary Se, results in the disease. Thus, Schwarz[168] found that administration of Se stimulated growth in two children with kwashiorkor. There is no evidence indicating abnormalities in Se metabolism in that or any other of these diseases.

Salonen et al.[29] found that low serum Se levels in Finnish subjects were associated with increased risk to cardiovascular disease. The more recent study of Luoma et al.[186] supports this hypothesis. Luoma et al.[186] conducted a double blind study in which Se (as a Se-enriched yeast product) or a placebo were given to a total of 26 healthy Finnish adults. They found that Se supplementation for 2 weeks resulted in increased activities of SeGHSpx (by 20%) and increased concentrations of Se (by 58%) and high density lipoprotein-bound cholesterol (HDLC) (by 43%) in serum. The increase in HDLC level was interpreted as possibly related to the decrease in cardiovascular disease risk observed by Salonen et al.[29]

Virtamo et al.[187] found, in a cohort of 1100 Finnish males of 55-74 years of age, that the adjusted relative risk of death to all causes was 1.4 (95% confidence interval: 1.0-2.0, $p > 0.05$) and to cardiovascular disease was 1.6 (95% confidence interval: 1.1-2.3, $p > 0.05$) among men with serum Se levels less than 45 ppb in comparison to those with higher serum levels of the element. Among men free of stroke at entry to the 5-year study, the adjusted relative risk to death to stroke of subjects with serum Se levels less than 45 ppb was 3.7 (95% confidence interval: 1.0-13.1, $p > 0.05$) in comparison to subjects with higher serum levels.

Low Se status, indicated by very low concentrations of the mineral in blood cells and/or plasma, has been identified in infants with the inborn errors of amino acid metabolism, maple syrup urine disease, or phenylketonuria.[38,39,169] These children have been found to have serum Se levels as low as 5 ppb[39] and erythrocyte SeGSHpx activities of only 10-20% of those of healthy children.[39,169] The basis of the low Se status of these patients, however, does not involve impairments in their abilities to assimilate Se; rather, it involves the use of parenteral nutrition fluids that have contained neglible amounts of Se in the management of these patients. Bratter et al.[38] found that infants (1-30 days, mostly newborns) maintained using a total parenteral feeding solution showed decreases in serum Se to ca. 50% of initial concentrations in 3-4 weeks and to ca. one-third of initial concentrations by 5 weeks.

Parenteral nutrition fluids, particularly those based upon amino acid mixtures, can be very low in Se if they are not supplemented with the element. Zabel et al.[170] found that amino acid-based total parenteral nutrition (TPN) solutions available in the USA provided less than 5 μg Se/1000 kcal, whereas TPN solutions based on casein hydrolysates provided 16-95 μg Se/1000 kcal (see Table 3.4). Similar findings have been reported in New Zealand[171] and Sweden.[172] Therefore, it is not surprising that several investigators have observed low Se status of patients maintained with TPN for extended periods of time.[165,172-180,198] Clinical signs have been reported in association with Se-deficiency in some of those individuals. Van Rij et al.[173] described one TPN-fed patient whose muscle pains, tenderness of the thighs, and resulting inability to walk responded within 1 week to Se supplementation. Kien and Ganther[178] reported the case of a boy who, after receiving TPN for about 1½ years, developed intermittant leg muscle pains and tenderness, with elevated serum enzyme activities (i.e., glutamic oxaloacetic transaminase, glutamic-pyruvic transaminase, creatine kinase). Six months later he developed whitened fingernail beds. His serum Se concentration at this time was later found to be only 3 ppb; intravenous supplementation with Se (42 μg Se/day as H_2SeO_3) raised this level to 20 ppb within 1 month and caused decreases in serum enzyme activities and improvement in nail bed condition. Although creatine kinase activities were increased in the serum, cardiologic evaluation revealed no evidence of impaired cardiac function.

Three cases of fatal cardiomyopathy have been reported in patients receiving long-term TPN.[161,174,176] Johnson et al.[175] reported the case of an adult male who, having been maintained with parenteral alimentation for 2 years, was found to be Se-deficient (i.e., 33 μg Se/g Hb) and of low vitamin E status (i.e., plasma level 0.40 mg/dl). On the third day after surgery for cholecystectomy, he experienced ventricular fibrillation that was followed by frequent ventricular extrasystoles and bursts of nonsustained ventricular tachycardia for several days. The patient developed pulmonary edema within 19 days; he died 29 days later. Post-mortem examination revealed an enlarged heart with irregular focal areas of myocyte loss and fibrous replacement scattered throughout the ventricular subepicardium. The authors, two of whom were thoroughly experienced in the pathology of Keshan disease, concluded that this cardiomyopathy resembled that disease.[175] Another case of a fatal cardiomyopathy associated with Se deficiency was reported in an adult male maintained for 6 years with home parenteral nutrition.[177] That patient had a whole blood Se concentration of only 12 ppb and had been found to have dilation of the left ventricle of the heart with poor left ventricular function. Post-mortem examination revealed widespread mulitfocal myocytolysis and replacement fibrosis similar to that described in Keshan disease. The third case was reported by Quercia et al.[161]; it involved a 42-year-old white male with Crohn's disease who had been maintained on total parenteral nutrition (TPN) for 8 years. After 6 years of TPN, he developed a gradual onset of thrombosis of the superior vena cava and was given anticoagulation therapy. After 7 years, he developed chest pains and occasional dyspnea; a chest roentgenogram showed some obstructive pulmonary disease but no cardiac enlargement. Three months later, he was hospitalized for severe chest pain and dyspnea. Electrocardiographic examination revealed sinus tachycardia with diffuse nonspecific ST- and T-wave changes. Chest roentgenograms revealed mild cardiomegaly and pulmonary edema with right pleural effusion. Six days after hospitalization, he developed ventricular fibrillation and died. At autopsy, the heart weighed 500 g; all chambers were dilated and the myocardium was found to be grossly flabby. Histological examination revealed multifocal myocardial necrosis with extensive fibrosis, particularly throughout the interventricular septum. The Se concentrations of the tissues were very low (i.e., plasma, <10 ppb; heart, 34 ppb; liver, 27 ppb; kidney, 102 ppb).

Levander[181] has discussed the importance of Se in TPN with regard to the potential for Se-deficiency in patients managed with this means for long periods of time. He recommended that TPN solutions should be supplemented with Se at appropriate concentrations to provide 25-30 μg Se/day, and that blood Se levels should be monitored to enable adjustments in the level of Se supplementation in such a way as to keep them in the normal range. He also suggested that the appropriate levels of Se-supplementation may be different for certain patients (e.g., those with compromised renal function, or losses of the gastric mucosa; Se-depleted patients). Levander[181] did not specify the most appropriate Se compound for use in the supplementation of TPN solutions; however, he did discuss the relative merits of the three most logical choices: selenites (i.e., sodium selenite, selenious acid, selenium dioxide), sodium selenate, and selenomethionine. Despite the fact that most current knowledge concerning the biological utilization of Se has employed Na_2SeO_3, the selenite form is known to be highly reactive and may, thus, be unstable in certain formulations. Selenomethionine is known to be well utilized; however, it may not serve as well for immediate metabolic demands for Se, as it is used rather indiscriminately in metabolism as its S-containing analog methionine. Selenate, with greater stability and good biological availability, would appear to be the form of choice for the supplementation of TPN solutions. Unfortunately, relatively little research has been conducted to date with this form; therefore, questions of relevance to this application (e.g., what is its metabolic utilization after intravenous delivery?) are unanswered at present.

V. OTHER FACTORS AFFECTING SELENIUM STATUS

Changes in Se status have been associated with exposure to several different types of drugs. Table 8.23 presents a summary of the results of studies that have examined the Se status in various groups of users of specific drugs with reference to appropriate controls. Mottonen et al.[182] found that patients using aurothiomalate for the treatment of rheumatoid arthritis had slight but significant increases (ca. 10%) in serum Se concentrations.* The use of steroid-type oral contraceptive agents has been associated with modest (ca. 9%) but significant increases in the Se levels of plasma and whole blood, apparently without affecting the Se or SeGSHpx levels of erythrocytes.[3,69] The consumption of ethanol has been associated with reduced Se status. Lloyd et al.[69] found that daily consumers of ethanol showed small (ca. 6%) but significant reductions of plasma Se; however, these individuals showed normal levels of Se in whole blood and of Se and SeGSHpx in erythrocytes. Alcoholics, on the other hand, have been found to have plasma Se concentrations reduced to as little as 40% of normal.[66] Dutta et al.[78] found that the urinary excretion of Se (as indicated by urine Se concentration) by alcoholics can be reduced to only about half of normal levels. Dworkin and Rosenthal[66] found that while alcoholics with severe liver disease showed levels of Se in whole blood, plasma, and erythrocytes of only 40-52% of those of healthy controls, well nourished symptom-free detoxified alcoholics also showed abnormally low values, although less severe (e.g., 68-73% of controls), for each of these parameters. The latter investigators concluded that Se should be added to the list of potential nutritional deficiencies in the alcoholic. Cigarette smokers have been found to have reduced blood Se levels in comparison to nonsmokers.[27,69] Ellis et al.[27] found that British smokers had significantly lower levels of Se in plasma and whole blood, and of SeGSHpx in erythrocytes, than nonsmokers. This was true of both drinking and nondrinking populations. These effects were also observed by Lloyd et al.,[69] but only in the older segment (i.e., 31-85 years.) of the population.

Selenium has been reported to have medical benefits in certain conditions that do not apparently involve reduced Se status. These include positive responses in the treatment of acne vulgaris,[185] arthritis,[187] and color vision loss in early diabetic retinopathy.[197] In addition Se, as ^{75}Se-selenomethionine, has been employed in the radiographic visualization of the pancreas.[189-191] In this use, ^{75}Se serves only as a convenient gamma-radiation emmitter (^{35}S emits less penetrating beta particles); it is readily taken up by the pancreas after intravenous administration by virtue of its innate tendency to take

---

*This observation is of interest as Chaudiere and Tappel[183] have demonstrated that aurothiomalate and other gold compounds to be potent in vitro inhibitors of SeGSHpx. Mercurio and Combs[183] found that a related antiarthritic drug, aurothioglucose, both inhibited SeGSHpx and exacerbated the Se- and vitamin E-deficiency disease exudative diathesis in the chick.

Table 8.23

Effects of Selected Drugs, Alcohol, and Tobacco on Se Status

Factor	Country	Group	Whole blood Se (ppb)	Plasma/serum Se (ppb)	Erythrocyte Se		Reference
					ppb	μg/g Hb	
Chlorthalidone[b]	Sweden	Controls	—	190±60 (10)[c]	—	—	(59)
		Before treatment	—	170±50 (10)	—	—	
		5 days treatment	—	190±50 (10)	—	—	
	Sweden	Before treatment	—	170±50 (4)	—	—	(61)
		6 months treatment	—	180±70 (4)	—	—	
Aurothiomalate[d]	Finland	Before treatment	—	75±9 (18)	—	—	(181)
		3 months treatment	—	88±13 (18)[e]	—	—	
		6 months treatment	—	93±18 (18)[e]	—	—	
Oral contraceptives[f]	England	Controls	136±17 (61)	113±16 (61)	—	0.504±0.078 (61)	(69)
		Users	143±18 (45)	121±17 (45)[e]	—	0.514±0.081 (45)	
	Belgium	Controls	122±14 (30)	93±12 (29)	168±29 (28)	—	(3)
		Users	126±17 (23)	101±10 (23)	157±30 (23)	—	
Alcohol	England	Nondrinkers	139±23 (43)	120±16 (43)	0.485±0.085 (43)	—	(69)
		"Weekend" drinkers	139±14 (58)	120±13 (58)	—	0.477±0.070 (58)	
		Daily drinkers	137±17 (48)	112±16 (48)[e]	—	0.490±0.074 (48)	
	USA	Controls	—	131±10 (12)	—	0.679±0.05 (12)	(78)
		Alcoholics	—	111±50 (9)[h]	—	0.630±0.05 (9)	
	USA	Control	109±14 (27)	95±16 (27)	126±22 (27)	—	(66)
		Detoxified alcoholics	76±10 (30)[i]	65±12 (30)[i]	92±16 (30)[i]	—	
		Alcoholics with liver disease	47±6 (16)[i]	38±7 (16)[i]	66±12 (16)[i]	—	

Tobacco	England	Nonsmokers	134 ± 20 (66)	115 ± 16 (66)	—	(27)
		Cigarette smokers	115 ± 11 (41)[i]	98 ± 11 (41)[i]	—	(27)
		Pipe, cigar smokers	122 ± 21 (9)	106 ± 13 (9)	—	
		Nondrinkers				
		Nonsmokers	133 ± 17 (15)	112 ± 12 (15)	—	(27)
		Cigarette smokers	115 ± 9 (7)[e]	102 ± 10 (7)	—	
		Daily drinkers				
		Nonsmokers	138 ± 23 (29)	114 ± 19 (29)	—	(27)
		Cigarette smokers	114 ± 12 (18)[i]	95 ± 10 (18)[i]	—	
	England	18-30 yrs				
		Nonsmokers	135 ± 15 (60)	114 ± 14 (60)	.477 ± 0.065 (60)	(69)
		Smokers	137 ± 18 (29)	113 ± 14 (29)	.490 ± 0.081 (29)	(69)
		31-85 yrs				
		Nonsmokers	141 ± 19 (93)	120 ± 16 (93)	.489 ± 0.086 (93)	(69)
		Smokers	122 ± 13 (26)[j]	108 ± 13 (26)[i]	.411 ± 0.54 (26)[j]	(69)

(continues)

Table 8.23 (*Continued*)

Factor	Country	Group	Erthrocyte glutathione peroxidase[a] (μmoles NADPH/min/g Hb)	Urinary Se (μg/24 hr)	Reference
Chlorthalidone[b]	Sweden	Controls	—	30 ± 14 (16)	(59)
		Before treatment	—	36 ± 14 (16)	
		5 days treatment	—	32 ± 11 (61)	
	Sweden	Before treatment	—	38 ± 12 (5)	
		6 months treatment	—		
Aurothiomalate[d]	Finland	Before treatment	—	—	(181)
		3 months treatment	—	—	
		6 months treatment	—	—	
Oral contraceptives[f]	England	controls	19.1 ± 4.3 (61)	—	(69)
		Users	19.1 ± 5.0 (45)	—	
	Belgium	Controls	—	—	(3)
		Users	—	—	
Alcohol	England	Nondrinkers	20.7 ± 5.8 (43)	—	(69)
		"Weekend" drinkers	20.3 ± 4.9 (58)	—	
		Daily drinkers	20.1 ± 5.3 (48)	—	
	USA	Controls	—	53 ± 11 (12)[g]	(78)
		Alcoholics	—	29 ± 3 (9)[gh]	
	USA	Control	—	—	(66)
		Detoxified alcoholics	—	—	
		Alcoholics with liver disease	—	—	

Tobacco	England	Nonsmokers	17.9 ± 3.5 (66)	—	(27)
		Cigarette smokers	$16.5 \pm 3.6 (41)^e$	—	
		Pipe, cigar smokers	18.4 ± 4.4 (9)	—	
		Nondrinkers			(27)
		Nonsmokers	19.1 ± 3.9 (15)	—	
		Cigarette smokers	$15.7 \pm 2.2 (7)^e$	—	
		Daily drinkers			(27)
		Nonsmokers	17.9 ± 3.7 (29)	—	
		Cigarette smokers	17.3 ± 3.9 (18)	—	
	England	18-30 yrs			(69)
		Nonsmokers	19.6 ± 4.6 (60)	—	
		Smokers	20.7 ± 5.1 (29)	—	
		31-85 yrs			(69)
		Nonsmokers	20.7 ± 5.6 (93)	—	
		Smokers	17.8 ± 4.4 (26)		

[a] Measured using t-butyl hydroperoxide as the acceptor substrate.

[b] An antihypertensive drug.

[c] Mean $\pm$ SD (n).

[d] An anti-arthritic drug.

[e] Significantly different from control group, $p < 0.05$.

[f] Steroid type.

[g] Estimated from the authors' report.

[h] Significantly different from control group, $p < 0.005$.

[i] Significantly different from control group, $p < 0.001$.

[j] Significantly different from control group, $p < 0.0001$.

385

Table 8.24

Selenium Status of Chinese Subjects after 8 Months of Consumption of Selenium-Supplements[a]

Supplemental Se[b] (μg/person/day)	Whole blood Se (ppb)	Hair Se (ppb)	Toenail Se (ppb)	Urinary Se (μg/24 hr)
0	29 ± 1[c]	164 ± 19	169 ± 19	4.8 ± 1.7
10	50 ± 2	252 ± 14	241 ± 30	8.7 ± 1.8
30	89 ± 13	373 ± 40	396 ± 30	15.9 ± 3.8
60	118 ± 39	503 ± 77	618 ± 102	25.7 ± 4.1
90	178 ± 6	591 ± 22	796 ± 163	39.3 ± 9.4

[a]Data of Yang et al.[6]

[b]Provided as DL-selenomethionine, April–November 1983, with a diet that provided an additional 10 μg Se/person/day.

[c]Mean ± SE (n = 8 or 9).

up methionine and its inability to descriminate between the S- and Se-containing analogs of this amino acid.

VI. DIETARY REQUIREMENTS FOR SELENIUM

The dietary requirements of humans have been reviewed by Levander[199,200] and Yang et al.,[6] and in 1980 the Food and Nutrition Board of the National Research Council, U. S. National Academy of Sciences, identified ranges of "safe and adequate" intakes of Se for the U. S. population.[195] As discussed by Levander,[199] the approach used by the Food and Nutrition Board in delineating those ranges was to extrapolate from nutritional experiments with animals on the basis of dietary concentrations that were adequate to prevent overt signs of nutritional Se-deficiency. According to this approach, because dietary levels of 0.1-0.2 ppm are adequate for most animals, intakes in the range of 50-100 μg/day are indicated as adequate for humans consuming an average of 500 g of food (dry matter) per day. Appropriate adjustments were made for individuals at different life cycle stages; slightly higher upper limits were used to allow for possible beneficial effects of high levels of Se intake, while still providing a caution against the potential hazards of toxicity at high levels. While it is not clear whether this kind of extrapolation from animals to humans is appropriate, the ranges so derived are compatible with the levels of Se found experimentally (e.g., 66-70 μg per person per day) to maintain Se balance in Americans.[67,74] These ranges of intake also specify minimal levels of Se at which human Se-related disorders (e.g., Keshan disease, Kaschin-Beck disease) have not been associated. It is apparent, therefore, that the "safe and adequate" ranges of the 1980 Food and Nutrition Board are sufficient to support good Se nutrition of the general U. S. population.

Another approach to the estimation of the dietary requirements of humans for Se is to evaluate the results of human nutritional studies and dietary surveys. The results of the available studies of this type are summarized in Tables 8.24 and 8.25. These results show that estimates of human dietary Se needs vary directly with the general Se status of the target population; i.e., lower Se levels have been identified among the known low-Se people (Chinese, Finns, New Zealanders) than among those of higher general Se exposure (e.g., Americans, English). A portion, but not all, of this effect appears to be due to regional differences in average body size. Another contributor to this apparent discrepancy is the difference in parameters of Se adequacy that have been used in different circumstances; thus, prevention from overt Se-related disease appears to be achieved with daily intakes of ca. 0.3 µg Se/kg body weight (i.e., 20 µg Se/day for a 70-kg man) while optimal levels of SéGSHpx are not maintained at levels of Se intake less than ca. 0.7 µg Se/kg body weight/day (i.e., ca. 50 µg Se/day for a 70 kg man). And individuals with greater previous rates of Se intake (e.g., Americans consuming 80-200 µg Se/day) have greater needs to maintain Se balance at that level. The present authors consider the minimal dietary requirement for Se to be that level of intake that prevents overt clinical problems (e.g., cardiomyopathy); that level is estimated to be ca. 0.3 µg/kg body weight/day. However, because biochemical indications of subadequate Se deficiency (i.e., SeGSHpx deficiency) may have subtle but important deleterious metabolic consequences, such as enhanced sensitivity to oxidant stress in infection or xenobiotic exposure, the present authors consider 0.7 µg Se/kg body weight/day to be a minimal healthy level of Se intake. A daily allowance of ca. 0.85 µg Se/kg body weight should provide an adequate margin (of 20%) to accommodate the individual variation in healthy populations. The present authors, therefore, propose that daily allowances of ca. 50-60 µg Se* support adequate Se nutriture in healthy adults of Eastern and Western populations.†

---

*Calculated on the basis of average body weights of 58-70 kg.

†These allowances do not take into account the putative relationship of higher Se status and reduction in cancer risk (see Chapter 10). Should the results of current randomized double blind Se-intervention trials indicate that higher intakes of Se may reduce cancer risk, then these allowances will need re-evaluation.

Table 8.25

Estimates of Minimum Daily Selenium Needs of Adults in Several Countries

Country	Estimated Se need[a]		Method/rationale	Reference
	μg/person/day	μg/kg body weight/day		
China	16-20	0.3[b]	Apparently adequate natural intake in "safety islands" from Keshan disease	(6)
	40	0.7[b]	Amount needed to maintain optimal levels of SeGSHpx in plasma after 5 months of feeding	(6)
	17-30	0.3-0.5[b]	Intake associated with prevention of Keshan disease in Se-intervention studies	(7)
	30	0.5[b]	Apparently adequate natural intake in areas unaffected by Keshan disease	(13)
England	60	0.9[c]	Natural level of intake associated with no apparent ill health effects	(192)
Finland	30	0.5[c]	Natural level of intake associated with no apparent ill health effects	(193)
New Zealand	30	0.5[c]	Natural level of intake associated with no apparent ill health effects	(53)
	28	0.4[c]	Natural level of intake associated with no apparent ill health effects	(102)
	20	0.3[c]	Amount needed to maintain Se balance experimentally	(194)
USA	70	1.1[c]	Amount needed to maintain Se balance in a depletion-repletion study	(67)
	66	1.0[c]	Amount needed to maintain Se balance experimentally	(74)

[a] In general, values represent averages for both sexes.
[b] Assumed average body weight for both sexes to be ca. 58 kg.
[c] Assumed average body weight for both sexes to be ca. 65 kg.

REFERENCES

1. Pearn, J., and McCrary, C. W. R., Blood selenium in chronic spinal muscular dystrophy, J. Neurol. Sci., 42, 199, 1979.
2. Verlinden, M., Van Sprundel, M., Van der Auwera, J. C., and Eylenbosch, W. J., The selenium status of Belgian population groups. II. Newborns, children, and the aged, Biol. Trace Elem. Res., 5, 103, 1983.
3. Verlinden, M., van Sprundel, M., Van der Auwera, J. C., and Eylenbasch, W. J., The selenium status of Belgian population groups. I. Healthy adults, Biol. Trace Elem. Res., 5, 91, 1983.
4. Neve, J., Molle, L., Hanocq, M., Sinet, P. M., and Van Geffel, R., Erythrocyte and plasma trace element levels in clinical assessments. Zinc, copper and selenium in normals and patients with Down's Syndrome and cystic fibrosis, Biol. Trace Elem. Res., 5, 75, 1983.
5. Dickson, R. C., and Tomlison, R. H., Selenium in blood and human tissues, Clin. Chim. Acta, 16, 311, 1967.
6. Yang, G. Q., Zhu, L. Z., Liu, S. J., Gu, L. Z., Qian, P. C., Huang, J. H., and Lu, M. D., Studies of human selenium requirements in China, in *Proceedings of the Third International Symposium on Selenium in Biology and Medicine*, Combs, G. F., Jr., Spallholz, J. E., Levander, O. A., and Oldfield, J. E., eds., Avi Publ. Co., Westport, Conn., 1986.
7. Yang, G., Research on Se-related problems in human health in China, in *Proceedings of the Third International Symposium on Selenium in Biology and Medicine*, Combs, G. F., Jr., Spallholz, J.E, Levander, O. A., and Oldfield, J. E., eds., Avi Publ. Co., Westport, Conn., 1986.
8. Yang, G. Q., Wang, G. Y., Yin, T. A., Sun, S. Z., Zhou, R. H., Man, R. E., Zhai, F. Y., Guo, S. H., Wang, H. Z., and You, D. Q., Relationship between distribution of Keshan disease and selenium status, Acta Nutr. Sinica, 3, 199, 1982.
9. Mo, D., Pathology and selenium deficiency in Kaschin-Beck disease, in *Proceedings of the Third International Symposium on Selenium in Biology and Medicine,* Combs, G. F., Jr., Spallholz, J. E., Levander, O. A., and Oldfield, J. E., eds., Avi Publ. Co., Westport, Conn., 1986.
10. Yin, J. A., Sun, S. Z., Wang, T. Z., You, D. Q., and Yang, Q. Q., The difference between selenium excretion of children in Keshan Disease endemic and nonendemic areas, Chin. J. Med., 13, 207, 1979.
11. Li, J., Ren, S., Chen, D., Wan, H., Liang, S., Zhang, F., and Gao, F., The distribution of selenium in microenvironment related to Kaschin-Beck Disease, in *Proceedings of the Third International Symposium on Selenium in Biology and Medicine*, Combs, G. F., Jr., Spallholz, J. E., Levander, O. A., and Oldfield, J. E., eds., Avi Publ. Co., Westport, Conn., 1986.
12. Wang, G. Y., Zhou, R. H., Sun, S. Z., Yin, T. A., Wang, H. Z., You, D. Q., and Yang, G. Q., The difference of blood and hair selenium content in residents of Keshan Disease endemic and non-endemic areas — correlation between blood and hair Se, Chin. J. Prev. Med., 13, 204, 1979.
13. Keshan Disease Research Group of the Chinese Academy of Medical Sciences, Epidemiological studies on the etiologic relationship of selenium and Keshan disease, Chin. Med. J., 92, 477, 1979.
14. Li, J., Ren, S., and Cheng, D., A study on relationship between Kaschin-Beck Disease and selenium from Se contents in human hair of various natural environments in Shaanxi Province, Huanjing Kexue, 2, 5, 1981.

15. Li, J., Ren, S., and Cheng, D., A study of selenium associated with Kaschin-Beck disease in different environments in Shaanxi, Acta Scientnae Circumstantiae, 2, 1, 1982.

16. Zhang, F., Ji, L., Wu, T., and Deng, J., Relationship between Se in hair and cancers of the digestive tract and a new method for determining Se in hair, in *Proceedings of the Third International Symposium on Selenium in Biology and Medicine*, Combs, G. F., Jr., Spallholz, J. E., Levander, O. A., and Oldfield, J. E., eds., Avi Publ. Co., Westport, Conn., 1986.

17. Chen, X. S., Yang, G. Q., Chen, J. S., Chen, X. C., Wen, Z. M., and Ge, K. Y., Studies on the relations of selenium and Keshen disease, Biol. Trace Elem. Res., 2, 91, 1980.

18. Environmental and endemic disease sections, Institute of Geography, Chinese Academy of Sciences, Geographical distribution of selenium content in human hair in Keshan-disease and non-disease areas in China, Acta Geogr. Sinica, 37, 1, 1982.

19. Cheng, Y. Y., Studies on the relationships between selenium and Keshan disease in Sichuan, in *Proceedings of the Third International Symposium on Selenium in Biology and Medicine*, Combs, G. F., Jr., Spallholz, J. E., Levander, O. A., and Oldfield, J. E., eds., Avi Publ. Co., Westport, Conn., 1986.

20. Wen, Z. M., Chen, X. S., Fu, P., Qian, P. C., Liu, R. W., and Huang, J. H., Effect of long-term selenium supplementation on the incidence of Keshan Disease, in *Proceedings of the Third International Symposium on Selenium in Biology and Medicine*, Combs, G. F., Jr., Spallholz, J. E., Levander, O. A., and Oldfield, J. E., eds., Avi Publ. Co., Westport, Conn., 1986.

21. Sun, S. Z., Yin, T. A., Wang, T. A., You, D. Q., and Yang, G. Q., The relation between the high incidences and the selenium content of human hair, Chin. J. Prev. Med., 14, 171, 1980.

22. Yang, G. Q., Yin, T. A., Sun, S. Z., Wang, H. Z., and You, D. Q., The selenium status of Keshan Disease susceptible population, Chin. J. Prev. Med., 14, 14, 1980.

23. The group of environmental and endemic disease, Institute of Geography, Academica Sinica, The relation of Keshan Disease to the natural environment and the background of selenium nutrition, Acta Nutr. Sinica, 4, 175, 1982.

24. Chu, Y., Liu, Q., Hou, C., and Yu, S., Blood selenium concentration in residents of areas in China having a high incidence of lung cancer, Biol. Trace Elem. Res., 6, 133, 1984.

25. Liu, B. S., and Li, S. S., Primary study of relationship between endemic selenosis and fluorosis, in *Proceedings of the Third International Symposium on Selenium in Biology and Medicine*, Combs, G. F., Jr., Spallholz, J. E., Levander, O. A., and Oldfield, J. E., eds., Avi Publ. Co., Westport, Conn., 1986.

26. Jensen, G. E., and Clausen, J., Glutathione peroxidase and reductase, glucose-6-phosphate dehydrogenase and catalase activities in multiple sclerosis, J. Neurol. Sci., 63, 45, 1984.

27. Ellis, N., Lloyd, B., Lloyd, R. S., and Clayton, B. E., Selenium and vitamin E in relation to risk factors for coronary heart disease, J. Clin. Pathol., 37, 200, 1984.

28. Westermarck, T., Selenium content of tissues in Finnish infants and adults with various diseases, and studies on the effects of selenium supplementation in normal ceroid lipofuscinosis patients, Acta Pharmacol. Toxicol., 41, 121, 1977.

29. Salonen, J. T., Alfthan, G., Huttunen, J. K., Pikkarainen, J., and Puska, P., Association between cardiovascular death and myocardial infarction and serum selenium in a matched-pair longitudinal study, Lancet, 2, 175, 1982.

30. Westermarck, T., Raunu, P., Kirjarinta, M., and Lappalainen, L., Selenium content of whole blood and serum in adults and children in different ages from different parts of Finland, Acta Pharmacol. Toxicol., 40, 465, 1977.

31. Westermarck, T., Rahola, T., Suomela, M., and Salmi, A., distribution of [75]Se- selenite in patients with progressive muscular dystrophy, N. Zealand Workshop in Trace Elem., 117, 1981.

32. Jaakola, K., Tummavuari, J., Pirineu, A., Kurkela, P., Tolonen, M., and Arstila, A. U., Selenium levels in whole blood of Finnish volunteers before and during organic and inorganic selenium supplementation, Scand. J. Clin. Lab. Invest., 43, 473, 1983.

33. Arvilommi, H., Poikonen, K., Jokinen, I., Muukkonen, O., Rasenen, L., Foreman, J., and Huttenen, J. K., Selenium and immune functions in humans, Infect. Immun., 41, 185, 1983.

34. Levander, O. A., Alfthan, G., Arilommi, H., Gred, C. G., Huttunen, J. K., Kataja, M., Koivistoinen, P., and Pikkarainen, J., Bioavailability of selenium to Finnish men as assessed by platelet glutathione peroxidase activity and other blood parameters, An. J. Clin. Nutr., 37, 887, 1983.

35. Salonen, J. T., Alfthan, G., Huttenen, J. K., and Puska, P., Association between serum selenium and the risk of cancer, Am. J. Epidemiol., 120, 342, 1984.

36. Neve, J., Sinet, P. M., Molle, L., and Nicole, A., Selenium, zinc and copper in Down's syndrome (trisomy 21): blood levels and relations with glutathione peroxidase and superoxide dismutase, Clin. Chim. Acta, 133, 209, 1983.

37. Sinet, P. M., Neve, J., Nicole, A., and Molle, L., Low plasma selenium in Down's syndrome (trisomy 21), Acta Pediatr. Scand., 73, 275, 1984.

38. Bratter, P., Negretti, S., and Rosick, V., The development of Se deficiency with total parenteral nutrition of infants, in *Proceeding of the Third International Symposium on Selenium in Biology and Medicine*, Combs, G. F., Jr., Spallholz, J. E., Levander, O. A., and Oldfield, J. E., eds., Avi Publ. Co., Westport, Conn., 1986.

39. Lombeck, I., Kasperek, K., Feinendegen, L. E., and Bremer, H. J., Serum-selenium concentrations in patients with maple syrup urine disease and phenylketonuria under dieto-therapy, Clin. Chim. Acta, 64, 57, 1975.

40. Behne, D., and Wolters, W., Selenium content and glutathione peroxidase activity in the plasma and erythrocytes of non-pregnant and pregnant women, J. Clin. Chem. Clin. Biochem., 17, 133, 1979.

41. Burk, R. F., Jr., Pearson, W. N., Wood, R. P., and Viteri, F., Blood-selenium levels and *in vitro* red blood cell uptake of ^{75}Se in Kwashiorkor, Am. J. Clin. Nutr., 20, 723, 1967.

42. Vernie, L. N., DeVries, M., Benckhuijsen, C., DeGoeij, J. J. M., and Zegers, C., Selenium levels in blood and plasma, and glutathione peroxidase activity in blood of breast cancer patients during adjuvant treatment with cyclophosphamide, methotrexate and 5-fluorouracil, Cancer Letts., 18, 283, 1983.

43. Mazella, G. L., Sinfurianai, E., Savoldi, F., Allegrini, M., Lanzola, E., and Scelsi, R., Blood cells glutathione perxodiase activity and selenium in multiple sclerosis, Exp. Neurol., 22, 442, 1983.

44. Schrauzer, G. N., Schrauzer, T., Mead, S., Kuehn, K., Yamamoto, H., and Araki, E., Selenium in the blood of Japanese and American women with and without breast cancer and fibrocystic disease, in *Proceeding of the Third International Symposium on Selenium in Biology and Medicine*, Combs, G. F., Jr., Spallholz, J. E., Levander, O. A., and Oldfield, J. E., eds., Avi Publ. Co., Westport, Conn., 1986.

45. Aihara, K., Nishi, Y., Hatano, S., Kihara, M., Yoshimitsu, K., Takeichi, N., Ito, T., Ezaki, H., and Usui, T., Zinc, copper, manganese and selenium metabolites in thyroid disease, Am. J. Clin. Nutr., 40, 25, 1984.

46. Hatano, S., Nishi, Y., and Usui, T., Plasma, selenium concentration in healthy Japanese children and adults determined by flameless atomic absorption spectrophotometry, J. Pediatr. Gastroenterol. Nutr., 3, 426, 1984.

47. Van Rij, A., Thomson, C. D., McKenzie, J. M., and Robinson, M. F., Selenium deficiency in total parenteral nutrition, Am. J. Clin., Nutr., 32, 2076, 1979.
48. Robinson, M. F., and Thomson, C. D., Se status of the food supply and residents of New Zealand, in *Proceeding of the Third International Symposium on Selenium in Biology and Medicine*, Combs, G. F., Jr., Spallholz, J. E., Levander, O. A., and Oldfield, J. E., eds., Avi Publ. Co., Westport, Conn., 1986.
49. Griffiths, N. M., and Thomson, C. D., Selenium in whole blood of New Zealand residents, N. Zealand Med. J., 80, 199, 1974.
50. Thomson, C. D., Robinson, M. F., Campbell, D. R., and Rea, H. M., Effect of prolonged supplementation with daily supplements of selenomethionine and sodium selenite on glutathione peroxidase activity in blood of New Zealand residents, Am. J. Clin. Nutr., 36, 24, 1982.
51. Thomson, C. D., Rea, H. M., Doesburg, V. M., and Robinson, M. F., Selenium concentrations and glutathione peroxidase activities in whole blood of New Zealand residents, Br. J. Nutr., 37, 457, 1977.
52. Rea, H. M., Thomson, C. D., Campbell, D. R., and Robinson, M. F., Relation between erythrocyte selenium concentrations and glutathione peroxidase (EC 1.11.1.9) activities of New Zealand residents and visitors to New Zealand, Br. J. Nutr., 42, 201, 1979.
53. Watkinson, J. H., Changes in blood selenium in New Zealand adults with time and importation of Australian wheat, Am. J. Clin. Nutr., 34, 9365, 1981.
54. Watkinson, J. H., The selenium status of New Zealanders, N. Zealand Med. J., 80, 202, 1974.
55. Aaseth, J., Aadland, E., and Thomassen, Y., Serum selenium in patients with short bowel syndrome, in *Proceedings of the Third International Symposium on Selenium in Biology and Medicine*, Combs, G. F., Jr., Spallholz, J. E., Levander, O. A., and Oldfield, J. E., eds., Avi Publ. Co., Westport, Conn., 1986.
56. Masiak, M., and Herzyk, D., Behaviour of microelements in lung cancer patients, Fresenius Z. Anal. Chem., 317, 661, 1984.
57. Akesson, B., and Johansson, U., Selenium status in patients with liver cirrhosis, in *Proceedings of the Third International Symposium on Selenium in Biology and Medicine*, Combs, G. F., Jr., Spallholz, J. E., Levander, O. A., and Oldfield, J. E., eds., Avi Publ. Co., Westport, Conn., 1986.
58. Ahlrot-Westerlund, B., Plantin, L. O., Savic, I., Siden, A., and Svensson, J., Selenium in plasma, erythrocytes and platelets from patients with multiple sclerosis, in *Proceedings of the Third International Symposium on Selenium in Biology and Medicine*, Combs, G. F., Jr., Spallholz, J. E., Levander, O. A., and Oldfield, J. E., eds., Avi Publ. Co., Westport, Conn., 1986.
59. Wester, P. O., Trace elements in serum and urine from hypertensive patients before and during treatment with chlorthalidone, Acta Med., Scand., 194, 505, 1973.
60. Gebre-Medhin, M., Ewald, U., Platin, L. O., and Tuvemo, T., Elevated serum selenium in diabetic children, Acta Pediatr. Scand., 73, 109, 1984.
61. Wester, P. O., Trace elements in serum and urine from hypertensive patients treated for six months with chlorthalidone, Acta Med. Scand., 196, 489, 1974.
62. Schrauzer, G. N., and Rhead, W. J., Interpretation of the methylene blue reduction test of human plasma and the possible cancer protecting effect of selenium, Experientia, 27, 1069, 1971.
63. Lane, H. W., Dudrick, S., and Warren, D. C., Blood selenium levels and glutathione-peroxidase activities in university and chronic intravenous hyperalimentation subjects, Proc. Soc. Exp. Biol. Med., 167, 383, 1981.
64. Kuhnlein, H. V., Levander, O. A., King, J. C., Sutherland, B., and Riskie, L., Dietary selenium and fecal mutagenicity in young men, Nutr. Res., 3, 203, 1983.

65. Schroeder, H. A., Frost, D. V., and Balassa, J. J., Essential trace metals in men: selenium, J. Chron. Dis., 23, 227, 1979.
66. Dworkin, B. M., and Rosenthal, W. S., Selenium and the alcoholic, Lancet, May 5, 1984.
67. Levander, O. A., Sutherland, B., Morris, V. C., and King, J. C., Selenium balance in young men during selenium depletion and repletion, Am. J. Clin. Nutr., 34, 2662, 1981.
68. Morris, J. S., Stampfer, M. J., and Willett, W., Dietary selenium in humans. Toenails as an indicator, Biol. Trace Elem. Res., 5, 529, 1983.
69. Lloyd, B., Lloyd, R. S., and Clayton, B. E., Effect of smoking, alcohol, and other factors on the selenium status of a healthy population, J. Epidemiol. Commun. Health, 37, 213, 1983.
70. McConnell, K. P., Jager, R. M., Bland, K. I., and Blotcky, A. J., The relationship of dietary selenium and breast cancer, J. Surg. Oncol., 15, 67, 1980.
71. Collipp, P. J., and Chen, S. Y., Cardiomyopathy and selenium deficiency in a two-year-old girl, N. Eng. J. Med., 304, 1304, 1981.
72. Sundstrom, H., Yrjanheikki, E., and Kauppila, A., Serum selenium in patients with ovarian cancer during and after therapy, Carcinogenesis, 5, 731, 1984.
73. Feldman, D. S., and Smith, D. K., Selenium status in multiple sclerosis resembles that of healthy normal subjects in Georgia, USA, a geochemical region of low soil selenium, in *Proceedings of the Third International Symposium on Selenium in Biology and Medicine*, Combs, G. F., Jr., Spallholz, J. E., Levander, O. E., and Oldfield, J. E., eds., Avi Publ. Co., Westport, Conn., 1986.
74. Levander, O. A., and Morris, U. C., Dietary selenium levels needed to maintain balance in North American adults consuming self-selected diets, Am. J. Clin. Nutr., 39, 809,1984.
75. Miller, L., Mills, B. J., Blotcky, A. J., and Lindeman, R. D., Red blood cell and serum selenium concentrations as influenced by age and selected diseases, J. Am. Coll. Nutr., 4, 331, 1983.
76. Allaway, W. H., Kubota, J., Losee, F., and Roth, M., Selenium, molybdenum and vanadium in human blood, Arch. Environ. Health, 16, 34, 1968.
77. Lane, H. W., Warren, D. G., Taylor, B. J., and Stool, E., Blood selenium and glutathione peroxidase levels and dietary selenium of free-living and institutionalized elderly subjects, Proc. Soc. Exp. Biol. Med., 173, 87, 1983.
78. Dutta, S. K., Miller, P. A., Greenberg, L. B., and Levander, O. A., Selenium and acute alcoholism, Am. J. Clin. Nutr., 38, 713, 1983.
79. Shamburger, R. J., Rukovena, E., Longfield, A. K., Tytko, S. A., Deodhar, S., and Willis, C. E., Antioxidants and cancer. I. Selenium in the blood of normals and cancer patients, J. Nat. Cancer Inst., 50, 863, 1973.
80. Schrauzer, G. N., and White, D. A., Selenium in human nutrition: dietary intakes and effects of supplementation, Bioinorg. Chem., 8, 303, 1978.
81. Sartiano, G. P., Lynch, W. E., Hopkins, C. B., and Darby, T. D., Erythrocyte and plasma selenium measurements in congestive cardiomyopathy, N. Eng. J. Med., 305, 558, 1982.
82. Butler, J. A., Whanger, P. D., and Tripp, M. J., Blood selenium and glutathione peroxidase activity in pregnant women: comparative assays in primates and other animals, Am. J. Clin. Nutr., 36, 15, 1982.
83. Schultz, T. D., and Leklem, J. E., Selenium status of vegetarians, nonvegetarians, and hormone-dependent cancer subjects, Am. J. Clin. Nutr., 37, 114, 1983.
84. Sullivan, J. F., Blotcky, A. J., Jetton, M. M., Hahn, H. K.J., and Burch, R. E., Serum levels of selenium, calcium, copper, magnesium, manganese, and zinc in various human diseases, J. Nutr., 109, 1432, 1979.

85. McConnell, K. P., Broghamer, W. L., Jr., Blotcky, A. J., and Hurt, O. J., Selenium levels in human blood and tissues in health and disease, J. Nutr., 105, 1026, 1975.
86. Stead, N. W., Bishop, S. L., and Carrol, R. M., Selenium (Se) balance in the dependent elderly, Am. J. Clin. Nutr., 39, 677, 1984.
87. Lane, H. W., Warren, D. C., Martin, E., and McCowan, J., Selenium status of industrial worker, Nutr. Res., 3, 805, 1983.
88. Lewko, W. M., and McConnell, K. P., Observations on selenium in human breast cancer, in *Proceedings of the Third International Symposium on Selenium in Biology and Medicine*, Combs, G. F., Jr., Spallholz, J.E, Levander, O. A., and Oldfield, J. E., eds., Avi Publ. Co., Westport, Conn., 1986.
89. Clark, L. C., Graham, G. F., Crounse, R., Turnbull, B. W., Bray, J., Hulka, B., and Shy, C. M., Nonmelanoma skin cancer and plasma selenium: a prospective cohort study, in *Proceedings of the Third International Symposium on Selenium in Biology and Medicine*, Combs, G. F., Jr., Spallholz, J. E., Levander, O. A., and Oldfield, J. E., eds., Avi Publ. Co., Westport, Conn., 1986.
90. McAdam, P.A., Smith, D.K., Feldman, E.B., and Hames, C., Effects of age, sex and race on selenium status of healthy residents of Augusta, Georgia, Biol. Trace Elem. Res., 6, 3, 1984.
91. Gallagher, M.L., Webb, P., Crounse, R., Bray, R., Webb, A., and Settle, E.A., Selenium levels in new growth hair and in whole blood during ingestion of a selenium supplement for six weeks, Nutr. Res., 4, 577, 1984.
92. Guseinova, L. M., Kuliev, M. K., and Dzhafarova, E. R., Selenium content in the blood of healthy children in relaton to age, Azerb. Med. Zh., 61, 70, 1984.
93. Jaffe, W. G., Ruphael, M., Mondragon, M. C., and Cuevas, M. A., Estudio clinico y bioquimico en ninos escolares de una zona selenifera, Arch. Latinamer. Nutr., 22, 595, 1972.
94. Ziesler, R., Harrison, S. H., and Wise, S. A., Trace elements in human livers using quality control in the complete analytical process, Biol. Trace Elem. Res., 6, 31, 1984.
95. Diskin, C. J., Tomasso, C. L., Alper, J. C., Glaser, M. L., and Gliegel, S. E., Long-term selenium exposure, Arch. Int. Med., 139, 824, 1979.
96. El-Yazizi, A., Al-Saleh, I., and Al-Mefty, O., Concentrations of Ag, Al, Au, Bi, Cd, Cu, Pb, Sb, and Se in cerebrospinal fluid of patients with cerebral neoplasms, Clin. Chem., 30, 1358, 1984.
97. Hadjimarkos, D. M., and Sheareu, T. R., Selenium concentrations in human saliva, Am. J. Clin. Nutr., 24, 1210, 1971.
98. Sundstrom, H., Karpela, H., Viinikka, L., and Kauppila, A., Serum selenium and glutathione peroxidase, and plasma lipid peroxides in uterine, ovarian or vulvar cancer, and their responses to antioxidants in patients with ovarian cancer, Cancer Letts., 24, 1, 1984.
99. Steiner, G., Menzel, H., Lombeck, I., Ohnesorge, F. K., and Bremer, H. J., Plasma glutathione peroxidase after selenium supplementation in patients with reduced selenium state, Eur. J. Pediatr., 138, 138, 1982.
100. Collins, B. J., Bell, P. M., McMaster, D., and Love, A. H.G., Selenium coeliac disease, Br. Med. J., 289, 439, 1984.
101. Szeinber, A., Golan, R., Ben-Ezzer, J., Sarova-Pinhas, I., and Kindler, D., Glutathione peroxidase activity in various types of blood cells in multiple sclerosis, Acta Neurol. Scand., 63, 67, 1981.
102. Thomson, C. D., and Robinson, M. F., Selenium in human health and disease with emphasis on those aspects peculiar to New Zealand, Am. J. Clin. Nutr., 33, 303, 1980.
103. Bjorksten, B., Marklund, S., and Hagglof, B., Enzymes of leukocyte oxidative metabolism in Down's syndrome, Acta Pediatr. Scand., 73, 97, 1984.

104. Lane, H. W., and Warren, D. C., Selenium status of industrial worker, Nutr. Res., 3, 805, 1983.

105. Rudolph, N., and Wong, S. L., Selenium and glutathione peroxidase activity in maternal and cord plasma and red cells, Pediatr. Res., 12, 789, 1978.

106. Beutler, E., and West, C., Red cell glutathione peroxidase polymorphism in Afro-Americans, Am. J. Hum. Genet., 26, 255, 1974.

107. Beutler, E., West, C., and Beutler, B., Electrophoretic polymorphism of glutathione peroxidase, Ann. Hum. Genet., 38, 163, 1974.

108. Khan, P. M., Verma, C., Wijnen, L. M.M., and Jairaj, S., Red cell glutathione peroxidase (GPX1) variation in Afro-Jamaican, Asiatic Indian, and Dutch populations, Hum. Genet., 66, 352, 1984.

109. Beutler, E., and Matsumoto, F., Ethnic variation in red cell glutathione peroxidase activity, Blood, 46, 103, 1975.

110. Cornelius, R., Speecke, A., and Hoste, J., Neutron activation analysis for bulk and trace elements in urine, Anal. Chin. Acta, 78, 317, 1975.

111. Lalonde, L., Jean, Y., Roberts, K. D., Chapdelaine, A., and Bleau, G., Fluorometry of selenium serum or urine, Clin. Chem., 28, 172, 1982.

112. Thomson, C., Recovery of large doses of selenium given as sodium selenite with or without vitamin E, N. Z. Med. J., 80, 163, 1974.

113. Cadell, P. B., and Cousins, F. B., Urinary selenium and dental caries, Nature, 185, 863, 1960.

114. Tsongas, J. A., and Fergerson, S. W., Human health effects of selenium in a rural Colorado drinking water supply, in *Trace Substances in Environmental Health*, Hemphill, D. A., ed., Univ. Missouri, Columbia, Vol. 11, p.30, 1977.

115. Robberecht, H. J., and Deelstra, H. A., Selenium in human urine. Determination, speciative and concentration levels, Talanta, 31, 497, 1984.

116. Robberecht, H. J., and Deelstra, H. A., Selenium in human urine: concentration level and medical implications, Clin. Chim. Acta, 136, 107, 1984.

117. Valentine, J. L., Kang, H. K., and Spivey, G. H., Selenium levels in human blood, urine and hair in response to exposure via drinking water, Environ. Res., 17, 347, 1978.

118. Clementi, G. F., Rossi, L. C., and Santarmi, G. P., Trace element intake and excretion in the Italian population, J. Radioanal. Chem., 37, 549, 1977.

119. Palmquist, D. L., Moxon, A. L., and Cantor, A. H., Pattern of urinary selenium excretion in normal adults, Federation Proc., 38, 391, 1979.

120. Griffiths, N. M., Dietary intake and urinary excretion of selenium in some New Zealand women, Proc. Univ. Otago Med. Sch., 51, 8, 1973.

121. Thomson, C. D., Burton, C. E., and Robinson, M. F., On supplementing the selenium intake of New Zealanders. 1. Short experiments with large doses of selenate or selenomethionine, Br. J. Nutr., 39, 579, 1978.

122. Van Rij, A. M., Thomson, C. D., McKenzie, J. M., and Robinson, M. F., Selenium deficiency in total parenteral nutrition, Am. J. Clin. Nutr., 32, 2076, 1979.

123. Robinson, M. F., Rea, H. M., Friend, G. M., Stewart, R. D. H., Snow, P. G., and Thomson, C. D., On supplementing the selenium intake of New Zealanders. 2. Prolonged metabolic experiments with daily supplements of selenomethionine, selenite or fish, Br. J. Nutr., 39, 589, 1978.

124. Morris, J. S., Stampfer, M. J., and Willett, W., Dietary selenium in humans. Toenails as an indicator, Biol. Trace Element Res., 5, 529, 1983.

125. Kauppila, A., Makila, U. M., Korpela, H., Viinikka, L., and Yrjanheikki, E., Decreased serum selenium does not correlate with increased lipid peroxidation in pre-eclampsia, in *Proceedings of the Third International Symposium in Biology and Medicine*, Combs, G. F., Jr., Spallholz, J. E., Levander, O. A., and Oldfield, J. E., eds., Avi Publ. Co., Westport, Conn., 1986.

126. Hyvonen-Dabek, M., Nikkinen-Vilkki, P., and Dabek, J. T., Selenium and other elements in human maternal and umbilical serum, as determined simultaneously by protein-induced X-ray emission, Clin. Chem., 30, 529, 1984.

127. Behne, D., von Berswordt-Wallrabe, R., Elger, W., and Wolters, W., Glutathione peroxidase in erythrocytes and plasma of rats during prenancy and lactation, Experientia, 34, 986, 1978.

128. Korpela, H., Loueniva, R., Yrjanheikki, E., and Kauppila, A., Selenium concentration in materal and umbilical cord blood, placenta and amniotic membranes, Int. J. Vit. Nutr. Res., 54, 257, 1984.

129. Gross, S., Hemolytic anemia in premature infants: relationship to vitamin E, selenium, glutathione peroxidase and erythrocyte lipids, Sem. Hematol., 13, 187, 1976.

130. Haga, P., and Lunde, G., Selenium and vitamin E in cord blood from preterm and full-term infants, Acta Pediat. Scand., 67, 735, 1978.

131. Amin, S., Chen, S. Y., Collipp, P. J., Castro-Magana, M., Maddaiah, V. T., and Klein, S. W., Selenium in premature infants, Nutr. Metab., 24, 331, 1980.

132. Rudolph, N., Preis, O., Bitzos, E.1., Reale, M. M., and Wong, S. L., Hematologic and selenium status of low-birth-weight infants fed formulas with and without iron, J. Pediatr., 99, 57, 1981.

133. Pleban, P. A., Numerof, B., Chrenka, B. A., and Wirth, F., Monitoring trace element concentrations in blood from premature infants in a neonatal intensive care unit, Chem. Toxicol. Clin. Chem. Metabl., Proc. 2nd Int. Conf., p.343, 1983.

134. Westermarck, T., Selenium content of tissues in Finnish infants and adults with various diseases, and studies on the effects of selenium supplementation in neuronal ceroid lipofuscinosis patients, Acta Pharmacol. Toxicol., 41, 121, 1977.

135. Gutcher, G. R., Raynor, W. J.. amd Farrel, P. M., An evaluation of vitamin E status in premature infants, Am. J. Clin. Nutr., 40, 1078, 1984.

136. Money, D. F.L., Vitamin E and selenium deficiencies and their possible aetiological role in the Sudden Death in Infants Syndrome, N. Zealand Med. J., 71, 32, 1970.

137. Money, D. F.L., The vitamin E/selenium responsive diseases of animals and the Sudden Infant Death Syndrome: common findings, N. Zealand Med. J., 45, 990, 1983.

138. Rhead, W. J., Cary, E. E., Allaway, W. H., Saltzstein, S. L., and Schrauzer, G. N., The vitamin E and selenium status of infants and the Sudden Infant Death Syndrome, Bioinorg. Chem., 1, 289, 1972.

139. Money, D. F.L., Vitamin E, selenium, iron, and vitamin A content of livers from Sudden Infant Death Syndrome cases and control children: interrelationships and possible significance, N. Zealand J. Sci., 21, 41, 1978.

140. Cowgill, V. M., Selenium and neonatal death, Lancet, Apr. 10, 816, 1976.

141. Ge, K., Xue, A., Bai, J., and Wang, S., Keshan disease - an endemic cardiomyopathy in China, Virchows Arch., 401, 1, 1983.

142. Apei, I. I., Report of etiological survey on Keshan disease, Res. Reps. Cent. Acad., 1, 1, 1937.

143. Tan, J. A., The Keshan disease in China: a study of ecological chemico-geography, Nat. Georg. J. Ind., 28, 15, 1982.

144. Tan,J. A., Zheng, D. Z., Hou, S. F., Zhu, W. Y., Li, R. B., Zhu, Z. Y., and Wang, W. Y., Selenium ecological chemico-geography and endemic Keshan disease and Kaschin-Beck's disease in China, in *Proceedings of the Third International Symposium on Selenium in Biology and Medicine*, Combs, G. F., Jr., Spallholz, J. E., Levander, O. A., and Oldfield, J. E., eds., Avi Publ. Co., Westport, Conn., 1986.

145. Environment and Endemic Disease Section, Institute of Geography, Chinese Academy of Sciences, Geographical distribution of selenium content in human hair in Keshan-disease and non-disease zones in China, Acta Geogr. Sin., 37, 136, 1982.

146. Chen, J., personal communication, 1982.

147. Chong, Y., Hang, J., and Liu, R., Analysis of 1,000 children cases of Keshan disease in Sichuan province, Symp. Third Conf. Etiol. Keshan Dis., p.94, 1979.

148. Chen, J. S., and Yang, G. Q., personal communication, 1984.

149. Sun, J., Lin, Y., Wu, G., and Teng, R., A survey of the epidemic of Keshan disease in the north of China, Chin. J. Epidemiol., 1, 2, 1982.

150. Chen, X. S., Meng, G. S., Li, W. X., Xie, Y. H., and Chen, X. C., Histochemical observation related to Keshan disease, in *Proceedings of the Third International Symposium on Selenium in Biology and Medicine*, Combs, G. F., Jr., Spallholz, J. E., Levander, O. A., and Oldfield, J. E., eds., Avi Publ. Co., Westport, Conn., 1986.

151. Ge, K., personal communication, 1982, 1984.

152. Su, C., Gong, C., Li, J., Cheng, C., Zhou, D., and Jin, Q., Preliminary results of viral etiological study of Keshan disease, Nat. Med. J. China, 59, 466, 1979.

153. Bai, J., Ge, K. Y., Deng, X. J., Wu, S. Z., Wang, S. Q., Xue, A. N., and Su, C. Q., Effects of selenium intake on myocardial necrosis induced by coxsackie viral infection in mice, Yingyang Xuebao, 4, 235, 1982.

154. Ge, K. Y., Bai, J., Deng, X. J., Su, S. Z., Wang, S. Q., Xue, A. N., and Su, C. Q., The protective effect of selenium against viral myocarditis in mice, in *Proceedings of the Third International Symposium on Selenium in Biology and Medicine*, Combs, G. F., Jr., Spallholz, J. E., Levander, O. A., and Oldfield, J. E., eds., Avi Publ. Co., Westport, Conn., 1986.

155. Wang, F., Li, G. S., Li, C., An, R. G., Yang, T. S., and Zhu, P., Experimental studies on pathogenic factors of Keshan disease in the grains cultivated in endemic areas, in *Proceedings of the Third International Symposium on Selenium in Biology and Medicine*, Combs, G. F., Jr., Spallholz, J. E., Levander, O. A., and Oldfield, J. E., eds., Avi Publ. Co., Westport, Conn., 1986.

156. Ren, H. Z., Zhu, T. Y., Li, G. Z., Wei, F. Q., Meng, L. Y., Cheng, B., Guan, J. Y., Zhao, Y. H., and Jin, Q., An experimental pathological study of the causation of Keshan disease, Chin. J. Endemic Dis., 1, 172, 1982.

157. The Research Group of Keshan Disease of Chinese Academy of Medical Science, Research on the relation between selenium and Keshan disease, Acta Acad. Med. Sin., 1, 75, 1979.

158. Keshan Disease Research Group of the Chinese Academy of Medical Sciences, Observations on effect of sodium selenite in prevention of Keshan disease, Chin. Med. J., 92, 471, 1979.

159. Johnson, R. A., Baker, S. S., and Fallon, J. T., An occidental case of cardiomyopathy and selenium deficiency, N. Eng. J. Med., 30, 1210, 1981.

160. King, W. W.K., Michel, L., and Wood, W. C., Reversal of selenium deficiency with oral selenium, N. Eng. J. Med., 304, 1305, 1981.

161. Quercia, R. A., Korn, S., O'Neill, D., Dougherty, J. E., Ludwig, M., Schweizer, R., and Sigman, R., Selenium deficiency and fatal cardiomyopathy in a patient receiving long-term home parenteral nutrition, Clin. Pharm., 3, 531, 1984.

162. Kaschin-Beck Disease Prevention and Therapy Research Team, Ning County, Gansu Province, curing Kaschin-Beck disease with selenium and vitamin E in 224 patients with x-ray observation and causation research, Chin. Med. J., 59, 169, 1979.

163. Liang, S. T., Zhang, J. C., Shang, X., Mu, S. Z., and Zhang, F. J., Effects of selenium supplementation in prevention and treatment of Kaschin-Beck disease, in *Proceedings of the Third International Symposium on Selenium in Biology and Medicine*, Combs, G. F., Jr., Spallholz, J. E., Levander, O. A., and Oldfield, J. E., eds., Avi Publ. Co., Westport, Conn., 1986.

164. Hou, S. F., Zhu, Z. Y., and Tan, J. A., The relationship between the selenium dynamics in the course of human body growth and the Kaschin-Beck disease epidemiology, Acta Geogr. Sinica, 39, 75, 1984.

165. Li, C., Huang, J., and Li, C., Observational report on the effects of taking sodium selenite for six years continuously as a preventative for Kaschin-Beck disease as shown in X-ray studies, in *Proceedings of the Third International Symposium on Selenium in Biology and Medicine*, Combs, G. F., Jr., Spallholz, J. E., Levander, O. A., and Oldfield, J. E., eds., Avi Publ. Co., Westport, Conn., 1986.

166. Fleming, C. R., McCall, J. T., O'Brien, J. F., Forsman, R. W., Ilstrup, D. M., and Petz, J., Selenium status in patients receiving home parenteral nutrition, J. Parent. Ent. Nutr., 8, 258, 1984.

167. Moore, J. A., Noiva, R., and Wells, I. C., Selenium concentrations in plasma of patients with arteriographically defined coronary atherosclerosis, Clin. Chem., 30, 1171, 1984.

168. Schwarz, K., Selenium and Kwashiorkor, Lancet, 1, 1335, 1966.

169. Steiner, G., Menzel, H., Lombeck, I., Ohnesorge, F. K., and Bremer, H. J., Plasma glutathione peroxidase after selenium supplementation in patients with reduced selenium state, Eur. J. Ped., 138, 138, 1982.

170. Zabel, N. L., Harland, J., Garmican, A. T., and Ganther, H. E., Selenium content of commercial formula diets, Am. J. Clin. Nutr., 31, 850, 1978.

171. McKenzie, J. M., van Rij, A. M., Robinson, M. F., and Guthrie, B. E., Trace element studies during total parenteral nutrition, in *Trace Substances in Environmental Health - X*, Hemphill, D. D., ed., Univ. Mo. Press, Columbia, p.481, 1976.

172. Jacobson, S., and Wester, P. O., Balance study of twenty trace elements during total parenteral nutrition in man, Br. J. Nutr., 37, 107, 1977.

173. Van Rij, A., Thomson, C. D., McKenzie, J. M., and Robinson, M. F., Selenium deficiency in total parenteral nutrition, Am. J. Clin. Nutr., 32, 2076, 1979.

174. King, W. W. K., Michel, L., Wood, W. C., Malt, R. A., Baker, S. S., and Cohen, H. J., Reversal of selenium deficiency with oral selenium, N. Eng. J. Med., 304, 1305, 1981.

175. Johnson, R. A., Baker, S. S. Fallon, J. T., Maynard, E. P., Ruskin, J. N., Wen, Z., Ge, K., and Cohen, H. J., An accidental case of cardiomyopathy and selenium deficiency, N. Eng. J. Med., 304, 1210, 1981.

176. Baker, S. S., Lerman, R. H., Krey, S. H., Crocker, K. S., Hirsh, E. F., and Cohen, H., Selenium deficiency with total parenteral nutrition: reversal of biochemical and functional abnormalities by selenium supplementation: a case report, Am. J. Clin. Nutr., 38, 769, 1983.

177. Fleming, C. R., Lie, J. T., McCall, J. T., O'Brien, J. F., Baillie, E. E., and Thistle, J. L., Selenium-deficiency and fatal cardiomyopathy in a patient on home parenteral nutrition, Gastroenterol., 83, 684, 1983.

178. Kien, C. L., and Ganther, H. E., Manifestation of chronic selenium deficiency in a child receiving total parenteral nutrition, Am. J. Clin. Nutr., 37, 319, 1983.

179. Baptista, R. J., Bistrian, B. R., Blackburn, G. L., Miller, D. G., Champagne, C. D., and Buchanan, L., Utilizing selenious acid to reverse selenium deficiency in total parenteral nutrition patients, Am. J. Clin. Nutr., 39, 816, 1984.

180. Friel, J. K., Gibson, R. S., Peliowski, A., and Watts, J., Serum zinc, copper, and selenium concentrations in preterm infants receiving enteral nutrition or parenteral nutrition supplemented with zinc and copper, J. Pediatr., 104, 763, 1984.

181. Levander, O. A., The importance of selenium in total parenteral nutrition, Bull. N. Y. Acad. Sci., 60, 144, 1984.

182. Mottonen, T., Hannonen, P., Seppala, O., Alfthan, G., and Oka, M., Glutathione and selenium in rheumatoid arthritis, Clin. Rheumatol., 3, 195, 1984.

183. Chaudiere, J., and Tappel, A. L., Interaction of gold (I) with the active site of selenium-glutathione peroxidase, J. Inorg. Biochem., 20, 313, 1984.
184. Mercurio, S. D., and Combs, G. F., Jr., Drug-induced changes in selenium-dependent glutathione peroxidase activity in the chick, J. Nutr. 115, 1459, 1985.
185. Michaelsson, G., and Edquist, L. E., Erythrocyte glutathione peroxidase activity in acne vulgaris and the effect of selenium and vitamin E treatment, Acta Derm. Venereol. (Stockh.), 64, 9, 1984.
186. Luoma, P. V., Sotaniemi, E. A., Korpela, H., and Kumpalainen, J., Serum selenium, glutathione peroxidase and high density lipoprotein cholesterol-effect of selenium supplementation, Res. Commun. Chem. Pathol. Pharmacol., 46, 469, 1984.
187. Virtamo, J., Valkeila, E., Alfthan, G., Punsar, S., Hattanen, J. K., and Karvonen, M. J., Serum selenium and the risk of coronary heart disease and stroke, Am. J. Epidemiol., 122, 276, 1985.
188. Kondo, M., A combination therapy for chronic rheumatoid arthritis with selenium and allogenic lymphocytes, in *Proceedings of the Third International Symposium on Selenium in Biology and Medicine*, Combs, G. F., Jr., Spallholz, J. E., Levander, O. A., and Oldfield, J. E., Avi Publ. Co., Westport, Conn., 1986.
189. Blau, M., and Manske, R. F., The pancreas specificity of Se[75]-selenomethionine, J. Nucl. Med., 2, 102, 1961.
190. Zuidema, G. D., Kirsh, M., Turcotte, U. G., Gaisford, W. D., Powers, W., and Kowalczyk, R. S., Pancreatic uptake of Se[75]-selenomethionine, Annls. Surg., 158, 401, 1963.
191. Goel, Y., Dubousky, E., and McDonald, M., Pancreatic visualization with ^{75}Se-selenomethionine after surgery, J. Nucl. Med., 13, 765, 1972.
192. Thorn, J., Robertson, J., Buss, D. H., and Bunton, N. G., Trace nutrients. Selenium in British food, Br. J. Nutr., 39, 391, 1978.
193. Varo, P., and Koivistoinen, P., Mineral element composition of Finnish foods. XII. General discussion and nutritional evaluation, Acta Agric. Scand., 22, 165, 1980.
194. Stewart, R. D.H., Griffiths, N. M., Thomson, C. D., and Robinson, M. F., Quantitative selenium metabolism in normal New Zealand women, Br. J. Nutr., 40, 45, 1978.
195. Food and Nutrition Board, *Recommended Dietary Allowances, Ninth Revised Edition*, National Academy of Sciences, Washington, D. C., 1980.
196. Wahlstrom, R. C., Goehring, T. B., Johnson, D. D., Libal, G. W., Olson, O. E., Palmer, I. S., and Thaler, R. C., The relationship of hair color to selenium content of hair and selenosis in swine, Nutr. Rep. Intern., 29, 143, 1984.
197. Eckhert, C. D., Breskin, M. W., Wise, W. W., and Knopp, R. H., Association between low serum selenium and diminished visual function in diabetic women, Federation Proc., 44, 1670 (abstract #7365), 1985.
198. Neve, J., Vertogen, F., Thonnart, N., and Carpentier, Y. A., Assessment of selenium status in patients receiving long-term total parenteral nutrition, Trace Elem.-Anal. Chem. Med. Biol., 3, 139, 1984.
199. Levander, O. A., Clinical consequences of low selenium intake and its relationship to vitamin E, Ann. N. Y. Acad. Sci., 355, 70, 1982.
200. Levander, O. A., Recent developments in selenium nutrition, Nutr. Uptake, 1, 147, 1983.

9

SELENIUM IN IMMUNITY AND INFECTION

Suboptimal intakes of Se in animals and humans may have undesirable effects that are less overt than those that characterize the frank deficiency diseases reviewed in Chapter 7. Among these potential effects are those that impair the development or function of the immune system and, hence, compromise resistance to infection. Such effects may not be apparent in the absence of challenges to the immune system and may have deleterious consequences that are not immediately associated with nutritional Se status. Therefore, the topic of the role of Se in support of normal immune function and disease resistance is appropriate to the full consideration of the role of Se in nutrition. In recent years, this topic has been addressed by several investigators. Much of this literature was reviewed by Spallholz.[1]

I. EFFECTS OF SELENIUM
ON B CELL-DEPENDENT IMMUNE FUNCTIONS

Selenium was not known to affect humoral immunity (i.e., the antibody-producing functions of bursa-derived lymphocytes, i.e., B cells) until Berenshtein[2] demonstrated that, when administered with vitamin E, it potentiated the antibody titers that were produced in response to typhoid vaccine in rabbits. This effect was produced by the administration of 50 μg Se (as Na_2SeO_3) per kilogram body weight, but did not occur in response to vitamin E (30 μg/kg) alone. Because the elevation in antibody titers persisted for 2 months after antigen challenge, it is apparent that Berenshtein[2] had measured an effect of Se primarily on the production of immunoglobulin G (IgG). Similar results were subsequently reported by Spallholz et al.[3]; they found that supplementation with high levels (1.75-2.25 ppm Se) of Na_2SeO_3 to a commercial diet significantly increased IgG titers in mice after challenge with sheep red blood cells (SRBC). In studies with dogs, Sheffy and Schultz[4] also found that correction of Se deficiency increased the production of IgG in response to SRBC challenge. Knight[5] observed the same effect in Shetland ponies.

Several investigators have demonstrated that the primary immune response can be affected by nutritional Se status. Spallholz et al.[6] showed that Se supplementation of either a commercial laboratory rodent diet or an Se-deficient *Torula* yeast-based diet resulted in enhancement of the immediate production of anti-SRBC antibody titers in mice. This occurred as the result of simply correcting Se deficiency in mice fed the semi-purified diet, but only after high-level supplementation (i.e., 2.8 ppm Se) in mice fed the practical type diet. Similar results were observed by Shakelford and Martin,[7] who found the administration of Se (1 ppm, as Na_2SeO_3) in the drinking water significantly enhanced anti-SRBC antibody titers in mice. By administering Se parenterally, Spallholz et al.[8] found that Se treatment enhanced the primary immune response in the mouse only when it was administered before or at the same time as the SRBC challenge. Other investigators have found that nutritional levels (i.e., 0.1-0.5 ppm) of Se added as dietary supplements have enhanced antibody production to *Leptospira pomona* in calves,[9] to bacterial antigens in mice and rabbits,[10] and to SRBC in chicks[11,12] and mice.[13]

The effect of Se in relation to vitamin E on the primary and secondary immune responses of mice given either tetanus toxoid or SBRC was investigated by Spallholz et al.[14] They found synergistic effects of Se and vitamin E on antibody production in response to either antigen; however, the nutrient effects were different for each antigen. Whereas Se and vitamin E treatments enhanced both primary and secondary immune responses to SRBC, these treatments enhanced only the secondary immune response to tetanus toxoid. Studies in the young chick by Marsh et al.[11] showed that the influences of Se and vitamin E on humoral immunity may change during the course of development of immunocompetence. They found that nutritional levels of both Se (0.10 ppm as Na_2SeO_3) and vitamin E (100 IU, as dl-alpha-tocopheryl acetate, per kilogram) were required in the 2-week-old chick for optimal production of anti-SRBC antibody, but that after ca. 3 weeks of age either Se or vitamin E were each fully capable of supporting the primary immune response. Sheffey and Schultz[4] found that combined Se- and vitamin E-deficiency in developmentally immunocompetent dogs resulted in depressed antibody titers in response to vaccination with a mixed canine distemper, infectious hepatitis virus vaccine.

Dietary supplementation with Se has been shown to increase the number of spleen plaque-forming cells (B cells) in mice.[6,13,15,16] Marsh et al.[17] have found that correction of combined Se/vitamin E-deficiency in the chick results in the prevention of depletion of lymphoid cells from the bursa of Fabricius that occurs in deficient animals (see Fig. 7.9). These results suggest that depletion of B lymphocyte numbers, rather than simply impaired antibody production by those cells, may be the basis of impaired humoral immunity in Se- and vitamin E-deficiency.

Selenium treatment at levels greater than those generally accepted as being in the nutritional range (i.e., 0.10-0.20 ppm) may depress the humoral immune response. Shakelford and Martin[7] found that a supplement of 3 ppm Se (as Na_2SeO_3) in the drinking water of mice resulted in marked decreases in anti-SRBC antibody production. Marsh et al.[11] showed that dietary concentrations of Se greater than ca. 0.20 ppm produced marked decreases in anti-SRBC antibody titers in the chick; this inhibitory effect was observed among males, but not among females.

Although these several investigations have demonstrated effects of Se on humoral immunity in several species, very little information has been developed concerning the mechanisms for these effects. Burton et al.[18] have found that selenite can react with purified human and goat immunoglobulins without altering their abilities to bind antibodies, but it is unlikely that this reaction occurs in vivo due to the scarcity of that species of Se in the body. And because optimal B cell function (particularly IgG synthesis) is dependent upon the optimal functioning of both T cells and macrophages, it is likely that some effects of Se on humoral immunity may be secondary to its effects on T cells and/or macrophages. The role of Se and related nutritional factors in the support of optimal humoral immunity must await further research for its elucidation.

II. EFFECTS OF SELENIUM
ON T CELL-MEDIATED IMMUNE FUNCTIONS

Several studies have been made of the effects of Se on immune functions of thymus-derived lymphocytes (T cells). Martin and Spallholz[19] found that supranutritional levels (e.g., 1 or 3 ppm) of dietary Se increased the sensitivity of guinea pigs to dinitrochlorobenzene-induced erythema and induration. This delayed-type hypersensitivity is known to be dependent on T cell reactivity, indicating that T cell function was affected at these high levels of Se. Evidence of effects of Se on T cell-dependent graft versus host reactions was reported by Aleksondrovicz,[10] who found that supplements of Se (22 μg Se as Na_2SeO_3 per kilogram body weight per day) decreased skin allograft rejection times in mice and rabbits. Sheffey and Shultz[4,20] showed that the lymphoproliferative response was impaired by combined Se- and vitamin E-deficiency in the dog. This was measured by the lymphocyte blastogenesis test to T cell mitogens (e.g., concanavalin A, phytohemagglutinin); deficient individuals were unresponsive to each of these mitogens. Bendrich et al.[21] have produced similar results (i.e., decreased mitogenic responses of splenic lymphocytes to T cell mitogens) due to vitamin E deficiency in the guinea pig; however, Se was not considered as a variable in those studies. These investigations would indicate that severe Se-deficiency may be expected to compromise T cell-dependent immune functions; however, Arvilommi et al.[22] found that human subjects from a population (in Finland) with moderately low serum Se concentrations (i.e., 74 ± 9 ng/ml) showed no significant differences in phytohemagglutinin- or concanavalin A-induced lymphocyte blastogenesis when compared to an Se-supplemented treatment group (i.e., blood Se level 169 ± 19 ng/ml). This finding would suggest that a Se deficiency more severe than that observed in Finland may be required to affect T cell function.

Karle et al.[23] found that phytohemagglutinin-stimulated lymphocytes took up ^{75}Se whether it was provided as selenite, selenate, selenocystine, selenomethionine, or bound to serum proteins. In confirmation of earlier work by the same group,[24] the organic forms were found to be taken up, in marked preference to the inorganic forms, by a process independent of energy or protein synthesis but inhibitable by sulfhydryl blocking reagents (e.g., N-ethylmaleamide, iodoacetamide, p-chloromercuribenzoate). Studies by Clausen and Tranum[25] have shown that the process of selenite uptake by lymphocytes is spontaneous and involves the metabolism of selenite during uptake. The uptake of Se by lymphocytes was shown to correlate with increases in the activity of SeGSHpx, apparently due to de novo synthesis of the enzyme by those cells; lymphocytes that were not exposed to Se showed low activities of SeGSHpx.[23] Parnham et al.[26] found that low lymphocytic activities of SeGSHpx (resulting from dietary deficiency of Se) were associated with enhancement of the adjuvant-induced chronic inflammatory response in the rat. They suggested that the inability, due to reduced activities of SeGSHpx, to metabolize peroxides produced at inflamed sites resulted in enhancement of inflammation. Support for this hypothesis comes from observations of increased concentrations of peroxides in rheumatoid synovial fluid and experimentally produced inflammatory exudates[27-30] and of the efficacy of antioxidants and free radical scavengers in inhibition of inflammation in model systems.[31-33] The peroxide metabolizing activity of SeGSHpx may thus explain the earlier results of Roberts,[34,35] which showed Se to have acute anti-inflammatory properties as measured by the Selye granuloma pouch assay in the rat. In unpublished studies by Roberts and Schwarz and cited by Spallholz,[1] this anti-inflammatory effect of Se was potentiated by dietary vitamin E, which was itself inactive. Spallholz[1] has discussed the patenting and subsequent development of Se as an acute anti-inflammatory agent.

III. EFFECTS OF SELENIUM
ON THE FUNCTIONS OF PHAGOCYTIC CELLS

Changes in nutritional Se status have been shown to affect the functions of the phagocytic cells (i.e., macrophages and neutrophils). Macrophages have been found to contain SeGSHpx, which is localized in lysosome-like subcellular structures,[36,37] and nutritional deprivation of Se results in decreases in macrophage SeGSHpx.[38,39] Parnham et al.[26] have demonstrated that macrophages from Se-deficient rats (which show reduced SeGSHpx activities) have enhanced H_2O_2 release upon stimulation with opsonized zymosan. In contrast, macrophages from Se-deficient rats released less hydrogen peroxide (H_2O_2) upon stimulation with phorbol myristic acetate; this finding was interpreted as indicating an increase in the cellular damage to the Se-depleted cells by the phorbol ester.[26] Macrophage function is known to be markedly impaired in vitamin E-deficiency,[40] but the possibility of an interactive effect of Se and vitamin E on macrophage function has not been addressed experimentally.

Neutrophils isolated from Se-deficient rats[41] and cattle[42] have been shown to have impaired ability to kill ingested *Candida albicans* although the ability to phagocytize the yeast cells was not significantly different from that of neutrophils from Se-fed control animals. Similar results were reported by Gyang et al.,[43] who found that the ability to kill ingested *Staphylococcus aureus*, but not to phagocytize the bacteria, was decreased in polymorphonucleated leukocytes (PMNs) from Se-deficient cows. Aziz et al.[44] showed that PMNs from Se-deficient goats had impaired phagocytosis of opsonized zymosan, and that replacement of Se by incubating the cells in the presence of Na_2SeO_3 was effective in restoring their normal phagocytic function. The restoration of phagocytosis by Se corresponded to a restoration of SeGSHpx activities of the PMNs.[44] In spite of the fact that most parameters of immune function were found to be normal in Finnish subjects with moderately low concentrations of Se in the serum, the phagocytic activity of human granulocytes against *S. aureus* was reduced by a small (9%) but significant amount in comparison to cells from Se-supplemented subjects.[22]

The effects of Se on the immune functions of phagocytic cells can be understood with regard to the metabolic events that attend the process of phagocytosis. During phagocytosis, these cells show a rise in nonmitochondrial respiration (the so-called respiratory burst), which involves the generation of large amounts of superoxide (O_2^-) by myeloperoxidase with the subsequent production of H_2O_2 and, perhaps, other highly reactive oxygen radicals.[45-48] This results in considerable oxidative stress in the internal and immediate external environment of the phagocytizing cell, a condition that can lead to cellular injury via the oxidation of critical elements within the cell (e.g., soluble thiols, protein-SH groups).[49,50] Cellular protection against this oxidative stress is effected in part by factors that either quench the deleterious radicals (e.g., vitamin E,[51,52] thiols[53]) or decrease their production by reducing O_2^- to H_2O_2 (i.e., super oxide dismutases[47,54-56]). Hydrogen peroxide so produced subsequent to the respiratory burst is metabolized by the phagocyte via catalase or SeGSHpx. Of these, the role of catalase is questionable, as catalase-deficient PMNs from patients with hereditary acatalasia show normal functions (i.e., chemotaxis, respiratory bursts after zymosan ingestion, bacterial killing).[57]

Experiments by Baker and Cohen[58] demonstrated the importance of SeGSHpx in protection of the phagocyte from the destructive effects of H_2O_2. They showed that a nutritional Se-deficiency in the rat (such that SeGSHpx activities in peritoneal granulocytes were reduced to 11% of those of Se-fed controls) resulted in a marked increase in the sensitivity of those cells to H_2O_2. Degranulation was greater for Se-deficient cells upon incubation in the presence of a H_2O_2-generating system; this effect was reflected by a more rapid loss of phagocytic ability of Se-deficient cells. These responses indicate that the reduction, due to Se deficiency, of SeGSHpx activity resulted in the loss of cellular protection from H_2O_2 and, probably, other toxic peroxides. Arthur et al.[59] and Boyne and Arthur[42] showed that neutrophils from Se-deficient cattle showed less production of hydroxyl radical adducts during phagocytosis, and decreased superoxide dismutase-sensitive reduction of both cytochrome c and tetrazolium salt. They interpreted these results as indicating increased oxidative damage to neutrophil enzymes with consequent impairment in the metabolic and microbicidal activities of the cell. Human PMNs have been found to contain glutathione S-transferase activity[60]; however, it is not known whether this enzyme may have glutathione peroxidase activity in that cell. Therefore, the Se-dependent enzyme SeGSHpx appears to have vital importance in the support of normal phagocytic function in immunity. Changes in phagocyte SeGSHpx activities occur as the result of changes of nutritional Se status of the host animal[38,39,41,42,58,59] and have been reported to be decreased in the diabetic state.[61]

Talcott et al.[62] found that Se may also have an enhancing effect on natural killer (NK) cell cytotoxicity. They found, in rats exposed to Se, a dose-dependent enhancement in splenic NK cell cytotoxicity at dietary levels of Se less than 5.0 ppm (as Na_2SeO_3). The mechanism of this effect is not clear.

IV. EFFECTS OF SELENIUM ON INFECTION

In view of the findings outlined above concerning effects of nutritional Se status on immunity, it may be anticipated that resistance to infectious disease is also affected. Relatively few investigations have undertaken to test that hypothesis; however, the results of those that have done so indicate that Se-deficiency reduces disease resistance in animals. Yarrington et al.[63] found that Se and vitamin E appeared to have a nonspecific influence in minimizing the severity of avian malarial (*Plasmodium spartani*) infection in ducks. However, the usefulness of that observation was compromised due to the high virulence of the infectious agent used, which resulted in high mortality and loss of sensitivity in those experiments. Colnago et al.[64,65] studied the effects of dietary Se and vitamin E in chickens infected with the intestinal coccidium *Eimeria tenella*. They found that dietary supplements of Se significantly increased the blood leukocyte count and produced generally improved survival and gains in body weight in animals innoculated with the coccidia. Tiege et al.[66-69] have shown that the Se-deficient pig has enhanced susceptibility to dysentery resulting from infection with *Treponema hyodysenteriae*. Although the mechanism is unclear for the protection by dietary Se against swine dysentery, the effect is seen upon first exposure of pigs to *T. hyodysenteriae*; therefore, Tiege et al.[69] have suggested that Se may act by stimulating nonspecific immunity of the colonic mucosa. It is likely that the role of Se in providing therapy for the so-called "Se-responsive unthriftiness" in sheep[70-72] and calves[70,71] may also be due to its effects on resistance to low-grade infections in those animals. Clearly, the fundamental information concerning the involvement of Se in immunity suggest that further studies on the role of dietary Se in resistance to infectious disease are very likely to be fruitful. Knowledge gained from such studies will have practical importance in animal and human health.

REFERENCES

1. Spallholz, J. E., Anti-inflammatory, immunologic and carcinostatic attributes of selenium in experimental animals, in *Diet and Resistance of Disease*, Phillips, M., and Baetz, A., eds., Plenum, New York, p.43, 1981.
2. Berenshstein, T. F., Effect of selenium and vitamin E on antibody formation in rabbits, Zdra Wookhr. Boloruss., 18, 34, 1972.
3. Spallholz, J. E., Martin, J. L., Gerlach, M. L., and Heinzerling, R. H., Enhanced IgM and IgG titers in mice fed selenium, Infect. Immunity, 8, 841, 1973.
4. Sheffy, B. E., and Schultz, R. D., Influence of vitamin E and selenium on immune response mechanisms, Cornell Vet., 68, Suppl. 7, 89, 1978.
5. Knight, D. A., The effect of selenium supplementation on the humoral antibody response in the equine, Ph.D. Thesis, Ohio State Univ., Columbus, Ohio, 87 pp., 1984.
6. Spallholz, J. E., Martin, J. L., Gerlach, M. L., and Heinzerling, R. H., Immunological responses of mice fed diets supplemented with sodium selenate, Proc. Soc. Exp. Biol. Med., 143, 685, 1973.

7. Shakelford, J., and Martin, J., Antibody response of mature male mice after drinking water supplemented with selenium, Federation Proc., 39, 339, 1980.

8. Spallholz, J. E., Martin, J. L., Gerlack, M. L., and Heinzerling, R. H., Injectable selenium: effect on the primary immune response of mice, Proc. Soc. Exp. Biol. Med., 148, 37, 1975.

9. Norman, B. B., and Johnson, W., Selenium responsive disease, Animal Nutr. Health, 31, 6, 1976.

10. Aleksondrovicz, J., Wazewska-Czyzewska, M., Bodzon, A., Dolezol, M., and Dubis, K., Effects of food enrichment with various doses of sodium selenite on some immune responses in laboratory animals, Rocz. Nauk. Zootech., 4, 113, 1977.

11. Marsh, J. A., Dietert, R. R., and Combs, G. F., Jr., Influence of dietary selenium and vitamin E on the humoral immune response of the chick, Proc. Soc. Exp. Biol. Med., 166, 228, 1981.

12. Abdel-Ati, K. A., and Latshaw, J. D., Distribution of selenium in chicken tissues as affected by bursectomy, Poultry Sci., 63, 518, 1984.

13. Schrauzer, G. N., Trace elements in carcinogenesis, in *Advances in Nutritional Research*, Volume 2, Draper, H. H., ed., Plenum, New York, p.219, 1979.

14. Spallholz, J. E., Heinzerling, R. H., Gerlach, M. L., and Martin, J. L., The effect of selenite, tocopheryl acetate and selenite: tocopheryl acetate on the primary and secondary immune responses of mice administered tetanus toxoid or sheep red blood cell antigen, Federation Proc., 33, 694 (abstract #2736), 1974.

15. Koller, L. D., Issacson-Kerkuliet, N., Exon, J. H., Brauner, J. A., and Patton, N. M., Synergism of methylmercury and selenium producing enhanced antibody formation in mice, Arch. Environ. Health, 39, 248, 1979.

16. Chandra, R. K., *Trace Elements, Immunity and Infection*, Wiley, New York, 1983.

17. Marsh, J. A., Dietert, R. R., and Combs, G. F., Jr., unpublished research, 1983.

18. Burton, R. M., Higgins, P. J., and McConnell, K. P., Reaction of selenium with immunoglobulin molecules, Biochim. Biophys. Acta, 493, 323, 1977.

19. Martin, J. L. and Spallholz, J. E., Selenium in the immune response, Proc. Symp. Se-Te Environ., P. 204, 1976.

20. Sheffey, B. E., and Schultz, R. D., Influence of vitamin E and selenium on immune response mechanisms, Federation Proc., 38, 2139, 1979.

21. Bendrich, A., D'Apolito, P., Garbiel, E., and Machlin, L. J., Interaction of dietary vitamin C and vitamin E on guinea pig immune responses to mitogens, J. Nutr., 114, 1588, 1984.

22. Arvilommi, H., Poilonen, K., Jokinen, I., Muukkonen, O., Rasenen, L., Foreman, J., and Huttunen, J. K., Selenium and immune functions in humans, Infec. Immunity, 41, 185, 1983.

23. Karle, J. A., Kull, F. J., and Shrift, A., Uptake of selenium-75 by PHA-stimulated lymphocytes. Effect on glutathione peroxidase, Biol. Trace Elem. Res., 5, 17, 1983.

24. Porter, E. K., Karle, J. A., and Shrift, A., Uptake of selenium-75 by human lymphocytes *in vitro*, J. Nutr., 109, 1901, 1979.

25. Clausen, J., and Tranum, J., Kinetics of selenite uptake by mononuclear cells from peripheral human blood, Biol. Trace Elem. Res., 4, 245, 1982.

26. Parnham, M. J., Winkelmann, J., and Leyck, S., Macrophage, lymphocytes and chronic inflammatory responses in selenium-deficient rodents. Association with decreased glutathione peroxidase activity, Int. J. Immunopharmacol., 5, 455, 1983.

27. Lunec, J., and Dormandy, T. L., Fluorescent lipid-peroxidation products of synovial fluid, Clin. Sci., 56, 53, 1979.

28. Bragt, P. C., Schenkelaars, E. P. M., and Bonta, I. L., Dissociation between prostaglandin and malondialdehyde formation in exudate and increased levels of malondialdehyde in plasma and liver during granulomatous inflammation in the rat, Prostaglandin Med., 2, 51, 1979.

29. Lunec, J., Halloran, S. P., White, A. G., and Dormandy, T. L., Free-radical oxidation (peroxidation) products in serum and synovial fluid in rheumatoid arthritis, J. Rheumatol., 8, 233, 1981.

30. Nishikaze, O., Furuya, E., Takita, H., Kosugi, T., and Imai, A., Lipid peroxide, a newly discovered protease, and three other enzymes in carrageenan induced inflammation in rats, IRCS Med. Sci., 9, 424, 1981.

31. Stuyvesant, V. W., and Jolley, W. B., Anti-inflammatory activity of alpha-tocopherol (vitamin E) and linoleic acid, Nature, 216, 585, 1967.

32. Bragt, P. C., Bransberg, J. I., and Bonta, I. L., Antiinflammatory effects of free radical scavenger and antioxidants. Further support for proinflammatory roles of endogenous hydrogen peroxide and lipid peroxides, Inflammation, 4, 289, 1980.

33. Hirschelmann, R., and Bekemeir, H., Effects of catalase, peroxidase, superoxide dismutase and 10 scavengers of oxygen radicals in carrageenan edema and in adjuvant arthritis of rats, Experientia, 37, 1313, 1981.

34. Roberts, M. E., Antiinflammation studies. I. Antiinflammatory properties of liver fractions, Toxicol. Appl. Pharm., 5, 485, 1963.

35. Roberts, M. E., Antiinflammation studies II. Antiinflammatory properties of selenium, Toxicol. Appl. Pharm., 5, 500, 1963.

36. Muraskoshi, M., Osmaura, Y., Yoshimura, S., and Watanabe, K., Immunohistocytochemical localization of glutathione peroxidase (GSH-PO) in the rat testis, Acta Histochem. Cytochem., 16, 335, 1983.

37. Murakoshi, M., Osamura, Y., Yoshimura, S., and Watanabe, K., Characteristic immunocytochemical localization of glutathione-peroxidase (GSH-PO) in rat testicular interstitial macrophages, Acta Histochem. Cytochem., 16, 588, 1983.

38. Novelli, R., and Spallholz, J. E., Incorporation of ^{75}Se-selenite into peritoneal exudate cells of mice: separation and glutathione peroxidase assay of adherent and nonadherent cells, in *Proceedings of the Third International Symposium on Selenium in Biology and Medicine*, Combs, G. F., Jr., Spallholz, J. E., Levander, O. A., and Oldfield, J. E., eds., Avi Publ. Co., Westport, Conn., 1986.

39. Serfass, R. E., and Ganther, H. E., Effects of dietary selenium and tocopherol in glutathione peroxidase and superoxide dismutase activities in rat phagocytes, Life Sci., 19, 1139, 1976.

40. Gebreimichael, A., Levy, E. M., and Cerwin, L. M., Adherent cell requirement for the effect of vitamin E on *in vitro* antibody synthesis, J. Nutr., 114, 1297, 1984.

41. Serfass, R. E., and Ganther, H. E., Defective microbicidal activity in glutathione peroxidase-deficient neutrophils of selenium-deficient rats, Nature, 255, 640, 1975.

42. Boyne, R., and Arthur, J. R., Alterations of neutrophil function in selenium-deficient cattle, J. Comp. Pathol., 89, 151, 1979.

43. Gyang, E. O., Stevens, J. B., Olson, W. G., Tsitsamis, S. D., and Usenik, E. A., Effects of selenium-vitamin E injection on bovine polymorphonucleated leukocytes phagocytosis and killing of *Staphylococcus aureus*, Am. J. Vet. Res., 45, 175, 1984.

44. Aziz, E. S., Klesius, P. H., and Frandsen, J. C., Effects of selenium on polymorphonuclear leucocyte function in goats, Am. J. Vet. Res., 45, 1715, 1984.

45. Sbarra, A. J., and Karnovsky, M. L., The biochemical basis of phagocytosis. I. Metabolic changes during the ingestion of particles by polymorphonuclear leukocytes, J. Biol. Chem., 234, 1355, 1959.

46. Iyer, G. Y.N., Islam, M. F., and Quastel, J. H., Biochemical aspects of phagocytosis, Nature, 192, 535, 1961.

47. Babior, B. M., Kipnes, R. S., and Curnutte, J. T., Biological defense mechanisms. The production by leukocytes of superoxide, a potential bactericidal agent, J. Clin. Invest., 52, 741, 1973.

48. Hamers, M. N., Lutter, R., VanZwieten, R., and Roos, D., Characterization of the O_2^-/H_2O_2-generating system in human neutrophils, in *Oxygen Radicals in Chemistry and Biology*, Bors, W., Saran, M., and Tait, D., eds., Walter de Gruyter, New York, p.843, 1984.

49. Klebanoff, S. J., Oxygen metabolism and the toxic properties of phagocytes, Ann. Intern. Med., 93, 480, 1980.

50. Weiss, S. J., and LoBuglio, A. F., Biology of disease. Phagocyte-generated oxygen metabolites and cellular injury, Lab. Invest., 47, 5, 1982.

51. Littarru, G. P., Lippa, S., DeSole, P., Oradei, A., Torre, F. D., and Macri, M., Quenching of singlet oxygen by D-alpha-tocopherol in human granulocytes, Biochem. Biophys. Res. Commun., 119, 1056, 1984.

52. Lafuze, J. E., Weisrnan, S. J., Ingraham, L. M., Butterick, C. J., Alpert, L. A., and Baehner, R. L., The effect of vitamin E on rabbit neutrophil activation, Ciba Found Symp., 101, 130, 1983.

53. Rajkovic, I. A., and Williams, R., Enhancement of neutrophil response by SH-containing compounds, modulation of superoxide and hydrogen peroxide production, Biochem. Pharmacol., 33, 1249, 1984.

54. Rister M., and Baehner R. L. The alteration of superoxide dismutase, catalase, glutathione peroxidase and NAD(P)H cytochrome c reductase in guinea pig polymorphonuclear leukocytes and alveolar macrophages during hyperoxia, J. Clin. Invest., 58, 1174, 1976.

55. Pasquier, C., Laoussadi, S., and Amor, B., Superoxide production in rheumatoid arthritis (R. A.), and ankylosing spondylitis (A. S.), in *Oxygen Radical in Chemistry and Biology*, Bors, W., Saran, M., and Tait, D., eds., Walter de Gruyter, New York, p.947, 1984.

56. Baret, A., Jadot, G., and Michelson, A. M., Pharmacokinetic and anti-inflammatory properties in the rat of superoxide dismutases (CuSODs and MnSOD) from various species, Biochem. Pharmacol., 33, 2755, 1984.

57. Roos, D., Weening, R. S., Wyss, S. R., and Aebi, H. E., Protection of human neutrophils by endogenous catalase, J. Clin. Invest., 65, 1515, 1980.

58. Baker, S. S., and Cohen, H. J., Increased sensitivity to H_2O_2 in glutathione peroxidase deficient rat granulocytes, J. Nutr., 114, 20 03, 1984.

59. Arthur, J. R., Boyne, R., Hill, H. A. O., and Okalow-Zubkowska, M. J., The production of oxygen-derived radicals by neutrophils from selenium-deficient cattle, FEBS Lett., 135, 187, 1981.

60. Seidegard, J., DePierre, J. W., Birberg, W., Pilotti, A., and Pero, R. W., Characterization of soluble glutathione transferase activity in resting mononuclear leukocytes from human blood, Biochem. Pharmacol., 33, 3053, 1984.

61. Chari, S. N., Nath, N., and Rathi, A. B., Glutathione and its redox system in diabetic polymorphonuclear leukocytes, Am. J. Med. Sci., 287, 14, 1984.

62. Talcott, P. A., Exon, J. H., and Koller, L. D., Attraction of natural killer cell-mediated cytotoxicity in rats treated with selenium, diethylnitrosamine and ethylnitrosourea, Cancer Letts., 23, 313, 1984.

63. Yarrington, J. T., Whitehair, C. K., and Corwin, R. M., Vitamin E-selenium deficiency and its influence on avian malarial infection in the duck, J. Nutr., 103, 231, 1973.

64. Colnago, G.L., Jensen, L.S., and Long, R.L., Effecto of selenium on peripheral blood leukocytes of chickens infected with *Eimeria*, Poultry Sci., 63, 896, 1984.

65. Colnago, G. L., Jensen, L. S., and Long, P. L., Effect of selenium and vitamin E on the development of immunity to coccidiosis in chickens, Poultry Sci., 63, 1136, 1984.
66. Tiege, J., Jr., Nordstoga, K., and Avrsjo, J., Influence of diet on experimental swine dysentery. 1. Effects of a vitamin E and selenium-deficient diet supplemented with 6.8% cod liver oil, Acta Vet. Scand., 18, 384, 1977.
67. Tiege, J., Jr., Saxegaard, F., and Froslie, A., Influence of diet on experimental swine dysentery. 2. Effects of a vitamin E- and selenium-deficient diet supplemented with 3% cod liver oil, vitamin E or selenium, Acta Vet. Scand., 19, 133, 1978.
68. Tiege, J., Jr., Swine dysentery: the influence of dietary vitamin E and selenium on the clinical and pathological effects of *Treponema hyodysenterial* infection in pigs, Res. Vet. Sci., 32, 95, 1982.
69. Tiege, J., Jr., Larsen, H. J., and Tollersrud, J., Swine dysentery: the influence of dietary selenium in clinical and pathological effects of *Treponema hyodysenterial* infection, Acta Vet. Scand., 25, 1, 1984.
70. Andrews, E. D., Hartley, W. J., and Grant, A. B., Selenium-responsive disease of animals in New Zealand, N. Z. Vet. J., 16, 3, 1968.
71. Hartley, W. J., and Grant, A. B., A review of selenium responsive diseases of New Zealand livestock, Federation Proc., 20, 679, 1961.
72. Drake, C., Grant, A. B., and Hartley, W. J., Selenium and animal health. Part 1. The effect of alpha-tocopherol and selenium in the control of field outbreaks of white muscle disease, N. Z. Vet. J., 8, 4, 1960.

10

SELENIUM AND CANCER

Selenium compounds were suggested for cancer chemotherapy more than 70 years ago,[1] i.e., 42 years before any role of the mineral in normal metabolism was recognized. However, it was not until 1949, when Clayton and Baumann[2] demonstrated that a high level of dietary Se (5 ppm as Na_2SeO_3) protected the rat from 3-methyl-4-dimethylaminobenzene-induced carcinogenesis of the colon, that scientific support for the notion of a relationship between Se and cancer could be cited. This notion was not only strengthened but also popularized in 1969 by Shamberger and Frost,[3] who suggested that cancer mortality rates in the USA were inversely associated with local Se status, as indicated by the Se contents of forage crops mapped by Kubota et al.[4] When Allaway et al.[5] showed that the geographic trends in Se contents that appeared in forage crops also tended to be manifest in the blood of resident populations (as estimated from analyses of samples from blood banks in 19 American cities), Shamberger and Willis[6] found a strong inverse association of blood Se level and cancer death rate in the same communities. This and other geographic observational studies[7-10] provided impetus for further investigation of the relationship of Se and cancer in both experimental animal models and in human populations.

I. EFFECTS OF SELENIUM ON CARCINOGENESIS IN EXPERIMENTAL ANIMAL MODELS

A. Early Questions of Selenium as a Carcinogen

In 1943, Nelson et al.[11] reported finding tumors (i.e., adenoma or low-grade carcinoma) in 11 of 53 Osborne-Mendel strain rats that had developed hepatic cirrhosis during the course of 18-24 months of feeding a low-protein diet supplemented with high levels (i.e., 5, 7, or 10 ppm) of Se provided largely by seleniferous feedstuffs. Four other Se-fed rats were found to have advanced adenomatoid hyperplasia within that period of time, but no tumors were found in any livers that were not cirrhotic nor in any animals within the first 18 months of the study. Some questions must be raised concerning the descriptions of tumors in this study, as Nelson *et al.*[11] reported no encapsulation or metastases, and pointed out their own difficulty in discriminating between hyperplasia and tumor.*

In order to address the questions raised by the Nelson *et al.*[11] study in an unequivocal way, a larger study was undertaken by investigators at Oregon State University.[12,13] That study included a total of 1191 Wistar strain rats, of which 274 were fed no supplemental Se, 829 were fed the basal diet supplemented with 0.15-16 ppm Se as either Na_2SeO_3 or Na_2SeO_4, and 88 were treated with a known liver carcinogen (2-aminofluorene). During the course of the study (more than 2 years), 1161 animals were autopsied and neoplasms were found in a total of 63 rats. Of that number, 11 were from the negative control group, 9 were from the Se-treatment groups, and 43 were from the 2-aminofluorene-treated group (i.e., the tumor incidences of these groups were 4, 1 and 49%, respectively). Among the Se-treated rats, no hepatic neoplasms were noted, although hyperplasia was observed in approximately one-half of the number of animals that lived at least 282 days. Other signs were noted: mottled and hypertrophic livers, hydrothorax, ascites, hydropericardium, icterus. The investigators[12,13] concluded that, although the levels of Se employed had been toxic (as indicated by changes in the liver and other organs), there was no evidence of carcinogenicity. Because the Nelson and Oregon State University studies used different strains of rats and forms of Se, their apparently discrepant results required further investigations to resolve the question of whether Se compounds may be carcinogenic. Two such studies sought to provide such information. Volgarev and Tscherkes[14] reported tumors among rats from high levels of Se in uncontrolled trials; however, when a controlled experiment was conducted, no tumors were observed in either Se-fed or control rats. Schroeder and Mitchner[15] maintained a total of 418 Long-Evans strain rats using a semi-purified diet with no supplemental Se (105 rats) or with Se added (2 ppm as either Na_2SeO_3 or Na_2SeO_4) to the drinking water (313 rats). After 1 year, the level of Se supplementation was increased to 3 ppm. Unfortunately, the rats experienced an epidemic of virulent pneumonia during the course of the study; therefore, the numbers of animals

---

*Nelson *et al.*[11] discussed the "difficulty of deciding just when the borderline between nonmalignant and malignant tumor has been passed, and also just when hyperplasia has passed into tumor."

available for autopsy at 21 months of age were greatly reduced (i.e., 73 controls, 75 selenate-treated, and 51 selenite-treated). Upon autopsy, tumors were observed in 20 control rats (i.e., 27% incidence), 30 selenate-treated rats (i.e., 40% incidence) and 4 selenite-treated rats (i.e., 8% incidence). According to Schroeder and Mitchner,[15] these results indicated no significant effect ($p > .05$) of selenite on tumor incidence, but a significant ($p < .05$) increase in tumor incidence due to selenate. They explained the apparent discrepancy between these results and those of Tinsley et al.[12] and Harr et al.[13] on the basis that rats in the latter studies did not survive as long due to the toxicity of the levels of Se fed; therefore, they did not reach "the tumor bearing age of 24-39 months" as had the Schroeder-Mitchner rats which had been fed a less toxic form (selenate) of the element. Scott[16] interpreted the Schroeder and Mitchner[15] study in a similar manner, i.e., that the increased longevity afforded by selenate relative to selenite placed treated animals at greater risk, by virtue of age, to tumorigenesis. It should be noted that selenate treatment was associated with greater longevity; those rats did not show 50% mortality until 125 days after that point was reached by the control group.

Selenium, as an element, cannot be considered carcinogenic any more than the element carbon can be. Therefore, implicit in any consideration of potential carcinogenicity of Se must be an understanding concerning the nature of the Se compounds or groups of Se compounds in question. It is only in this light that the question of possible carcinogenicity of Se in feedstuffs or discrete inorganic or organic compounds can be addressed. In view of the questionable interpretation of the histological findings of Nelson et al.[11] and the absence of clear confirmation of their conclusions, evidence for carcinogenic activities of Se in feedstuffs, selenite, and selenate must be considered very weak. In the opinion of the present authors, these sources of Se cannot be considered carcinogenic.

B. Anticarcinogenic Effects of Selenium

Several Se compounds have been demonstrated to inhibit or retard carcinogenesis in a variety of experimental animal models. These studies have been discussed in several recent reviews.[17-25] In considering the prospective role(s) of Se compounds as anti-carcinogenic agents, it is necessary to discriminate between levels of exposure to the element as being either in the nutritional range (i.e., levels resulting in the correction of a physiological or biochemical abnormality, such as prevention of a deficiency disease or increase in tissue Se-dependent glutathione peroxidase activity) or in the pharmacological range (i.e., levels above saturation of tissue Se-dependent glutathione peroxidase activities, but that result in increased tissue accumulation of Se and increased production of potentially biologically active intermediates of Se metabolism such as methylated forms of Se). An examination of the available information concerning experimental carcinogenesis as affected by either nutritional or pharmacological levels of Se reveals different general effects, which may relate to dose-related differences in Se metabolism.

The results of 55 studies that have evaluated the effects of pharmacological levels of Se on experimental carcinogenesis using several systems, including chemical, viral, and transplantable tumor models, are summarized in Table 10.1[26-62]. Of those studies, some 49 found that high-level Se treatment reduced the development of tumors at least moderately (i.e., by 15-35% from control levels) and, in two-thirds of the cases, very substantially (i.e., by more than 35%). Only seven studies found Se treatments of animals to be without effect on tumor outcome, and two of those[32,39] employed levels of Se that may be regarded as being only slightly above or perhaps within the nutritional range. A study by Ankerst and Sjoegren,[64] not summarized in that table, found Se treatment of rats to be associated with increased incidences of 1,2-dimethylhydrazine (DMH) -induced small intestinal tumors and of viral-induced (i.e., adenovirus type 9) mammary tumors. The same study[64] found Se treatment to reduce DMH-induced tumors of the large intestine. Other investigators have found Se treatment to result in only slight reductions in azo dye-induced hepatic tumors[65] or in L-azaserine-induced preneoplastic pancreatic acinar cell nodules[66] in rats. (This effect was only apparent when rats were fed a diet containing 20% corn oil.)

The overwhelming majority of investigations in this area has found that high levels of Se reduce the incidence of tumors in experimental animal models, presumably by inhibition or retardation of tumorigenesis. Furthermore, reduction in tumorigenesis by Se in these systems has been observed in many cases at levels of Se intake that are not overtly toxic. (Note absence of changes in gross body weights in Table 10.1.) Nevertheless, the results summarized in Table 10.1 provide some indication that Se (in almost all cases studied given as Na_2SeO_3) is less effective as an antitumorigenic agent when used at levels less than the equivalent of 1 ppm in the diet. When Se intakes are estimated on a dietary equivalency basis (i.e., for Se administered in drinking water by assuming that animals consume ca. 1.5 ml water per 1.0 g feed), those studies indicate the following relationship between dietary intake levels and average reduction in tumor incidence from control levels: <1 ppm Se, 19% reduction (8 studies); 1-2 ppm Se, 42% reduction (12 studies); 2-4 ppm Se, 45% reduction (18 studies); 4-8 ppm Se, 41% reduction (24 studies), >8 ppm Se, 58% reduction (8 studies). While this kind of analysis cannot be interpreted to demonstrate a dose-response relationship between Se level and tumorigenesis, it does

Table 10.1

Summary of Studies That Have Evaluated Effects of High Levels of Selenium on Carcinogenesis in Experimental Animal Models

Organ site	Species	Carcinogenic agent	Se treatment Dietary (ppm)	Drinking water (ppm)	Other	Tumor response [a] (% control)	Growth response (% control)	Reference
Colon	Rat	1,2-Dimethylhydrazine	⎰	0^c	—	100^c	100^c	(28)
				4^d		27^e	100	
	Rat	1,2-Dimethylhydrazine	0.183	0^c	—	100^c	100^c	(29)
				4^d		93^e	94^e	
	Rat	1,2-Dimethylhydrazine	0.183	0^c	—	100	100^a	(30)
				4^d		83^e	91^g	
	Rat	Methylazoxymethanol acetate	⎰	0^c	—	100^c	100^c	(28)
				4^d		54^e	100	
	Rat	Bis-(2-oxypropyl) nitrosamine	0.17^c	—	—	100^c	100^c	(31)
			2.07^d	—		66^e	101	
Intestine	Rat	Azoxymethane	0.04^b	0^c	—	100^c	⎰	(26)
				2^d		83^e	⎰	
	Rat	Azoxymethane	0.04^b	0^c	—	100^c	⎰	(27)
				2^d		85^e	⎰	
Liver	Rat	2-Acetylaminofluorene	0.04^{bc}	—	—	100^c	100^c	(32)
			0.54^h	—		100	100	
	Rat	2-Acetylaminofluorene	⎰	0^c	—	100^c	100^c	(33)
				4^d		41^e	97^e	
	Rat	2-Acetylaminofluorene	0.10^c	—	—	100^c	—	(34)
			0.50	—		100	—	
			2.50	—		67^e	—	

(continues)

Table 10.1 *(Continued)*

Organ site	Species	Carcinogenic agent	Se treatment Dietary (ppm)	Se treatment Drinking water (ppm)	Se treatment Other	Tumor response [a] (% control)	Growth response (% control)	Reference
	Rat	3-Methyl-4-dimethyl aminobenzene	0.1^c	—	—	100^c	∫	(2)
			5	—	—	52^e	—	
	Rat	3-Methyl-4-dimethyl aminobenzene	0.1^{bc}	—	—	100^c	100^c	(35)
			6^i	—	—	51^j	97^e	
				6^d	—	70^g	96^f	
Lung	Rat	bis-(2-oxypropyl) nitrosamine	0.17^c	—	—	100^c	100^c	(31)
			2.07^d	—	—	0	101	
Mammary	Mouse	7,12-Dimethylbenz(a) anthracene^e	0.15^h	0^c	—	100^c	∫	(36)
				6^a	—	47^p		
	Mouse	7,12-demethylbenz(a) anthracene^m	0.15	0^c	—	100^c	∫	(36)
				6^a	—	27^p		
	Mouse	7,12-Dimethylbenz(a) anthracene	0.002	0^c	—	100^c	∫	(37)
				2^a	—	39^p		
				4^a	—	48^p		
	Mouse	7,12-Dimethylbenz(a) anthracene	0.15	0^c	—	100^c	100^c	(38)
			0.15	7^d	—	30^e	96^g	
	Mouse	7,12-Dimethylbenz(a) Anthracene	0.35^c	—	—	100^c	∫	(38)
			2.15^h	—	—	28^e		
	Mouse	7,12-Dimethylbenz(a) anthracene	0.1^{cd}	—	—	100^c	∫	(39)
			1^d	—	—	51^e		
			0.1^k	—	—	69^e		

(continues)

418

Table 10.1 (*Continued*)

Organ site	Species	Carcinogenic agent	Se treatment			Tumor response [a] (% control)	Growth response (% control)	Reference
			Dietary (ppm)	Drinking water (ppm)	Other			
Mammary	Mouse	7,12-Dimethylbenz(a)anthracene	0.2^c 0.5^d 1.0^d 2.0^d	— — — —	— — — —	100^c 54° 44° 28°	$\checkmark^f$	(40)
	Mouse	7,12-Dimethylbenz(a)anthracene	0.2^d	0^c 8^d	— —	100^c 64^p	100^c 100	(41)
	Rat	7,12-Dimethylbenz(a)anthracene[l]	0.15^{ch} 1.05^h 2.06^h	— — —	— — —	100^c 100 88^e	$\checkmark^f$	(42)
	Rat	7,12-Dimethylbenz(a)anthracene[m]	0.15^{ch} 1.05^h 2.06^h	— — —	— — —	100^c 86^e 79^e	$\checkmark$	(43)
	Rat	7,12-Dimethylbenz(a)anthracene	$—^f$	0^c 5	— —	100^c 31^e	$\checkmark$	(43)
	Rat	7,12-Dimethylbenz(a)anthracene	0.3^{ch} 4.3 4.3^{hn}	— — —	— — —	100^c 51^e 8^e	$\checkmark$	(44)
	Rat	7,12-Dimethylbenz(a)anthracene	0.1^{cq} 2.5^{dq} 5.0^{dq}	— — —	— — —	100^c 45^p 21°	100^c 96^e 88^e	(45)
	Rat	7,12-Dimethylbenz(a)anthracene	0.1^{cr} 2.5^{dr} 5.0^{dr}	— — —	— — —	100^c 63^g 34°	100^c 104^e 87^e	(45)

(continues)

Table 10.1 (*Continued*)

Organ site	Species	Carcinogenic agent	Se treatment Dietary (ppm)	Drinking water (ppm)	Other	Tumor response [a] (% control)	Growth response (% control)	Reference
Mammary	Rat	7,12-Dimethylbenz(a)anthracene	0.1^c	—	—	100^{cs}	100^{cs}	(46)
			2.5^d	—	—	75^{es}	99^{es}	
	Rat	7,12-Dimethylbenz(a)anthracene	0.1^q	—	—	100^c	100^c	(47)
			2.5^{dq}	—	—	71^e	99^e	
	Rat	7,12-Dimethylbenz(a)anthracene	0.1^{cr}	—	—	100^c	100^c	(47)
			2.5^{dr}	—	—	52^e	98^e	
	Rat	7,12-Dimethylbenz(a)anthracene[l]	0.15^{ch}	—	—	100^c	100^c	(48)
			1.05^h	—	—	73^p	98^p	
			2.06^h	—	—	63^p	90^p	
	Rat	7,12-Dimethylbenz(a)anthracene	0.15^{eh}	—	—	100^c	—[f]	(48)
			1.05^h	—	—	90^g		
			2.06^h	—	—	65^g		
	Rat	2-Acetylaminofluorene	0.1^{cdt}	—	—	100^c	100^c	(49)
			0.5^{dt}	—	—	13^p	107	
			2.5^{dt}	—	—	0	109	
	Rat	2-Acetylaminofluorene	0.1^{cdt}	—	—	100^c	—[f]	(34)
			0.5^{dt}	—	—	85^e		
			2.5^{dt}	—	—	85^e		
	Rat	N-Methyl-N-nitrosourea	0.2^{cd}	—	—	100^c	100^c	(50)
			4^d	—	—	77^p	94^e	
	Rat	N-Methyl-N-nitrosourea	0.2^{cdh}	—	—	100^c	100^c	(50)
			4^{dh}	—	—	70^p	98^e	

(*continues*)

Table 10.1 (*Continued*)

Organ site	Species	Carcinogenic agent	Se treatment Dietary (ppm)	Se treatment Drinking water (ppm)	Se treatment Other	Tumor response[a] (% control)	Growth response (% control)	Reference
Mammary	Rat	N-Methyl-N-nitrosourea	0.1^{cd}	—	—	100^c	100^c	(51)
			4^d	—	—	100	95^g	
			5^d	—	—	106	93^p	
			6^d	—	—	100	96^g	
			5^u	—	—	106	97^g	
			6^u	—	—	89^g	93^p	
	Rat	N-Methyl-N-nitrosourea	0.5^{cd}	—	—	100^c	100^c	(52)
			5^d	—	—	58^p	92^p	
	Mouse	Virus	$\{$	0^c	—	100^c	$\{$	(53)
				2^d	—	59^e		
				6^d	—	9^e		
	Mouse	Virus	0.2^d	0^c	—	100^c	100^c	(41)
				8^d	—	65^p	100	
	Mouse	Virus	$\{$	0^c	—	100^c	100^c	(54)
				2^d	—	12^v	91^e	
				5^d	—	44^v	88^e	
				15^d	—	40^v	76^e	
	Mouse	Virus	0.15^d	—	—	100^c	$\{$	(56)
			1.0^d	—	—	60^p		
	Mouse	Virus	$\{$	0^c	—	100^c	$\{$	(53)
				2^d	—	59^e		
				6^d	—	9^e		
	Mouse	Virus	$\{$	0^c	—	100	$\{$	(55)
				2^d	—	12^p		
	Mouse	Transplants (6 preneoplastic outgrowth lines)	$\{$	0^c	—	100^{cw}	$\{$	(53)
				4^d	—	95^{cgw}		

(continues)

Table 10.1 (Continued)

Organ site	Species	Carcinogenic agent	Se treatment Dietary (ppm)	Se treatment Drinking water (ppm)	Se treatment Other	Tumor response [a] (% control)	Growth response (% control)	Reference
Mammary	Mouse	Transplants (MT-W9B cells)	0.1^{cd} 2^d	—	—	100^{cx} 53^{ex}	∫	(57)
	Mouse	Transplants (CMT-14B cells)	∫^{f}	—	0^c $2\ \mu g/g$ BW, s.c.	100^c 40^e	100^c 92^p	(58)
Skin	Mouse	Benzo(a)pyrene^y	0.2^{cd} 2^d	—	—	100^c 56^e	∫	(59)
	Mouse	7,12-Dimethylbenz(a)anthracene^z	0.04^c	—	0 0.0005% Na$_2$Se, topical	100^{cx} 53^{ex}	∫	(39)
	Mouse	7,12-Dimethylbenz(a)anthracene	0.04^c 0.14^h 1.04^h 0.1^k	—	—	100^c 153^e 60^e 120^e	∫	(39)
Trachea	Hamster	N-Methyl-N-nitrosourea	0.04^c 1.04^h 5.04^h	—	—	100^c 93^g 90^g	∫	(60)
Erhlich acites	Mouse	Transplants	∫^{f}	—	0^c $2\ \mu g/g$, p.o. $2\ \mu g/g$ i.p.	100^c 100 85^g	100^c 79^g 41°	(61)
	Mouse	Transplants	∫	—	0^c $10\ \mu g$ Se/g, i.p.	100^c 10	100^c 57^e	(22, 63)

(continues)

Table 10.1 (*Continued*)

Organ site	Species	Carcinogenic agent	Se treatment Dietary (ppm)	Se treatment Drinking water (ppm)	Se treatment Other	Tumor response [a] (% control)	Growth response (% control)	Reference
Erlich acites	Mouse	Transplants			$0.125\ \mu g/g$, i.p.[bb]	20^e	83^g	
					$0.25\ \mu g/g$, i.p.[bb]	0^e	77^g	

[a] Based on numbers of tumors per animal or where those data were not reported, incidence of tumor-bearing animals.

[b] Estimated by present authors.

[c] Control treatment; tumor and growth responses arbitrarily assigned values of 100%.

[d] Supplemental Se provided as Na_2SeO_3.

[e] Significance of treatment effect not tested.

[f] Data not given in original report.

[g] Treatment effect not significant ($p > 0.05$).

[h] Total Se level includes amount of Se in basal diet plus that amount supplemented as Na_2SeO_3.

[i] Supplemental Se provided as a high-Se yeast product.

[j] Treatment effect significant ($p < 0.01$).

[k] Supplemental Se provided as N_2Se.

[l] Animals given a relatively high dose of the carcinogen.

[m] Animals given a relatively low dose of the carcinogen.

[n] Administered with retinoic acid (250 ppm)

[o] Treatment effect significant ($p < 0.02$).

[p] Treatment effect significant ($p < 0.05$).

[q] 5% Dietary fat (as corn oil).

[r] 25% Dietary fat (as corn oil).

[s] Average results of two studies with high (1050 IU/kg) and adequate (50 IU/kg) dietary vitamin E.

[t] Added to basal diet, which contained 0.018 ppm Se.

[u] Supplemental Se provided as DL-selenomethionine.

[v] Treatment effect significant ($p < 0.005$).

[w] Average results of six experiments.

[x] Average results of two experiments.

[y] Promoted with 12-O-tetradecanoylphorbol acetate.

[z] Promoted with croton oil.

[aa] Supplemental Se provided as SeO_2.

[bb] Supplemental Se provided as Na_2SeO_4.

[cc] Supplemental Se provided as DL-selenocystine.

Table 10.1 *(Continued)*

Organ site	Species	Carcinogenic agent	Se treatment Dietary (ppm)	Se treatment Drinking water (ppm)	Se treatment Other	Tumor response [a] (% control)	Growth response (% control)	Reference
Erhlich acites	Mouse	Transplants	—[f]	—	0[c]	100	100	(22, 62)
					0.25 µg/g, i.p.[aa]	25[e]	58[p]	
					1 µg/g, i.p.[aa]	0[e]	58[p]	
					0.25 µg/g, i.p.[d]	0[e]	64[p]	
					1 µg/g, i.p.[d]	0[e]	48[p]	
					0.25 µg/g, i.p.[bb]	40[e]	43[p]	
					1 µg/g, i.p.[bb]	0[e]	38[p]	
					0.25 µg/g, i.p.[v]	100[e]	103[g]	
					1 µg/g i.p.[v]	100	103[g]	
					0.25 µg/g, i.p.[cc]	60[e]	65[p]	
					1 µg/g i.p.[cc]	0[e]	51[p]	
	Mouse	Transplants	—	—	0[c]	100[c]	100[c]	(22)
					0.0625 µg/g i.p.[bb]	40[e]	79[g]	

raise questions concerning the effect of dietary Se level on the efficacy of the element in reduction of experimental carcinogenesis. Because these investigations appear to show that the lowest level of Se intake is the least protective against carcinogenesis, it is appropriate to consider specifically the effect of nutritional levels of Se in this regard.

Relatively few studies have evaluated the effect of nutritional levels and, particularly, nutritionally deficient levels of Se on carcinogenesis in experimental animal models. The results of these are summarized in Table 10.2.[67-69] The 18 studies presented in that table indicate that, in general, dietary deficiencies of Se may not affect carcinogenesis of the colon or liver in the rat, or of the mammary gland in the mouse; however, Se-deficiency appears to result in enhanced carcinogenesis of the mammary gland in the rat and of the skin in the mouse. Unfortunately, the significance of the effect of Se was not adequately tested by appropriate statistical means in many of these studies. It must also be pointed out that the severity of nutritional Se deficiency is difficult to determine in many of these studies because specific indicators of Se status were not measured. Therefore, while the available information suggests that nutritional Se-deficiency may exacerbate carcinogenesis under some circumstances, this conclusion must remain a tentative one until more definitive data are produced in a variety of animal model systems.

C. Mechanisms of Selenium as an Anticarcinogenic Agent

Selenium may be active in the inhibition of carcinogenesis in various tumor model systems in any of several ways. One of these, pertinent to Se inhibition of chemical carcinogenesis, is the possibility that the metabolism of chemical carcinogens may be affected by Se status. Research addressing this possibility is summarized in Table 10.3.[70-84] Studies that have determined the effects of Se treatment on the activities of carcinogen-metabolizing enzymes have been restricted mainly to hepatic microsomal aryl hydrocarbon hydroxylase (AHH). Although there is some evidence that constitutive (i.e., noninduced) AHH activities may be enhanced by Se,[73,74] the induced levels of the enzyme appear not to be affected. This conforms to findings with other hepatic microsomal cytochrome P450-dependent mixed function oxidases, i.e., that changes in Se status may not affect a particular activity (see Chapter 6).

Other studies, however, have been concerned with aspects of carcinogen metabolism that can be assessed by the production of metabolites capable of forming covalent adducts with intracellular macromolecules (e.g., DNA). Such studies have found varied effects of Se treatment on DNA-adduct formation. In fact, Combs' group found that supranutritional levels (i.e.,

Table 10.2

Summary of Studies That Have Evaluated Effects of Nutritionally Deficient Levels of Selenium on Carcinogenesis in Experimental Animal Models

Organ site	Species	Carcinogenic agent	Se treatment Dietary (ppm)	Drinking water (ppm)	Tumor response^a (% control)	Growth response (% control)	Reference
Colon	Rat	1,2-Dimethylhydrazine	<0.02	—	109^d	93^e	(67)
			0.10^{bc}	—	100^c	100^c	
Liver	Rat	2-Acetylaminofluorene	0.018	—	100	101^d	(49)
			0.1^{bc}	—	100^c	100^c	
	Rat	2-Acetylaminofluorene	0.018	—	50^f	—^{g}	(34)
			0.1^{bc}	—	100^c		
Mammary	Mouse	7,12-Dimethylbenz(a)anthracene^h	0.02^i	—	83^f	—^{g}	(39)
			0.1^{bc}	—	100^c		
			0.1^j	—	69^f		
	Mouse	Virus	0.02^i	—	119^d	122^f	(54)
			0.1^{ci}	—	100^c	100^c	
	Rat	2-Acetylaminofluorene	0.018	—	92^f	—^{g}	(34)
			0.1^{bc}	—	100^c		
	Rat	7,12-Demethylbenz(a)anthracene	<0.02	—	258^e	—^{g}	(68)
			0.1^{bc}	—	100^c		
	Rat	7,12-Dimethylbenz(a)anthracene	0.05	—	97^f	—^{g}	(42)
			0.15^{bc}	—	100^c		
	Rat	7,12-Dimethylbenz(a)anthracene	0.05	—	123^f	—^{g}	(42)
			0.15^{bc}	—	100^c		

Species	Compound	Dose				Ref.
Rat	7,12-Dimethylbenz(a) anthracene[k]	[k] <0.02	—	139[f]	—[g]	(69)
		0.1[bc]		100[c]		
Rat	7,12-Dimethylbenz(a)[l] anthracene	<0.02	—	132[f]	—[g]	(69)
		0.1[bc]		100[c]		
Rat	7,12-Dimethylbenz(a) anthracene[m]	<0.02	—	160[f]	—[g]	(69)
		0.1[bc]		100[c]		
Rat	7,12-Dimethylbenz(a) anthracene[n]	<0.02	—	122[f]	—[g]	(69)
		0.1[bc]		100[c]		
Rat	7,12-Diemthylbenz(a) anthracene[o]	0.05	—	83[d]	99[d]	(48)
		0.15[bc]		100[c]	100[c]	
Rat	7,12-Diemthylbenz(a) anthracene[p]	0.05	—	125[d]	—[g]	(48)
		0.15[bc]		100[c]		
Rat	N-Methyl-N-nitrosourea	0.01	—	141[d]	98[d]	(52)
		0.10[bc]		100[c]	100[c]	
Rat	Transplants	<0.02	—	106[d]	—[g]	(57)
		0.1[bc]		100[c]		
Skin						
Mouse	7,12-Demethylbenz(a) anthracene	0.04	—	65[e]	—[g]	(39)
		0.14		100[c]		

(continues)

427

Table 10.2 *(Continued)*

Organ site	Species	Carcinogenic agent[q]	Se treatment		Tumor response[a] (% control)	Growth response (% control)	Reference
			Dietary (ppm)	Drinking water (ppm)			
	Mouse	Benzo(a)pyrene[q]	<0.01	0	250[f]	—[g]	(59)
			<0.01	0.02[b]	175[f]		
			<0.01	0.2[bc]	100[c]		

[a] Based on numbers of tumors per animal or, where those data were not reported, incidence of tumor-bearing animals.
[b] Added to basal diet as Na_2SeO_3.
[c] Control treatment.
[d] Treatment effect not significant ($p > 0.05$).
[e] Treatment effect significant ($p < 0.05$).
[f] Significance of treatment effect not tested.
[g] Data not given in original report.
[h] Promoted with croton oil.
[i] Level in basal diet estimated by present authors.
[j] Added to basal diet as Na_2Se.
[k] Basal diet contained 1% corn oil.
[l] Basal diet contained 5% corn oil.
[m] Basal diet contained 25% corn oil.
[n] Basal diet contained 1% corn oil and 24% coconut oil.
[o] Carcinogen administered at relatively low dose.
[p] Carcinogen administered at relatively high dose.
[q] Promoted with 12-O-tetradecanoylphorbol acetate.

428

Table 10.3

Summary of Studies of Selenium and Carcinogen Metabolism

Type of effect	Species	Se treatments		Findings	Reference
		Negative control	+Se		
Activities of carcinogen-metabolizing enzymes	Rat	Diet: 0.1^a ppm	Diet: 5^b ppm	No significant differences in constitutive aryl hydrocarbon hydroxylase (AHH) activities in liver or mammary tissue.	(70)
	Rat	Diet: 0.02 ppm	Diet: $0.2–6^{bc}$ ppm	No significant differences in constitutive AHH activities in liver.	(71)
	Rat	Diet: 0.02 ppm	Diet: 2^b ppm	No significant differences in the constitutive or PCB^d-induced AHH activities in liver.	(72)
	Rat	Diet: 0.02 ppm	Diet: 2^b ppm	Se significantly ($p < 0.05$) increased constitutive AHH activity in liver, but did not affect PCB^d-induced activities in that organ.	(73)
	Rat	Diet: 0.02^{ef} ppm	Diet: $0.1–0.4^{cg}$ ppm	Se significantly ($p < 0.05$) increased constitutive AHH activities in liver.	(74)
	Rat	Diet: 0.02 ppm Water: 0	Diet: 0.02 ppm Water: 0.2^b ppm	Se significantly ($p < 0.05$) decreased dimethylnitrosamine methylase in liver.	(75)
DNA-binding	Rat	Diet: 0.1^a ppm	Diet: 2.5, 5^b ppm	The highest level of Se appeared to cause increased (by two-fold) formation of 7,12-dimethylbenz(a)-anthracene (DMBA)-DNA adducts by 6 hrs after DMBA treatment, but significantly less (by 46%) adduct formation by 24 hrs, indicating enhanced DNA repair.	(70)
	Rat	Diet: 0.02^{ef} ppm	Diet: $0.1–0.4^{cg}$ ppm	No significant differences in benzo(a)pyrene-DNA adduct formation.	(74)

(continues)

Table 10.3 *(Continued)*

Type of effect	Species	Se treatments Negative control	+Se	Findings	Reference
DNA-binding	Rat	Diet: 0.02[e] ppm	Diet: 0.5[b] pm	No significant differences in 2-acetylaminofluorene (AAF)- DNA adduct formation; but Se significantly ($p < 0.05$) reduced AAF-induced repairable DNA single-strand breakage.	(76)
	Chick	Diet: 0.02 ppm	Diet: 0.2-20[bc] ppm	Se, at levels of 0.2 ppm and greater, significantly ($p < 0.05$) reduced aflatoxin B_1 (AFB_1)-DNA adduct formation (to 75% of low-Se group) both at 2 and 24 hrs after AFB_1 treatment.	(77)
	Rat	Diet: 0.02 ppm	Diet: 0.2-6[bc] ppm	Se, at levels of 0.2 and 2 ppm, significantly ($p < 0.05$) increased (by almost two-fold) the formation of aflatoxin B_1 (AFB_1)- DNA adducts; the highest level of Se (ppm) reduced AFB_1-DNA adduct formation to 43% of that of low Se group.	(71)
Metabolite production	Rat	Diet: 0.02 ppm	Diet: 0.5b ppm	Se significantly ($p < 0.05$) increased the *in vitro* production of 3-OH-acetylaminofluorine (by 53%) by liver microsomes incubated with 2-acetylaminofluorene (AAF), but did not affect ($p > 0.05$) the production of 7-OH-AAF, 5-OH-AAF, or N-OH-AAF. Se treatment significantly ($p < 0.05$) reduced the urinary excretion of both nonconjugated and glucuronic acid-conjugated N-OH-AAF.	(78)

Rat	Diet: [h] Water: 0	Diet: [h] Water: 4^b ppm	Se significantly ($p < 0.05$) increased ring hydroxylation but significantly ($p < 0.05$) decreased N-hydroxylation of 2-acetylaminofluorene (AAF).	(33)
Rat	Diet: 0.02 ppm Water: 0	Diet: 0.02 ppm Water: 0.2 ppm	Se did not affect ($p > 0.05$) the C-oxygenation of N,N-dimethylaniline, but significantly ($p < 0.05$) increased its N-oxygenation by hepatic microsomes in vitro. Se reduced ($p < 0.05$) the in vitro formation by microsomes of metabolites of dimethylnitrosamine that were mutagenic in Chinese hamster V79 cells.	(75)
Rat	Diet: 0.02^e ppm	Diet: 0.1-5^{bc} ppm	No significant differences ($p > 0.05$) on the in vitro production by hepatic microsomes of metabolites of aflatoxin B_1 that were mutagenic to Salmonella typhimurium.	(79)
Rat	Diet: 0.15^a ppm Water: 0	Diet: 0.15^a ppm Water: 5^b ppm	Se significantly ($p < 0.05$) reduced the in vitro production by hepatic microsomes of metabolites of 7,12-dimethylbenz(a)anthracene that were mutagenic to S. typhimurium.	(80)
Rat	Diet: 0.05 ppm	Diet: 2.5 ppm	Dietary Se reduced ($p < 0.05$) ring oxidation of 7,12-dimethylbenz(a)anthracene, but increased its 12-methyloxidation by hepatic microsomes in vitro.	(84)
Rat	Diet: 0.02^e ppm	Diet: 0.1-5^{bc} ppm	Se significantly ($p < 0.05$) reduced the in vitro production by hepatic microsomes of metabolites of 7,12-dimethylbenz(a)anthracene that were mutagenic to S. typhimurium.	(80)

(continues)

Table 10.3 (Continued)

Type of effect	Species	Se treatments		Findings	Reference
		Negative control	+Se		
Metabolite production	Rat	Diet: 0.02 ppm	Diet: 1^b ppm	The *in vitro* production by hepatic microsomes of metabolites that were mutagenic to *S. typhimurium* from 2-aminofluorene was increased ($p < 0.05$) by Se, but from 2-acetylaminofluorene was decreased ($p < 0.05$) by Se.	(72,73)
	Rat	Diet: $-^h$	Diet: $-^h$ Water: 20^b ppm	Se significantly ($p < 0.05$) reduced the capacity of hepatic microsomes to transform 7,12-dimethylbenz(a)anthracene to forms that were mutagenic to *S. typhimurium*.	(81)
Carcinogen acute toxicity	Turkey poults	Diet: 0.1^a ppm	Diet: $5,10^b$ ppm	No significant ($p > 0.05$) effects on the acute toxicity of alflatoxin B_1 as measured by growth and liver weight.	(82)
	Rat	Diet: $-^h$	Diet: $-^h$ +0.5 mg Se^{bi}/kg, i.p.	Se enhanced the acute toxicity of dimethylnitrosamine, as evidenced by significant ($p < 0.05$) increases in plasma aspartate aminotransferase.	(83)

[a]Value given in original report; probably includes only that amount of Se that was added as Na_2SeO_3 in the preparation of the basal diet and not the Se intrinsic to the feed ingredients.

[b]Provided as a supplement of Na_2SeO_3.

[c]Graded levels were employed.

[d]Polychlorinated biphenyls.

[e]Estimated by the present authors.

[f]Rats were maintained on this diet for 6 months prior to the study to deplete the Se stores.

[g]Rats were fed Se-supplemented diets for 4 weeks after the 6-month Se-depletion period.

[h]Se content of diet not indicated.

[i]Injection given 48 hrs before administration of DMN.

0.2-2.0 ppm) of Se (as Na_2SeO_3) reduced the formation of aflatoxin B_1-DNA adducts in the chick[70] but had the opposite effect in the rat.[71] Direct study of the metabolism of several chemical carcinogens has been accomplished. Two groups[33,78] have demonstrated that Se supplementation of the rat increases the ring-hydroxylation but decreases the N-hydroxylation of 2-acetylamino-fluorene, thereby reducing the activation and enhancing the detoxification of this carcinogen. Other studies have shown that the metabolites of N,N-dimethylanaline,[75] 7,12-dimethylbenz(a)anthracene[80,81,84,88,89] 2-aminofluorene,[72,73] and benzo(a)pyrene[90] produced by hepatic microsomes prepared from Se-supplemented rats are less mutagenic as determined in the Ames-type *Salmonella typhimurium* tester system. Therefore, the limited information presently available indicates that, while high-level Se supplementation can result in alterations in the metabolism of certain chemical carcinogens, this effect is not universal with respect to either host animal species or carcinogen. The more widespread effects of Se on carcinogenesis in experimental animal models must involve mechanisms in addition to or other than those involved in carcinogen metabolism.

Griffin[19] suggested that Se may be involved in carcinogenesis in the protection against oxidative damage by virtue of its role in Se-dependent glutathione peroxidase (SeGSHpx). This hypothesis is supported by the demonstration by Shamberger et al.[85] that malonaldehyde, a product of the peroxidative degradation of linoleic acid, is carcinogenic when applied to mouse skin and mutagenic when assayed in the Ames *Salmonella typhimurium* tester system. The hypothesis that the anticarcinogenic action of Se may be due to the function of SeGSHpx in the general antioxidant protection of cells seems plausible to explain the increases in tumor incidence observed among nutritionally Se-deficient animals (see Table 10.2). However, it is not supported in the case of 7,12-dimethylbenz(a)anthracene-induced mammary carcinogenesis in the studies of Horvath and Ip,[46] who found that the antitumorigenic activity of Se, administered at levels in the nutritional range, could not be accounted for by suppression of tissue lipid peroxidation. In addition, most experimental animal studies have found Se supplementation to be effective against carcinogenesis at levels above those required to support maximal tissue activities of SeGSHpx. Therefore, it is very unlikely that the anticarcinogenic mechanism(s) of action of high levels of Se involve the oxidation-protection function of SeGSHpx.

LeBoeuf and Hoekstra[86,87] proposed that the anticarcinogenic activities of high levels of Se may be due to the toxicity of Se metabolites to proliferating cells. They pointed out that, with only a few exceptions, the anticarcinogenic effects in animal model systems have been seen when selenite was the species of Se used, and that the reductive metabolism of high levels of selenite may be expected to result in the catalytic oxidation of large amounts of glutathione from its reduced (GSH) to oxidized (GSSG) forms, as described by Tsen and Tappel.[88] LeBoeuf and Hoekstra[86,87] suggested that high levels of selenite may perturb normal intracellular concentrations of GSH, GSSG, and their mixed disulfides, which are required for normal cell function. In experimental work, they then demonstrated that prolonged feeding of a high level of Se (i.e., 6 ppm Se fed as Na_2SeO_3 for 6 weeks) resulted in increases in the hepatic concentrations of GSH and GSSG, and that the ratio of GSSG:GSH increased in comparison to rats fed an Se-adequate (i.e., 0.1 ppm Se as Na_2SeO_3) diet.[86] Because these changes were observed with concomitant increases in the hepatic activities of glutathione reductase and glucose-6-phosphate dehydrogenase, they concluded that selenite-induced GSH oxidation resulted in an adaptive response of the liver to reduce intracellular concentrations of GSSG towards the restoration of a more nearly normal GSSG:GSH ratio. LeBoeuf and Hoekstra[87] found that high levels (i.e., 50 μM and 100 μM) of Na_2SeO_3 caused a significant dose-dependent increase in the population doubling time of H-4-II-C3 "minimal deviation" hepatoma cells in culture. The inhibition was lost upon replacement of the growth medium with one that was Se-free, and the cell cycle inhibition pattern caused by Se resembled those of known inhibitors of protein synthesis. The hepatoma cells showed the same kinds of biochemical changes in response to selenite treatment (e.g., dose-dependent increases in the concentrations of GSH and GSSG, and in GSSG:GSH ratio; increased glutathione reductase activity) that were observed in high-Se-fed rat liver. The investigators suggested that, because GSSG is known to activate a protein kinase that inactivates, via phosphorylation, eukaryotic initiation factor 2 (eIF-2),[89,91] the antiproliferative effect of selenite was due to its effect in increasing GSSG levels. This hypothesis is supported by the findings of Safer et al.[92] that selenite can inactivate eIF-2 through a mechanism mediated by a protein kinase.

Thus, several studies[86,87,93-94] indicate that high levels of Se can inhibit cell proliferation and that the likely mechanism of action involves decreased protein synthesis. The effects of Se on tumor cells in vitro have been studied by several investigators, whose results are summarized in Tables 10.4[95-98] and 10.5.[99-103] Most of the these studies have demonstrated selenite to inhibit the growth and/or viability of tumor cells in culture (see Table 10.4) and have shown that these effects are associated with changes in tumor cell metabolism, which include, in various systems, decreased mitochondrial oxidative metabolism, increased levels of cAMP, and reduced synthesis of RNA (see Table 10.5). Selenite-induced reductions in the rates of synthesis of DNA and protein have been reported.[96,103] Similar results were observed

Table 10.4

In Vitro Effects of Selenium on Tumor Cell Growth and Viability

Cell line	Se treatment	Growth[a] (% control)	Viability[b] (% control)	Reference
MCF-7 human mammary tumor	0	—	100[c]	(22)
	Na_2SeO_3, 2.7 μM Se	—	100[c]	
	Na_2SeO_3, 5.4 μM Se	—	47[cd]	
	Na_2SeO_3, 8.1 μM Se	—	39[cd]	
MDA-MB-231 human mammary tumor	0	—	100[c]	(22)
	Na_2SeO_3, 2.7 μM Se	—	62[cd]	
	Na_2SeO_3, 5.4 μM Se	—	57[cd]	
	Na_2SeO_3, 8.1 μM Se	—	20[cd]	
MRC-5 nonneoplastic human lung	0	—	100[c]	(22)
	Na_2SeO_3, 2.7 μM Se	—	100[c]	
	Na_2SeO_3, 5.4 μM Se	—	100[c]	
	Na_2SeO_3, 8.1 μM Se	—	90[cd]	
YN-4 murine mammary cells	0	100[c]	—	(96)
	Na_2SeO_3 0.05 μM Se	153[ce]	—	
	Na_2SeO_3, 5 μM Se	66[ce]	—	
	Na_2SeO_3, 50 μM Se	19[ce]	—	
L 1210 leukemic cells	0	—	100[fg]	(97)
	Na_2SeO_3, 0.01 μM Se	—	0[ef]	
	Na_2SeO_3, 0.06 μM Se	—	0[ef]	
	Na_2SeO_3, 0.13 μM Se	—	0[ef]	
	0	—	100[f]	
	Na_2SeO_3, 0.006 μM Se	—	40[ef]	
	Na_2SeO_4, 0.006 μM Se	—	87[ef]	
	SeO_2, 0.006 μM Se	—	11[ef]	
	Se-cystine, 0.006 μM Se	—	75[ef]	

(continues)

Table 10.4 (*Continued*)

Cell line	Se treatment	Growth[a] (% control)	Viability[b] (% control)	Reference
Ehrlich ascites tumor cells	0	—	100[h]	(62)
	Na$_2$SeO$_3$, 0.03 μM Se	—	86[dh]	
	Na$_2$SeO$_3$, 0.06 μM Se	—	70[dh]	
	Na$_2$SeO$_3$, 0.13 μM Se	—	19[dh]	
	Na$_2$SeO$_4$, 0.03 μM Se	—	96[dh]	
	Na$_2$SeO$_4$, 0.06 μM Se	—	87[dh]	
	Na$_2$SeO$_4$, 0.13 μM Se	—	82[dh]	
	SeO$_2$, 0.03 μM Se	—	59[dh]	
	SeO$_2$, 0.06 μM Se	—	33[dh]	
	SeO$_2$, 0.13 μM Se	—	11[dh]	
	Se-methionine, 0.03 μM Se	—	71[dh]	
	Se-methionine, 0.06 μM Se	—	81[dh]	
	Se-methionine, 0.13 μM Se	—	70[dh]	
	Se-cystine, 0.03 μM Se	—	78[dh]	
	Se-cystine, 0.06 μM Se	—	73[dh]	
	Se-cystine, 0.13 μM Se	—	55[dh]	
CMT-13 canine mammary tumor	0	100[f]	—	(98)
	Na$_2$SeO$_3$, 10 μM Se	48[ef]	—	
	Se-methionine 10 μM Se	94[ef]	—	
	Se-cystine 10 μM Se	69[ef]	—	
	Se-diglutathione 10 μM Se	5[ef]	—	

436

CMT-11 canine mammary tumor	0	100[f]	—	(98)
	Na$_2$SeO$_3$, 10 µM Se	58[ef]	—	
	Se-methionine, 10 µM Se	87[ef]	—	
	Se-cystine, 10 µM Se	94[ef]	—	
	Se-diglutathione, 10 µM Se	24[ef]	—	
Canine mammary cells, nonneoplastic	0	100[f]	—	(98)
	Na$_2$SeO$_3$, 10 µM Se	97[ef]	—	
	Se-methionine, 10 µM Se	101[ef]	—	
	Se-cystine, 10 µM Se	104[ef]	—	
	Se-diglutathione, 10 µM Se	99[ef]	—	

[a]Determined by cell counts.
[b]Determined by trypan blue exclusion.
[c]Determined 72 hrs after the addition of Se.
[d]Significance of treatment effect not tested.
[e]Significantly different ($p < 0.05$) from control.
[f]Determined 3 days after addition of Se.
[g]Viability of controls was 75%.
[h]Determined 4 days after addition of Se.

437

Table 10.5

Reported Effects of Selenium on Tumor Cell Metabolism

Type of effect	Tumor system	Treatment		Findings	Reference
		Control	Se		
Mitochondrial respiration	Erhlich ascites tumor cells	None	Na_2SeO_3, 1 mM	Se decreased glutamate and pyruvate oxidation ($p < 0.05$) but had no effects ($p > 0.05$) on the oxidation of malate, NADPH, or succinate.	(99)
	Hepatoma cells	None	Na_2SeO_3, 1 mM	Se did not affect ($p > 0.05$) the oxidation of glutamate, succinate, or ascorbate, and had no effect ($p > 0.05$) on phosphorylation (i.e., P:O ratio); however, Se stimulated ($p < 0.05$) glutamate, succinate, and ascorbate oxidation in normal liver mitochondria. Se (10^{-6} to 10^{-3} M) increased ($p < 0.05$) mitochondrial ATPase activity in normal liver cells, but did not have this effect ($p > 0.05$) in hepatoma cells.	(100)
cAMP levels	Murine hepatoma cells	None	Na_2SeO_3, 1 mg Se/kg, i.p.	Se treatment of host mice increased cAMP levels by 3.7-fold ($p < 0.05$) in hepatoma cells but decreased cAMP levels by 36% ($p < 0.05$) in host hepatocytes.	(101, 102)

	Cell type	Modifier	Treatment	Effect	Ref.
		None	Na_2SeO_3, 2 mg Se/kg, s.c.	Se treatment of host mice increased cAMP levels by 65% in hepatoma cells ($p < 0.05$), but decreased cAMP levels by 30% ($p < 0.05$) in host hepatocytes.	(101, 102)
RNA synthesis	SV 40-3T3 cells	None	Na_2SeO_3, 8 μM	Se treatment for 48 hrs reduced RNA synthesis by 24% ($p < 0.05$).	(22)
	CMT-13 canine mammary cells	None	$+^a$	Se treatment reduced RNA synthesis by 83% ($p < 0.05$).	(98)
	CMT-11 canine mammary cells	None	$+^a$	Effect of Se was not significant ($p > 0.05$).	(98)
DNA synthesis	SV 40-3T3 cells	None	Na_2SeO_3, 8 μM	Effect of Se was not significant ($p > 0.05$).	(22)
	CMT-13 canine mammary cells	None	$+^a$	Effect of Se was not significant ($p > 0.05$).	(98)
	CMT-11 canine mammary cells	None	$+^a$	Effect of Se was not significant ($p > 0.05$).	(98)
	YN-4 murine mammary cells	None	Na_2SeO_3, 0.05 or 5 μM	Se, at 0.05 μM, increased ($p < 0.05$) DNA synthesis by 23%; but at 5 μM, decreased DNA synthesis by 19% ($p < 0.05$).	(96)

(continues)

439

Table 10.5 (*Continued*)

Type of effect	Tumor system	Treatment		Findings	Reference
		Control	Se		
Protein synthesis	SV40-3T3 cells	None	Na_2SeO_3, 8 μM	Effect of Se was not significant ($p > 0.05$).	(22)
	CMT-13 canine mammary cells	None	$+^a$	Effect of Se was not significant ($p > 0.05$).	(22)
	CMT-11 canine mammary cells	None	$+^a$	Effect of Se was not significant ($p > 0.05$).	(22)
	L 1210 leukemic cells	None	Se-diglutathione, ≥ 40 μM	Se decreased ($p < 0.05$) leucine incorporation.	(103)

[a]Level or species not indicated in the report.

in vivo by Banner *et al.*,[104] who found that Se treatment of regenerating rat liver cells (after partial hepatectomy) significantly reduced RNA synthesis, but had no effect on DNA synthesis in rats given methylazoxymethanol acetate. However, similar effects have not been observed by all investigators. In fact, Milner and Fico[98] found selenite treatment to inhibit RNA synthesis in a line of cannine mammary tumor cells (CMT-13) but to have no effect on RNA synthesis in another cannine mammary tumor cell line (CMT-11). Selenite did not affect protein synthesis in either tumor cell line.[22] Thus, available evidence indicates that Se treatment does not uniformly affect aspects of tumor cell metabolism involved in cell growth and proliferation. Although tumors of the lung[105] and mammary gland[106] have been found to show lower SeGSHpx activities than nonneoplastic host tissue, and Ehrlich ascites tumor cells have been found to have a greater proportion of their intracellular Se associated with the nuclear fraction at the expense of the mitochondrial fraction,[107] little is known about the metabolism of Se, particularly at high levels of exposure, by neoplastic cells. Nevertheless, because Se has been shown to affect critical metabolic processes required for cell proliferation (e.g., energy metabolism, macromolecular synthesis) in certain neoplastic and nonneoplastic cell lines, it is possible that at least some of the anticarcinogenic effects of high levels of Se may involve metabolic inhibition of cell proliferation. Studies in the laboratories of Milner and Vernie indicate that antitumorigenic effects of high levels of selenite may be mediated by metabolites produced through the normal metabolism of that form of the element. Poirier and Milner[61] (also reviewed by Milner[24,98]) found that selenodiglutathione (GSSeSG), a reductive metabolite of selenite (see Chapter 5), was more effective in inhibiting the growth of Ehrlich ascites tumors than was Na_2SeO_3, Na_2Se, $(CH_3)_2Se$, Se-cystine, or Se-methionine when each source of Se was administered to the tumor cell-recipient mice. Also, pre-incubation of tumor cells with GSSeSG effectively increased the mean lifespan of mice subsequently innoculated with the cells; however, pretreatment with Na_2SeO_3 or $(CH_3)_2Se$ had no such effects. Evidence of the particular antitumorigenic efficacy of GSSeSG in this tumor model is supported by the findings of Vernie *et al.*[108] that GSSeSG was particularly effective in inhibiting tumor growth and increasing mean lifespan in mice treated with MBVIA strain malignant lymphoblasts. Vernie *et al.*[94,103,109] attributed the particularly strongly protective effect of GSSeSG to its action in the inhibition of protein synthesis, presumably in tumor cells. They found Se treatment to reduce *in vitro* amino acid incorporation in the livers of rats exposed to hepatocarcinogens,[110] and that reduced amino acid incorporation could also be effected by the addition of Na_2SeO_3 *in vitro*.[111] However, the *in vitro* inhibition occurred only when a thiol was present in the incubation mixture.[110]

They reasoned that selenite reacted with GSH in their incubation mixture to produce GSSG and GSSeSG as described by Ganther,[112] and they demonstrated that GSSeSG inhibited amino acid incorporation at micromolar concentrations.[110] The basis of this effect was a specific inhibition by GSSeSG of elongation factor 2 (EF-2) (i.e., GSSeSG did not inhibit peptidyl transferase, EF-1, or polyribosomes, etc.).[109] This effect appears to be specific for eukaryotic EF-2, as the analogous bacterial elongation factor, EF-G, was not inhibited by GSSeSG.[94]

The finding of specific inhibition of EF-2 by GSSeSG offers the basis for an attractive hypothesis for the antitumorigenic properties of high levels of selenite, i.e., that the reductive metabolism of excessive amounts of selenite results in production of an intermediate (GSSeSG) that inhibits protein synthesis, thus inhibiting the proliferative response. Although this would appear consistent with the findings of LeBoeuf and Hoekstra[86] of increased concentrations of both GSSG and GSH (the latter of which could react with selenite) in response to high-level selenite treatment, those investigators have challenged this hypothesis.[87] They have pointed out the finding of Ganther[112] that GSSeSG is unstable and, at GSH:GSSG ratios greater than ca. 4:1, it is rapidly reduced to GSSeH and H_2Se. Because the intracellular GSH:GSSG ratio is considerably greater than 4:1, even under conditions of excessive selenite exposure, LeBoeuf and Hoekstra[87] concluded that it is unlikely that intracellular concentrations of GSSeSG are ever great enough to affect protein synthesis. Therefore, it is presently unclear whether selenite, GSSeSG, or some other metabolite of Se is the active species in the inhibition of protein synthesis, although it is likely that this metabolic lesion, effected by some metabolite of Se, is the basis of at least some anticarcinogenic activities of Se.

Only a few studies have addressed the issue of Se anticarcinogenicity with respect to the temporal relationship between carcinogen exposure and Se administration. Clayton and Baumann[2] found Se to be effective against the development of azo dye-induced hepatomas in rats, even when it was not administered until after exposure to the carcinogen ceased. Griffen[19] found that Na_2SeO_3 was still effective in reducing hepatoma incidence when it was added only during the last 4 weeks to the drinking water of rats fed 3'-methyl-4-dimethylaminoazobenzene continuously for 9 weeks. Medina and Lane[38] found that Na_2SeO_3 was effective in the inhibition of 7,12-dimethylbenz(a)anthracene (DMBA)-induced mammary tumorigenesis in mice, even when the animals were given Se only after carcinogen exposure had been concluded. Ip[113] undertook to study the importance of time of Se administration on the efficacy of Na_2SeO_3 in the inhibition of DMBA-induced mammary carcinogenesis in rats. He demonstrated that Se can inhibit both the early (i.e., initiation) and late (i.e., promotion) phases of carcinogenesis in that model. He found that Se decreased tumor development in 24 weeks when it was given either around the time of DMBA administration (–2 to +2 weeks) or during the proliferation phase of tumor development (+2 to +24 weeks). The inhibitory effect of Se in the early promotion phase appeared to be reversible, as the antitumorigenic response was less when Se was administered only from +2 to +12 weeks. When Se was given from +12 to +24 weeks, it did not significantly affect tumorigenesis, indicating that the efficacy of Se is lost with time after carcinogen exposure. The results of these few studies indicate that Se may be effective in antitumorigenesis in both the initiation and promotion phases, and that best protection is achieved by continuous exposure to Se.

II. SELENIUM AND CANCER IN HUMANS

The impressive body of experimental animal carcinogenesis data that has accrued in recent years necessitates an evaluation of Se as a potential factor in the etiology of cancer in human populations. At the time of the early geographical correlational (i.e., ecological studies) studies of Shamberger and colleagues,[2,3] the authors' inferences appeared weak by virtue of the inherent limitations of that approach and the lack of strong supporting experimental data. Therefore, the subsequent development of supporting animal data both strengthens the rationale for epidemiological evaluation of Se as a risk factor in cancer and demands that appropriate epidemiological methodology be used in such evaluations in order to determine, with as much confidence as possible, whether Se is involved in human carcinogenesis. It is, therefore, necessary to go beyond ecological evaluations to other types of epidemiological approaches (e.g., cross sectional studies, case control studies, cohort studies) and, finally, to intervention experiments to understand the role, if any, of Se in human cancer.

Ecological studies by Shamberger et al.,[3,6-8] Schrauzer et al.,[9,10] Jansson et al.,[114] and Cowgill[115] reported that Se status and cancer mortality were inversely correlated. For example, Shamberger and Willis[6] found that cancer mortality for lymphomas and cancers of the gastrointestinal tract, peritoneum, lung, and breast were lower for both sexes in areas of the United States that were classified as either moderate-Se (i.e., 0.06-0.10 ppm) or high-Se (i.e., > 0.10 ppm) on the basis of the Se contents of locally produced forage crops.[4] Schrauzer et al.[9] estimated the average per capita Se intakes of 27 countries and found intake to correlate inversely with overall cancer mortality. They reported significant inverse correlations for estimated Se intake and age-corrected mortality rates for leukemia and for cancers of the colon, rectum, breast, ovary, and lung. Schrauzer *et al.*[9] also reported significant inverse correlations between whole blood Se concentrations (their data included those of Allaway *et al.*[5] and comprised 41 locations in the USA) and age-adjusted mortality rates for cancers of the breast, colon, rectum, and lung. Yu *et al.*[116] found a significant inverse correlation between whole blood Se level and age-adjusted total cancer mortality rates in a study of 24 regions in eight provinces of China. They also observed an inverse correlation between the regional distribution of liver cancer incidence and the Se contents of whole blood and grains within Qidong County, Jiangsu Province, P. R.C., an area of high risk to hepatoma. The interpretation of these studies, particularly the earlier ones, is not as clear as presented in most cases by these authors, however, due to methodological problems.[117] These include the use of crude (instead of age-adjusted) mortality rates, the exclusion of a number of locations from particular analyses, the estimation of national average Se intakes from "typical" Se contents of foods and national average food consumption data, the use of state-level (instead of county-level) exposure and mortality data, the failure to adjust for differences in urbanization, and the use of ordinary (instead of weighted) least-squares regression analyses.

An ecological study of Se status and cancer mortality in the USA was undertaken by Clark and associates[118] using methods appropriate to avoid the problems associated with the previous studies of this type. This study was described in Clark's review.[117] Those investigators analyzed the association of major site-specific cancers and county-based forage crop Se levels (estimated from the actual data of Kubota *et al.*[4] and extrapolations made from those data). Their use of county level data was undertaken to reduce the misclassification of Se exposure that would otherwise result in states with both high and low levels of Se; they restricted their analysis to counties with fewer than 50,000 residents (by 1960 census data) and, thus, minimized confounding effects of urbanization. They used U. S. cancer mortality data for 1950-1969[119] and adjusted for regional differences in cancer mortality by considering the USA in four broad geographic regions that were arbitrarily defined to include areas of low, moderate, and high forage Se status. They adjusted for urbanization, the presence of major ethnic groups, the presence of chemical and petroleum industrial activities, and mean annual sunlight. Their analysis employed weighted least-squares regression where weight was inversely proportional to the variance of the site- and sex-specific mortality rate. Clark[117] described the results of this analysis as indicating that intermediate- and high-Se counties had lower rates than low-Se counties of cancers of all sites combined and, specifically, in both sexes, of the lung, colon, rectum, bladder, esophagus, and pancreas. Inverse associations were also found for cancers of the breast, ovary, and cervix. Cancers of the liver and stomach, Hodgkin's disease, and leukemia showed positive associations with forage Se level in both sexes.

It is not within the power of ecological correlational studies to establish causality of associated effects, despite the tendencies of some to use them in this manner. Rather, the limitations of this approach render it useful only in establishing the plausibility of an hypothesis. Considered in this light, the ecological studies to date indicate that an hypothesis for Se status as a risk factor in human cancer is indeed plausible. In fully testing this hypothesis, experimental animal studies are necessary to address questions concerning biochemical mechanisms of action; however, more sophisticated epidemiological studies and, ultimately, Se-intervention experiments using humans at known risk to cancer are also required.

A number of case-control studies have been conducted; these are summarized in Table 10.6.[120-143] Most of these have been cross-sectional in nature and, as such, are valuable in generating hypotheses but can test only the plausibility of the hypothesis that Se status is related to cancer risk. The results of most of these studies suggest that many cancer patients may be of lower Se status than healthy controls. However, the proper interpretation of these studies must include two important considerations, i.e., whether the controls were drawn from the same populations as the cases, and whether Se metabolism and, therefore, status may be affected by the process of carcinogenesis. Because many cancer patients can be expected to have patterns of food consumption that are different from those of healthy individuals, case-control studies that examine Se status of prevalent cases, particularly of late stage and debilitating cancers, may yield associations which indicate effects attributable to cancer rather than causative of it. In the majority of the studies cited in Table 10.6, the latter distinction was not possible.

Four important case-control studies have been conducted in manners that avoid the problems of the confounding effects mentioned above and, thus, constitute useful tests of the hypothesis that Se status is related to cancer risk. Clark et al.[143] studied Se status (as indicated by plasma Se concentration) as a potential risk factor for skin cancer in residents of eastern North Carolina, USA. Skin cancer was selected for the study because its diagnosis is readily confirmed by histological examination, and its mortality and morbidity rates are very low, thus reducing the possibility of perturbation of either metabolism or food habits by the cancer process in ways that might affect Se status. Clark et al.[143] categorized their subjects (192 prevalent skin cancer patients and 60 current clinic controls) by decile of plasma Se level and compared the risk of disease between the strata. They found that the logistic estimate (adjusted for the effects of age, sex, sun damage, plasma retinol, and plasma total carotenoids) of the odds

Table 10.6

Summary of Studies of Se Status of Cancer Patients in Comparison to Healthy Subjects

Country	Subject group	Serum/plasma Se (ppb)	Whole blood Se (ppb)	Erythrocyte Se (ppb)	Cerebrospinal fluid Se (ppb)	Reference
China	Healthy controls	—	$88 \pm 1 \ (353)^a$	—	—	(120)
	Lung cancer	—	$62 \pm 2 \ (72)^{abc}$	—	—	
	Non cancer patients	—	$73 \pm 4 \ (24)^{ad}$	—	—	
Finland	Healthy female controls	—	$93 \pm 2 \ (56)^e$	—	—	(121)
	Endometrial cancer	—	$89 \pm 4 \ (20)^{ef}$	—	—	
	Cervical cancer	—	$86 \pm 7 \ (10)^{ef}$	—	—	
	Ovarian cancer	—	$81 \pm 7 \ (9)^{ef}$	—	—	
	Other gynecological cancer	—	$76 \pm 7 \ (5)^{eg}$	—	—	
	< 55 yrs:					(122)
	Healthy controls	$115 \pm 5 \ (12)^{em}$	—	—	—	
	Ovarian cancer	$98 \pm 6 \ (12)^{eg}$	—	—	—	
	< 55-64 yrs					(122)
	Healthy controls	$128 \pm 6 \ (17)^{em}$	—	—	—	
	Ovarian cancer	$99 \pm 6 \ (17)^{be}$	—	—	—	
	> 65 yrs:					(122)
	Healthy controls	$119 \pm 4 \ (11)^{em}$	—	—	—	
	Ovarian cancer	$77 \pm 4 \ (11)^{be}$	—	—	—	
	Healthy controls	$54 \pm 1 \ (128)^{am}$	—	—	—	(123)
	Cancer (all sites) patients	$51 \pm 1 \ (128)^{ag}$	—	—	—	
	Healthy controls	$54 \pm 1 \ (128)^{a}$	—	—	—	
	Gastrointestinal cancer	$49 \pm 3 \ (21)^{ah}$	—	—	—	
	Lung cancer	$49 \pm 2 \ (23)^{ah}$	—	—	—	
	Skin and skeletal cancer	$52 \pm 2 \ (32)^{ah}$	—	—	—	
	Urogenital cancer	$52 \pm 2 \ (27)^{ah}$	—	—	—	
	Hemophilia	$48 \pm 3 \ (13)^{ah}$	—	—	—	

Healthy control	$132 \pm 5 \ (37)^a$	—	—	(124)
	$129 \pm 5 \ (64)^a$	—	—	
	$122 \pm 3 \ (40)^a$	—	—	
Cervical cancer	$82 \pm 4 \ (37)^{ab}$	—	—	
Endometrial cancer	$101 \pm 5 \ (64)^{ab}$	—	—	
Ovarian cancer	$93 \pm 4 \ (40)^{ab}$	—	—	
Holland				
Healthy matched controls	$110 \pm 10 \ (7)^{em}$	$133 \pm 20 \ (7)^{em}$	$145 \pm 38 \ (7)^{em}$	(125)
Breast cancer patients	$110 \pm 5 \ (7)^{ef}$	$137 \pm 14 \ (7)^{ef}$	$162 \pm 29 \ (7)^{ef}$	
Italy				
Healthy controls	$79 \pm 30 \ (34)^e$	—	—	(126)
Chronic lymphocytic leukemia	$52 \pm 70 \ (4)^{el}$	—	—	
Hodgkin's disease	$79 \pm 30 \ (20)^{ef}$	—	—	
Non-Hodgkin's malignant lymphoma	$78 \pm 60 \ (14)^{ef}$	—	—	
Japan				
Healthy female controls	—	$285 \pm 32 \ (25)^e$	—	(127)
Breast cancer, new cases	—	$195 \pm 57 \ (79)^{be}$	—	
Breast cancer, recurrent cases	—	$188 \pm 61 \ (14)^{de}$	—	
New Zealand				
< 60 yrs				
Healthy controls	$48 \pm 11 \ (66)^e$	$59 \pm 13 \ (66)^e$	$74 \pm 17 \ (66)^e$	(128)
Cancer patients	$38 \pm 14 \ (30)^{be}$	$53 \pm 16 \ (30)^{ef}$	$71 \pm 20 \ (30)^{ef}$	
Noncancer patients	$45 \pm 14 \ (40)^{be}$	$57 \pm 14 \ (40)^{ef}$	$72 \pm 16 \ (4)^{ef}$	
> 60 yrs				
Healthy controls	$37 \pm 10 \ (47)^e$	$47 \pm 10 \ (47)^c$	$57 \pm 11 \ (47)^e$	(128)
Cancer patients	$35 \pm 15 \ (50)^{ef}$	$49 \pm 16 \ (50)^{ef}$	$64 \pm 16 \ (50)^{ef}$	
Noncancer patients	$34 \pm 11 \ (26)^{ef}$	$51 \pm 13 \ (26)^{ef}$	$65 \pm 14 \ (26)^{ef}$	
Poland				
Healthy controls	—	9 ± 47^i	—	(129)
Lung cancer patients	—	81 ± 13^{fi}	—	

(continues)

447

Table 10.6 (*Continued*)

Country	Subject group	Serum/plasma Se (ppb)	Whole blood Se (ppb)	Erythrocyte Se (ppb)	Cerebrospinal fluid Se (ppb)	Reference
Saudi Arabia	Hydrocephalus patients (controls)	—	—	—	$191 \pm 13 \ (10)^e$	(130)
	Astrocytoma patients	—	—	—	$238 \pm 16 \ (6)^{eh}$	
	Medulloblastoma patients	—	—	—	$851 \pm 135 \ (3)^{eh}$	
	Pinealblastoma patients	—	—	—	$154 \ (1)^j$	
	Chondrosarcoma patients	—	—	—	$157 \ (1)^j$	
United States	Healthy controls	$120 \pm 10 \ (37)^e$	—	—	—	(131)
	Cancer patients	$110 \pm 30 \ (20)^{ef}$	—	—	—	
	Healthy female controls	—	$112 \pm 50 \ (35)^e$	—	—	(132)
	Hormone-dependent, cancer patients^k	—	$110 \pm 46 \ (16)^{ef}$	—	—	
	Healthy controls	$148 \pm 70 \ (18)^e$	—	—	—	(133)
	Carcinoma patients	$127 \pm 3 \ (110)^{eh}$	—	—	—	
	Gastrointestinal cancer patients	$114 \pm 8 \ (16)^{eh}$	—	—	—	
	Reticuloendothelial cancer patients	$176 \pm 24 \ (36)^{eh}$	—	—	—	
	Healthy controls	—	$157 \pm 8 \ (27)^a$	—	—	(134)
	Breast cancer patients	—	$125 \pm 4 \ (35)^{ab}$	—	—	
	Healthy controls	$99 \pm 2 \ (92)^a$	—	$159 \pm 5 \ (84)^a$	—	(135)
	Liver cancer with metastases	$67 \pm 7 \ (12)^{ag}$	—	$110 \pm 19 \ (99)^{al}$	—	
	Liver cancer without metastases	$77 \pm 6 \ (14)^{ag}$	—	$139 \pm 15 \ (11)^{af}$	—	
	Healthy female controls	—	$183 \pm 24 \ (14)^e$	—	—	(127)
	Breast cancer, new cases	—	$164 \pm 39 \ (11)^{ef}$	—	—	
	Breast cancer, recurrent cases	—	$164 \pm 39 \ (10)^{ef}$	—	—	
	Healthy controls	103 ± 10^{an}	—	—	—	(136)
	Breast cancer patients	77 ± 3^{ahn}	—	—	—	
	Healthy controls	$89 \pm 4 \ (18)^{an}$	—	—	—	(137)

448

Group				Ref
Hodgkin's patients	146 ± 44 (12)[agn]	—	—	(138)
Lymphoreticular malignancy	84 ± 6 (29)[afn]	—	—	
Multiple myeloma	86 ± 11 (10)[afn]	—	—	
Myeloproliferative disorder	83 ± 9 (8)[afn]	—	—	
Healthy controls	89 ± 4 (18)[an]	—	—	(139)
Noncancer patients	90 ± 4 (34)[an]	—	—	
Cancer patients	76 ± 2 (110)[acgn]	—	—	
Healthy female controls	94 ± 5 (27)[an]	—	—	(139)
Breast cancer patients	75 ± 2 (35)[agn]	—	—	
Healthy controls		229 ± 35 (48)e	—	(140)
Colon cancer		158 ± 21 (28)[eh]	—	
Stomach cancer		153 ± 21 (12)[eh]	—	
Liver cancer		150 ± 26 (14)[eh]	—	
Pancreatic cancer		132 ± 29 (4)[eh]	—	
Rectal carcinoma		207 ± 51 (23)[eh]	—	
Breast cancer		245 ± 48 (11)[eh]	—	
Lymphoma		229 (2)[j]	—	
Bladder cancer		214 (2)[j]	—	
Cervical cancer		243 (1)[j]	—	
Face and neck cancer		221 ± 11 (7)[eh]	—	
Hodgkin's disease		162 ± 33 (6)[eh]	—	
Lung cancer		221 ± 66 (3)[eh]	—	
Ovarian cancer		166 (2)[j]	—	
Prostate cancer		240 (1)[j]	—	
Uterine cancer		238 (2)[j]	—	
Healthy controls	102 ± 18 (17)[e]	—	—	(141)
Noncancer controls	88 ± 21 (17)[ef]	—	—	
Cancer patients	70 ± 13 (8)[ceg]	—	—	

(continues)

449

Table 10.6 (*Continued*)

Country	Subject group	Serum/plasma Se (ppb)	Whole blood Se (ppb)	Erythrocyte Se (ppb)	Cerebrospinal fluid Se (ppb)	Reference
	Healthy controls	80 ± 10 (50)[a]	—	74 ± 40 (50)[a]	—	(142)
	Head and neck cancer patients	57 ± 60 (52)[ad]	—	110 ± 10 (52)[ab]	—	
	Healthy controls	150 (103)[j]	—	—	—	(143)
	Basal cell epithelioma only	141 (142)[j]	—	—	—	
	Squamous cell epithelioma only	141 (48)[j]	—	—	—	
	Both basal and squamous cell epithelioma	141 (50)[j]	—	—	—	

[a]Mean ± SE (*n*).
[b]Significantly different ($p < 0.001$) from healthy controls.
[c]Significantly different ($p < 0.05$) from noncancer patients.
[d]Significantly different ($p < 0.01$) from healthy controls.
[e]Mean ± SD (*n*).
[f]Not significantly different ($p > 0.05$) from healthy controls.
[g]Significantly different ($p < 0.05$) from healthy controls.
[h]Significance of difference from healthy controls not tested.
[i]Mean ± SD; *n* not specified.
[j]Mean (*n*).
[k]Includes ovarian, uterine and breast cancers.
[l]Significantly different ($p < 0.005$) from healthy controls.
[m]Age- and sex-matched controls.
[n]Recalculated from data (μg/g serum dry matter) presented in original report, assessing serum to confirm 6% solids.

ratios for the lowest (average plasma Se = 84 ppb) versus the highest (average plasma Se = 221 ppb) deciles was 3.91 ($p < 0.05$) for patients with basal cell epitheliomas, 3.03 ($p < 0.05$) for patients with squamous cell carcinomas, and 4.39 ($p < 0.05$) for all skin cancer cases combined. The unadjusted observed odds ratios were similar to the logistic estimates of the odds ratios. When cases and controls were stratified on high versus low plasma retinol and total carotenoids, results indicated that low plasma Se was associated with elevated risk of skin cancer in patients low with respect to either of those variables.

The second important test of the "Se and cancer" hypothesis was a prospective case-control study conducted by Salonen et al.[123] Those investigators evaluated the relationship of serum Se level and total cancer mortality in a random population sample of 8113 residents of two counties in eastern Finland. The subjects, all free of cancer at the beginning of the study, were examined in 1972 and were followed for a period of 6 years. Each case that developed during that time was matched to a single control according to age, sex, daily tobacco use, and serum cholesterol level. The results of the matched-pair analysis (n = 128) showed that the mean serum Se concentration was significantly ($p = 0.012$) lower in cases (50.5 ± 1.1 ppb) than in controls (54.3 ± 1.0 ppb). The logistic estimate of the odds ratio (adjusted for the four other effects) was 3.1 ($p < 0.01$).

The third important test was the nested case-control study of Willett et al.,[144] in which 111 subjects who developed cancer during a 5-year follow-up period were compared to 210 matched controls. This study was nested in the Hypertension Detection and Follow-up Program cohort; cancer cases were diagnosed after the serum samples were collected and frozen for future analysis. Willett et al.[144] found that the relative risk of subjects in the lowest quintile of serum Se (i.e., <115 ppb) versus those in the highest group (i.e., >154 ppb) was 2.0. In addition, the relative risk in low-Se subjects appeared to be greatest if those individuals were also in the lowest tertiles with respect to plasma retinol and alpha-tocopherol; however, the strength of this conclusion was limited due to the small sample sizes of some of the multi-factor subgroups.

Most recently Salonen et al.[145] reported a fourth important study, which was a prospective case-control analysis involving 51 terminal cancer cases, and an equal number of controls matched by sex, age, and smoking habits selected from a random sample of 12,155 subjects in eastern Finland. Their analysis showed that the cancer cases had mean serum Se concentrations that were 12% lower than those of the matched control (i.e., 53.7 ppb vs. 60.9 ppb, $p < 0.05$). The adjusted relative risk of death to cancer was 5.8 among subjects in the lowest tertile of serum Se concentration when compared with subjects in the highest tertile. A significant interaction of low Se status and low vitamin E status was also detected; subjects in the lowest tertiles with respect to serum concentrations of both nutrients had an adjusted relative risk of fatal cancer of 11.4 compared to subjects in the highest tertiles.

A recent report by Peleg et al.[146] does not support a general effect of Se nutriture on cancer incidence. In a retrospective study of 130 cancer cases and controls matched by race, sex, and age from a population of some 10,000 residents of Evans County, Georgia, USA, Peleg et al.[146] observed no significant differences in serum Se levels between cases and controls.

In summary, several ecological correlational studies and cross-sectional case-control studies have established the plausibility of an hypothesis that low Se status may increase the risk of cancer in several populations. This hypothesis is different from that derived from studies with tumor models in experimental animals, i.e., that pharmacologic levels of Se may be anticarcinogenic. In fact, experimental animal studies have indicated that there are likely to be multiple mechanisms by which Se affects carcinogenesis. Therefore, it is likely that the dose-response relationship between Se and tumor development will not be linear, i.e., that the nature of the low-Se status effect that is suggested by human epidemiological studies may be quite different from the high-dose Se effect indicated by the results of animal studies. This consideration is represented diagramatically in Fig. 10.1. Whereas the available experimental animal data indicate an inverse relationship between tumor incidence/risk at high levels of Se exposure, little information exists to describe this relationship at subadequate levels of Se exposure (Fig. 10.1A). The reverse situation exists with regard to the available epidemiological data: there is some indication of increased tumor risk at levels of Se intake and no information pertinent to this relationship at high levels of Se exposure (Fig. 10.1B). To infer, as some have, from the animal data that if high levels of Se protect somehow against carcinogenesis, low Se status must increase tumor risk, is not warranted by the data: i.e., this represents an extrapolation beyond the current range of observations (see Fig. 10.1C). To apply this kind of extrapolation to the human epidemiological data would support the hypothesis of low Se status as a risk factor for cancer. However, that approach is not correct, as it implies a consistency of action of Se between tumor models and human cancers and throughout a wide range of doses. Such a consistency is not supported by the available data. It can be inferred that, because Se may be involved in one or more of several ways in metabolic processes that relate to carcinogenesis, the nature of the relationship between Se status and cancer risks may be multi-phasic (for example, Fig. 10.1D). The nature of this relationship in human population remains to be elucidated.

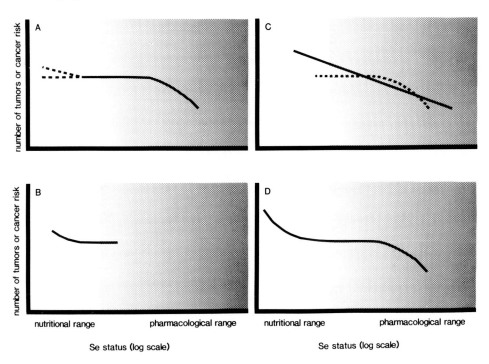

Fig. 10.1   Stylized observed and hypothetical relationships of Se status and cancer risk. (A)
General relationship between Se status and tumor production in experimental
animal models; note the dashed lines indicating the great uncertainty of the nature
of the relationship within the nutritional range of Se status due to the execution
of only very few studies in that range. (B) General relationship that appears to
be emerging from epidemiological studies of human populations; note the restricted
range of Se status in which these types of studies have been possible. (C) Linear
extrapolation based on most of the experimental animal tumor model data; this
would predict enhanced tumor risk of low Se status, an area largely outside of
the range of experimental observation. (D) General model for a biphasic relationship
between tumor risk and Se status.

The hypothesis of an effect of low Se status on human cancers has been
tested appropriately in only a few recent studies. While the results of most
of these studies support it, further testing is clearly needed to determine
whether low Se status is indeed a risk factor for at least some cancers
of humans. The most rigorous tests of this hypothesis will be, of course,
Se-intervention studies that will evaluate the cancer preventative effects
(or lack thereof) of treatments that increase Se status of subjects at known
risk to particular cancers.

REFERENCES

1. Walker, C. H., and Klein, E., "Selenium"—its therapeutic value—especially in cancer, Amer. Med., 628, Aug. 1915.
2. Clayton, C. C., and Baumann, C. A., Diet and azo dye tumors: effect of diet during a period when the drug is not fed, Cancer Res., 9, 575, 1949.
3. Shamberger, R. J., and Frost, D. V., Possible protective effect of selenium against human cancer, Can. Med. Assn. J., 104, 82, 1969.
4. Kubota, J., Allaway, W. H., Carter, D. L., Cary, E. E., and Lazar, U. A., Selenium in crops in the United States in relation to selenium-responsive diseases of animals, J. Agr. Food Chem., 15, 448, 1967.
5. Allaway, W. H., Kubota, J., Losee, F., and Roth, M., Selenium, molybdenum and vanadium in human blood, Arch. Environ. Health, 16, 342, 1968.
6. Shamberger, R. J., and Willis, C. E., Selenium distribution of human cancer mortality, CRC Crit. Rev.: Clin. Lab Sci., 2, 211, 1971.
7. Shamberger, R. J., Tytko, S., and Willis, C., Antioxidants and cancer. II. Selenium and human cancer mortality in the United States, Canada and New Zealand, Trace Sub. Environ. Health, 7, 35, 1974.
8. Shamberger, R. J., Tytko, S. A., and Willis, C. E., Antioxidants and cancer. Part VI. Selenium and age-adjusted human cancer mortality, Arch. Environ. Hlth., 26, 231, 1976.
9. Schrauzer, G. N., White, D. A., and Schneider, C. J., Cancer mortality correlation studies. III. Statistical association with dietary selenium intakes, Bioinorg. Chem., 7, 23, 1977.
10. Schrauzer, G. N., White, D. A., and Schneider, C. J., Cancer mortality correlation studies. IV. Associations with dietary intakes and blood levels of certain trace elements, notable Se-antagonists, Bioinorg. Chem., 7, 35, 1977.
11. Nelson, A. A., Fithugh, O. G., and Calvery, H. O., Liver tumors following cirrhosis caused by selenium in rats, Cancer Res., 3, 230, 1943.
12. Tinsley, I. J., Harr, J. R., Bone, J. F., Weswig, P. H., and Yamamato, R. S., Selenium toxicity in rats. I. Growth and longevity, in Selenium in Biomedicine, Muth, O. H., Ed., Avi Publ. Co., Westport, Conn., p.141, 1967.
13. Harr, J. R., Bone, J. T., Tinsley, I. J., Weswig, P. H., and Yamamoto, R. S., Selenium in rats. II. Histopathology, in Selenium in Biomedicine, Muth, O. H., ed., Avi Publ. Co., Westport, Conn., p.153, 1967.
14. Volgarev, M. N. and Tscherkes, L. A., Further studies in tissue changes associated with sodium selenate, in Selenium in Biomedicine, Muth, O. H., Ed., Avi Publ. Co., Westport, Conn., p.179, 1967.
15. Schroeder, H. A., and Mitchner, M., Selenium and tellurium in rats: effects on growth, survival and tumors, J. Nutr., 101, 1531, 1971.
16. Scott, M. L., The selenium dilemma, J. Nutr., 103, 803, 1973.
17. Schrauzer, G. N., Selenium and cancer: a review, Bioinorg. Chem., 5, 275, 1976.
18. Schrauzer, G. N., Trace elements in carcinogenesis, in Advances in Nutritional Research, Vol. 2, Draper, H. H., ed., Plenum, New York, p.219, 1977.
19. Griffin, A. C., Role of selenium in the chemoprevention of cancer, Adv. Cancer Res., 29, 419, 1979.
20. Jacobs, M. M., Effects of selenium on chemical carcinogens, Preventive Medicine, 9, 362, 1980.
21. Newberne, P. M., and Suphakarn, V., Nutrition and cancer: a review, with emphasis on the role of vitamins C and E and selenium, Nutr. Cancer, 5, 107, 1983.

22. Milner, J. A., Selenium and the transplantable tumor, J. Agric. Food Chem., 32, 436, 1984.
23. Ip, C., Selenium inhibition of chemical carcinogenesis, Federation Proc., 44, 2573, 1985.
24. Milner, J. A., The effect of selenium on virally-induced and transplantable tumors, Federation Proc., 44, 2568, 1985.
25. Milner, J. A., and Fico, M. E., Selenium and tumorigenesis, in *Proceedings of the Third International Symposium on Selenium in Biology and Medicine*, Combs, G. F., Jr., Spallholz, J. E., Levander, O. A., and Oldfield, J. E., eds., Avi Publ. Co., Westport, Conn., 1986.
26. Nigro, N. D., Bull, A. W., Wilson, P. S., Soullier, B. K., and Alousi, M. A., Combined inhibitors of carcinogenesis: effects on azoxymethane-induced intestinal cancer in rats, J. Nat. Cancer Inst., 69, 103, 1983.
27. Soullier, B. K., Wilson, P. S., and Nigro, N. D., Effect of selenium on azoxymethane-induced intestinal cancer in rats fed high fat diet, Cancer Lett., 12, 343, 1981.
28. Jacobs, M. M., Jansson, B., and Griffin, A. C., Inhibitory effects of selenium on 1,2-dimethylhydrazine and methylazoxymethanol acetate induction of colon tumors, Cancer Letters, 2, 133, 1977.
29. Jacobs, M. M., Forst, C. F., and Beams, F. A., Biochemical and clinical effects of selenium on dimethylhydrazine-induced colon cancer in rats, Cancer Res., 41, 4458, 1981.
30. Jacobs, M. M., Selenium inhibition of 1,2-dimethylhydrazine-induced colon carcinogenesis, Cancer Res., 43, 1646, 1983.
31. Birt, D. F., Lawson, T. A., Julius, A. D., Runice, C. E., and Salmasi, S., Inhibition by dietary selenium of colon cancer induced in the rat by bis(2- oxypropyl)nitrosamine, Cancer Res., 42, 4455, 1982.
32. Johnston, W. K., Effect of selenium on chemical carcinogenicity in the rat, M. S.. thesis, Oregon State Univ., Corvallis, Oregon, 88 pp., 1974.
33. Marshall, M. V., Arnott, M. S., Jacobs, M. M., and Griffin, A. C., Selenium effects on the carcinogenicity and metabolism of 2-acetylaminofluorene, Cancer Letts., 7, 331, 1979.
34. Harr, J. R., Exon, J. H., Whanger, P. D., and Weswig, P. H., Effect of dietary selenium on N-2-fluorenyl acetamide (FFA)-induced cancer in vitamin E- supplemented, selenium-depleted rats, Clin. Toxicol., 5, 187, 1972.
35. Griffin, A. C., and Jacobs, M. M., Effects of selenium on azo dye hepatocarcinogenesis, Cancer Letts., 4, 177, 1977.
36. Medina, D. and Shepard, F., Selenium-mediated inhibition of 7,12-dimethylbenz(a)anthracene-induced mouse mammary tumorigenesis, Carcinogenesis, 2, 451, 1981.
37. Welsch, C. W., Goodrich-Smith, M., Brown, C. K., Greene, H. D., and Hamel, E. J., Selenium and the genesis of murine mammary tumors, Carcinogenesis, 2, 519, 1981.
38. Medina, D., and Lane, H. W., Stage specificity of selenium-mediated inhibition of mouse mammary tumorigenesis, Biol. Trace Elem. Res., 5, 297, 1983.
39. Shamberger, R. J., Relationship of selenium to cancer. I. Inhibitory effect of selenium on carcinogenesis, J. Nat. Cancer Inst., 44, 931, 1970.
40. Lane, H. W., Butel, J. S., and Medina, D., Selenium, lipid peroxidation and murine mammary tumorigenesis, in *Proceedings of the Third International Symposium on Selenium in Biology and Medicine*, Combs, G. F., Jr., Spallholz, J. E., Levander, O. A., and Oldfield, J. E., eds., Avi Publ. Co., Westport, Conn., 1986.
41. Medina, D., and Shepherd, F. S., Selenium inhibition of the neoplastic transformation in preneoplastic mammary cell populations, Cancer Letts., 24, 227, 1984.

42. Thompson, H. J., Soule, R. A., and Becci, P. J., Inhibition of mammary tumorigenesis by graded levels of selenium. Federation Proc., 40, 929 (abstract), 1981.

43. Thompson, H. J., and Tagliaferro, A. R., Effect of selenium on 7,12-dimethylbenz(a)anthracene-induced mammary tumorigenesis, Federation Proc., 39, 1117 (abstract), 1980.

44. Ip, C., and Ip, M. M., Chemoprevention of mammary tumorigenesis by a combined regimen of selenium and vitamin A, Carcinogenesis, 2, 915, 1981.

45. Ip, C., Factors influencing the anticarcinogenic efficacy of selenium in dimethylbenz(a)anthracene-induced mammary tumorigenesis in rats, Cancer Res., 41, 2683, 1981.

46. Horvath, P. M., and Ip, C., Synergistic effect of vitamin E and selenium in the chemoprevention of mammary carcinogenesis in rats, Cancer Res., 43, 5335, 1983.

47. Ip, C., and Sinha, D., Anticarcinogenic effect of selenium in rats treated with dimethylbenz(a)anthracene and fed different levels and types of fat, Carcinogenesis, 2, 435, 1981.

48. Thompson, H. J., Meeker, L. D., Becci, P. J., and Kokoska, S., Effect on short-term feeding of sodium selenite on 7,12-dimethylbenz(a)anthracene-induced mammary carcinogenesis in the rat, Cancer Res., 42, 4954, 1982.

49. Harr, J. R., Exon, J. H., Weswig, P. H., and Whanger, P. D., Relationship of dietary selenium concentration, chemical cancer induction an tissue concentration of selenium in rats, Clin. Toxicol., 6, 487, 1973.

50. Thompson, J., Meeker, L. D., and Becci, P. J., Effect of combined selenium and retinyl acetate treatment on mammary carcinogenesis, Cancer Res., 41, 1413, 1981.

51. Thompson, H. J., Meeker, L. D., and Kokoska, S., Effect of an inorganic and organic form of dietary selenium on the promotional stage of mammary carcinogenesis in the rat, Cancer Res., 44, 2803, 1984.

52. Thompson, H. J. and Becci, P. J., Selenium inhibition of N-methyl-N-nitrosourea-induced mammary carcinogenesis in the rat, J. Nat. Cancer Inst., 65, 1299, 1985.

53. Medina, D., and Shepherd, F., Selenium-mediated inhibition of mouse mammary tumorigenesis, Cancer Letts., 8, 241, 1980.

54. Schrauzer, G. N., White, D. A., and Schneider, C. J., Inhibition of the genesis of spontaneous mammary tumors in C3H mice: effects of selenium and of selenium-antagonistic elements and their possible role in human breast cancer, Bioinorg. Chem., 56, 265, 1976.

55. Schrauzer, G. N. and Isshmael, D., Effects of selenium and of arsenic on the genesis of spontaneous mammary tumors in inbred C_3H mice, Ann. Clin. Lab. Sci. 4, 441, 1974.

56. Schrauzer, G. N., McGuinness, J. E., and Kuehn, K., Effects of temporary selenium supplementation on the genesis of spontaneous mammary tumors in inbred female C_3H/St mice, Carcinogenesis, 1, 199, 1980.

57. Ip, C., Ip, M. M., and Kim, U., Dietary selenium intake and growth of the MT-W9B transplantable rat mammary tumor, Cancer Letts., 14, 101, 1981.

58. Watrach, A. M., Milner, J. A., and Watrach, M. A., Effect of selenium on growth rate of canine mammary carcinoma cells in athymic nude mice, Cancer Letts., 15, 137, 1982.

59. Wilt, S., Pereira, M., and Couri, D., Selenium effect on initiation and promotion of tumors by benzo(a)pyrene and 12-O-tetradecanoylphorbol, Amer. Assoc. Cancer Res., 20, 21, 1979.

60. Thompson, H. J. and Becci, P. J., Effect of graded dietary levels of selenium on tracheal carcinomas induced by 1-methyl-1-nitrosourea, Cancer Letts., 7, 215, 1979.

61. Poirier, K. A., and Milner, J. A., Factors influencing the antitumorigenic properties of selenium in mice, J. Nutr., 113, 2147, 1983.

62. Poirier, K. A., and Milner, J. A., The effect of various seleno-compounds on Ehrlich ascites tumor cells, Biol. Trace Elem. Res., 1, 25, 1979.

63. Greeder, G. A., and Milner, J. A., Factors influencing the inhibitory effect of selenium on mice innoculated with Ehrlich ascites tumor cells, Science, 209, 825, 1980.

64. Ankerst, J., and Sjoegren, H. O., Effect of selenium on the induction of breast fibroadenomas by adenovirus type 9 and 1,2-dimethylhydrazine-induced bowel carcinogenesis in rats, Int. J. Cancer, 29, 707, 1982.

65. Daoud, A. H., and Griffin, A. C., Effect of retinoic acid, butylated hydroxytoluene, selenium and sorbic acid on azo-dye hepatocarcinogenesis, Cancer Lett., 9, 299, 1980.

66. O'Connor, T. P., and Cambell, C., Influence of dietary fat and selenium on L-azaserine-induced preneoplastic acinar cell nodules (AACN) development in rat pancreas, Federation Proc., 43, 794 (abstract), 1984.

67. Pence, B. C., and Buddingh, F., Effect of selenium deficiency on 1,2- dimethylhydrazine-induced colon cancer in rats, in *Proceedings of the Third International Symposium on Selenium in Biology and Medicine*, Combs, G. F., Jr., Spallholz, J. E., Levander, O. A., and Oldfield, J. E., eds., Avi Publ. Co., Westport, Conn., 1986.

68. Ip, C., Modification of mammary carcinogenesis and tissue peroxidation by selenium deficiency and dietary fat, Nutr. Cancer, 2, 136, 1981.

69. Ip, C., and Sinha, D. K., Enhancement of mammary tumorigenesis by dietary selenium deficiency in rats fed a high polyunsaturated fat intake, Cancer Res., 41, 31, 1981.

70. Thompson, H. J., Selenium as an anticarcinogen, J. Agric. Food Chem., 32, 422, 1984.

71. Chen, J., Goetchius, M. P., Cambell, C., and Combs, G. F., Jr., Effects of dietary selenium and vitamin E on hepatic mixed-function oxidase activities and *in vivo* covalent binding of aflatoxin B_1 in rats, J. Nutr., 112, 324, 1982.

72. Gairola, C., and Chow, C. K., Dietary selenium, hepatic arylhydrocarbon hydroxylase and mutagenic activation of benzo(a)pyrene, 2-aminoanthracene and 2-aminofluorene, Toxicol. Letts., 11, 281, 1982.

73. Chow, C. K., and Gairola, G. C., Influence of dietary vitamin E and selenium on metabolic activation of chemicals to mutagens, J. Agric. Food Chem., 32, 443, 1984.

74. Capel, I. D., Jenner, M., Darrell, H. M., and Williams, D. C., The influence of selenium on some hepatic carcinogen metabolizing enzymes of rats, IRCS Med. Sci. Libr. Compend., 8, 382, 1980.

75. Olsson, U., Onfelt, A., and Beije, B., Dietary selenium deficiency causes decreased N-oxygenation of N,N-diethylaniline and increased mutagenicity of dimethylnitrosamine in the isolated rat liver/cell culture system, Mutation Res., 126,73,1984.

76. Wortzman, M. S., Besbris, H. J., and Cohen, A. M., Effect of dietary selenium on the interaction between 2-acetylaminofluorene and rat liver DNA *in vivo*, Cancer Res., 40, 2670, 1980.

77. Chen, J., Goetchius, M. P., Combs, G. F., Jr., and Cambell, C., Effects of dietary selenium and vitamin E on covalent binding of aflatoxin to chick liver cell macromolecules, J. Nutr., 112, 350, 1982.

78. Besbris, H. J., Wortzman, M. S., and Cohen, A. M., Effect of dietary selenium on the metabolism and excretion of 2-acetylaminofluorene in the rat, J. Toxicol. Environ. Health, 9, 63, 1982.

79. Hughes, D. A., and Bjeldanes, L. F., Influence of selenium-supplemented torula yeast diets on liver-mediated mutagenicity of aflatoxin B_1, J. Food Sci., 48, 759, 1983.

80. Schillaci, M., Martin, S. E., and Milner, J. A., The effects of dietary selenium on the biotransformation of 7,12-dimethylbenz(a)anthracene, Mutation Res., 101, 31, 1982.

81. Martin, S. E., and Schillaci, M., Inhibitory effects of selenium on mutagenicity, J. Agric. Food Chem., 32, 426, 1984.

82. Burguera, J. A., Edds, G. T., and Osuna, 0., Influence of selenium on aflatoxin B_1 or crotalaria toxicity in turkey poults, Am. J. Vet. Res., 44, 1714, 1983.

83. Skaare, J. U. and Nafstad, I., Interaction of vitamin E and selenium with the hepatotoxic agent dimethylnitrosamine, Acta Pharmacol. Toxicol., 43, 119, 1978.

84. Grunau, J. A., and Milner, J. A., Selenium modification of 7,12-dimethylbenz(a)anthracene metabolism, Federation Proc., 42, 928 (abstract), 1983.

85. Shamberger, R. J., Corlett, C. L., Beaman, K. D., and Kastan, B. L., Antioxidants reduce the mutagenic effect of malonaldehyde and β-propiolactone, Mutation Res., 66, 349, 1979.

86. LeBoeuf, R. A., and Hoekstra, W. G., Acaptive changes in hepatic glutathione metabolism in response to excess dietary selenium, J. Nutr., 113, 845, 1983.

87. LeBoeuf, R. A., and Hoekstra, W. G., Changes in cellular glutathione levels: possible relation to selenium-mediated anti-carcinogenesis, Federation Proc., 44, 2563, 1985.

88. Tsen, C. C. and Tappel, A. L., Catalytic oxidation of glutathione and other sulfhydryl compounds by selenite, J. Biol. Chem., 233, 1230, 1958.

89. Jacobs, M. M., Matney, J. S., and Griffin, A. C., Inhibitory effects of selenium on the mutagenicity of 2-acetylaminofluorene (AAF) and AAF derivatives, Cancer Letts., 2, 319, 1977.

90. Teel, R. W., and Kain, S. R., Selenium modified mutagenicity and metabolism of benzo(a)pyrene in an S9-dependent system, Mutation Res., 127, 9, 1984.

91. Ernst, V., Levin, D. H., and London, I. M., Inhibition of protein synthesis initiation by oxidized glutathione: activation of a protein kinase that phosphorylates the subunit of eukaryotic initiation factor 2, Proc. Nat. Acad. Sci., USA, 75, 4110, 1978.

92. Safer, B., Jagus, B., and Crouch, D., Indirect inactivation of eukaryotic initiation factor 2 in reticulocyte lysates by selenite, J. Biol. Chem., 255, 6913, 1980.

93. Gruenwedel, D. W., and Cruikshank, M. K., The influence of sodium selenite on the viability and intracellular synthetic activity (DNA, RNA and protein synthesis) of HeLa S3 cells, Tox. Appl. Pharmacol., 50, 1, 1979.

94. Vernie, L. N., Collard, J. G., Eker, A. P.M., DeWildt, A., and Wilders, 1. T., Studies on the inhibition of protein synthesis by selenodiglutathione, Biochem. J., 180 213, 1979.

95. Lewko, W. M., and McConnell, K. P., Biphasic influence of selenium on cell growth and the synthesis of collagen in cultured mammary tumor cells, Federation Proc., 41, 623, 1982.

96. Medina, D., and Oborn, C. J., Selenium inhibition of DNA synthesis in mouse mammary epithelial cell line YN-4, Cancer Res., 44, 4361, 1984.

97. Milner, J. A. and Hsu, C. Y., Inhibitory effects of selenium on the growth of L1210 leukemic cells, Cancer Res., 41, 1652, 1982.

98. Milner, J. A., and Fico, M. F., Selenium and tumorigenesis, in *Proceedings of the Third International Symposium on Selenium in Biology and Medicine*, Combs, G. F., Jr., Spallholz, J. E., Levander, O. A., and Oldfield, J. E., eds., Avi Publ. Co., Westport, Conn., 1986.

99. Yu, S., Zhu, Y., Liu, Q., and Hou, C., Effect of selenium on Ehrlich ascitic tumor growth, mitochondrial respiration and oxidative phosphorylation, Zhonghua, Zhongliu Zazhi, 5, 8, 1983.

100. Yu, S., Zhu, Y., Hou, C., and Huang, C., Selective effects of selenium on the function and structure of mitochondria isolated from hepatoma and normal liver, in *Procedings of the Third International Symposium on Selenium in Biology and Medicine*, Combs, G. F., Jr., Spallholz, J. E., Levander, O. A., and Oldfield, J. E., eds., Avi Publ. Co., Westport, Conn., 1986.

101. Yu, S., and Wang L., Different biochemical effects of selenium on hepatoma and normal liver. I. Effects on cAMP level, Zhongguo Yixue Kexueyuan Xuebao, 5, 196, 1983.

102. Yu, S., and Wang, L., Different effects of selenium on cyclic AMP metabolism in hepatoma cells and normal liver cells, Biol. Trace Elem. Res., 5, 9, 1983.

103. Vernie, L. N., Inhibition of protein synthesis and anticarcinogenicity of selenium compounds, in *Proceedings of the Third International Symposium on Selenium in Biology and Medicine*, Combs, G. F., Jr., Spallholz, J. E., Levander, O. A., and Oldfield, J. E., eds., Avi Publ. Co., Westport, Conn., 1986.

104. Banner, W. P., Tan, Q. H., and Zedeck, M. S., Selenium and the acute effects of the carcinogens, 2-acetylaminofluorene and methylazoxymethanol acetate, Cancer Res., 42, 2985, 1982.

105. Capel, I., Antioxidant defense in hypoxic regions of tumors, Med. Biol., 62, 119, 1984.

106. Lane, H. W., and Medina, D., Selenium concentration and glutathione peroxidase activity in normal and neoplastic development of the mouse mammary gland, Cancer Res., 43, 1558, 1983.

107. Baumgartner, W. A., Hill, V. A., and Wright, E. T., Antioxidant effects in the development of Erhlich ascites carcinoma, Am. J. Clin. Nutr., 31, 457, 1978.

108. Vernie, L. N., Hamburg, C. J., and Bont, W. S., Inhibition of the growth of malignant mouse lymphoid cells by selenodiglutathione and selenocystine, Cancer Letts., 14, 303, 1981.

109. Vernie, L. N., Bont, W. S., Ginjaar, H. B., and Emmelot, P., Elongation factor 2 as the target of the reaction product between sodium selenite and gluathione (GSSeSG) in the inhibiting of amino acid incorporation *in vitro*, Biochim. Biophys. Acta, 414, 283, 1975.

110. Vernie, L. N., Bont, W. S., and Emmelot, P., Inhibition of *in vitro* amino acid incorporation by sodium selenite, Biochem., 13, 337, 1974.

111. Everett, G. A., and Holley, R. W., Effect of minerals on amino acid incorporation by a rat liver preparation, Biochim. Biophys. Acta, 46, 390, 1961.

112. Ganther, H. E., Reduction of the selenotrisulfide derivative of glutathione to a persulfide analog by glutathione reductase, Biochem., 10, 4089, 1971.

113. Ip, C., Prophylaxis of mammary neoplasia by selenium supplementation in the initiation and promotion phases of chemical carcinogenesis, Cancer Res., 41, 4386, 1981.

114. Jansson, B., Jacobs, M. M., and Griffen, A. C., Gastrointestinal cancer: epidemiologic and experimental studies, Adv. Exp. Med. Biol., 91, 305, 1978.

115. Cowgill, V. M., The distribution of selenium and cancer mortality in the continental US, Biol. Trace Elem. Res., 5, 345, 1983.

116. Yu, S. Y., Chu, Y. J., Gong, X. L., Hou, C., Li, W. G., Gong, H. M., and Xie, J. R., Regional variation of cancer mortality incidence and its relation to selenium levels in China, Biol. Trace Elem. Res., 7, 21, 1985.

117. Clark, L. C., The epidemiology of selenium and cancer, Federation Proc., 44, 2584, 1985.

118. Clark, L. C., Cantor, K. P., and Allaway, W. H., unpublished research, 1984.

119. Mason, T. J. and McKay, F. W., *Atlas of Cancer Mortality for US Countries: 1950-1969*, Dept. of Health, Education and Welfare, Washington, D. C., 1975.

120. Chu, Y. J., Liu, Q. Y., Hou, C., and Yu, S. Y., BloGd selenium concentration in residents of areas in China having a high incidence of lung cancer, Biol. Trace Elem. Res., 6, 133, 1984.

121. Sundstrom, H., Korpela, H., Viinikka, L., and Kauppila, A., Serum selenium and glutathione peroxidase and plasma lipid peroxides in uterine, ovarian or vulvar cancer, and their responses to antioxidant in patients with ovarian cancer, Cancer Lett., 24, 1, 1984.

122. Sundstrom, H., Yrjankeikki, E., and Kauppila, A., Serum selenium in patients with ovarian cancer during and after therapy, Carcinogenesis, 5, 731, 1984.

123. Salonen, J. T., Alfthan, G., Huttunen, J. K., and Puska, P., Association between serum selenium and the risk of cancer, Am. J. Epidemiol., 120, 342, 1984.

124. Kauppila, A., Sundstrom, H., Korpela, H., Viinikka, L., and Yrjanheikki, E., Serum selenium and gynecological cancer: effect of selenium supplementation on plasma malandialdehyde and serum glutathione peroxidase, in *Icosanoids and Cancer*, Thaler-Dao, H., ed., Raven Press, New York, 263, 1984.

125. Vernie, L. N., De Vries, M., Beckhuijsen, C., De Goeij, J. J. M., and Zegers, C., Selenium levels in blood and plasma, and glutathione peroxidase activity in blood of breast cancer patients during adjuvant treatment with cyclophosphamide, methotrexate and 5-fluorouracil, Cancer Letts., 18, 283, 1983.

126. Calautti, P., Moschini, G., Stievano, B. M., Tomio, L., Clazavara, F., and Perona, G., Serum selenium levels in malignant lymphoproliferative diseases, Scand. J. Haematol., 24, 63, 1980.

127. Schrauzer, G. N., Schrauzer, T., Mead, S., Kvehn, K., Yamamoto, H., and Arakl, E., Selenium in the blood of Japanese and American women with and without breast cancer and fibrocystic disease, in *Proceedings of the Third Internation Symposium on Selenium in Biology and Medicine*, Combs, G. F., Jr., Spallholz, J. E., Levander, O. A., and Oldfield, J. E., eds., Avi Publ. Co., Westport, Conn., 1986.

128. Robinson, M. F., Godfrey, P. J., Thomson, C. D., Rea, H. M., and van Rij, A. M., Blood selenium and glutathione peroxidase activity in normal subjects and in surgical patients with and without cancer in New Zealand, Am. J. Clin. Nutr., 32, 1477, 1979.

129. Masiak, M. and Herzyk, D., Behavior of microelements in lung cancer patients, Fresenius Z. Anal. Chem., 317, 661, 1984.

130. El-Yazigi, A., Al-Saleh, I., and Al-Mefty, O., Concentration of Ag, Al, Au, Bi, Cd, Cu, Pb, Sb and Se in cerebrospinal fluid of patients with cerebral neoplasms, Clin. Chem., 30, 1358, 1984.

131. Sullivan, J. F., Blotcky, A. J., Jetton, M. M., Hahn, H. K.J, and Burch, R. E., Serum levels of selenium, calcium, copper, magnesium and zinc in various human diseases, J. Nutr., 19, 1432, 1979.

132. Shultz, J. D., and Leklem, J. E., Selenium status of vegetarians, nonvegetarians, and hormone-dependent cancer subjects, Am. J. Clin. Nutr., 37, 114, 1983.

133. McConnell, K. P., Broghamer, W. L., Jr., Blotcky, A. J., and Hurt, O. J., Selenium levels in human blood and tissues in helath and in disease, J. Nutr., 105, 1026, 1975.

134. McConnell, K. P., Jager, R. M., Bland, K. I., and Blotcky, A. J., The relationship of dietary selenium and breast cancer, J. Surg. Oncol., 15, 67, 1980.

135. Miller, L., Mills, B. J., Blotcky, A. J., and Lincleman, R. D., Red blood cell and serum Selenium concentrations as influenced by age and selected diseases, J. Am. Coll. Nutr., 4, 331, 1983.

136. McConnell, K. P., Jager, R. M., Higgins, P. J., and Blotcky, A. J., Serum selenium levels in patients with and without breast cancer, in *Nutrition and Cancer*, Van Eys, J., Seelig, M. S., and Nichols, B. S., eds., S. P. Medical and Scientific Books, New York, p.145, 1978.

137. Broghamer, W. L., Jr., McConnell, K. P., Grimaldi, M., and Blotcky, A. J., Serum selenium and reticuloendothelial tumors, Cancer, 41, 1462, 1978.

138. Broghamer, W. L., Jr., McConnell, K. P., and Blotcky, A. J., Relationship between serum selenium levels and patients with carcinoma, Cancer, 37, 1384, 1976.

139. McConnell, K. P., Jager, R. M., Bland, K. I., and Blotcky, A. J., The relationship of dietary selenium and breast cancer, J. Surg. Oncol., 15, 67, 1980.

140. Shamberger, K. J., Rukovena, E., Longfield, A. K., Tytko, S. A., Deodhar, S., and Willis, C. E., Antioxidants and cancer. I. Selenium in the blood of normals and cancer patients, J. Nat. Cancer Inst., 50, 863, 1973.

141. Schrauzer, G. N., Rhead, W. J., and Evans, G. A., Selenium and cancer: chemical interpretation of a plasma "cancer test," Bioinorg. Chem., 2, 329, 1973.

142. Goodwin, W. J., Lane, H. W., Bradford, K., Marshall, M. V., Griffin, A. C., Geopfert, H., and Jesse, R. H., Selenium and glutathione peroxidase levels in patients with epidermoid carcinoma in the oral cavity and oropharynx, Cancer, 51, 110, 1983.

143. Clark, L. C., Graham, G. F., Crounse, R. G., Grimson, R., Hulka, B., and Shy, C. M., Plasma selenium and skin neoplasma: a case-control study, Nutr. Cancer, 6, 13, 1984.

144. Willett, W., Polk, B. F., and Hames, C., Prediagnostic serum selenium and risk of cancer, Lancet, 8342, 130, 1983.

145. Salonen, J. T., Salonen, R., Lappetelainen, R., Maenpaa, P. H., Althan, G., and Puska, P. Risk of cancer in relation to serum concentrations of selenium and vitamins A and E: matched case-control analysis of prospective data, Br. Med. J., 290,417,1985.

146. Peleg, I., Morris, S., and Hames, C. G., Is selenium a risk factor for cancer? Med. Oncol. Tumor Pharmacother., in press, 1985.

11

EFFECTS OF SELENIUM EXCESSES

Cases of poisonings of animals by what are now recognized to have been Se compounds long predated the systemmatic study of the roles of Se in biology. In fact, in the 1930s, the toxic effects of Se excesses were the first biological consequences of the element to be recognized. This early experience with Se compounds as toxicants, and the subsequent finding of the relatively narrow margin between the levels of Se that are nutritionally important and those that can be toxic, may have contributed to the popular view of Se as a nutrient that can be quite toxic if not used very carefully. This view is, in fact, overly cautious; it is the purpose of this chapter to review the evidence concerning the toxicity of Se compounds and to set this in perspective with current knowledge of the roles of Se in nutrition and health and of the normal exposures of animals and humans to Se compounds. Much of this information has been reviewed by previous authors.[1-20]

I. EARLY EXPERIENCES WITH SELENIUM TOXICITIES

The earliest written account of Se poisoning is thought to be the description by Marco Polo[21] of a necrotic hoof disease of horses that occurred in thirteenth-century China. Although the etiology of the disease was not known, Polo described its association with the consumption of a poisonous plant indigenous to the region of the disease. Of traders entering the region, he wrote, "They cannot venture amongst the mountains with any beasts of burden except those accustomed to the country on account of a poisonous plant growing there which, if eaten by them, has the effect of causing the hoofs of the animals to drop off. Those of the country, being aware of its dangerous quality, take care to avoid it." Six centuries later, this disease was to reappear on the American Great Plains as the so-called "alkali disease."

Benavides and Mojica[22] cited an account from 1560 by a Colombian priest in which corn and other vegetables grown in some regions of the country were described as being so poisonous that persons or animals consuming them would suffer hair losses. Of greater concern in this report is the association of human fetal malformations with consumption of the same poisonous foods. (This topic is addressed in Section III. C. of this chapter.)

Madison[23] reported the occurrence in 1856 of a fatal disease of horses resembling that mentioned earlier by Marco Polo.[21] United States Army horses allowed to graze freely in the vicinity of Fort Randall in northern Nebraska were described as suffering from losses of the long hair from the mane and tail, and from a debilitating necrotic hoof disease. Settlers of that region (i.e., northern Nebraska, South Dakota), who came by the 1890s, observed similar disorders in their livestock.[2] They associated the disease with alkali seeps and waters of high salt content; hence, it became known as "alkali disease." By the turn of the century, researchers in the northern Great Plains area proposed that alkali disease and the related "blind staggers disease" were caused by molded feed grains[24,25], but in 1931, Hutton[26] recognized an association of the endemic distribution of these livestock diseases with particular soil types now known to be seleniferous.

The recognition of Se compounds as toxic principles in alkali and blind staggers diseases came in the early 1930s. During that time, Kurt Franke at the South Dakota State Experiment Station was able to identify toxic feedstuffs using rat[27-31] or chick[32] bioassays. As the signs of intoxication were thought to resemble those of metallic poisoning, a systematic search for trace elements was made in grain samples that were found to be toxic in Franke's rat bioassay. Thus it was that Se was found to be present in the toxic grains.[33,34] Because seleniferous plants and soils were also found to contain appreciable levels of Mo, Te, and Cr,[35,36] the proof that Se was the active toxic factor was not firm until Franke and Potter[37] demonstrated the production in rats, by the feeding of Na_2SeO_3 or Na_2SeO_4, of toxic signs apparently identical with those produced by toxic grains. Subsequent studies[38] showed that the injection of inorganic Se compounds into eggs produced chick embryo malformations similar to those observed among progeny of hens fed toxic grains,[39,40] and that Se was the active factor associated with protein in toxic grain.[41]

II. SELENIUM TOXICITY IN ANIMALS

The classical description of Se toxicoses of animals was presented by Rosenfeld and Beath.[5] Those authors described three clinical types of Se intoxication: acute selenosis, sub-acute selenosis (i.e., blind staggers type), and chronic selenosis (i.e., alkali disease type).

A. Acute Selenosis

Acute selenosis is characterized by exposure to large doses of Se within a short period of time with severe signs of toxicity that are manifest with rapid onset. Generalizations concerning the acute toxicity of Se to animals are exceedingly difficult to make due to the large array of chemical forms of the element, species, routes of administration, and means of quantifying toxicity that have been used by various investigators. Studies that provide information concerning the acute lethalities of several Se compounds are summarized in Table 11.1.[43-47] In general, it is apparent that the acute lethalities of Se compounds are substantially less when they are administered orally than when they are given parenterally. This is best seen in the case of the most frequently studied form of Se, Na_2SeO_3; it shows an average oral LD_{50} value of ca. 5.9 mg Se/kg (body weight),* and an average parenteral LD_{50} value of only ca. 2.0 mg Se/kg b.w.,† i.e., one-third of the former value. Using LD_{50} values as indices of toxicity, various Se compounds can be categorized according to relative toxicity as shown in Table 11.2. By such general categorization, the common inorganic Se salts Na_2SeO_3 and Na_2SeO_4, selenomethionine, and selenodiglutathione appear among the more toxic species. However, it must be pointed out that the information base for such categorization is very limited and that comparative toxicological evaluations of series of Se compounds within species is limited to the single study of Palmer et al.[44] Those investigators were able to rank the toxicities of eight inorganic and organic Se compounds on the basis of their acute lethalities to 4-day-old chick embryos to which the test compounds were administered by injection into the air cell in ovo. Their results (see Table 11.3) showed that the toxicities of Na_2SeO_4 and selenomethionine were comparable but somewhat greater than that of Na_2SeO_3, and greater still than that of selenocystine. Cummins and Kimura[58] pointed out that two

*The oral LD_{50} values for different species have been reported to be as low as ca. 2.3 mg Se/kg b.w. for the guinea pig[49] and rabbit,[49] and as great as 13-18 mg Se/kg b.w. for the pig.[46]

†The parenteral LD_{50} values for different species have been reported to be as low as 0.46 mg Se/kg b.w. for the sheep[46] and as great as 5.7 mg Se/kg b.w. for the rat.[59]

Table 11.1
Acute Toxicities of Selenium Compounds in Experimental Animals

Se compound	Species	Route of administration	Criteria of toxicity (mg Se/kg body weight)				Reference
			LD$_{50}$	LD$_{75}$	MLD[a]	Other	
Na$_2$SeO$_3$	Cat	i.v.[b]			2–3		(43)
	Chick embryo	Air cell[cd]	0.7				(38)
		Air cell[ce]	0.3				(44)
		Air cell[cf]	0.5				(45)
	Cow	Oral			9.9–11.0		(46)
		i.m.[g]				1–2: Lethal	(47)
	Dog	s.c.[h]		1.5–2.0 (24 hrs)[i]			(48)
		i.v.[b]			2		(2)
	Guinea pig	Oral	2.3				(49)
	Horse	Oral			3.3		(46)
	Horse (pony)	Oral	6				(50)
	Mouse	Oral	3.2–3.5				(49)
		Oral	2.2 (7 days)[i]				(51)
		i.v.[b]	2.3 (24 hrs)[i]				(52)
		i.v.[b]			>3.3		(46)
		s.c.[a]				LD$_{80}$ = 3.2	(53)
	Pig	Oral	13–18				(46)
		i.m.[g]	1.4[j] 0.9–1.0[k]				(54)
	Rabbit	Oral	2.25	3			(43)
		Oral	2.85				(49)
		Oral			0.9–1.5		(56)
		i.v.[b]	0.9				(2)
		i.v.[b]			1.5		(43)
		i.v.[b]			1.5		(55)
		s.c.[h]		1.8			(57)

Rat		Oral	3.2 (10 days)[i]				(58)
		Oral	4.8-6.0				(49)
		i.v.[b]	5.7				(56)
		i.v.[b]			3-5.7		(2)
		i.v.[b]			3		(43)
		i.v.[b]		3 (2 days)[i]			(55)
		i.p.[l]		3.25-3.5 (48 hrs)[i]			(57)
	Sheep	s.c.[h]	3.2				(59)
		i.m.[g]	0.7 (8 days)[i]				(60)
		i.m.[g]	0.46 (7 days)[i]				(61)
HgSeO$_3$	Mouse	s.c.[h]	2.88				(53)
SeOCl$_2$	Rabbit	Topical				83 mg: Death, 5 hrs; 4 mg: Death, 24 hrs	(62)
Na$_2$SeO$_4$	Chick embryo	Air cell[ce]	0.13				(44)
		Air cell[cf]	1.8-2.0				(45)
	Rabbit	Oral	1.8				(56)
		i.v.[b]	1.1				(56)
		i.v.[b]			2-2.5		(55)
		i.v.[b] rat		4.3			(56)
		i.v.[b]			3		(55)
		i.p.[l]	5.25-5.75 (48 hrs)[i]	5.5-5.75 (48 hrs)			(63)
		i.p.[l]					(55)
SeF$_6$	Rat	Inhalation			>10 ppm		(64)
Elemental Se	Rat	Oral	6700 (10 days)[i]				(58)
		i.p.[l]			>1000		(65)
H$_2$Se	Guinea pig	Inhalation	0.001 ppm[m] (8 hrs)[i]				(66)
		Inhalation				0.2 ppm[m] lethal (60 min)	(67)

(continues)

Table 11.1 *(Continued)*

| Se compound | Species | Route of administration | Criteria of toxicity (mg Se/kg body weight) | | | Other | Reference |
			LD$_{50}$	LD$_{75}$	MLD[a]		
HgSe	Mouse	s.c.[h]	31.6				(53)
SeS$_2$	Mouse	Oral	2620				(68)
	Rat	Oral	76 (10 days)[i]				(58)
Dimethylselenide	Mouse	i.p.[l]	1300 (24 hrs)[i]				(69)
	Rat	i.p.[l]	1600 (24 hrs)[i]				(69)
Dimethylselenoxide	Chick embryo	Air cell[ce]	6.53				(44)
Trimethylselenonium chloride	Chick embryo	Air cell[ce]	15.7				(44)
	Rat	i.p.[l]	49.4 (4 hrs)[i]				(70)
Selenourea	Rat	Oral	32 (10 days)[i]				(58)
DL-Selenomethionine	Chick embryo	Air cell[ce]	0.13				(44)
	Mouse	i.v.[b]	8.9 (24 hrs)[i]				(46)
		i.c.[n]	5.3 (24 hrs)[i]				(66)
	Rat	i.p.[l]		4.25 (48 hrs)[i]			(71)
DL-Selenocystine	Chick embryo	Air cell[ce]	0.64				(44)
	Rat	i.p.[l]		4.0 (48 hrs)[i]			(72)
Se-methylseleno-cysteine	Chick embryo	Air cell[ce]	0.57				(44)
Selenodiglutathione	Mouse	i.v.[b]	1.8 (7 days)				(52)
Diphenylselenide	Rat	Oral	122 (10 days)				(58)
Bis-(β-N,N-dimorpholino) ethyl selenide	Rabbit	i.v.[b]	21 (14 days)				(73)
	Rat	i.v.[b]	103-206 (14 days)				(73)
		i.p.[l]	347-1606 (14 days)				(73)

Compound	Chick embryo	Air cell[ce]			
Methylseleninic acid			0.052		(44)
n-Propylseleninic acid	Rat	i.p.[l]		20-25 (48 hrs)	(74)
β-Seleninopropionic acid	Rat	i.p.[l]		25-30 (48 hrs)	(74)
β-selenodipropionic acid	Rat	i.p.[l]	>40 (48 hrs)		(74)
β,β'-diselenodipropionic acid	Rat	i.p.[l]		25-30 (48 hrs)	(74)
Selenium diphenylacetate	Rat	i.p.[l]		>30 (48 hrs)	(72)
Dimethylselenetindicarboxylic acid	Rat	i.p.		>30 (48 hrs)	(72)

[a] Minimal lethal dose.
[b] Administered by intravenous injection.
[c] Administered by injection through eggshell to surface of air cell.
[d] Treated prior to incubation.
[e] Treated after 4 days of incubation.
[f] Treated after 14 days of incubation.
[g] Administered by intramuscular injection.
[h] Administered by subcutaneous injection.
[i] Period of observation indicated parenthetically.
[j] Se-adequate individuals.
[k] Se-deficient individuals.
[l] Administered by intraperitoneal injection.
[m] Concentration in air.
[n] Administered by intracerebroventricular injection.

Table 11.2

Relative Acute Toxicities of Selenium Compounds[a]

Route of administration	Most toxic ($LD_{50} < 10$ mg Se/kg b.w.)	Moderately toxic (LD_{50}: 10–100 mg Se/kg b.w.)	Least toxic ($LD_{50} > 100$ mg Se/kg b.w.)
Oral	Na_2SeO_3 Na_2SeO_4	SeS_2 (rat) Selenourea	Elemental Se SeS_2 (mouse) Diphenylselenide
Parenteral	Na_2SeO_3 Na_2SeO_4 HgSe $HgSeO_3$ Se-methionine Selenodiglutathione	$(CH_3)_3SeCl$ BDMES (rabbit)[b]	$(CH_3)_2Se$ BDMES (rat)[b]

[a]Categorized according to LD_{50} values presented in Table 11.1.
[b]Bis-(beta-N,N-dimorpholino)ethylselenide.

Table 11.3

Relative Toxicities of Several Selenium Compounds for Chick Embryos[a]

Se compounds	LD_{50} (mg Se/kg egg contents)
CH_3SeO_2H	0.052
Se-DL-methionine	0.13
Na_2SeO_4	0.13
Na_2SeO_3	0.3
Se-methylselenocysteine	0.57
Se-DL-cystine	0.64
$(CH_3)_2SeO$	6.53
$(CH_3)_3SeCl$	15.7

[a]Data of Palmer et al.[44]

important determinants of the acute toxicities of Se compounds were the oxidation state and the aqueous solubility. For inorganic compounds, this is certainly true, i.e., the reduced and poorly soluble forms are the least toxic of the Se compounds.* The available evidence, taken somewhat generally, does not indicate that the acute toxicities of the common inorganic Se salts vary greatly from those of the two selenoamino acids thought to represent important sources of Se in foods and feedstuffs.

Reports of the signs of acute Se toxicity in livestock are summarized in Table 11.4.[75-84] These signs are similar to those described in the classic report of Franke and Moxon[63] of acute selenosis in dogs and rats. The most characteristic sign of acute selenosis is "garlic breath" due to the pulmonary excretion of volatile Se metabolites, e.g., dimethyl selenide. Other signs include lethargy, excessive salivation, vomiting, dyspnea, muscle tremors, and respiratory failure resulting in death. Pathological findings include congestion of the liver and kidney, fatty metamorphosis and focal necrosis of the liver, endocarditis and myocarditis, degeneration of the smooth musculature of the gastrointestinal tract, gall bladder, and bladder, and erosion of the long bones.

B. Subacute Selenosis

Rosenfeld and Beath[5] described subacute selenosis as resulting from exposure to large doses of Se over a longer period of time and as resulting in the manifestation of neurological signs (e.g., blindness, ataxia,

*In this respect, the toxicities and biological availabilities (i.e., utilization at nutritional levels of exposure) of inorganic Se compounds are related, probably because the major determinants of absorption are important affectors of both biological responses to the element.

Table 11.4

Toxic Responses to Single or a Few Doses (i.e., Acute Toxicity) of Selenium in Livestock

Species	Se source	Route	Response	Reference
Cattle	Na₂SeO₃	Drench	Although 7.0 mg Se/kg produced no ill effects, 10.1 mg Se/kg caused anorexia (2 days) and decreased milk production (5 days); levels above 11 mg Se/kg caused respiratory distress, garlic breath and death within 48 hrs.	(75)
		s.c.[a] or i.m.[b]	Does of ca. 0.5 mg Se/kg caused excessive salivation, respiratory or distress, hydrothorax, pulmonary edema, and 67% mortality within 2 hrs to 5 wks.	(76)
Horse	Na₂SeO₃	Drench	A dose of 2.7 mg Se/kg caused respiratory distress and anorexia for 1 day; 4.4 mg Se/kg caused respiratory distress, convulsions, and death within 26 hrs; 8.0 mg Se/kg caused hemorrhagic gastritis, fatty liver degeneration, and death within 18 hrs; 10.1 mg Se/kg caused cutaneous muscle spasms, pupil dilation, profuse sweating, respiratory distress, and death within 22 hrs; 12.1 mg Se/kg caused lethargy, tremors, garlic breath, and death within 24 hrs.	(75)
Pig	Na₂SeO₃	Drench	A single dose of 2.2 mg Se/kg had no ill effects, but a dose of 4.4 mg Se/kg caused anorexia and depression for 24 hrs and a dose of 8.8 mg Se/kg caused the same signs, which lasted for 5 days. Higher doses produced more severe effects, e.g., 17.4 mg Se/kg caused emesis, diarrhea, and fatty liver degeneration. A dose of 22.7 mg Se/kg caused vascular congestion, liver degeneration, and death within 72 hrs.	(75)
		s.c.[a]	A dose of 0.8 mg Se/kg had no ill effects; doses of 0.9-1.1 mg Se/kg produced slight increases in plasma GOT. Higher doses (1.2 or 2 mg Se/kg) caused ataxia, paresis, tremors, increased plasma GOT, muscular dystrophy, and death within 4 hrs.	(77)
	Se-methionine	i.v.[c]	A dose of 3 mg Se/kg caused pulmonary edema and death in 2.5 hrs.	(78)
		i.v.[c]	A dose of 3 mg Se/kg caused pulmonary edema and death within 14 hrs.	(78)

472

Species	Compound	Route	Effects	Ref.
Sheep	Na_2SeO_3	Drench	A dose of 6.4 mg Se/kg caused pulmonary congestion, mild diffuse fatty metamorphosis of liver, and 95% mortality within 15 days.	(79)
			Does to young lambs at ca. 2.2 mg Se/kg caused pulmonary hyperemia and edema, acute necrotizing nephrosis, diarrhea, and 35% mortality within 10-16 hrs.	(80)
			Doses of ca. 1.7 mg Se/kg caused hyperpnea, salivary frothing, hydrothorax, pulmonary edema, hepatic and renal degeneration, and 35% mortality within 12-48 hrs.	(81)
		i.m.[b]	A dose of 1 mg Se/kg to a yearling caused ataxia, dyspnea, hyperthermia, increased pulse and respiration, frequent urination, cyanosis, and death within 8 hrs.	(80)
			Doses of ca. 0.8 mg Se/kg caused 45% mortality in 6 hrs to 1 wk.	(82)
			Graded doses indicated an acute LD_{50} of 455 μg Se/kg; toxicity signs included pulmonary congestion and edema and hepatic and renal degeneration.	(61)
		i.m.[b]	Doses of 500-800 μg Se/kg body weight produced deaths within hours; before death, Se caused rapid weak pulses and increases in serum transaminases, creatine phosphokinase, lactate dehydrogenase, urea, and albumin. Necropsy revealed tracheo-bronchial-pulmonary edema and renal tubular degeneration and necrosis.	(83)
	SeO_2	i.v.[c]	Single doses of 4 mg Se/kg to adults caused hyperpnea, cyanosis, pulmonary edema, tremors, hypersensitivity, opisthotonus, paresis, and death in 20 min.	(84)
	Se-methionine	i.v.[c]	Three doses of 0.46 or 0.54 mg Se/kg depressed growth of lambs and caused macrocytic anemia. An adult given two doses of 1 mg Se/kg lost weight and showed macrocytic anemia and hypocythemia. Two adults given 3.4 mg Se/kg showed cyanosis and pulmonary edema and died in 10 hrs.	(84)
	Se-cystine	i.v.[c]	Three doses of 0.9-1.0 mg Se/kg reduced growth and caused anorexia, macrocytic anemia, and hypocythemia.	(84)
	Choline selenite	i.m.[b]	Responses similar to those obtained for Na_2SeO_3 were reported.	(83)

[a] Se administered by subcutaneous injection.
[b] Se administered by intramuscular injection.
[c] Se administered by intravenous injection.

473

disorientation) and respiratory distress. This condition is most frequently observed in grazing livestock that have consumed Se-accumulator plants, i.e., in "blind staggers." [44] Although Rosenfeld and Beath[5] considered blind staggers to result strictly from subacute selenosis, the finding that similar neurologic signs can be produced by giving animals aqueous extracts of Se-accumulator plants prompted Maag and Glenn[7] and Van Kampen and James[42] to suggest that some other factors (e.g., alkaloids) may be involved in the etiology of the disorder.

C. Chronic Selenosis

Chronic selenosis is characterized by exposure to more moderate levels of Se for periods of weeks or months; the major signs are dermatitic lesions involving alopecia, hoof necrosis* and loss, and emaciation, i.e., alkali disease. Other signs include anorexia with attendant weight loss, and increased serum transaminases and alkaline phosphatase. One study[98] found that blood SeGSHpx activity was reduced by 50% in chronically Se-intoxicated rats that showed no pathological signs of selenosis; this finding indicates the potential for false negative results from the diagnosis of nutritional Se status solely on the basis of SeGSHpx activity. Reports of chronic selenosis in domestic, laboratory, and livestock species are summarized in Tables 11.5[85-99] and 11.6.[100-121] While it would be useful to be able to cite a clinical predictor of chronic selenosis in various species, the available parameter is based only on observations from cattle. Reports by Dinkel et al.[122] and Maag et al.[123] indicate that signs of chronic selenosis may be expected among animals with whole blood Se concentrations of 2000-3000 ppb or more. This level corresponds to that indicated by Rosenfeld and Beath[5] to be associated with alkali disease; those authors gave blood Se levels of 1500-4000 ppb in association with blind staggers and of as much as 25,000 ppb in acute selenosis.

The relative chronic toxicities of Se compounds are of interest with regard to the selection of sources of Se for use in the supplementation of animal feeds and human foods. However, no studies have been conducted to date in which a series of Se compounds have been evaluated toxicologically in a chronic exposure design. Therefore, ranking of the chronic toxicities of Se compounds by direct comparison is not possible at the present time. It may be possible, however, to categorize their relative toxicities in a general manner by inference from the reports summarized in Tables 11.5 and 11.6

*Chronic selenosis results in abnormal hoof formation at the coronary band, which results in fracture of the hoof at that point. The lesion is obviously painful; affected animals show great reluctance to move, a factor contributing to the decreased feed intake and resultant wasting.

Table 11.5

Toxic Responses of Domestic and Laboratory Species to Selenium Administered Continuously in Feed or Water (i.e., Chronic Selenosis)

| Species | Se treatment | | Period | Response | Reference |
	Source	Route			
Dog	High-Se corn	Diet	189 days	7.2 ppm Se reduced gain and caused anorexia.	(85)
	Na_2SeO_3	Diet	150 days	10 ppm Se reduced gain and caused anorexia; 20 ppm caused weight loss, anorexia, severe ascites, and increased serum alkaline phosphatase; no mortality.	(85)
Hamster	Na_2SeO_3	Water	4 weeks	6 ppm Se reduced water intake (30%) without affecting gain; 9 or 12 ppm reduced water intake further (45 and 46%, respectively) and reduced gain (both ca. 18%) with no deaths.	(86)
Monkey[a]	Na_2SeO_3	Diet	40 days	10 ppm Se caused tail dermatosis, onychoptosis, anorexia, leukopenia, tongue erosions, but no deaths.	(87)
Mouse	Na_2SeO_3	Water	48 days	0.9 ppm Se reduced water intake by 21% during 30 days precoital period, but did not affect feed consumption during that period, or water and feed intake during 3–18 days of gestation; 1.8 ppm Se reduced total growth by 8%.	(88)
	Na_2SeO_3	Water	46 days	Body weight was reduced in mice given 10 ppm Se starting at 7 wks of age and 4 ppm Se starting at 18 wks; serum alkaline phosphatase and glutamic-oxaloacetic transaminase activities and mortality were increased at levels >32 ppm Se for mice of either age.	(51)
		Water	47 weeks	Levels up to 8 ppm Se increased survival, although the 8 ppm Se level reduced growth (by 44%) and white blood cell count, and increased serum alkaline phosphatase and glutamic-oxaloacetic transaminase.	(51)
Rat	High-Se Brazil nuts	Diet	4 weeks	8.3 ppm Se reduced growth by 35%, relative liver weight by 31%, and relative kidney weight by 29%.	(78)
	High-Se corn	Diet	4 weeks	8.6 ppm Se reduced growth by 45% and relative kidney weight by 28%.	(89)
	High-Se wheat	Diet	100 days	4.4 ppm Se caused reduced gain; 17.5 ppm Se caused weight loss but no deaths.	(90)
		Diet	21 days	10 ppm Se reduced gain by 59% with no mortality.	(91)
	High-Se wheat	Diet	21–32 days	10 ppm Se reduced growth by 94%,[b] relative liver weight by 46%,[b] and survival by 60%.	(92)

(continues)

Table 11.5 (*Continued*)

| Species | Se treatment | | Period | Response | Reference |
	Source	Route			
	High-Se wheat and oats	Diet	4 weeks	2.6 ppm Se reduced growth by 10%; 5.6 ppm Se reduced growth by 14% and increased relative liver weight by 19%.	(93)
	High-Se sesame meal	Diet	10 weeks	4.5 or 10 ppm Se in diets of dams caused increased incidence of liver lesions, increased serum transaminases and alkaline phosphatase, edema, and pancreatitis in pups fed 10 ppm Se.	(94)
	Se-methionine	Diet	4 weeks	8.3 pm Se reduced growth by 36% and relative kidney weight by 29%.	(91)
	K_2SeO_3	Diet	21 days	10 ppm Se reduced gain by 53%; no mortality.	(91)
	Na_2SeO_3	Diet	28 days	10 ppm Se reduced growth by 63%	(95)
		Diet	7 weeks	10 ppm Se reduced growth by 95%, survival by 67%, and caused liver damage.	(96)
		Diet[c]	26-29 days	10 ppm Se reduced growth by 84%, relative liver weight by 49%, and survival by 42%.	(92)
		Diet	4 weeks	8.2 ppm Se reduced growth by 44%, relative liver weight by 41%, and relative kidney weight by 36%.	(89)
		Diet	4 weeks	2.6 ppm Se increased relative liver weight by 20% without affecting growth; 5.6 ppm Se increased relative liver weight by 22% but reduced growth by 28%.	(93)
		Diet	21 days	10 ppm Se reduced gain by 56% with 11% mortality.	(91)
		Diet	359 days	22 ppm Se reduced gain with 56% mortality; liver degeneration noted.	(37)
		Water	63 days	3 ppm Se reduced gain (9%) and feed (99%) and water intake (23%); levels ≥6 ppm Se caused more severe decreases in gain and in feed and water intakes, with high mortality; water intakes most severely affected.	(97)
		Water	35 days	Rats first exposed to Se at 5 weeks of age showed reduced growth at 4 ppm Se and reduced survival at levels ≥8 ppm Se; rats first exposed to Se at 12 weeks of age showed reduced growth at 1 ppm, weight loss at levels ≥4 ppm, and reduced survival at levels ≥16 ppm. Serum alkaline phosphatase and glutamic-oxaloacetic transaminase activities increased at levels ≥8 ppm Se.	(98)

	Water	53 weeks	4 pm Se did not affect survival or growth but reduced SeGSHpx by 50%; no pathological signs.	(98)
Na₂SeO₄	Water	111 weeks	4 ppm did not affect survival, growth or pathological signs.	(98)
	Diet	28 days	10 ppm Se reduced growth by 54%.[b]	(95)
	Diet	8 weeks	10 ppm Se produced poor growth and moderate liver damage.	(99)
	Water	63 days	3 ppm Se reduced gain (13%) and feed (8%) and water intakes (31%); levels ≥6 ppm Se caused more severe decreases in gain and in feed and water intakes (water intake most severely affected), with high mortality.	(97)

[a] *Maccaca fasicularis*.
[b] Average value from several experiments.
[c] Authors did not state form of Se in original report; it is presumed to have been Na₂SeO₃.

Table 11.6

Toxic Responses of Livestock to Selenium Administered Continuously in Feed or Water (i.e., Chronic Selenosis)

Species	Se treatment Source	Route	Period	Response	Reference
Chicken (growing)	Na_2SeO_3	Diet	Several weeks	4 ppm Se had no adverse effects; 8 ppm Se reduced growth.	(90)
		Water	14 days	4 ppm Se reduced gain and feed intake, but not water intake, of Leghorn chicks; 4 or 8 ppm Se reduced gain, feed intake, feed/gain and water intake in broiler chicks; 2 ppm Se had no adverse effects in either strain, but reduced water intake in broilers.	(100)
		Diet[a]	14 days	Levels ≥10 ppm Se reduced growth; mortality was increased by 40 ppm Se.	(101)
		Diet[a]	4 weeks	25 ppm Se reduced growth and feed intake; survival was reduced at 25-50 ppm Se.	(102)
		Diet[a]	4 weeks	10 ppm Se reduced growth by 27%[b], 15 ppm Se reduced growth by 51% and caused garlic breath.	(92)
	SeO_2	Diet	2 weeks	5 ppm Se had no adverse effects; levels ≥10 ppm reduced growth; 40 ppm Se caused 36% mortality.	(103)
		Diet	5 weeks	Although 5 ppm Se did not affect growth, it increased mortality from *Salmonella gallinarum*; 10 or 20 ppm Se also decreased growth.	(104)
	Diphenyl Se	Diet	2 weeks	Levels ≥10 ppm Se reduced growth.	(103)
Chicken (Hen)	Mixed high-Se corn, barley, wheat	Diet	Several weeks	5 ppm Se reduced survival of progeny; 10 ppm Se reduced hatchability to 0% with embryonic deformities.	(90)
	Na_2SeO_3	Diet	28 weeks	Liver ≥5 pm Se reduced hatchability of fertile eggs, without affecting fertility, egg production, egg weight, feed consumption, etc.	(105)
		Diet	Several weeks	6.5 ppm Se reduced feed consumption and body weight and caused embryonic deformation; 26 ppm Se also reduced egg production.	(90)
		Diet	2 weeks	8 ppm Se caused embryonic deformation.	(106)
	H_2SeO_3	Diet	76 weeks	8 ppm Se reduced body weight, egg weight, egg production, hatchability, and growth of progeny.	(107)
	Cystine selenate	Water	40 days	10 ppm Se reduced growth and egg production, and produced anemia; histological lesions were noted in duodenum, lungs, kidney, and testes.	(108)

				Effects	Ref.
Horse	Na$_2$SeO$_3$	Diet	Up to 6.5 months	Levels ≥24 ppm Se caused alopecia, scaling of hooves, weight loss, listlessness, hemorrhagic and cirrhotic liver, and death.	(109)
Pig (growing)	High-Se corn	Diet	8 weeks	5 ppm Se caused no adverse effects; 10 ppm Se caused reduced gain, anorexia, dyspnea, but no deaths.	(110)
	High-Se wheat, oats	Diet	6 weeks	Levels ≤8.4 ppm Se did not affect growth, feed intake, or feed/gain; but 8.4 ppm increased relative liver weight by 17%.	(93)
	Se-methionine	Diet	39 days	Levels ≥20 ppm Se caused reduced gain, anorexia, dyspnea, vomiting and diarrhea. All pigs fed ≥45 ppm Se lost weight and died.	(78)
	Na$_2$SeO$_3$	Diet	108 days	Levels ≥7 ppm Se caused reduced gain, alopecia, cracked hooves.	(111)
		Diet	35 days	8 ppm Se reduced growth in white (12%), black (27%), and red (64%) pigs.	(112)
		Diet[a]	8-10 weeks	48 ppm Se in a practical pig grower diet was associated with afebrile paresis in 8% of a farm herd; half of the affected animals died acutely, and only 11% recovered.	(113)
		Diet	29 days	52 ppm Se caused paresis and paralysis in 2 of 5 pigs; histology showed focal symmetrical poliomegelomalacia of cervical and lumber/sacral spinal cord enlargements.	(113)
		Diet	5 weeks	Levels ≥8 ppm Se reduced gain and feed intake, and increased serum transaminase activities with no deaths with levels up to 20 ppm.	(114)
		Diet	37 days	Levels ≥5 ppm Se reduced gain and feed intake; 40 ppm Se caused complete feed refusal within a few days; alopecia was seen at ≥25 ppm Se within 17 days and at 5 ppm Se by 37 days; levels ≥20 ppm Se caused ataxia; levels ≥5 ppm Se caused abnormal hoof formation at the coronary band.	(115)
		Diet	39 days	Levels ≥20 ppm Se caused weight loss, anorexia, dyspnea, vomiting, diarrhea; mortality was seen in some pigs fed 20 or 45 ppm Se and in all pigs fed ≥60 ppm Se.	(78)
		Diet	8 weeks	No adverse effects.	(116)
		Diet	17 weeks	Levels ≤8.3 ppm Se did not affect growth, feed intake, or feed/gain; but 5.7 and 8.3 ppm increased relative liver weight by 16 and 7%, respectively.	(93)

(continues)

479

Table 11.6 *(Continued)*

Species	Se treatment				Response	Reference
	Source	Route	Period			
Pig (sow)	Na_2SeO_3	Diet	Several weeks		10 ppm Se reduced growth by 82% and feed intake by 53%.	(117)
		Diet	Several weeks		10 ppm Se reduced growth by 30% and feed intake by 22% of preweaning progeny.	(117)
			Through 2 litters		10 ppm Se reduced conception rate of sows, decreased live births, and reduced pig birth weights.	(118)
			4 months		Levels $\geq$24.5 ppm Se caused anorexia, alopecia, abnormalities of coronary band and cracking of hooves, diarrhea, liver degeneration, and death.	(119)
Rainbow trout	Na_2SeO_3	Diet	16 weeks		13 ppm Se reduced growth, feed intake, and feed/gain, and trout increased mortality.	(120)
		Diet	16 weeks		10 ppm Se reduced growth, feed intake, and feed/gain; liver Cu was increased by 10 ppm Se, and kidney Ca was increased by 5 ppm Se.	(121)

[a] Although the authors did not state the form of Se used, it is presumed that it was Na_2SeO_3.
[b] Average value of several experiments.

and from information about their acute toxicities. By this approach, various Se compounds appear to fall into three categories of chronic toxicity: the soluble inorganic salts (Na_2SeO_3 and Na_2SeO_4) appear to be among the more toxic species; the Se inherent in grains and the purified selenoamino acids (selenomethionine and selenocystine) appear to have relatively moderate chronic toxicities; the insoluble forms of Se (e.g., elemental Se, Na_2Se, SeS_2, and diphenyl selenide) appear to be among the least toxic species.

D. Effects of Selenium Excesses on Reproduction

Olson[124] suggested that the negative effects of excessive intakes of Se on reproductive performance (e.g., reduced rates of conception and progeny weaned) have greater economic impacts on animal agriculture than does the occurrence of overt selenosis. This conclusion is supported by observations in several species of impaired reproduction due to levels of Se insufficient to produce clinical signs of toxicity in exposed animals. Munsell et al.[125] found that female rats exposed to 3 ppm Se (as seleniferous wheat included in the diet) showed abnormally low rates of conception. Similar results were reported by Schroeder and Mitchener[126] in mice given 3 ppm Se (as Na_2SeO_4) in their drinking water. Impaired neonatal survival was observed by Halverson[127] in the third generation of rats fed diets containing 3.75 ppm Se (as Na_2SeO_3), and Schroeder and Mitchener[126] found that mice given 3 ppm Se (as Na_2SeO_4) in the drinking water produced litters with excessive incidences (70%) of runts. Wahlstrom and Olson[118] noted reduced birth weights in the progeny of gilts fed a diet supplemented with 10 ppm Se (as Na_2SeO_3). Rosenfeld and Beath[128] found that female rats given drinking water containing 2.5 ppm Se (as Na_2SeO_4) showed reductions by one-half of the number of young reared. The numbers of young weaned per dam was also reduced due to 10 ppm Se (as Na_2SeO_3) in the diets of gilts,[118] and due to pasturage of beef cattle on seleniferous range.[129]

Decreases in rates of conception have also been observed in rats fed 25 ppm Se (as seleniferous wheat included in the diet) for periods of at least 40 days,[130] in rats given 7.5 ppm Se (as Na_2SeO_4) in the drinking water,[128] in mice maintained for several generations with 3 ppm Se (as Na_2SeO_4) in the drinking water,[126] in pigs fed diets supplemented with 10 ppm Se (as Na_2SeO_3),[118] and in cattle grazing on seleniferous pastures.[129] Studies using rats by Franke and Potter[130] and Rosenfeld and Beath[128] showed that reductions in conception rates resulted from the exposure of females to high levels of Se; Se exposure of males did not affect this parameter. Although dietary Se levels of 5 or 10 ppm (as Na_2SeO_3) effectively reduced the hatchability (i.e., embryonic survival) of laying hens, Poley and Moxon[131] found no evidence of impairment of egg fertility or production by these levels of Se in that species.

Studies that describe the effects on progeny of high-level exposure of dams to Se are summarized in Table 11.7.[132] These reports indicate that Se in naturally seleniferous feedstuffs, Na_2SeO_3, or Na_2SeO_4 can be embryocidal in chickens[105,107,131] and fetocidal in mice,[133] pigs,[18] and rats,[130] and can reduce growth rates of chick embryos[106] or of fetal or neonatal mice[52,133] and pigs.[118] Malformations were observed in embryos of hens fed a diet supplemented with 8 ppm Se (as Na_2SeO_3)[106] and in chick embryos treated *in ovo* with Se salts.[38] In one report of exceptionally poor hatchability of chicken eggs from South Dakota, two farms indicated that three-quarters of unhatched eggs contained deformed embryos, implicating selenosis as a causative factor. However, teratogenic effects of Se have not been reported in other species. In studies in which embryonic or fetal development was specifically examined, Se was found not to be teratogenic when fed (at levels above 5 ppm as Na_2SeO_3) to hens,[105] when given parenterally (2 mg Se/kg b.w. as Na_2SeO_3) to hamsters,[132] or when given in the drinking water (at levels as great as 1.8 ppm Se as Na_2SeO_3) to mice.[133] Thus, it cannot be generalized that subacute exposure to Se compounds is teratogenic to all species, although this may be most likely for birds.

E. Cariogenic Effects of Selenium Excesses

High levels of Se can increase the incidence of dental caries in experimental animals if exposure occurs during the time of tooth development. Buttner[134] demonstrated a dose-dependent increase in both the number and extent of carious lesions in rats given 2.2 or 4.6 ppm Se (as Na_2SeO_3) in their drinking water. Navia *et al.*[135] found that the addition of 4 ppm (as Na_2SeO_3) to the diets of rats did not affect caries incidence, but the supplementation of drinking water with the same concentration resulted in a 12% increase in the incidence of lesions.* Bowen[136] treated monkeys (*Macaca irus*) with 2 ppm Se (as Na_2SeO_3) in their drinking water for 15 months before reducing the level to 1 ppm Se for another 45 months. By the end of that time, the second permanent molars and premolars of Se-treated individuals had developed a yellow chalky appearance, and the caries score of the Se-treated

---

*Because rats drink approximately 1.5 ml water per gram of food they consume, the supplementation of drinking water with the same concentration of Se would be expected to result in an approximate 50% increase in Se exposure by that route in comparison to that provided by feed supplementation.

Table 11.7

Toxic Effects of High Levels of Selenium on Progeny of Exposed Animals

Species	Se treatment		Response	Reference
	Source	Route		
Chicken	High-Se grains (corn, barley, wheat)	Diet	After 4 weeks, hatchability was not affected by 2.5 ppm Se, was slightly reduced by 5 ppm Se, and was reduced to 0% by 10 ppm Se.	(131)
	Na_2SeO_3	Diet[a]	8 ppm Se reduced egg production (by 31%), egg weight (by 3%), hatchability (by 41%), and progeny early growth (by 3%).	(107)
		Diet	8 ppm Se caused embryonic malformations (necrosis of local areas of the brain, spinal cord and eyes) with structural alterations in nearby areas and slight retardation of growth.[b]	(106)
		Diet	Levels ≥5 ppm Se reduced hatchability but had no effects on fertility and were not teratogenic. Levels of 7 or 9 ppm Se reduced egg weight (by 3 or 9%, respectively); egg production was decreased by 26% by 9 ppm Se.	(105)
Hamster	Na_2SeO_3	i.v.[c]	2 mg Se/kg was not teratogenic; when administered in combination with Cd or As, it reduced their teratogenicity.	(132)
Mouse	Na_2SeO_3	s.c.[d]	Dose-dependent fetocidal effects and fetal growth depression were observed in dams treated on day 12 of gestation (but not when they were treated on day 16). On day 12, 4.6 mg Se/kg caused abortion; on day 16, both 2.1 and 3.2 mg Se/kg also caused abortion.	(133)
		i.v.[c]	Levels up to 2.5 mg Se/kg were toxic to dams, but did not affect fetal implantations or survival; body weight of offspring was reduced at birth by 9-14% by Se treatment of dams.	(52)
		Water	Levels up to 1.8 ppm Se were not teratogenic or fetotoxic, but reduced growth by up to 8%; 0.9 ppm Se increased the embryocidal and teratogenic effects of CH_3Hg; 1.8 ppm Se reduced the latter effect.	(88)
	Na_2SeO_4	Water	3 ppm Se did not affect the first two generations, but the third generation showed reduced litter number and an excessive (70%) production of runts.	(126)
	Se-diglutathione	i.v.[c]	Levels up to 2.5 mg Se/kg were toxic to dams, but did not affect fetal implantations or survival; body weight of offspring was reduced at birth by 9-14% by Se treatment of dams.	(52)

(continues)

Table 11.7 *(Continued)*

| Species | Se treatment | | Response | Reference |
	Source	Route[a]		
Pig	Na$_2$SeO$_3$	Diet[a]	Progeny of dams fed 10 ppm Se showed reduced (by 21%) body weight at birth and reduced growth (by 30%) and feed efficiency (by 12%); however, progeny of Se-treated dams were less sensitive to toxic effects of 10 ppm Se in their own diet.	(117)
		Diet	10 ppm Se reduced conception rate, increased the number of still births (by 19%), decreased the number of pigs weaned (by 26), and decreased the average weaning body weights of progeny (by 22%).	(118)
Rat	High-Se sesame meal	Diet	Dams fed 4.5 ppm Se produced pups that did not accumulate as much hepatic Se as did progeny of dams fed 0.5 ppm Se.	(94)
	High-Se wheat	Diet	24.6 ppm Se fed to females mated to control-fed males resulted wheat in still births or in pups being eaten by the dam shortly after birth.	(130)
	Na$_2$SeO$_3$	Diet	Se levels up to 2.5 ppm did not affect performance through three successive generations; but 3.75 ppm Se reduced neonatal survival.	(127)
		Water	2.5 ppm Se decreased the number of young reared by treated dams (by 50%).	(128)

[a]The authors did not indicate the form of Se used; it is presumed to have been Na$_2$SeO$_3$.
[b]Embryos were observed only through 5 days of incubation.
[c]Se was administered by intravenous injection.
[d]Se was administered by subcutaneous injection.

group was almost twice that of controls. The author noted that the first permanent molars, formed prior to the period of Se exposure, did not show discoloration or increased caries.

Bowen[136] concluded, therefore, that Se has a cariogenic effect when administered prior to eruption. Several studies in which high levels of Se have been administered to post-eruptive rats have found no cariogenic effects of the mineral,[137-141] supporting this conclusion. The conclusion is also supported by the finding by Shearer[137] that the uptake of Se from either Na_2SeO_3 or selenomethionine (provided in the drinking water) was greater in rat pups undergoing dental development than in their dams with fully developed teeth, suggesting that the cariogenic effect of Se may involve a direct action of the element in dental enamel.

F. Cataractogenic Effects of Selenium Excesses

In 1978, Ostadalova et al.[142] found that bilateral lens cataracts could be produced, without other signs of toxicity, in 10-day-old rats by subcutaneous injection of 20-30 +moles Na_2SeO_3 (i.e., 1.6-2.3 mg selenite-Se) per kilogram of body weight. Since that report, several investigators[143-155] have studied cataractogenesis due to excesses of Se as a model for cataracts in humans, which has been associated with increased levels of Se in affected lenses.[157-159] Rats, rabbits, and guinea pigs are susceptible to Se-induced cataracts, but there appears to be a window of susceptibility to high doses of selenite during lens development. Ostadalova and Babicky[149] demonstrated that the Se-cataractogenic period in the rat occurs from 2 to 17 days post partum. High doses of selenite given shortly after this period (e.g., at 18-19 days) may induce rare cataracts[149]; similar doses given later in development do not produce nuclear cataracts.[143,149] In fact, the window of susceptibility may actually commence at about the time of parturition, inasmuch as changes outside of the lens nucleus are observable (by slit lamp examination) at least two days prior to nuclear cataract formation.[151]

Selenite-induced cataracts are associated with increases by as much as five-fold of lens Ca concentrations,[148,154] two-fold increases in lens inorganic P,[154] and small (8-19%) increases in lens Mg concentrations.[148] These changes do not appear to result from general changes in lens permeability, as the Na, K, and water contents of Se-cataractous lenses have been found to be normal.[148,154] Shearer and David[148] found by electron microprobe microanalysis that the accumulation of Ca was specific for the nuclear lens. Concentrations of Ca similar to those (i.e., 1.2 mM) found in the selenite cataractous lens were shown to increase the light scattering of soluble rat lens proteins in vitro in a manner that was promoted by phosphate.[148] This suggested that the basis of the selenite-induced lesion involves the calcium phosphate bridging of lens proteins, thus altering their solubilities. Because high level selenite treatment does not affect plasma Ca in young rats, nor does it affect lens Ca levels in older rats not susceptible to the cataract, Shearer and David[148] considered the lens accumulation of Ca to be a general aspect of cataract formation not specifically associated with Se intoxication.

The onset of the selenite-induced cataract is rapid, its signs being detectable within 72 hrs of the subcutaneous injection of Na_2SeO_3.[154] After an injection of ^{75}Se-selenite, the radiolabel is even more rapidly accumulated in the lens, reaching maximum concentrations within 24 hrs,[144,147,158] but declining rapidly thereafter to have virtually disappeared by 120 hrs.[144,147] Radioselenium administered in this manner has been found to be accumulated in both soluble and insoluble proteins of the lens[147,155] and not to be concentrated in the nuclear cataract.[147] The greatest portion of lens Se is found in association with the soluble proteins, as this class comprises more than 90% of the total lenticular proteins in the neonatal rat.[147] However, Se is taken up substantially less (e.g., one-eighth to one-fifth) by the soluble lens proteins[147] than by the insoluble ones, which are increased in the selenite-induced cataract.[144] Shearer et al.[155] found that while injected selenite-Se was taken up into all three crystalline lens proteins in both normal and cataractous lenses, the latter did not take up the element into one of the soluble proteins that served as a major repository of Se in the normal lens. They found Se in the gamma-crystalline fraction to be associated with an unusual and unidentified acidic amino acid. Shearer et al.[155] proposed that the uptake of Se by critical structural or enzymatic proteins in the peripheral regions of the lens results in transient opacities and leads, through subsequent reactions in the lens, to the nuclear opacities noted as the selenite-induced cataract.

The molecular basis for the selenite-induced cataract appears to involve the pro-oxidant character of selenite, according to which it tends to undergo reduction in aerobic systems using reducing equivalents of protein and nonprotein sulfhydryls. Selenite injection has been found to produce a fall in lens total reducing capacity (i.e., decreases in GSH, NADPH, and protein-SH),[144,145] an increase in the H_2O_2 content of the aqueous humor,[145] and decreases in the activities of catalase and superoxide dismutase in lens,[145] with no changes in the lenticular activities of SeGSHpx.[145] This lack of antioxidant protection is associated with substantial increases in the malondialdehyde contents of affected lens.[145,153] Thus, it appears that the mode of action of parenteral selenite in cataractogenesis is through its stimulation of lipid peroxidation, which leads, through its propagation of highly reactive free radical species, to the oxidation of lenticular reductants and of critical soluble lenticular proteins. The resulting protein oxidation involves structural alterations that are manifest as losses of solubility of lens proteins, seen on a gross scale as the nuclear cataract. It should be noted that, according to this hypothesis, the selenite-induced cataract results from the tendency of Se^{+4} to undergo reduction *in vivo* to Se^{-2}; thus, the lesion cannot be considered an aspect of Se toxicity in the strictest sense. Nevertheless, this phenomenon illustrates the potential hazards of parenteral administration of selenite and indicates that prudence would dictate the selection of forms of Se that either are reduced (e.g., the selenoamino acids) or are less readily reduced (e.g., selenates) for such use.

III. SELENIUM TOXICITY IN HUMANS

Recent reviews of the toxicities of Se compounds for humans[17-19,159,160] show that the information currently available on the subject concerns only a few chemical forms and natural sources of the element. In addition, many of the reports in the scientific and medical literature fail to document quantitatively Se exposure in ways that would render them useful for the establishment of appropriate safety standards. Nevertheless, that body of literature is very useful for establishing the symptomology of human selenosis and, when it is considered in its entirety, it should be possible to draw inferences for the establishment of standards of safety.

A. Acute Selenosis

With a few exceptions, documented cases of acute Se toxicity in humans have involved the occupational exposure of workers in Cu smelting or Se rectifier plants. Several of these cases have involved the inhalation of Se fumes from fires or from heated metals in those plants.[160-164] Whereas most of the airborne Se in such cases can be expected to be elemental Se and SeO_2 aerosols, an actual toxic species to the victim would be H_2SeO_3 formed on the exposed skin or mucous membranes by the hydration of SeO_2 with tissue moisture. Several other cases of acute Se toxicity have involved the inhalation of H_2Se.[165-171] Other cases have involved the accidental consumption of H_2SeO_3[172] or the voluntary consumption of Na_2SeO_4[173] and high-Se nuts.[174]

Reports of acute selenosis in humans are summarized in Table 11.8.[175] They show that the acute exposure to high levels of these Se compounds by inhalation results immediately in irritation to mucous membranes of the upper respiratory tract with the symptoms of tearing and burning sensations of the eyes, running nose, hoarseness, coughing, and sneezing. Patients may complain of headache, dizziness, dyspnea, fatigue, nausea

Table 11.8

Reports of Acute Selenosis in Humans

Form of Se	Route of exposure	Situation	Major signs and symptoms	Recovery	Reference
Se fumes[a]	Inhalation	Smelting workers	Congestion of mucous membranes of nose and throat, with lung involvement.	Complete in a few days	(160)
Se fumes[a]	Inhalation	Smelting workers	Soreness and burning of nose and throat; dyspnea; headache, dizziness, burning eyes; substernal burning, inflammation of nasal mucosa.	Complete in 10 days	(161)
Se fumes[a]	Inhalation	Workers in rectifier factory	Immediately: burning of nose and throat; violent coughing, gagging with nausea and vomiting, transient loss of consciousness; bitter acid taste in mouth. After 6-12 hrs: generalized chills, nausea, vomiting, diarrhea, malaise, dyspnea, headache. After 24 hrs: bronchitis or pneumonia.	Most victims complete in 1 week	(163)
SeO_2[a]	Eyes	Chemist	Immediate severe burning sensation of eyes; vision blurred for 24 hrs.	Complete in 10 days	(175)
SeO_2[b]	Inhalation	Metal workers	Acute eye pain, hoarseness, painful cough, dyspnea, acute conjunctivitis, larygotracheitis, bronchitis, some fever.	Complete in 5-7 days	(163)
SeO_2[b]	Inhalation	Metal workers	Irritation of eyes and mucous membranes of nose and throat; nasal secretions, dry coughing; headache, vertigo, nausea, vomiting, garlic breath and skin odor, generalized weakness; loss of consciousness.	Symptoms gone by 2 wks, but contact allergy to Se was observed	(164)
H_2SeO_3[c]	Peroral	Accidental consumption by a 3-yr-old boy	Bradycardia, slight cyanosis of extremities, bright red lips, excessive salivation; garlic breath noted immediately prior to death.	Terminal in a few hours	(172)
H_2Se	Inhalation	Metal workers	Nausea, vomiting, metallic taste in mouth, garlic breath, dizziness, lassitude, fatigue.	Complete	(165)
H_2Se	Inhalation	Metal workers	Immediate: tearing, running nose. Within a few hours: hoarseness, increasing dyspnea, erythema of the skin, conjunctivitis, pulmonary edema, abnormal EKG, porphyrinuria.	Complete in 10 days	(166)

Compound	Route	Subject	Symptoms	Outcome	Ref.
H_2Se	Inhalation	Metal workers	Immediate: dyspnea, coughing, tears, burning of nose. Within 4-5 hrs: severe cough, dyspnea, fever. By 24 hrs: irritating cough, bronchitis.	Complete in 9 days	(167)
H_2Se	Inhalation	Metal workers	Within 5 hrs: dyspnea, painful cough, yellow sputum. By 24 hrs: cyanosis, severe expiratory dyspnea, rhinitis, conjunctivitis.	Complete in 4 days	(168)
H_2Se	Inhalation	Metal worker	Immediate: burning of eyes and throat. Within a few hours: coughing, wheezing. By 18 hrs: recurrent cough, progressive dyspnea, bronchitis.	Slow improvement	(169)
H_2Se	Inhalation	—	Immediate: irritation of mucous membranes (i.e., tearing, running nose, cough, sneeze). Within a few hours: dyspnea, By several hours: pulmonary edema.	Complete	(170)
H_2Se	Inhalation	—	Nausea, vomiting, fatigue, bronchitis, conjunctivitis; one of five cases developed pulmonary edema.	Four cases showed complete recovery in a few days; one case showed signs of myocardial damage 7 wks later.	(171)
Na_2SeO_4	Peroral[d]	Intentional consumption by a 15-yr-old girl	Loose, gray stools; garlic breath; minor aches and pains, irritability.	Complete	(173)
Coco De Munco nuts[e]	Peroral	Voluntary consumption	Nervousness, chills, diarrhea, anorexia, asthenia, dyspepsia, streaked nails, general loss of hair.	Complete	(174)

[a]Fumes expected to by comprised of Se^0 aerosols and SeO_2.
[b]The active species is likely to be H_2SeO_3 formed by the hydration of SeO_2 by the moisture of mucous membranes, skin, etc.
[c]Consumed in the form of a liquid gun-blueing preparation that contained ca. 1.8% H_2SeO_3.
[d]Intake estimated to be ca. 9.3 mg Se/kg body weight.
[e]*Lecythis ollaria*; main form of Se thought to be Se-cystathionine.

and vomiting, and a bitter taste in the mouth. Some may have a garlic-type odor of the breath. Clinical signs of conjunctivitis, rhinitis, and bronchitis follow. After several hours, pulmonary edema may develop; Hamiton[176] has suggested that this condition may result from the local toxic effects in the lung of dimethylselenide produced during the metabolism of such high doses of Se and excreted from that organ. It is difficult to evaluate the relative toxicities of the primary forms of Se to which industrial workers may be exposed by inhalation (i.e., SeO_2, H_2Se, and elemental Se aerosols); however, it is apparent that each is absorbed via that route. Studies by Weissman et al.[177] using the dog have modeled the pharmacokinetics of Se from H_2SeO_3 or elemental Se after exposure by inhalation; their results indicate that the long-term retention of Se in the lung is much greater after exposure to elemental Se aerosols than to H_2SeO_3, but that the long-term retention of Se in liver was greater for H_2SeO_3.* This finding might suggest that elemental Se from aerosols may be relatively poorly metabolized locally or systemically and, hence, may have relatively more severe effects as a local irritant.

Other compounds of Se are known to be rather well absorbed enterically. The few documented cases of sublethal acute selenosis involving peroral exposure to such compounds (i.e., Na_2SeO_4[173] and high-Se Coco De Munco nuts[174]†) show gastrointestinal disturbances as the major signs (e.g., dyspepsia, diarrhea, anorexia, garlic odor of the breath) but with some neurological signs (e.g., irritability, nervousness, asthenia, minor aches and pains) and changes in hair and nails. These signs and symptoms resemble those resulting from chronic exposure to high levels of Se and may be indicative of the quantitatively greater exposure of victims of acute peroral selenosis than of those of acute selenosis by inhalation. The relatively high enteric absorption of high doses of H_2SeO_3 is demonstrated by the most unfortunate case of a 3-year-old boy who died within a few hours of drinking a liquid gun-blueing preparation that contained ca. 1.8% H_2SeO_3. Each of the reports of nonfatal acute selenosis indicates that the signs and symptoms of the toxicity are readily reversible upon cessation of exposure to the toxicant, and that complete recovery with no sequelae can be expected within 7-10 days.

The dermal absorption of Se compounds is largely unknown except for the reports of Dudley[178] and Dutkiewicz et al.,[179] which showed that SeOCl and Na_2SeO_3 were absorbed through the skin of rabbits and rats,

---

*At 128 days after exposure, dogs treated with elemental Se had 6.2% of the total body burden in lung and 7.4% in liver, whereas dogs treated with H_2SeO_3 had 1.3% in lung and 11.4% in liver.[177]

†The major form of Se in the nuts of this plant (*Lecythis ollaria*) is thought to be selenocystathionine.

respectively.* Cases of contact exposure to SeO_2,[180-182] $SeOCl$,[178] and Na_2SeO_3[183] have shown these compounds to be contact irritants producing painful burning skin reactions, erythema, and, on occasion, allergic dermatitis, the severities of which vary according to the degree of exposure.

B. Chronic Selenosis

Cases of Se intoxication due to chronic exposure to high levels of the element have been encountered in both occupation-related and -unrelated situations. Reports of chronic selenosis in humans are summarized in Table 11.9.[184-187] Each of these cases has involved occupational exposure to Se by inhalation of Se fumes (i.e., elemental Se aerosals, SeO_2, or H_2Se), accompanied, in some cases, by apparent topical exposure to Se-containing materials. The signs and symptoms include those observed in cases of acute inhalatory selenosis (i.e., inflammation of the upper respiratory mucosa, rhinitis, chronic bronchitis) but also include more severe gastrointestinal effects (e.g., nausea, vomiting, dyspepsia, epigastric pain), as well as irritability, sleeplessness, anorexia, lassitude, extreme fatigue, headaches, dizziness, metallic taste in the mouth, and garlic breath odor.

Chronic peroral exposure to high levels of Se has been observed in several populations in seleniferous geographic regions† (e.g., the northern Great Plains of the USA, parts of Venezuela and Colombia, and one county in China‡). These reports, a few of which are anecdotal, are summarized in Table 11.10.[188-200] Selenium exposure was documented in 10 of these reports, eight of which gave measures of urinary Se as indicators of the magnitude of Se exposure. These studies show that signs of toxicity were observed in populations with urinary Se concentrations in excess of 200 ppb, with individual values as great as 3900 ppb. In the high-Se populations studied, signs or symptoms of toxicity have generally not been found unless urinary Se levels exceeded ca. 600 ppb, although in 1940 Lemley[192] reported selenosis in a South Dakota family with urine Se levels of 200-600 ppb. The most frequently reported signs and symptoms of chronic selenosis include lassitude, depression, fatigue, and dermatological lesions (e.g., brittleness and loss of hair; white streaking, brittleness, and breakage of nails; scaly dermatitis).

---

*The only data available concerning the quantitative dermal absorption of water-soluble Se compounds are those of Dutkiewicz *et al.*[179] for Na_2SeO_3. They found that ca. 10% of a dose of 0.1 M Na_2SeO_3 was absorbed by rats within 1 hour after topical application.

†See Chapter 2, Section V, Geo-Botanical Mapping of Areas of Selenium Deficiency and Excess

‡Enshi County, Hubei Province, P. R. C.

Table 11.9

Reports of Chronic Selenosis in Humans by Occupational Exposure

Form of Se	Route of exposure	Situation	Major signs and symptoms	Reference
Se fumes[a]	Inhalation, topical	Worker in a Se refinery for 50 yrs	Red hair and finger nails; autopsy[b] showed numerous noncaseating granulomas in lung, high Se levels in lung, hair, and nails but not in other tissues.	(184)
Se fumes[a]	Inhalation	Worker in a Cu smelter	Cough, coryxza, bronchitis.	(176)
In electrode slimes	Topical	Worker in a Cu smelter[c]	Garlic breath, nervousness, pallor, gastrointestinal disturbances.	(185)
Se fumes[a]	Inhalation	Worker in a Se rectifier plant	Amnestic difficulties, headaches, sleeplessness, irritability, tachycardia, anorexia, substernal burning; inflammation of nasal mucosa.	(186)
Se fumes[a]	Inhalation	Female workers in Se rectifier plant	Irregular menses, menostasis.	(187)
Se fumes[a]	Inhalation	—	Rhinitis, nasal bleeding, headaches, weight loss, irritability, pain in extremities.	(161)
Se fumes[a]	Inhalation	Workers in Se rectifier plant	Irritability, sleeplessness, anorexia, nausea, headaches, conjunctivitis, slight tracheal bronchitis; a few workers showed impaired liver functions.	(186)
SeO$_2$	Inhalation	Se rectifier workers exposed 3-16 yrs	Pain in right hypochondrium, dyspepsia, fatigue, sleeplessness, toxic hepatitis, dyskinesis of gall bladder, cholecystitis, spastic colitis, chronic bronchitis or moderate emphysema, hyperthyroidism.	(163)
SeO$_2$	Inhalation	Workers in Se rectifier plant[d]	Dyspepsia, epigastric pain, lassitude, irritability, garlic breath.	(170)
H$_2$Se	Inhalation	Workers	Nausea, vomiting, metallic taste in the mouth, dizziness, extreme lassitude, fatigue.	(165)

[a]Fumes expected to be comprised of SeO$_2$ and elemental Se aerosols; a toxic species was likely to be H$_2$SeO$_3$ formed by the hydration of SeO$_2$ by tissue moisture.
[b]Subject died at age 76 of massive myocardial infarction not believed to be related to his exposure to Se.
[c]Urinary Se excretion was estimated to be 150 μg/24 hr; this value appears to be too low to be consistent with Se intoxication.
[d]Urinary Se concentration was 500-1000 ppb in this 3-yr study.

Table 11.10

Reports of Chronic Selenosis in Humans by Exposure via Food and Water[a]

Country	Major findings	Reference
USA	Residents of a seleniferous part of Colorado (with urinary Se excretion of ca. 158 μg/24 hr) had no significant health differences from residents of North Dakota (with urinary Se excretion of ca. 80 μg/24 hr).[b]	(188)
USA	A survey of 111 families of Nebraska, Wyoming, and South Dakota revealed urine Se concentrations of 200-1330 ppb, and 127 individuals reported "bad" teeth, icteroid skin, dermatitis, arthritis, gastrointestinal disturbances, pathological nails.	(189)
USA	A study of 50 families in South Dakota and Nebraska showed urine Se concentrations of 200-1980 ppb with complaints of gastrointestinal disturbances and hepatic distress.	(190)
USA	A family in Wyoming whose drinking water contained 9 ppm Se experienced hair loss, weakened nails, and listlessness; hair loss was also reported for the family dog.	(191)
USA	Five members of a family had urine Se concentrations of 200-600 ppb and showed lassitude, depression, and excessive fatigue. Symptoms responded to treatment with bromobenzene.	(193)
USA	Four members of a family in South Dakota had urine Se concentrations of 255-336 ppb (i.e., 246-383 μg Se excreted/24 hr) and an average blood Se concentration of 340 ppb with no associated health problems.	(192)
Mexico	It was implied that symptoms attributed to Hg poisoning may actually involve Se poisoning inasmuch as they occurred in a region with relatively high levels of Se in soil, vegetables, and milk.	(194)
Venezuela	School children in two high-Se parts of the country had average urine Se concentrations of 150 ppb (n = 1055), with the highest village averaging 630 ppb[c] with no apparent associated health problems.	(195)
Venezuela	Symptoms of nausea, dermatitis, loose hair, and pathological nails were slightly more common among 110 school children from a high-Se part of the country (this group showed urine Se = 636 μg/g creatinine and blood Se = 810 ppb)[d] than among 50 children from Caracas (urine Se = 224 μg/g creatinine, blood Se = 360 ppb).	(196)
Venezuela	No correlation was formed between the incidence of congenital malformations and Se intake.	(197)
Venezuela	Residents of a high-Se part of the country had blood Se = 420 ppb and hair Se = 1560 ppb, but few reports of dermatitis, pathological nails, or loose hair.	(198)
Columbia	It was suggested that high Se content of plant foods was associated with hair loss of many residents.	(199)
Columbia	Anecdotal report of elevated incidences of hair and nail losses and birth defects in a high-Se region.	(22)
China	A study of five villages in Enshi County, Hubei Province, with a total of 248 residents indicated that 49.2%[e] showed hair loss, pathological nails, hepatomegaly, and/or blistering and erythema of skin, with some paralysis and hemiplegia, and mottled teeth. One death was attributed to Se intoxication.	(200)

[a]Exposure to Se is presumed to have been through food and drinking water, although this was not quantified.

[b]The difference in Se excretion is compared to the difference in the Se contents of the respective water supplies (i.e., Colorado, 50-125 ppb; North Dakota, not detectable to 16 ppb).

[c]One individual had a urinary Se concentration of 3900 ppb.

[d]One subgroup had blood Se of 1320 ppb.

[e]In one village, this rate was 82.5%, i.e., all residents except three breast-fed infants and one 82-year-old man.

The best documented report of naturally occurring chronic selenosis in humans is that of Yang et al.[200] They described an endemic disease in a particular mountainous locale (Enshi County, Hubei Province) of China, which showed high prevalence in 1961-1964 and which was ultimately diagnosed as chronic selenosis. During the years of peak prevalence* among the 248 residents of the five most heavily affected villages, morbidity was ca. 50%, and one death was attributed to Se poisoning. Signs of selenosis were observed in almost all residents of one village; the only individuals free of signs were three nursing infants and an 82-year-old man. The most common signs were losses of hair and nails, but other signs and symptoms were also noted: skin lesions (e.g., affected skin became red and swollen, then blistered and eruptive with intense itching), hepatomegaly, polyneuritis (e.g., peripheral anesthesia, acroparesthesia, pain in the extremities, convulsions, partial paralysis, motor impairment, hemiplegia), and gastrointestinal disturbances. Almost one-third of 66 cases examined had mottled teeth; however, the area is also known to have endemic fluorosis,[201] so that this sign cannot be attributed to selenosis on the basis of this report.

The endemic selenosis in Enshi County appears to result from the exceedingly high concentrations of Se in that environment. Yang et al.[200] found very great concentrations of Se in the local soils (7.87 ppm), foods (e.g., corn: 6.33 ppm; rice: 1.48 ppm), and water (54 ppb); these levels are one to two orders of magnitude greater than those found in most areas of the world. Enshi County coal was found to contain more than 300 ppm Se (one sample was found to contain more than 84,000 ppm Se); the local use of this as fuel in the home and of its ash as an agent to amend agricultural soils is the probable ultimate source of the abundant Se in this area. Yang et al.[200] estimated the Se intakes of Enshi County residents†: six adults in six households from a village with a history of high prevalence of selenosis were estimated to have consumed 3200-6690 μg/person/day (average: 4990 μg/person/day), and adults in three households from a village with low prevalence of selenosis were estimated to have consumed 240-1510 μg/person/day (average: 750 μg/person/day).

---

*The "outbreak" of selenosis occurred during years of drought (1961-1964). In those years, water was not plentiful enough to grow the traditional staple grain of the area, rice. Instead, corn was grown. The latter, requiring a minimum of irrigation, apparently accumulated Se from the soil much better than rice, which is grown for part of its production period in an excess of water. It is likely that the irrigation water, when available, reduced the uptake of Se by the plant, thus affording the residents protection from selenosis.

†Yang et al.[200] were not able to estimate the Se intakes of affected villagers during the period of peak prevalence of selenosis (i.e., 1961-1964) but were able to make these estimates of Se intake some 10 years later. Because these estimates were made at a time of no reported human selenosis, it is possible that Se intakes at the time of the "outbreak" were even greater than these values.

Chronic selenosis has been reported in humans as the result of the use of various oral supplements which provided Se. These reports are summarized in Table 11.11.[202-207] The consumption of Na_2SeO_3 at rates as great as 1 mg Se/person/day for at least short periods of time appear to produce no toxic signs or symptoms.[202] However, clear signs of selenosis were reported by Yang et al.[200] in the case of a 62-year-old man after having taken 900 mg Se as Na_2SeO_3 daily for 2 years. That individual had garlic breath odor, and thickened and fragile nails; these signs subsided when he stopped taking the Se supplement. However, Westermarck[203] found no signs of Se toxicity among patients with neuronal ceroid lipofuscinosis to whom he had administered a higher level of Se (23 μg/kg b.w., equivalent to ca. 1600 μg/day for a 70-kg male). Thirteen cases of selenosis were identified among consumers of a commercial vitamin-trace element supplement, individual tablets of which were found to contain ca. 27 mg Se.[205] Although the form of Se in the preparation was not identified, 90% of the total was found to be water-soluble and may have been an inorganic salt (e.g., Na_2SeO_3 or Na_2SeO_4). The individual cases reported showed variable signs that correlated with the number of tablets of the supplement that they consumed.* The most commonly observed signs were changes in hair and nails. The individual that consumed the greatest amount of total Se in this group developed total alopecia, severe nausea and vomiting, severe diarrhea, and garlic breath odor, but had normal liver and kidney function. Some individuals had experienced irritability, fatigue, and paresthesias.

Ransome et al.[208] reported the case of selenosis in an adult female who had used an SeS_2-containing shampoo two to three times weekly for 8 months. Within 1 hr after using the shampoo for an eruptive scalp condition, she developed mild nonrhythmical tremors of the arms and hands; this progressed to generalized tremors of increasing severity. Within 2 hrs, she experienced a metallic taste of the mouth and had garlic breath odor. Two days later, she was weak and anorexic; the lethargy persisted for a couple of days, during which time she was nauseous and had porphyrinuria. She recovered gradually thereafter; recovery was complete in 2 weeks.

C. Other Disorders Linked to Selenium Excesses

Several reports have linked excessive intakes of Se with increased incidences of dental caries,[189,209-216] amyotrophic lateral sclerosis (ALS),[217] and birth defects.[22,188,218] Scrutiny of the available information on each of

---

*This ranged from 1 to 77 tablets and resulted in a range of individual Se intakes of 30-2000 mg.

Table 11.11

Reports of Chronic Selenosis in Humans by Exposure through Oral Supplementation

Form of Se	Situation	Major signs and symptoms	Reference
Na$_2$SeO$_3$	Voluntary consumption, five female subjects in New Zealand	No ill effects were noted as the result of consuming 1 mg Se/day for 5 days.	(202)
	Voluntary consumption, 20 subjects in New Zealand	No ill effects were noted as the result of consuming 0.5 mg Se/day for 20 days.	(202)
	Neuronal ceroid lipofuscinosis patients in Finland	23 μg Se/kg b.w. given for 1 yr produced no apparent signs of toxicity.	(203)
	Voluntary consumption, 62-yr-old male subject in China	Consumption of 900 μg Se/day for 2 yrs resulted in garlic breath, thickened, fragile nails, blood Se of 179 ppb, and hair Se of 828 ppb. Recovery of symptoms occurred after Se supplementation was stopped.	(200)
	Voluntary consumption, four subjects	2 mg Se/day for 20-40 days produced no apparent signs of toxicity.	(204)
Not identified[a]	Mistaken consumption, 13 adult subjects	Signs and symptoms were dose-related and included (in order of decreasing frequency) pathological nails, hair changes (e.g., dryness to total alopecia), severe fatigue, gastrointestinal disturbances (i.e., nausea, vomiting), severe watery diarrhea, macular rash, paresthesias, garlic breath. All biochemical tests of liver and renal function were normal.	(205)
Selenocystine	Four leukemic patients given ca. 50 mg Se/day for 10-57 days	Nausea, vomiting, diarrhea, alopecia, nail damage.	(206)
High-Se yeast	Voluntary consumption by two subjects for 18 months	One subject consumed 200 μg Se/day as Se yeast supplement (i.e., ca. 350 μg total Se/day) and second subject consumed 450 μg supplemental Se/day (i.e., ca. 600 μg total Se/day). Neither showed clear signs or symptoms of toxicity, but serum transaminases were borderline high.	(207)

[a]The predominant form was water-soluble, probably Na$_2$SeO$_3$, comprising ca. 89% of the total Se contained in the supplement (the balance is presumed to have been elemental and/or organic).

these proposed relationships indicates that the incidences of dental caries is frequently elevated in populations residing in seleniferous areas, but that no firm evidence supports associations of Se excesses and ALS or birth defects.

Smith et al.[189] first reported "bad teeth" as prevalent among rural populations in the seleniferous areas of South Dakota, Nebraska, and Wyoming. Others have made similar observations for populations living in the seleniferous areas of the American Northern Great Plains,[212,213] Oregon,[209,211,214] the Ukraine[215], and Enshi County, Hubei Province, China.[200] In these areas, high incidences of dental caries have been positively associated with the Se contents of food and drinking water,[214] of urine,[210,212] and of teeth themselves.[215] Tank and Starvick[213] were unable to detect any consistent relationships between the estimated Se intake and caries incidence or between urinary Se level and caries incidence among Wyoming residents. Cadell and Cousins[219] detected no association of urinary Se concentration and caries incidence among New Zealanders, but that population was of relatively low Se status and would not be expected to show effects related strictly to Se excesses. The reported association of dental caries and high Se intakes in humans is supported by controlled studies with experimental animals in which Se compounds have been found to be cariogenic if exposure occurs during the period of dental development (see Section I,E, this chapter). Thus, it appears that childhood exposure to high levels of Se may affect dental development such that caries susceptibility is increased.

Kilness and Hochberg[217] reported a cluster of four cases of ALS in rural males living in a seleniferous area of the American Northern Great Plains. They suggested that excessive intakes of Se may have been contributing factors to the rare disease. Schwarz[220] pointed out that the incidence of ALS was at least as great in geographic areas of lower Se status, and Kurland[221] suggested that the clustering observed by Kilness and Hochberg[217] was likely due to chance alone. The finding of Norris and Sang[222] that 19 of 20 known ALS patients were of subnormal Se status, as indicated by their urinary Se levels, suggested that high Se intake is not a factor in the etiology of this disease.

Benavides and Mojica[22] cited a Colombian tradition dating back at least four centuries that birth defects were associated with an endemic dermatological disease now thought to be due to selenosis. More recently, Robertson[218] reported that among 6 women who prepared microbiological media containing Na_2SeO_3, at least 4 of 6 certain pregnancies ended in spontaneous abortion. Tsongas and Ferguson[188] reported a positive association of Se intake in drinking water and history of miscarriage. These reports suggest a possible teratogenic risk of exposure to excessive amounts of Se. Although the available evidence from animal studies lends plausibility to this hypothesis, the available human data support only its plausibility and do not confirm the hypothesis itself. In a survey of high- and low-Se areas of Venezuela, Jaffe and Velez[197] detected no relationship between the incidence of infant mortality due to congenital malformations and apparent Se status as indicated by the urinary Se concentrations of school children in the same areas. Jaffe[216] concluded that the available evidence does not indicate that excessive levels of Se are teratogenic in humans.

IV. TREATMENT OF SELENIUM TOXICITY

No good therapy for Se toxicity has been identified; however, some acute signs can be treated, and a variety of treatments may promote the excretion of Se from the body after high level exposure. Glover[170] emphasized the need for oxygen therapy of patients with inhalatory Se intoxication; such treatment is important in preventing or minimizing the extent of development of pulmonary edema in those cases. Glover[223] also recommended the use of a reductant-containing bathing solution or ointment (e.g. 10% sodium thiosulphate) to prevent pain and necrosis in cases of burns due to topical exposure to SeO_2 or H_2SeO_3.

Treatment with p-bromobenzene has been shown to increase the urinary excretion of Se in cattle[224] and dogs,[225] although Westfall and Smith[226] did not find it to be effective in rabbits. Lemley reported it to be beneficial in the treatment of human selenosis[192,227,228]; however, its hepatotoxicity should preclude its use for humans. Administration of Ca- or Na_2-EDTA* has been shown to ameliorate acute Se toxicity in the rat if given within 15 minutes of Se exposure,[229] but the nephrotoxicity of this treatment would render it unsuitable for human cases. The reduced form of glutathione, GSH, has been shown to reduce the toxicity of Se in the rat,[230] apparently by increasing its biliary excretion.[231,232] Feeding the sulfhydryl reagent D-penicillamine (0.1% of diet) has been shown to offer partial protection against chronic selenosis in the rat; subcutaneous administration of the compound was ineffective against acute Se toxicity.[233]

However, another sulfhydryl reagent effective in the treatment of As toxicity, British Anti-Lewisite,† has been found to enhance the toxicity of Na_2SeO_3 in the rat[234,235]; dithiothreitol had similar effects.[233] Several dietary factors have been shown effective in altering the chronic toxicities of Se compounds in experimental animals. These are discussed in Section VI of this chapter.

*Ethylenediaminetetraacetic acid.
†2,3-Dimercapto-1-propanol.

V. METABOLIC BASES OF SELENIUM TOXICITY

The proximal biochemical lesion(s) of Se toxicity are not clear at the present time; however, it is thought that these involve the oxidation of and/or binding to critical sulfhydryl groups by Se species present in excessive concentrations. Dickson and Tappel[236] proposed that the signs of Se toxicity are related to changes in intracellular concentrations of reduced glutathione (GSH) and/or other nonprotein sulfhydryls. Studies by Anundi et al.[237] and LeBoeuf and Hoekstra[238] confirm that Se intoxication causes decreases in the intracelluar ratios of the reduced and oxidized (i.e., GSSG) forms of glutathione. Such perturbations of intracellular GSH:GSSG ratios would be expected to result in the loss of GSSG from the cell and a compensatory stimulation in GSH synthesis. Hence, LeBoeuf and Hoekstra[238] observed increases in hepatic GSH concentrations in rats fed diets containing 6 ppm Se (as Na_2SeO_3) for 6 weeks.

Csallany et al.[239] reported that mice maintained with a modest amount of Se (0.10 ppm) provided as Na_2SeO_3 in the drinking water developed increased hepatic concentrations of lipofuscin-type pigments by 9 months.* Although it is not at all clear that hepatic lipofuscinosis has any negative health implications, this finding has been taken as evidence of a negative metabolic effect of chronic supplementation with Na_2SeO_3. The accumulation of lipofuscin pigments would indicate lipid peroxidation having occurred as a result of the selenite treatment; this is consistent with the character of selenite as an oxidizing species (by virtue of its ready reduction to selenide). However, it is unlikely that healthy animals would absorb nutritional levels of selenite, such as those used by Csellany et al.,[239] without reducing it to the selenide state en route to the liver and other tissues. If the reduction were to occur in the gut, then it is likely that any peroxy and hydroperoxy lipids formed would have been reduced by peroxidases of the intestinal mucosa before reaching the liver. The observation by Csallany et al.,[239] therefore, suggests that, at least under some circumstances, relatively low levels of selenite may be absorbed and may react post-absorptively as pro-oxidants. If this report can be confirmed, the chronic use of Na_2SeO_3 as a feed or food supplement may require reevaluation; it may prove wiser to use other forms of Se (e.g., organic Se compounds, Na_2SeO_4) for such applications.

Reports of metabolic responses to high doses of Se are summarized in Table 11.12.[240-245] These include alterations in the metabolism of methionine in the mouse[241] and chromosomal changes in several in vitro systems.[244-246]

---

*The mice were fed a semi-purified diet that was said to have contained ca. 0.05 ppm Se, presumably from Torula yeast.

Table 11.12

Metabolic Responses to High Doses of Selenium

Species	Se treatment			Response	Reference
	Source	Route	Period		
				In vivo effects	
Rat	Na_2SeO_3	Gavage	20 hrs	Levels of 8-31 μg Se/g body weight did not affect O_2 consumption, but reduced glucose oxidation by liver and kidney minces *in vitro*.	(240)
	Na_2SeO_3	Gavage	30-96 days	Levels of 32-50 μg Se/g body weight did not affect O_2 consumption by liver or kidney minces *in vitro*; 82 μg Se/g b.w. increased O_2 consumption by 32-42% by liver minces *in vitro* with no effects on kidney minces.	(240)
	Na_2SeO_3	Diet	6 weeks	6 ppm Se caused increases in hepatic levels of GSH, GSSG, and in GSSG:GSH ratios.	(238)
Mouse	Na_2SeO_3	Diet	9 months	Se (ca. 0.05 ppm in diet plus 0.10 ppm in water) did not affect growth, but increased hepatic lipofuscin contents.	(239)
	Na_2SeO_3	i.p.[a]	Immediate	2 μg Se/g body weight caused rapid decreases in hepatic S-adenosyl methionine, increases in hepatic S-adenosyl homocysteine, and reductions (by 57%) in hepatic methionine adenosyltransferase activities.	(241)
Guinea pig	Na_2SeO_3	i.p.[a]	24 hrs	1 mg Se/kg body weight caused selective disruption of pig myocardial mitochondria with no ultrastructural changes observed in liver or kidney.	(242)
				In vitro effects	
Rat hepatocytes	Na_2SeO_3			Concentrations >4 ppm Se decreased intracellular GSH levels, increased GSSG levels, and produced lysis in freshly isolated hepatocytes.	(237)

Cell/Tissue	Se compound	Effect	Ref.
Mouse tracheae	Na_2SeO_3	Levels >40 ppm Se reduced ciliary activity, ATP contents, and protein synthesis.	(243)
Chinese hamster V79 cells	Na_2SeO_3	Treatment with Se induced sister chromatid exchanges.	(244)
	Na_2Se	Treatment with Se induced sister chromatid exchanges; this was enhanced by the presence of S9 (microsomal) fractions.	(244)
Human fibroblasts	Na_2SeO_3	Levels of 6-237 ppm Se induced DNA fragmentation, DNA-repair synthesis, chromosome abberations, and inhibition of mitosis. These effects were enhanced by incubation in the presence of mouse liver S9 fraction.	(245)
	Na_2SeO_3	8 ppm Se induced unscheduled DNA synthesis.	(246)
	Na_2SeO_4	Levels of 6-237 ppm Se induced small amounts of DNA repair synthesis; this effect was not altered by the presence of mouse liver S9 fraction.	(244)
	Na_2SeO_4	0.8-24 ppm Se induced unscheduled DNA synthesis	(245)
	Na_2Se	0.8-79 ppm Se induced unscheduled DNA synthesis.	(246)
	Se-cystine	0.8-79 ppm Se induced a low level of unscheduled DNA synthesis. Other organic Se compounds (Se-methionine, Se-cystamine) were without effect.	(246)

501

[a]Se administered by intraperitoneal injection.

VI. FACTORS AFFECTING SELENIUM TOXICITY

The toxicity of Se is affected by several factors related to diet, gender, and previous exposure to the element. These factors have been reviewed by Levander[233] and Kalouskova et al.[247] Among the diet-related factors that can affect Se toxicity are level and type of protein, and levels of heavy metals and trace elements, inorganic sulfur, methyl group donors, and antioxidants. Reports of these effects are summarized in Table 11.13.[261,262]

A. Dietary Factors

Gortner[248] first showed that Se toxicity in rats could be reduced by feeding high levels of protein. Subsequently, differences in the protective effects of major dietary proteins were observed[248-251]; protection from Se toxicity in experimental animals was oberved for casein,[248] lactalbumin,[248] linseed oil meal,[94,99,249-252] and *Torula* yeast.[102] The protective factor associated with linseed oil meal was found to be nonproteinaceous and extractable in hot ethanol.[251] It appears to reduce the toxicity of Se by facilitating the binding of the element in tissue in a less toxic form[232]; hence, animals fed diets containing linseed oil meal show increased tissue Se levels yet reduced toxic responses.[232,253] Reports by Palmer et al.[254] and Smith et al.[255] indicate that the active factor in linseed oil meal appears to be a cyanogenic glycoside; cyanide has been shown to ameliorate Se toxicity in the rat.[256] The protective factor in *Torula* yeast has not been characterized, but the studies of El-Begearmi and Combs[102] indicate that, unlike the linseed oil meal factor, it is retained in the ash fraction.

In 1938, Moxon[257] reported that the growth-depressing effects of feeding seleniferous grains to rats could be reduced by adding sodium arsenite to their drinking water. Since that time, several investigators have demonstrated protective effects of As against Se toxicity in several species.[92,107,117,118] The basis for this protective effect has been shown to reside in the ability of As to enhance the biliary elimination of Se.[258-260] However this may not be effective in the detoxification of certain Se metabolites, as Obermeyer et al.[70] has shown that As can potentiate the acute toxicity of trimethylselenonium ion. Selenium toxicity (i.e., that of SeO_2 or Na_2SeO_3) has also been reduced by feeding high levels of Ag,[262] Cu,[103,262] or Fe.[103] Hill[103] reported a significant protective effect of dietary Cd (57 ppm, as $CdSO_4$), but his results show that effect to be minimal.

Supplemental methionine has been shown to protect against Se toxicity when vitamin E is in adequate supply in the diet.[92,99,249,263-266] Levander and Morris[99] demonstrated that the interaction of methionine and vitamin E in facilitating protection from Se toxicity was related to their combined ability to reduce tissue (i.e., liver and kidney) levels of the element. They found that neither the sulfur-containing amino acid cystine nor the methyl

Table 11.13

Dietary Factors Affecting Selenium Toxicity in Experimental Animals

Factor	Species	Se treatment Form	Route	Observation	Reference
Protein sources Linseed oil meal	Rat	Na_2SeO_3	Diet	A dietary level of 43% linseed oil meal alleviated much of the depressed growth and liver damage due to 10 ppm Se.	(96)
	Rat	High-Se corn	Diet	Linseed oil meal or a water-soluble extract protected rats from the growth-depressing effect of up to 13 ppm Se.	(254)
	Rat	Na_2SeO_3	Diet	Linseed oil meal or a water-soluble extract protected rats from lethality and growth depression due to 10 ppm Se.	(254)
	Chick	$Na_2SeO_3{}^{a}$	Diet	20% Linseed oil meal reduced the growth depression and hepatic Se accumulation due to 10–40 ppm Se.	(101)
	Chick	Na_2SeO_3	Diet	A factor that protected against growth depression due to 20 ppm Se was extractable in ethanol, but was destroyed by ashing.	(252)
Torula yeast	Chick	Na_2SeO_3	Diet	Inclusion of Torula yeast in the diet reduced the mortality, growth depression, hepatic Se accumulation, and hepatic steatosis due to 50 ppm Se. The protective factor was present in the ash fraction of Torula yeast.	(102)
	Casein Rat	Na_2SeO_3	Diet	A dietary level of 30% casein alleviated much of the growth depression due to 35 ppm Se.	(248)
Lactalbumin	Rat	Na_2SeO_3	Diet	A dietary level of 24% lactalbumin alleviated part of growth depression due to 35 ppm Se.	(248)
Heavy metals As	Chicken (hen)	Na_2SeO_3	Diet	15 ppm As (as Na_2AsO_3) reduced the oppressions in growth, egg production, egg weight, and feed efficiency and prevented the drop in hatchability caused by 8 ppm Se.	(107)
	Pig	Na_2SeO_3	Diet	34.5 ppm As [as (4-aminophenyl)arsonic acid] reduced the depressions, due to 10 ppm Se, in numbers of live pigs farrowed and body weight at weaning but did not affect the Se-induced reduction in birth weight.	(118)
	Pig	Na_2SeO_3	Diet	34.5 ppm As [as (4-aminophenyl)arsonic acid] fed to weanling pigs overcame 45% of the growth depression and all of the reduction in feed efficiency; when fed to sows, that level restored one-third of the reduction in birth weight of progeny.	(117)

(continues)

Table 11.13 (*Continued*)

Factor	Species	Se treatment		Observation	Reference
		Form	Route		
	Chick	Na_2SeO_3	Diet	The addition of 0.04% (4-aminophenyl)arsonic acid did not affect the response to 0.3% betaine in reducing growth retardation due to 10 ppm Se.	(92)
Cd	Chick	SeO_2	Diet	The growth retardation due to 40 ppm Se was reduced by 57 ppm Cd (as $CdSO_4$), although this effect was weak.	(103)
Hg	Chick	SeO_2	Diet	The growth-depression effect of 40 ppm Se was eliminated by 500 ppm Hg (as $HgCl_2$); Hg did not affect survival.	(103)
	Chick	SeO_2	Diet	The growth retardation due to 20 ppm Se was eliminated by 25 ppm Hg as phenylmercuryacetate.	(103)
	Chick	Diphenyl Se	Diet	The mild growth retardation due to levels up to 20 ppm Se was not affected by 50 ppm Hg as either $HgCl_2$ or phenylmercuryacetate.	(103)
	Japanese quail	Na_2SeO_3	Diet	Addition of 5-15 ppm Hg (as CH_3Hg) overcame quail the reduced hatchability produced by 12 ppm Se.	(261)
Ag	Chick	Na_2SeO_3	Diet	1000 ppm Ag (as $AgNO_3$) reduced the growth depression and prevented the lethality of 5-40 ppm Se.	(263)
Trace elements Cu	Chick	SeO_2	Diet	500 ppm Cu (as $CuSO_4 \cdot 5H_2O$) reduced growth inhibition due to 40 ppm Se by ca. 20% and completely prevented its lethality.	(103)
	Chick	Na_2SeO_3	Diet	1000 ppm Cu (as $CuSO_4 \cdot 5H_2O$) reduced the growth depression and prevented the lethality of 5-40 ppm Se.	(262)
Fe	Chick	SeO_2	Diet	500 ppm Fe (as $FeSO_4 \cdot 7H_2O$) did not affect either the growth depression or lethality of 40 ppm Se.	(103)
Zn	Chick	SeO_2	Diet	500 ppm Zn (as $ZnSO_4$) did not affect the growth depression or lethality of 40 ppm Se.	(103)

	Compound	Species	Route	Description	Ref.
Inorganic sulfur compounds					
Sulfate	Na_2SO_4	Rat	Diet	0.29% Na_2SeO_4 reduced by 16% the growth depression due to 10 ppm Se; K_2SO_4 at 0.29–0.87% caused dose-dependent reduction in growth depression due to 10 ppm Se by as much as 39%.	(95)
	K_2SeO_4	Rat	Diet	Addition of 2% Na_2SO_4 reduced the growth depressing effects, mortality, and hepatic Se accumulation due to 10 ppm Se; 1.11% $Na_2S_2O_3$ also reduced Se-induced growth impairment.	(91)
	Na_2SeO_3	Rat	Diet	Neither Na_2SO_4 (2%) or $Na_2S_2O_3$ (1.11%) affected the growth depression or mortality due to 10 ppm se.	(91)
	Na_2SeO_3	Rat	Diet	Supplements of 0.29% Na_2SO_4 did not affect the growth depression due to 10 ppm Se.	(95)
	High-Se wheat	Rat	Diet	Levels of Na_2SO_4 up to 2% did not affect the growth depression or mortality due to 10 ppm Se.	(91)
Sulfite	K_2SO_4	Rat	Diet	1.78% Na_2SO_3 reduced slightly the growth impairment due to 10 ppm Se.	(91)
	Na_2SeO_3	Rat	Diet	1.78% Na_2SO_3 did not affect the growth depression or mortality due to 10 ppm Se.	(91)
Methyl group donors					
Methionine	Na_2SeO_3	Rat	Diet	1% DL-Methionine added to a low-methionine corn-casein-yeast basal diet reduced the growth-depressing effect of 10 ppm Se by more than half. Addition of at least 0.3% DL-methionine or L-methionine to a low-methionine soy protein-corn starch based diet reduced the growth retardation due to 10 ppm Se by ca. 15%.	(92)
	Na_2SeO_3	Chick	Diet	Supplements of as much as 1% DL-methionine to a corn-soy diet did not affect the growth retardation due to 10 ppm Se.	(92)
	Na_2SeO_3	Rat	Diet	A dietary supplement of 0.5% DL-methionine gave little protection against liver damage due to 10 ppm Se, unless the supplement was given with 0.01–0.05% vitamin E,[b] 0.05% DPPD,[c] 0.05% ethoxyquin,[d] or 0.05% BHT.[e]	(99)

(continues)

505

Table 11.13 (*Continued*)

| Factor | Species | Se treatment | | Observation | Reference |
		Form	Route		
	Rat	High-Se wheat	Diet	Dietary supplements to a low-methionine diet of 1 or 2% DL-methionine gave variable results in reducing growth retardation caused by 10 ppm Se.	(92)
Homocystine	Rat	Na_2SeO_3	Diet	Supplements of up to 1.62% homocystine did not affect the growth-depressing effect of 10 ppm Se.	(92)
Betaine	Rat	Na_2SeO_3	Diet	Supplements of up to 0.67% betaine reduced the growth-depressing effect of 10 ppm Se by up to 14%.	(92)
	Chick	Na_2SeO_3	Diet	0.3% Betaine reduced the growth-depressing effect of 10 ppm Se by 22%.	(92)
Choline	Rat	Na_2SeO_3	Diet	Supplements of as much as 0.8% choline chloride reduced the growth depression due to 10 ppm Se by up to 26%.	(92)
	Chick	Na_2SeO_3	Diet	0.3% Choline reduced the growth-depressing effect of 10 ppm Se by 30%.	(92)
Creatine	Rat	Na_2SeO_3	Diet	2% Creatine reduced the growth-depressing effect of 10 ppm by 13%.	(92)
N-Amidinoglycine[f]	Rat	Na_2SeO_3	Diet	Supplements of as much as 1% N-Amidinoglycine did not affect the growth retardation of 10 ppm Se.	(92)
	Chick	Na_2SeO_3	Diet	Supplements of 0.5% N-amidinoglycine reduced the growth retardation of 10 ppm Se when administered with 0.5% DL-methionine; this combination was not effective vs. 15 ppm Se.	(92)
Antioxidants Vitamin E[b]	Mouse	Na_2SeO_3	s.c.[g]	Five daily injections of 50 mg vitamin E[b]kg prevented abortion and maternal death due to 4.6 mg Se/kg, s.c., but did not affect Se-induced fetal growth retardation.	(133)

506

	Rat	Na_2SeO_3	Diet	A dietary supplement of 0.01-0.05% vitamin E[b] potentiated the protective effect of 0.5% DL-methionine against 10 ppm Se as indicated by growth and liver histology.	(99)
DPPD[c]	Rat	Na_2SeO_3	Diet	A dietary supplement of 0.05% DPPD[c] potentiated the protective effect of 0.5% DL-methionine against 10 ppm Se, as indicated by growth and liver histology.	(99)
Ethoxyquin[d]	Rat	Na_2SeO_3	Diet	A dietary supplement of 0.05% ethoxyquin[d] potentiated the protective effect of 0.5% DL-methionine against 10 ppm Se, as indicated by growth and liver histology.	(99)
BHT[e]	Rat	Na_2SeO_3	Diet	A dietary supplement of 0.05% BHT[e] potentiated the protective effect of 0.5% DL-methionine against 10 pm Se, as indicated by growth and liver histology.	(99)
Glutathione, reduced form[h]	Mouse	Na_2SeO_3	s.c.[g]	2-5 mmoles GSH/kg s.c. administered 20 min before s.c. injection of 4-6 mg Se/kg exacerbated Se-induced maternal death and abortion, but did not affect body weight of pups or number of live pups born.	(133)
Other Glucose	Rainbow trout	Na_2SeO_3	Diet	25% Glucose monohydrate added in replacement of 14% cellulose and 11% capelin oil increased the hepatic Se accumulation, mortality, and growth depression, and reduced hepatic Cu accumulation due to dietary levels of Se as great as 11-12 ppm.	(121)

[a] Authors did not state, in the original report, the form of Se used; it is presumed to have been Na_2SeO_3.
[b] All-*rac*-alpha-tocopheryl acetate.
[c] *N*-*N*-Diphenyl-*p*-phenylenediamine.
[d] 1,2-Dihydro-6-ethoxy-2,2,4-trimethylquinoline.
[e] Butylated hydroxytoluene, i.e., 2,6-bis(1,1-dimethylethyl)-4-methylphenol.
[f] Glycocyamine.
[g] Administered by subcutaneous injection.
[h] GSH.

group donor betaine could replace methionine in this protection; a methyl group acceptor, guanidoacetic acid, reduced the protective effect of methionine. Further, other structurally unrelated antioxidant compounds (e.g., ethoxyquin, BHT,* and DPPD†) also potentiated the protective effect of methionine. Levander and Morris[99] concluded that methionine reduced Se toxicity by providing labile methyl groups for the production of readily excreted methylated metabolites (e.g., dimethylselenide, trimethylselenonium ion) (see Chapter 5, Section II), and that vitamin E served as a lipid-soluble antioxidant in this process to increase in some manner the availability of the methionine-methyl group. Other studies have shown protection in varying degrees by inorganic sulfur compounds[91,95] other methyl group donors,[92] vitamin E,[133] and reduced glutathione.[133]

B. Sex-Related Effects

Studies with rats have shown males to be less sensitive than females to intoxication with selenite, but more sensitive to intoxication with dimethylselenide or trimethylselenonium ion.‡[247,267] In addition, males have been shown to be able to adapt to high Se intakes better than females: i.e., previous exposure to high levels of Se reduces the toxicity of selenite in males more so than in females. This effect is associated with a sex-related increase in the production of volatile Se metabolites (presumably dimethylselenide).[247] Kalouskova et al.[247] found that the retention of ^{75}Se in the whole body and various organs (particularly kidneys) of rats given radiolabeled dimethylselenide or trimethylselenonium ion was greater in males than in females. They found this sex-related difference to be evident by 35 days post partum; however, the sex-related difference in the acute toxicity of dimethylselenide did not appear until ca. 60 days.** Castration did not abolish these differences; treatment of females with androgens did not affect their sensitivities to the toxic effects of the methylated Se compounds.[269] Even though males produce more volatile Se metabolites, the biological half-lives of the methylated Se compounds are longer in males. These observations indicate that the sex-related difference in sensitivity to Se intoxication must involve differences at the level of the biochemical lesion(s) (i.e., target differences) in addition to differences in Se metabolism.

*Butylated hydroxytoluene.

†N,N'-Diphenyl-p-phenylenediamine.

‡This is in contrast with the greater sensitivity of males to nutritional Se deficiency.[268]

**At 35 days, dimethylselenide had LD_{50} values of 2.1 ml/kg b.w. in males and 1.9 ml/kg b.w. in females; after 90 days, it had LD_{50} values of 2.2 ml/kg b.w. in males and 0.5 ml/kg b.w. in females.

C. Differences Between Genetic Strains

Genetic factors affecting sensitivity to Se intoxication are indicated by the report of Stowe and Miller,[279] who were able to generate by selective breeding two strains of pigs that maintained different blood Se levels when fed the same diet. Their hyposelenemic strain maintained blood Se concentrations of ca. 75 ppb, whereas their hyperselenemic strain maintained blood Se at ca. 109 ppb; these levels were maintained whether each strain was fed 0.1 or 0.3 ppm dietary Se. LaVorgna and Combs[280,281] developed two genetic strains of chickens with different sensitivities to Se-deficiency. The sensitivities of each of these genetic models to selenosis has not been evaluated but may prove of interest relative to the possibility of the adaptation by species to local conditions of Se exposure.

D. Adaptation to Selenium Excesses

Some evidence suggests that animals are able to adapt to high-level exposures to Se. Ermakov and Koval'skij[270] demonstrated that the incremental increases in Se contents of most organs (except liver) that occurred as the result of feeding 2 mg Se (as Na_2SeO_3) daily to sheep were less in animals from seleniferous regions than from animals from regions of lower Se status. Sheep from the lower Se area showed much greater increases in the activities of alkaline phosphatase and acid phosphatase in serum in response to the Se treatment than did sheep from the seleniferous area; this indicated that those animals previously exposed to a higher level of Se were less susceptible to selenosis. Jaffe and Mondragon[271] presented evidence that rats exposed chronically to Se reduce their tissue storage of the element. They found that feeding young rats a diet containing 4.5 ppm Se (as seleniferous sesame meal) resulted in progressive decreases in hepatic Se concentrations among progeny of dams fed the same seleniferous diet; the progeny of dams fed a nonseleniferous diet showed progressive increases in hepatic Se levels when fed the seleniferous diet. Jaffe and Mondragon[94] confirmed these findings and found that this kind of adaptation conferred protection of rats from Se toxicity. Wahlstrom and Olson[117] made similar observations in pigs: 4.5 ppm Se (as Na_2SeO_3) in the diets of weanling pigs caused a greater reduction in growth rate and a greater incidence of toxic signs in animals that had no access to high-Se diets previous to weaning than in the progeny of sows that received Se during growth, gestation, and lactation. Adaptation to high-Se environments has been observed in microorganisms[272-274] by developing the ability to reduce Se. Animals may adapt to high Se exposures by increasing their metabolic production of methylated Se compounds (i.e., dimethylselenide and trimethylselenonium ion), which are readily excreted (across the lung and kidney, respectively), thus decreasing the whole body retention of the element.[275-277] Exposure to high levels of Se can also reduce the toxicity of the methylated selenides, although the mechanism of this effect is not clear.[269,278]

VII. SAFE LEVELS OF SELENIUM

Because the toxicities of Se compounds vary according to their identity, route, and duration of administration with various species, guidelines for safe levels must include considerations of these variables, something that current information does not permit with great confidence. Exposure of animals and humans to Se, in most circumstances, occurs primarily by way of the diet. Thus, while it is possible to set safe levels for several Se compounds based on their acute peroral or parenteral LD_{50} values (these can be estimated from the data summarized in Tables 11.1 and 11.4), most questions concerning the safety of Se are presented in the context of dietary levels in animal feeds or daily intakes of humans. Therefore, these considerations pertain chiefly to those Se compounds that occur naturally in feedstuffs and foods (e.g., seleniferous grains, meats), as well as to those that may be candidates for use as nutritional and/or medical supplements (e.g., Na_2SeO_3, Na_2SeO_4, selenomethionine, selenocystine, Se-enriched yeasts). In this context, it should be kept in mind that Se is an essential nutrient; thus, guidelines for protection against the possibility of Se intoxication must accommodate levels of intake that satisfy the needs of sound nutrition and good health.

Depressions in the rates of growth of young animals have been shown to be the most sensitive parameters of Se intoxication. Animals do not show depressed growth at dietary levels of less than 2 ppm Se when it is provided in the common feeding forms mentioned above. Animals of some species and stages of development may not be adversely affected by dietary levels as great as 5-10 ppm Se. In consideration of the fact that the dietary requirements of most species for Se are in the range of 0.05-0.20 ppm,* the ratio of safety between potentially toxic and nutritionally required levels of Se is 10-20.

Although present knowledge of the toxicology of Se in humans is very incomplete, available evidence indicates that dermatological (including pathological changes in hair and nails) and gastrointestinal (including

---

*In general, animals fed diets containing adequate levels of all other known nutrients (particularly vitamin E and cystine) show no needs for Se at levels above those found in most practical and semi-purified diets (i.e., 0.05 ppm) for protection from deficiency syndromes and impaired production (i.e., growth, efficiency of feed utilization, reproductive success, etc.). Dietary levels of 0.10-0.20 ppm Se are usually needed for the maintenance of optimal activities of SeGSHpx in the tissues.

nausea) signs may be the earliest indicators of Se intoxication. The lowest Se dosage that has been documented to be associated with the manifestation of these signs is 1000 μg Se (as Na_2SeO_3) per day.* This level was achieved by the daily use of an oral supplement of 900 μg Se (as 2 mg Na_2SeO_3) and a daily intake of ca. 100 μg Se from other dietary sources. This level may, in fact, be very near a threshold dose for toxic responses; signs of toxicity that occurred as the result of that dose level were mild and did not become manifest for nearly 2 years.[200] In addition, others have found chronic oral intakes of much higher levels of Se to be without toxicity.[203] The present authors suggest that a level of 550 μg Se per day† may be a realistic upper limit of safety for chronic oral consumption of Se predominantly from inorganic Se salts. The upper safe limit of Se intake from seleniferous foods and/or certain organic Se compounds can be expected to be greater than this level, inasmuch as the forms of Se in foods and the selenoamino acids (presumed to resemble those naturally occurring Se species) are apparently less toxic than the inorganic Se salts when given orally. Therefore, the present authors suggest an upper safe limit of 775 μg Se per person per day‡ for chronic oral consumption of Se from seleniferous foods and/or organic Se compounds.

The present recommended upper safe limits of Se intake are intended to be conservative. Levels of Se as great as ca. 1000 μg per person per day probably offer no risk if consumption is limited to days (for the inorganic

---

*Chen[282] reported that one case of selenosis was identified in an Enshi county village that had no history of the condition and for which the typical per capita Se intake was estimated to be ca. 750 +g Se per day. In consideration of the error associated with this estimate (it was based on the variable apparent intakes of three families that consumed 240-1510 +g/person/day), it must be inferred that the actual Se intake of the individual showing signs of selenosis was probably much greater than 750 +g per day. This conclusion is supported by the observation of Yang et al.[200] of average daily Se intakes of almost 5 mg per person for healthy residents of a village with a history of selenosis. If the latter individuals could consume such a high level of Se without ill effects, then it is likely that the actual Se intake of the single selenosis case from the former village was substantially greater than the estimated intake level of Se given for that village. Therefore, the present authors do not consider the report of Yang et al.[200] to indicate a significant risk for individuals of an actual intake of 750 +g per day.

†This figure was derived from the lowest chronically toxic Se intake reported by Yang et al.[200] The Se estimated to have been consumed from the subject's normal diet (i.e., 100 +g Se per day) was added to that consumed in the form of daily Na_2SeO_3 supplements after the latter figure was corrected by a 50% safety factor.

‡This figure was derived from the lowest chronically toxic level of Se intake as reported by Yang et al.[200] The Se estimated to have been consumed from the subject's normal diet (i.e., 100 +g Se per day) was added to that consumed in the form of daily Na_2SeO_3 supplements, except in this case the latter figure was corrected by a 75% safety factor, i.e., assuming that organic Se compounds are generally two-thirds as toxic as the inorganic Se salts.

Se salts) or weeks (for seleniferous foods or organic Se compounds); nevertheless, such a level cannot be recommended for general use on the basis of present information. These recommendations are somewhat higher than those of Sakurai and Tsuchiya[283] (500 μg/person/day) and Olson[159] (350 μg/person/day), and fall well above the upper limit of the range called "safe and adequate" by the Food and Nutrition Board, National Research Council[284] (200 μg/person/day). These latter estimates, however, did not consider the differential toxicity of the inorganic Se salts and the organic forms of Se including those in foods. The present authors believe that a realistic consideration of present knowledge of the toxicology of Se supports the present recommended guidelines.

Under normal circumstances outside of certain kinds of industrial sites (e.g., Cu smelters, Se-rectifier plants), the Se content of the air averages less than 10 ng Se/m[311] and represents a negligible source of the total Se exposure of humans or animals.[285] Although water very seldom contains more than 10 μg Se/l, a few cases of greater Se concentrations have been reported, which may constitute significant sources of Se to humans and animals using those water supplies. One such recent case was that of the waters of the Kesterson National Wildlife Refuge, Fresno and Merced Counties, California, which receive agricultural drainage waters from the San Luis Drain. Water samples were found to contain 140-1400 ppb Se.[286] Were such waters to be consumed by humans (assuming a daily per capita intake of 2 l), the daily Se intake from that source alone would be 280-2800 μg. In order to maintain daily human Se intakes not greater than the upper safe limit recommended above, water Se concentrations less than ca. 175 ppb should represent no risk for individuals consuming ca. 200 μg Se per day from their normal diets. In situations where individuals consume only ca. 100 μg dietary Se daily, water Se levels as great as 225 ppb should pose no risk.* These levels are substantially greater than the drinking water standard currently set by the U. S. Environmental Protection Agency, i.e., 10 ppb Se.[287] However, that standard was set with the assumption that water should contribute no more than 10% of the daily Se intake of a normal American. That logic is certainly questionable in view of the growing appreciation of the role of Se in nutrition and health. There may be situations of limited food Se intake (e.g., vegetarian diets in low-Se areas) wherein water-borne Se, should it exist, would constitute an important nutritional resource and, as such, would be valuable in contributing more than 10% of the total ingested Se. Lafond and Calabrese[288] have also challenged the current Se drinking water standard.

---

*These projections were made by allowing water-borne Se to contribute no more than the difference between each level of dietary Se consumed and the upper safe limit for chronic consumption of predominantly inorganic forms of Se.

REFERENCES

1. Painter, E. P., The chemistry and toxicity of selenium compounds, with special reference to the selenium problem, Chem. Rev., 28, 179, 1941.
2. Moxon, A. L., and Rhian, M. A., Selenium poisoning, Physiol. Rev., 23, 305, 1943.
3. Amor, A. J., and Pringle, P., A review of selenium as an industrial hazard, Bull. Hygiene, 20, 239, 1945.
4. Cerwenka, E. A., Jr. and Cooper, W. C., Toxicology of selenium and tellurium and their compounds, Arch. Environ. Health, 3, 189, 1961.
5. Rosenfeld, I., and Beath, O. A., *Selenium: Geobotany, Biochemistry, Toxicity and Nutrition*, Academic Press, New York, 1964.
6. Muth, O. H., and Binns, W., Selenium toxicity in domestic animals, Ann. New York Acad. Sci., 111, 583, 1964.
7. Maag, D. D., and Glenn, M. W., Toxicity of selenium: farm animals, in *Symposium: Selenium in Biomedicine*, Muth, O. H., Oldfield, J. E., and Weswig, P. H., eds., Avi Publ. Co., Westport, Conn., 1967, 127.
8. Cooper, W. C., Selenium toxicity in man, in *Symposium: Selenium in Biomedicine*, Muth. O. H., Oldfield, J. E., and Weswig, P. H., Eds., Avi Publ. Co., Westport, Conn., 1967, 185.
9. Harr, J. R. and Muth, O. H., Selenium poisoning in domestic animals and its relationship to man, Clin. Toxicol., 5, 175, 1972.
10. Shapiro, J. R., Selenium compounds in nature and medicine. C. Selenium and human biology, in *Organic Selenium Compounds: Their Chemistry and Biology*, Klagman, D. L., and Gunther, W. H. H., eds., Wiley, New York, 1973, 693.
11. Committee on Medical and Biological Effects of Environmental Pollutants, National Academy of Sciences, *Selenium*, National Academy of Sciences, Washington, D.C., 1976.
12. Burk, R. F., Selenium in man, in *Trace Elements in Human Health and Disease*, Vol. II, Prasad, A. S., and Oberleas, D., eds., Academic Press, New York, 1976, 105.
13. Prasad, A. S., Selenium, in *Trace Elements and Iron in Human Metabolism*, Plenum Medical, New York, 1978, 215.
14. Doyle, J. J., and Spaulding, J. E., Toxic and essential trace elements in meat — a review, J. Anim. Sci. 47, 398, 1978.
15. Task Force on Metal Interaction, Factors influencing metabolism and toxicity of metals: a concensus report, Environ. Health Perspect., 25, 3, 1978.
16. Subcommittee on Mineral Toxicity in Animals, Committee on Animal Nutriton, National Research Council, *Mineral Tolerance of Domestic Animals*, National Academy of Sciences, Washington, D.C., 1980.
17. Lo, M. T., and Sandi, E., Selenium: occurrence in food and its toxicological significance — a review, J. Environ. Pathol. Toxicol., 4, 193, 1980.
18. Subcommittee on Selenium, Committee in Animal Nutrition, National Research Council, *Selenium in Nutrition, Revised Edition*, National Academy Press, Washington, D. C., 1983.
19. Buell, D. N., Potential hazards of selenium as a chemopreventative agent, Seminars Oncol., X, 311, 1983.
20. Shamberger, R. J., *Biochemistry of Selenium*, Plenum, New York, 1983.
21. Polo, M., *The Travels of Marco Polo*, translated by Latham, R., Penguin Books, New York, 1958.

22. Benavides, J. T., and Mojica, R. F. S., Selenosis: occurrencia de selenio en rocas, svelos y plantas. Intoxicacion por selenio en animales y en humanos, Publicacion IT-3, Instituto Geografico de Columbia, Bogota, Columbia, 1959.

23. Madison, T. C., Sanitory report — For Randall, in Coolidge, R. H., *Statistical Report on Sickness and Mortality in the Army of the United States. Jan. 1855 to Jan. 1860*, Washington, D.C., G. W. Bowman, 1860 (US) Cong. 36th, 1st Session, Senate Ex. Doc. 52, 37, 1860.

24. Mayo, N. S., Enzootic cerebritis, or "staggers," of horses, Kansas Agr. Exp. Stat. Bull., 24, 107, 1891.

25. Peters A. T. A fungus disease of corn Nebr. Agr. Exp. Sta., 17th Ann. Rep., 13, 1904.

26. Hutton, J. G., The correlation of certain lesions in animals with certain soil types, J. Am. Soc. Agron., 23, 1076, 1931.

27. Franke, K. W., A new toxicant occurring naturally in certain samples of plant foodstuffs. I. Results obtained in preliminary feeding trials, J. Nutr., 8, 597, 1934.

28. Franke, K. W., A new toxicant occurring naturally in certain samples of plant foodstuffs. II. The occurrence of the toxicant in the protein fraction, J. Nutr., 8, 609, 1934.

29. Franke, K. W., and Potter, V. R., A new toxicant occurring naturally in certain samples of plant foodstuffs. III. Hemoglobin levels observed in rats which were fed toxic wheat, J. Nutr., 8, 615, 1934.

30. Franke, K. W., A new toxicant occurring naturally in certain samples of plant foodstuffs. X. The effect of feeding toxic foodstuffs in varying amounts and for different time periods, J. Nutr., 10, 223, 1935.

31. Franke, K. W., A new toxicant occurring naturally in certain samples of plant foodstuffs. XI. The effect of feeding toxic and control foodstuffs alternately, J. Nutr., 10, 233, 1935.

32. Tully, W. C., and Franke, K. W., A new toxicant occurring naturally in certain samples of plant foodstuffs. VI. A study of the effect of affected grains on growing chicks, Poultry Sci., 14, 280, 1935.

33. Robinson, W. O., Determination of selenium in wheat and soils, J. Assoc. Offic. Anal. Chem., 16, 423, 1933.

34. Franke, K. W., and Painter, E. P., Selenium in proteins from toxic foodstuffs. 1. Remarks in the occurrence and nature of the selenium present in a number of foodstuffs or their derived products, Cereal Chem., 13, 67, 1936.

35. Beath, O. A., Eppson, H. F., and Gilbert, C. S., Annual Report, Wyoming Agr. Exp. Sta. Bull., 206, 1935.

36. Byers, H. G., Selenium, vanadium, chromium and arsenic in one soil, Ind. Eng. Chem., News Ed., 12, 122, 1934.

37. Franke, K. W., and Potter, W. R., A new toxicant occurring naturally in certain samples of plant foodstuffs. IX. Toxic effects of orally ingested selenium, J. Nutr., 10, 213, 1935.

38. Franke, K. W., Moxon, A. L., Poley, W. E., and Tully, W. C., Monstrosities produced by the injection of selenium salts into hen's eggs, Anat. Rec., 65, 15, 1936.

39. Franke, K. W., and Tully, W. C., A new toxicant occurring naturally in certain samples of plant foodstuffs. V. Low hatchability due to deformities in chicks, Poultry Sci., 14, 273, 1935.

40. Franke, K. W., and Tully, W. C., A new toxicant occurring naturally in certain samples of plant foodstuffs. VII. Low hatchability due to deformities in chicks produced from eggs obtained from chickens of known history, Poultry Sci., 15, 316, 1936.

41. Franke, K. W., and Painter, E. P., Selenium in proteins from toxic foodstuffs. IV. The effect of feeding toxic proteins, toxic protein hydrolysates and toxic protein hydrolysates from which the selenium has been removed, J. Nutr., 10, 599, 1935.

42. Van Kampen, K. R., and James, L. F., Manifestations of intoxication by selenium-accumulating plants, in *Effects of Poisonous Plants on Livestock*, Keeler, R. F., Van Kampen, K. R., and James, L. E., eds., Academic Press, New York, 1978, 135.

43. Smith, M. I., Stohlman, E. F., and Lillie, R. D., The toxicity and pathology of selenium, J. Pharmacol. Exp. Therap., 60, 449, 1937.

44. Palmer, I. S., Arnold, R. L., and Carlson, C. W., Toxicity of various selenium derivatives to chick embryos, Poultry Sci., 52, 1841, 1973.

45. Halverson, A. W., Jerde, L. G., and Hills, C. L., Toxicity of sodium selenite to chick embryos, Toxicol. Appl. Pharmacol., 7, 675, 1965.

46. Ammar, E. M. and Couri, D., Acute toxicity of sodium selenite and selenomethionine in mice after ICV or IV administration, Neurotoxicol., 2, 383, 1981.

47. MacDonald, D. W., Christian, R. G., Strauz, K. I., and Raff, J., Acute Selenium toxicity in neonatal calves, Can. Vet. J., 22,279, 1981.

48. Anderson, H. D., and Moxon, A. L., The excretion of selenium by rats on a seleniferous wheat ration, J. Pharmacol. Exp. Therap., 76, 343, 1942.

49. Pletnikova, I. P., Biological effect and safe concentration of selenium in drinking water, Hygiene Sanit., 35, 16, 1970.

50. Stowe, H. D., Effects of copper pretreatment upon the toxicity of selenium in ponies, Am. J. Vet. Res., 41, 1925, 1980.

51. Jacobs, M., and Forst, C., Toxicological effects of sodium selenite in Swiss mice, J. Toxicol. Environ. Hlth, 8, 587, 1981.

52. Yonemoto, J., Hongo, T., Suzuki, T., Naganuma, A., and Imura, N., Toxic effects of selenodiglutathione on pregnant mice, Toxicol. Lett., 21, 35, 1984.

53. Taylor, T. J., Reiders, F., and Kocsis, J. J., Toxicological interactions of mercury and selenium, Toxicol. Appl. Pharmacol., 45, 347 (abstract), 1978.

54. Van Vleet, J. F., Meyer, K. B., and Olander, H. J., Control of selenium-vitamin E deficiency in growing swine by parenteral administration of selenium-vitamin E preparations to baby pigs or to pregnant sows and their baby pigs, J. Am. Vet. Med. Assoc., 165, 543, 1974.

55. Smith, M. I. and Westfall, B. B., Further field studies on the selenium problem in relation to public health, U. S. Public Health Rep., 52, 1375, 1937.

56. Muehlberger, C. W., and Schrenck, H. H., The effect of the state of oxidation on the toxicity of certain elements, J. Pharmacol., 33, 270, 1928.

57. Levine V. E., and Flaherty R. A. Hypoglycemia induced by sodium selenite, Proc. Soc. Expt. Biol. Med., 24, 251, 1926.

58. Cummins, L. M., and Kimura, E. T., Safety evaluation of selenium sulfide antidandruff shampoos, Toxicol. Appl. Pharmacol., 20, 89, 1971.

59. Ostadalova, I., Babicky, A., and Obenberger, J., Cataract induced by administration of a single dose of sodium selenite to suckling rats, Experientia, 34, 222, 1978.

60. Blodgett, D. J., Acute selenium toxicosis in sheep, Ph. D. Thesis, University of Illinois, Urbana-Champaign, 132 pp., 1983.

61. Caravaggi, C., Clark, F. L., and Jackson, A. R. B., Acute selenium toxicity in lambs following intramuscular injection of sodium selenite, Res. Vet. Sci., 11, 146, 1970.

62. Dudley, H. C., Toxicology of selenium. V. Toxic and vesicant properties of selenium oxychloride, US Public Health Rep., 53, 94, 1938.

63. Franke, K. W., and Moxon, A. L., A comparison of the minimum fatal doses of selenium, tellurium, arsenic and vanadium, J. Pharmacol. Exp. Ther., 58, 454, 1936.

64. Wilbur, C. G., Toxicology of selenium: a review, Clin. Toxicol., 17, 171, 1980.

65. Hall, R. H., Laskin, S., Frank, P., Maynard, E. A., and Hodge, H. C., Preliminary observations on toxicity of elemental selenium, Arch. Indus. Hygiene Occupat. Med., 4, 458, 1951.

66. Dudley, H. C., and Miller, J. W., Toxicology of selenium. VI. Effect of subacute exposure to hydrogen selenide, J. Indus. Hyg. Toxicol., 23, 470, 1941.
67. Dudley, H. C., and Miller J. W., Toxicology of selenium. IV. Effects of exposure to hydrogen selenide, US Public Health Rep., 52, 1217, 1937.
68. Henschler, D., and Kirshner, U., Zur Resorption und Toxizitat von Selensulfid, Arch. Toxikol., 24, 341, 1961.
69. McConnell, K. P., and Portman, O. W., Toxicity of dimethyl selenide in the rat and mouse, Proc. Soc. Exp. Biol. Med., 79, 230, 1952.
70. Obermeyer, B. D., Palmer, I. S., Olson, O. E., and Halverson, A. W., Toxicity of trimethylselenonium chloride in the rat with and without arsenite, Toxicol. Appl. Pharmacol., 20, 135, 1971.
71. Klug, H. L., Peterson, D. F., and Moxon, A. L., The toxicity of selenium analogues of cystine and methionine, Proc. S. Dak. Acad. Sci., 28, 117, 1949.
72. Moxon, A. L., Toxicity of selenium-cystine and some other organic selenium compounds, J. Am. Pharmacol. Assoc., 29, 249, 1940.
73. Kostyniak, P. J., Preliminary toxicity studies on bis-(beta-(N,N- dimorpholino)ethyl) selenide (MOSE), a new radioimaging agent, Drug Chem. Toxicol., 7, 41, 1984.
74. Moxon, A. L., Anderson, H. D., and Painter, E. P., The toxicity of some organic selenium compounds, J. Pharmacol. Expt. Therap., 63, 357, 1938.
75. Miller, W. T., and Williams, K. T. Minimum lethal doses of selenium, as sodium selenite, for horses, mules, cattle and swine, J. Agric. Res., 60, 163, 1940.
76. Shortridge, E. H., O'Hara, P. J., and Marshall, P. M., Acute selenium poisoning in cattle, N. Z. Vet. J., 19, 47, 1971.
77. Orstadius, K., Toxicity of a single subcutaneous dose of sodium selenite in pigs, Nature, 188, 117, 1960.
78. Herigstad, R. R., Whitehair, C. K., and Olson, O. E., Inorganic and organic selenium toxicosis in young swine: comparison of pathologic changes with those in swine with vitamin E-selenium deficiency, Am. J. Vet. Res., 34, 1337, 1973.
79. Gabbedy, B. J., and Dickson, J., Acute selenium poisoning in lambs, Aust. Vet. J., 45, 470, 1969.
80. Morrow, D. A., Acute selenite toxicosis in lambs, J. Am. Vet. Med. Assoc., 152, 1625, 1968.
81. Lamborne, D. A., and Mason, R. W., Mortality in lambs following overdosing with sodium selenite, Aust. Vet. J., 45, 208, 1969.
82. Caravaggi, C., and Clark, F. L., Mortality in lambs following intramuscular injection of sodium selenite, Aust. Vet. J., 45, 383, 1969.
83. Soffietti, M. G., Nebbia, C., Valenza, F., Cagnasso, A., and Guglielmino, R., Studio comparativo sulla tossicita del selenito di sodio e del selenito di colina nelle pecore, Arch. Vet. Ital., 34, 65, 1983.
84. Neethling, L. P., Brown, J. M. M., and DeWet, P. J., The toxicology and metabolic fate of selenium in sheep, J S. Afr. Vet. Med. Assoc., 39, 25, 1968.
85. Rhian, M., and Moxon, A. L., Chronic selenium poisoning in dogs an its prevention by arsenic, J. Pharmacol. Exp. Therap., 78, 249, 1943.
86. Hadjimarkos, D. M., Toxic effects of dietary selenium in hamsters, Nutr. Rep. Int., 1, 175, 1970.
87. Loew, F. M., Olfert, E. D., and Schiefer, B., Chronic selenium toxicosis in cynomolgus monkeys, Lab. Primate Newsl., 14, 7, 1975.
88. Nobunaga, T., Satoh, H., and Suzuki, T., Effects of sodium selenite on methylmercury embryotoxicity and teratogenicity in mice, Toxicol. Appl. Pharmacol., 47, 79, 1979.
89. Palmer, I. S., Herr, A., and Nelson, T., Toxicity of selenium in Brazil nuts to rats, J. Food Sci., 47, 1595, 1982.

90. Moxon, A. L., Alkali disease or selenium poisoning, S. Dakota Agric. Exp. Stn. Bull. No. 311, S. Dakota State College of Ag. and Mechanic Arts, Brookings, 91 pp., 1937.

91. Halverson, A. W., Guss, P. L., and Olson, O. E., Effect of sulfur salts on selenium poisoning in the rat, J. Nutr., 77, 459, 1962.

92. Olson, O. E., Carlson, C. W., and Leitis, E., Methionine and related compounds and selenium poisoning, Tech. Bull. 20, S. Dakota State College of Ag. and Mechanic Arts, Brookings, 15 pp., 1958.

93. Goebring, T. B., Palmer, I. S., Olson, O. E., Libal, G. W., and Wahlstrom, R. C., Effects of seleniferous grains and inorganic selenium on tissue and blood composition and growth performance of rats and swine, J. Anim. Sci., 59, 725, 1984.

94. Jaffe, W. G., and Mondragon, C., Effects of ingestion of organic selenium in adapted and non-adapted rats, Br. J. Nutr., 33, 387, 1975.

95. Halverson, A. W., and Monty, K. J., An effect of dietary sulfate on selenium poisoning in the rat, J. Nutr., 70, 100, 1960.

96. Levander, O. A., Young, M. L., and Meeks, S. A., Studies on the binding of selenium by liver homogenates from rats fed diets containing either casein or casein plus linseed oil meal, Toxicol. Appl. Pharmacol., 16, 79, 1970.

97. Palmer, I. S., and Olson, O. E., Relative toxicities of selenite and selenate in the drinking water of rats, J. Nutr., 104, 306, 1974.

98. Jacobs, M., and Forst, C., Toxicological effects of sodium selenite in Sprague-Dawley rats, J. Toxicol. Environ. Hlth., 8, 575, 1981.

99. Levander, O. A., and Morris, V. C., Interactions of methionine, vitamin E and antioxidants in selenium toxicity in the rat, J. Nutr., 100, 1111, 1970.

100. Cantor, A. H., Nash, D. M., and Johnson, T. H., Toxicity of selenium in drinking water of poultry, Nutr. Rep. Int., 29, 683, 1984.

101. Jensen, L. S., Werho, D. B., and Leyden, D. E., Selenosis, hepatic selenium accumulation, and plasma glutathione peroxidase activity in chicks as affected by a factor in linseed meal, J. Nutr., 107, 391, 1977.

102. El-Begearmi, M. M., and Combs, G. F., Jr., Dietary effects on selenite toxicity in the chick, Poultry Sci., 61, 770, 1982.

103. Hill, C. H., Reversal of selenium toxicity in chicks by mercury, copper and cadmium, J. Nutr., 104, 593, 1974.

104. Hill, C. H., Interrelationships of selenium with other trace elements, Federation Proc., 34, 2096, 1975.

105. Ort, J. F., and Latshaw, J. D., The toxic level of sodium selenite in the diet of laying chickens, J. Nutr., 108, 11 14, 1978.

106. Gruenwald, P., Malformations caused by necrosis in the embryo. Illustrated by the effect of selenium compounds on chick embryos, Am. J. Pathol., 34, 77, 1958.

107. Thapar, N. T., Grenthner, E., Carlson, C. W., and Olson, O. E., Dietary selenium and arsenic addition to diets for chickens over half a cycle, Poultry Sci., 48, 1988, 1969.

108. Soffieti, M. G., Nebbia, C., and Valenza, F., Tossicita cronica sperimentale del selenato di custina nel polio. Rilievi clinici ed anatomo-istopatolgici. Nutr. Clin. Vet., 106, 97, 1983.

109. Miller, W. T., and Williams, K. T., Minimum lethal doses of selenium, as sodium selenite, for horses, mules, cattle and swine, J. Agr. Res., 60, 163, 1940.

110. Schoening, H. W., Production of so-called alkali disease in hogs by feeding corn grown in affected area, N. Am. Vet., 17, 22, 1936.

111. Wahlstrom, R. C., Kamstra, L. D., and Olson, O. E., Preventing selenium poisoning in growing and fattening pigs, S. Dak. Agric. Exp. Stn. Bull. No. 456, S. Dakota State College, Brookings, 15 pp., 1956.

112. Wahlstrom, R. C., Goehring, T. B., Johnson, D. D., Libal, G. W., Olson, O. E., Palmer, I. S., and Thaler, R. C., The relationship of hair color to selenium content of hair and selenosis in swine, Nutr. Rep. Int., 29, 143, 1984.

113. Wilson, T. M., Scholz, R. W., and Drake, T. R., Selenium toxicity and porcine focal symmetrical poliomyelomalacia: description of a field outbreak and experimental reproduction, Can. J. Comp. Med., 47, 412, 1983.

114. Goehring, T. B., Palmer, I. S., Olson, O. E., Libal, G. W., and Wahlstrom, R. C., Toxic effects of selenium on growing swine fed corn-soybean meal diets, J. Anim. Sci., 59, 733, 1984.

115. Mahan, D. C., and Moxon, A. L., Effect of inorganic selenium supplementation on selenosis in post-weaning swine, J. Anim. Sci., 58, 1216, 1984.

116. Grace, A. W., Ullrey, D. E., Miller, E. R., Ellis, D. J., and Keahey, K. K., Selenium and vitamin E in practical swine diets, J. Anim. Sci., 33, 230, 1971.

117. Wahlstrom, R. C., and Olson, O. E., The relation of pre-natal and pre-weaning treatment to the effect of arsenilic acid on selenium poisoning in weanling pigs, J. Anim. Sci., 18, 578, 1959.

118. Wahlstrom, R. C., and Olson, O. E., The effect of selenium on reproduction in swine, J. Anim. Sci., 18, 141, 1959.

119. Miller, W. T., and Schoening, H. W., Toxicity of selenium fed to swine in the form of sodium selenite, J. Agric. Res., 56, 831, 1938.

120. Hilton, J. W., Hodson, P. V., and Slinger, P. V., The requirement and toxicity of selenium in rainbow trout (*Salmo gairdneri*), J. Nutr., 110, 2527, 1980.

121. Hilton, J. W., and Hodson, P. V., Effect of increased dietary carbohydrate on selenium metabolism and toxicity in rainbow trout (*Salmo gairdneri*), J. Nutr., 113, 1241, 1983.

122. Dinkel, C. A., Mingard, J. A., Whitehead, E. I., and Olson, O. E., Agricultural Research at the Reed Substation, S. Dakota Agr. Exp. Sta., Circ. No. 135, 1957.

123. Maag, D. D., Orsborn, J. S., and Clopton, J. R., The effect of sodium selenite on cattle, Am. J. Vet. Res., 21, 1049, 1960.

124. Olson, O. E., Selenium as a toxic factor in animal nutrition, Proc. Georgia Nutr. Conf., 68, 1969.

125. Munsell, H. E., Devaney, G. M., and Kennedy, M. H., Toxicity of food containing selenium as shown by its effect on the rat, U.S.D.A., Tech. Bull. No. 534, U.S.D.A., Washington, D.C., 25 pp., 1936.

126. Schroeder, H. A., and Mitchener, M., Selenium and tellurium in mice. Effects on growth, survival and tumors, Arch. Environ. Health, 24, 66, 1972.

127. Halverson, A. W., Growth and reproduction with rats fed selenite-Se, Proc. S. Dakota Acad. Sci., 53, 167, 1974.

128. Rosenfeld, I., and Beath, O. A., Effect of selenium on reproduction in rats, Proc. Soc. Exp. Biol. Med., 87, 295, 1954.

129. Dinkel, C. A., Minyard, J. A., and Ray, D. E., Effects of season of breeding on reproductive and weaning performance of beef cattle grazing on seleniferous range, J. Anim. Sci., 22, 1043, 1963.

130. Franke, K. W. and Potter, V. R., The effect of selenium containing foodstuffs on growth and reproduction of rats at various ages, J. Nutr., 12, 205, 1936.

131. Poley, W. E., and Moxon, A. L., Tolerance levels of seleniferous grains in laying hens, Poultry Sci., 17, 72, 1938.

132. Holmberg, R. E., and Ferm, V. H., Interrelationships of selenium, cadmium and arsenic in mammalian teratogenesis, Arch. Environ. Hlth., 18, 873, 1969.

133. Yonemoto, J., Satoh, H., Hommeno, S., and Suzuki, T., Toxic effects of sodium selenite on pregnant mice and modification of the effects by vitamin E or reduced glutathione, Teratol., 28, 333, 1983.

134. Buttner, W., Action of trace elements on the metabolism of fluoride, J. Dent. Res., 42, 453, 1963.

135. Navia, J. M., Menaker, L., Seltzer, J., and Harris, R. S., Effect of Na_2SeO_3 supplemented in the diet or the water on dental caries of rats, Federation Proc., 27, 676, 1968.

136. Bowen, W. H., The effects of selenium and vanadium on caries activity in monkeys (*M. irus*), J. Irish Dent. Assoc., 18, 83, 1972.

137. Shearer, T. R., Developmental and post-developmental uptake of dietary organic and inorganic selenium into the molar teeth of rats, J. Nutr., 105, 338, 1975.

138. Wheatcraft, M. G., English, J. A., and Schlack, C. A., Effects of selenium on the incidence of dental caries in white rats, J. Dent. Res., 30, 523, 1951.

139. Muhler, J. C., and Shafer, W. G., The effect of selenium on the incidence of dental caries in rats, J. Dent. Res., 36, 895, 1957.

140. Claycomb, C. K., Summers, G. W., and Jump, E. B., Effect of dietary selenium on dental caries in Sprague-Dawley rats, J. Dent. Res., 44, 826, 1965.

141. Kaqueler, J. C., Maloigne, E., and Bonifay, P., Effects of sodium selenate on caries incidence in the rat, J. Dent. Res. Special Issue D56, D151, 1977.

142. Ostadalova, I., Babicky, A., and Obenberger, J., Cataract induced by administration of a single dose of sodium selenite to suckling rats, Experientia 34, 222, 1978.

143. Ostadalova, I., Babicky, A., and Obenberger, J., Cataractogenic and lethal effect of selenite in rats during postnatal ontogenesis, Physiol. Bohemoslov., 28, 393, 1979.

144. Bunce, G. E., and Hess, J. L., Biochemical changes associated with selenite-induced cataract in the rat, Exp. Eye Res., 33, 505, 1981.

145. Bhuyan, K. C., Bhuyan, D. K., and Podos, S. W., Selenium-induced cataract an its biochemical mechanism, in *Proceedings of the Third International Symposium on Selenium in Biology and Medicine*, Combs, G. F., Jr., Spallholz, J. E., Levander, O. A., and Oldfield, J. E., eds., Avi Publishing Co., Westport, Conn., 1986.

146. Ostadalova, I., Babicky, A., and Kopoldova, J., Ontogenic changes in selenite metabolism in rats, Arch. Toxicol., 49, 247, 1982.

147. Shearer, T. R., Anderson, R. S., and Britton, J. L., Uptake and distribution of radioactive selenium in cataractous rat lens, Curr. Eye Res., 2, 561, 1982/1983.

148. Shearer, T. R., and David, L. L., Role of calcium in selenium cataract, Curr. Eye Res., 2, 777, 1982/1983.

149. Ostadalova, I., and Babicky, A., Delimitation of the period of sensitivity to the cataractogenic action of selenite in rats, Physiol. Bohemoslov., 32, 324, 1983.

150. Shearer, T. R., Anderson, R. S., and Britton, J. L., Influence of selenite and fourteen trace elements on cataractogenesis in the rat, Invest. Ophthalmol. Vis. Sci., 24, 417, 1983.

151. Shearer, T. R., Anderson, R. S., Britton, J. L., and Palmer, E. A., Early development of selenium-induced cataract: slit lamp evaluation, Exp. Eye Res. 36, 781, 1983.

152. Hess, J. L., Wisthoff, F., and Funce, G. E., Impact of selenite on rat lens metabolism, Invest. Ophthalmol. Vis. Sci., 24, 31, 1983.

153. Bhuyan, K. C., and Bhuyan, D. K., Molecular mechanism of cataractogenesis. II. Evidence of lipid peroxidation and membrane damage, in *Oxy Radicals, Their Scavenger Systems, Proceedings of the Third International Conference on Superoxide Dismutase*, Cohen, G. and Greenwald, R. A., eds., Elsevier, New York, 349, 1983.

154. Bunce, G. E., Hess, J. L., and Batra, R., Lens calcium and selenite-induced cataract, Curr. Eye Res., 3, 315, 1984.

155. Shearer, T. R., Ridlington, J. W., Goeger, D. E., and Whanger, P. D., Uptake of ^{75}Se in cataractous rat lens proteins, Biol. Trace Elem. Res., 6, 195, 1984.

156. Swanson, A. A., and Truesdale, A. W., Elemental analysis in normal and cataractous human lens tissues, Biochem. Biophys. Res. Commun., 45, 1488, 1971.

157. Lakomaa, E. L. and Eklund, P., Trace element analysis of human cataractous lenses by neutron activation analysis and atomic absorption, Proceedings Series — Nuclear Activation Techniques in Life Sciences, Int'l. Atomic Energy Agency - SM 227,333,1979.

158. Bhuyan, R. C., Baxter, T., and Morris, J. S., Selenium status in the eye: Increased level in cataract in the human and its distribution in eye tissues of animals, Invest. Ophthalmol. Vis. Sci., 22, 35, 1982.

159. Olson, O. E., Selenium toxicity in animals, with emphasis on man, presented at workshop on Strategies for the Development of Selenium Compounds as Cancer Chemopreventative Agents, Nat. Cancer Inst., Feb. 7, 8, 1985.

160. Clinton, M., Jr., Selenium fume exposure, J. Ind. Hyg. Toxicol., 29, 225, 1947.

161. Izraelson, Z. I., Mogilevska, O. J., and Suvorov, S. W., (Selenium), in *(Problems of Occupational Hygiene and Occupational Pathology Connected with Work with Toxic Metals)*, Medicine Publ. House, Moscow, 1973, 245 (in Russian).

162. Wilson, H. M., Selenium oxide poisoning, N. Carolina Med. J., 23, 73, 1962.

163. Monaenkova, A. M. and Glotova, K. V., (Selenium intoxication), Gig. Sanit., 6, 41, 1963 (in Russian).

164. Skornjakova, L. V., Buchanov, A. I., and Salechov, M. I., (On the acute manifestations of selenium poisoning), Gig. Truda I. Prof. Sabol., 11, 45, 1969 (in Russian).

165. Buchan, R. F., Industrial selenosis, Occup. Med., 3, 439, 1947.

166. Senf, H. W., (A case report of poisoning by hydrogen selenide), Dtsch. Med. Wochenschr., 67, 1094, 1941 (in German).

167. Symanski, H., (A case of hydrogen selenide poisoning), Dtsch. Med. Wochenschr., 75, 1730, 1950 (in German).

168. Bonard, E. C., and Koralink, K. D., Intoxication aigue par vapeurs d'hydrogene selenide, Proxis, 47, 533, 1958.

169. Schecter, A., Shanske, W., Stenzler, A., Quintilian, H., and Steinberg, H., Acute hydrogen selenide intoxication, Chest; 77, 554, 1980.

170. Glover, J. R., Selenium and its industrial toxicology, Ind. Med. Surg., 39, 50, 1970.

171. Lazarev, N. V., and Gadaskina, I. D., *(Noxious Substances in Industry)*, Chimija Publ. House, Leningrad, 1977 (in Russian).

172. Carter, R. F., Acute selenium poisoning, Med. J. Australia, 1, 525, 1966.

173. Civil, I. D., and McDonald, M. J., Acute selenium poisoning: case report, N. Zealand Med. J., 87, 354, 1978.

174. Kerdal-Vegas, F., Generalized hair loss due to the ingestion of "coco de mono" *(Lecythis ollaria)*, J. Invest. Dermatol., 42, 91, 1964.

175. Middleton, J. M., Selenium burn of eye; report of case, with review of literature, Arch. Ophthalmol., 38, 806, 1947.

176. Hamilton, A., *Industrial Poisons in the United States*, Macmillan Co., New York, 1925.

177. Weissman, S. H., Cuddihy, R. G., and Burkstaller, M. A., Distribution and retention of inhaled selenious acid and selenium metal aerosols in beagle dogs, in *Trace Substances in Environmental Health XIII*, Hemphill, D. D., ed., Univ. Missouri, Columbia, 1979, 477.

178. Dudley, H. C., Toxicology of selenium. VI. Toxic acid vesicant properties of selenium oxychloride, U. S. Publ. Health Rep., 53, 94, 1938.

179. Dutkiewicz, T., Kutkiewicz, B., and Balcerska, T., Dynamics of organ and tissue distribution of selenium after intragastric and dermal administration of sodium selenite, Bromatol. Chem. Toksykol., 4, 475, 1972.

180. Duvoir, M., Pollett, L., and Herrenschmidt, J. L., Eczema professionel du an selenium, Bull. Soc. Franc. Dermatol. Syphil., 44, 88, 1937.

181. Pringle, P., Occupational dermatitis following exposure to organic selenium compounds, Br. J. Dermatol. Syphil., 54, 54, 1942.

182. Hogger, D., and Bohn, C., On dermal injury produced by selenite, Dermatologica, 90, 217, 1944.
183. Halter, K., (Selenium poisoning, especially skin changes accompanied by secondary porphyria), Arch. Dermatol., 178, 340, 1938 (in German).
184. Diskin, D. J., Tomasso, C. L., and Alper, J. C., Long-term selenium exposure, Arch. Intern. Med., 139, 824, 1979.
185. Dudley, H. C., Toxicology of selenium. II. The urinary excretion of selenium, Amer. J. Hyg., 23, 181, 1936.
186. Kinnigkeit, Q., (Studies on workers exposed to selenium in a rectifier plant), Z. Gesamte Hyg. Ihre Grenzgeb., 8, 350, 1962 (in German).
187. Nagai, I., (An experimental study of selenium poisoning), Igaku Kenkyu, 28, 105, 1959 (in Japanese).
188. Tsongas, T. A., and Ferguson, S. W., Human health effects of selenium in a rural Colorado drinking water supply, in *Trace Substances in Environmental Health, XI*, Hemphill, D. D., ed., Univ. Missouri, Columbia, 1977, 30.
189. Smith, M. I., Franke, K. W., and Westfall, B. B., The selenium problem in relation to public health. A preliminary survey to determine the possibility of selenium intoxication in th rural population living on seleniferous soil, U. S. Pub. Health Rep., 51, 1496, 1936.
190. Smith, M. I., and Westfall, B. B., Further field studies on the selenium problem in relation to public health, U. S. Pub. Health Rep., 52, 1375, 1937.
191. Anonymous, Selenium poisons Indians, Sci. News Lett., 81, 254, 1962.
192. Lemley, R. E., Selenium poisoning in the human, Lancet, 60, 528, 1940.
193. Palmer, I. S., Olson, O. E., Ketterling, L. M., and Shank, C. E., Selenium intake and urinary excretion in persons living near a high selenium area, J. Amer. Dietetic Assoc., 82, 511, 1983.
194. Byers, H. G., Selenium in Mexico, Ind. Eng. Chem., 29, 1200, 1937.
195. Mondragon, M. C. and Jaffe, W. G., (Selenio en alimentos y en orino de escolares de differentes zonas de Venezuela), Arch. Latinoamer. Nutr., 21, 185, 1971 (in Spanish).
196. Jaffe, W. G., Ruphael, M. D., Mondragon, M. C., and Cuevas, M. A., Clinical and biochemical studies on school children from a seleniferous zone, Arch. Latinoamer. Nutr., 22, 595, 1972.
197. Jaffe, W. G., and Velez, B. F., Selenium intake and congenital malformations in humans, Arch. Latinoamer. Nutr., 23, 514, 1973.
198. Bratter, P., Negretti, V. E., Rosick, V., Jaffe, W. G., Mendez, H., and Tovar, G., Effects of selenium intake in man at high dietary levels of seleniferous areas of Venezuela, Trace Elem. Anal. Chem. Med. Biol., 3, 29, 1984.
199. Ancizar-Sordo, J., Occurrence of selenium in soils and plants of Columbia, South America, Soil Sci., 63, 437, 1947.
200. Yang, G. Q., Wang, S., Zhou, R., and Sun, R., Endemic selenium intoxication of humans in China, Amer. J. Clin. Nutr., 37, 872, 1983.
201. Liu, B. S., and Li, S. S., Primary study of the relationship between endemic selenosis and fluorosis, in *Proceedings of the Third International Symposium on Selenium in Biology and Medicine*, Combs, G. F., Jr., Spallholz, J. E., Levander, O. A., and Oldfield, J. E., eds., Avi Publ. Co., Westport, Conn., 1986.
202. Thomson, C. D., Burton, C. E., and Robinson, M. F., On supplementing the selenium intake of New Zealanders. I. Short experiments with large doses of selenite or selenomethionine, Br. J. Nutr., 39, 579, 1978.
203. Westermarck, T., Selenium content of tissues in Finnish infants and adults with various diseases, and studies on the effects of selenium supplementation in neuronal ceroid lipofuscinosis patients, Acta Pharmacol. Toxicol., 41, 121, 1977.

204. Perona, G., Guide, G. C., Piga, A., Cellerino, R., Menna, R., and Zatti, M., *In vivo* and *in vitro* variations of human erythrocyte glutathione peroxidase activity as result of cells aging, selenium availability and peroxide activation, Br. J. Haematol., 39, 399, 1978.
205. Helslzour, K., Case study of Se toxicity in humans presented at Workshop on Strategies for the Development of Selenium Compounds as Cancer Chemopreventative Agents, Nat. Cancer Inst., Feb. 7,8, 1985.
206. Weisberger, A. S., and Suhrland, L. G., Studies on analogues of L-cysteine and L-cystine. III. The effect of selenium cystine on leukemia, Blood, 11, 19, 1956.
207. Schrauzer, G. N., and White, D. A., Selenium in human nutrition: dietary intakes and effects of supplementation, Bioinorg. Chem., 8, 303, 1978.
208. Ransome, J. W., Scott, N. M., Jr., and Knoblock, E. C., Selenium sulfide intoxication, N. Eng. J. Med., 264, 384, 1961.
209. Hadjimarkos, D. M., and Storvick, C. A., Geographic variations of dental caries in Oregon. IV. Am. J. Pub. Health, 40, 1552, 1950.
210. Hadjiinarkos, D. M., Storvick, C. A., and Remmert, L. F., Selenium and dental caries. An investigation among school children of Oregon, J. Pediatr., 40, 451, 1952.
211. Hadjimarkos, D. M., Geographic variation of dental caries in Oregon. VII. Caries prevalence among children in the blue mountains regions, J. Pediatr., 48, 195, 1956.
212. Hadjimarkos, D. M., and Bonhorst, C. W., The trace element selenium and its influence on dental caries susceptibility, J. Pediatr., 52, 274, 1958.
213. Tank, G., and Starvick, C. A., Effect of naturally occurring selenium and vanadium on dental caries, J. Dent. Res., 39, 473, 1960.
214. Hadjimarkos, D. M., and Bonhorst, C. W., The selenium content of eggs, milk and water in relation to dental caries in children, J. Pediatr., 59, 256, 1961.
215. Suchkov, B. P., Kacap, I. M., and Gulgasenko, A. I., (Affection of the population of the Chernovitsi region with caries in association with selenium content in the teeth), Stomatologia, 52, 21, 1973 (in Russian).
216. Jaffe, W. G., Effect of selenium intake in humans and rats, in *Proceedings of the Symposium on Selenium-Tellurium in the Environment*, Industrial Health Found., Pittsburgh, 1976, 188.
217. Kilness, A. W., and Hochberg, F. H., Amyotrophic lateral sclerosis in a high selenium environment, J. Am. Med. Assoc., 237, 2843, 1977.
218. Robertson, D. S. F., Selenium, a possible teratogen? Lancet, 1, 518, 1970.
219. Cadell, P. B., and Cousins, F. B., Urinary selenium and dental caries, Nature, 185, 863, 1960.
220. Schwarz, K., Amyotrophic lateral schlerosis and selenium, J. Am. Med. Assoc., 238, 2365, 1977.
221. Kurland, L. T., Amyotrophic lateral sclerosis and selenium, J. Am. Med. Assoc., 238, 2365, 1977.
222. Norris, F. H., and Sang, K., Amyotrophic lateral sclerosis and low urinary selenium levels, J. Am. Med. Assoc., 239, 404, 1978.
223. Glover, J. R., Some medical problems concerning selenium in industry, Trans. Assoc. Ind. Med. Off., 4, 94, 1954.
224. Moxon, A. L., Schaefer, A. E., Lardy, H. A., Dubos, K. P., and Olson, O. A., Increasing the rate of excretion of selenium from selenized animals by the administration of *p*-bromobenzene, J. Biol. Chem., 132, 785, 1940.
225. McConnell, K. P., Kreamer, A. E., and Roth, D. M., Presence of selenium-75 in the mercapturic acid fraction of dog urine, J. Biol. Chem., 234, 2932, 1959.
226. Westfall, B. B., and Smith, M. I., Further studies on the fate of selenium in the organism, J. Pharmacol. Exp. Ther., 72, 245, 1941.

227. Lemley, R. E., and Merryman, M. P., Selenium poisoning in the human, Lancet, 61, 435, 1941.

228. Lemley, R. E., Observations on selenium poisoning in South and North America, Lancet, 63, 257, 1943.

229. Sivjakov, K. I., and Braun, H. A., The treatment of acute selenium, cadmium, and tungsten intoxication in rats with calcium disodium ethylenediaminetetra acetate, Toxicol. Appl. Pharmacol., 1, 602, 1959.

230. DuBois, K. P., Rhian, M., and Moxon, A. L., The effect of glutathione on selenium toxicity, Proc. S. Dakota Acad. Sci., 19, 71, 1939.

231. Levander, O. A., and Baumann, C. A., Selenium metabolism. VI. Effect of arsenic on the excretion of selenium in the bile, Toxicol. Appl. Pharmacol., 9, 106, 1966.

232. Levander, O. A., Young, M. L., and Meeks, S. A., Studies on the binding of selenium by liver homogenates from rats fed diets containing either casein or casein plus linseed oil meal, Toxicol. Appl. Pharmacol., 16, 79, 1970.

233. Levander, O. A., Metabolic interrelationships and adaptation in selenium toxicity, Ann. N. Y. Acad. Sci., 192, 181, 1972.

234. Braun, H. A., Lusky, L. M., and Calvery, H. O., Efficacy of 2,3-dimercaptopropanol (BAL) in therapy of poisoning by compounds of antimony, bismuth, chromium, mercury, and nickel, J. Pharmacol. 87, Suppl. 119, 1946.

235. Belogorsky, J. B., and Slaughter, D., Administration of BAL in selenium poisoning, Proc. Soc. Exp. Biol. Med., 72, 196, 1949.

236. Dickson, R. C. and Tappel, A. L., Reduction of selenocystine by cysteine or glutathione, Arch. Biochem. Biophys., 130, 547, 1969.

237. Anundi, I., Hogberg, J., and Stahl, A., Involvement of glutathione reductase in selenite metabolism and toxicity, studied in isolated rat hepatocytes, Arch. Toxicol., 50, 113, 1982.

238. LeBoeuf, R. A., and Hoekstra, W. G., Adaptive changes in hepatic metabolism in response to excess selenium in rats, J. Nutr., 113, 845, 1983.

239. Csallany, A. S., Su, L. C., and Menken, B. Z., Effect of selenite, vitamin E and N,N'-diphenyl-p-phenylenediamine on liver organic solvent-soluble lipofuscin pigments in mice, J. Nutr., 114, 1582, 1984.

240. Caravaggi, C., Oxygen consumption and $^{14}CO_2$ production in tissue of rats with chronic and acute selenite poisoning, Experientia, 27, 369, 1971.

241. Hoffman, J. L., Selenite toxicity, depletion of liver S-adenosylmethionine, and inactivation of methionine adenosyltransferase, Arch. Biochem. Biophys., 179, 136, 1977.

242. Dini, G., Franconi, F., and Martini, F., Mitochondrial alterations induced by selenium in guinea pig myocardium, Exp. Mol. Pathol., 34, 226, 1981.

243. Lag, M., Paulsen, G., and Jonsen, J., Effect of sodium selenite in the ciliary activity, adenosine triphosphate, and protein synthesis in mouse trachea organ cultures, J. Toxicol. Environ. Hlth., 13, 857, 1984.

244. Sirianni, S. R., and Huang, C. C., Induction of sister chromatid exchange by various selenium compounds in Chinese hamster cells in the presence and absence of S9 mixture, Cancer Lett., 18, 109, 1983.

245. Lo, L. W., Koropatnick, J., and Stich, H. F., The mutagenicity and cytotoxicity of selenite, "activated" selenite and selenate for normaland DNA repair-deficient human fibroblasts, Mutat. Res., 49, 305, 1978.

246. Whiting, R. F., Wei, L., and Stich, H. F., Unscheduled DNA synthesis and chromosome abberations by inorganic and organic selenium compounds in the presence of glutathione, Mutat. Res., 78, 159, 1980.

247. Kalouskova, J., Korunova, V., Zouchova, Z., Pavlik, L., and Styblo, M., Factors influencing selenium metabolism and toxicity, Spurenelementsymposium (KMU Leipzig, FSU Jena), 254, 1983.

248. Gortner, R. A., Jr., Chronic selenium poisoning of rats as influenced by dietary protein, J. Nutr., 19, 105, 1940.

249. Smith, M. E., and Stohlman, E. F., Further observations on the influence of dietary protein on the toxicity of selenium, J. Pharmacol. Exp. Therap., 70, 270, 1940.

250. Moxon, A. L., The influence of some proteins on the toxicity of selenium, Ph. D. Thesis, Univ. of Wisconsin, Madison, 1941.

251. Halverson, A. W., Hendrick, C. M., and Olson, O. E., Observations on the protective effect of linseed oil meal and some extracts against chronic selenium poisoning in rats, J. Nutr., 56, 51, 1955.

252. Jenson, L. S., and Chang, C. H., Fractionation studies on a factor in linseed meal protecting against selenosis in chicks, Poultry Sci., 55, 594, 1976.

253. Olson, O. E., and Halverson, A. W., Effect of linseed oil meal and arsenicals on selenium poisoning in the rat, Proc. S. Dakota Acad. Sci., 33, 90, 1954.

254. Palmer, I. S., Olson, O. E., Halverson, A. W., Miller, R., and Smith, C., Isolation of fractions in linseed oil meal protective against chronic selenosis in rats, J. Nutr., 110, 145, 1980.

255. Smith, C. R., Jr., Weisleder, D., Miller, R. W., Palmer, I. S., and Olson, O. E., Linostatin and neolinustatin: cyanogenic glycosides of linseed meal that protect animals against selenium toxicity, J. Org. Chem., 45, 507, 1980.

256. Palmer, I. S., and Olson, O. E., Partial prevention by cyanide of selenium poisoning in rats, Biochem. Biophys. Res. Commun., 90, 1379, 1979.

257. Moxon, A. L., The effect of arsenic on the toxicity of seleniferous grain, Science, 88, 81, 1938.

258. Ganther, H. E. and Baumann, C. A., Selenium metabolism. I. Effects of diet arsenic and cadmium, J. Nutr., 77, 210, 1962.

259. Levander, O. A., and Baumann, C. A., Selenium metabolism. V. Studies on the distribution of selenium in rats given arsenic, Toxicol. Appl. Pharmacol., 9, 98, 1966.

260. Levander, O. A., and Baumann, C. A., Selenium metabolism. VI. Effect of arsenic on the excretion of selenium in the bile, Toxicol. Appl. Pharmacol., 9, 106, 1966.

261. El-Begearmi, M. M., Sunde, M. L., and Ganther, H. E., A mutual protective effect of mercury and selenium in Japanese quail, Poultry Sci., 56, 313, 1977.

262. Jensen, L. S., Modification of a selenium toxicity in chicks by dietatry silver and copper, J. Nutr., 105, 769, 1975.

263 Sellers, E. A., You, R. W., and Lucas, C. C., Lipotropic agents in liver damage produced by selenium or carbon tetrachloride, Proc. Soc. Exp. Biol. Med., 75, 118, 1950.

264. Lewis, H. B., Schultz, J., and Gortner, R. A., Jr., Dietary protein and the toxicity of sodium selenite in the rat, J. Pharmacol. Exp. Therap., 68, 292, 1940.

265. Klug, H. L., Harshfield, R. D., Pengra, R. M., and Moxon, A. L., Methionine and selenium toxicity, J. Nutr., 48, 409, 1952.

266. Witting, L. A., and Horwitt, M. K., Effects of dietary selenium, methionine, fat level and tocopherol on rat growth, J. Nutr., 84, 351, 1964.

267. Parizek, J., Ostadalova, I., Kalouskova, J., Babicky, A., and Benes, J., The detoxifying effects of selenium. Interrelationships between compounds of selenium and certain metals, in *Newer Trace Elements in Nutrition*, Mertz, W., and Cornatzer, W. E., eds., Marcell Dekker, New York, 1971, 85.

268. Siami, G., Schulbert, A. R., and Neal, R. A., A possible role for the mixed-function oxidase system in the requirement for selenium in the rat, J. Nutr., 102, 857, 1972.

269. Parizek, J., Kalouskava, J., Benes, J., and Pavlik, L., Interactions of selenium-mercury and selenium-selenium compounds, Ann. NY Acad. Sci., 355, 347, 1980.

270. Ermakov, V. V., and Koval'skij, V. V., (The geochemical ecology of organisms at high selenium levels in the environment), in *Trudy*, Biogeochimickleskaj laboratorii, Nauka Publ. House, Moscow, Vol. 12, 204, 1968 (in Russian).

271. Jaffe, W. G., and Mondragon, M. C., Adaptation of rats to selenium intake, J. Nutr., 97, 431, 1969.

272. Shrift, A., and Kelly, E., Adaptation of *Escherichia coli* to selenate, Nature, 195, 732, 1962.

273. Koval'skij, V. V., Ermakov, V. V., and Letunova, S. V., (Geochemical ecology of microorgansisms under conditions of different selenium content in soils), Mikrobiologiya, 37, 122, 1968 (in Russian).

274. Koval'skij, V. V., Ermakov, V. V., and Letunova, S. V., (Selenite reduction by *Bacillus magaterium* strains isolated from soils with a different selenium content), Zh. Obshchei Biol., 28, 724, 1976 (in Russiam).

275. Ganther, H. E., Metabolism of hydrogen selenide and methylated selenides, Adv. Nutr. Res., 2, 107, 1979.

276. Ewan, R. C., Pope, A. L., and Bauman, C. A., Elimination of fixed selenium by the rat, J. Nutr., 91, 547, 1967.

277. Burke, R. F., Seeley, R. J., and Kiker, K. W., Selenium: dietary threshold for urinary excretion in the rat, Proc. Soc. Exp. Biol. Med., 142, 214, 1973.

278. Parizek, J., Kalouskova, J., Korunova, V., Benes, J., and Pavlik, L., The protective effect of pretreatment with selenite in the toxicity of dimethyl selenide, Physiol. Bohemoslov., 25, 573, 1976.

279. Stowe, H. D., and Miller, E. R., Genetic predisposition of pigs to hypo- and hyperselenemia, J. Anim. Sci., 60, 200, 1985.

280. LaVorgna, M. W., and Combs, G. F., Jr., Evidence of a hereditary factor affecting the chick's response to uncomplicated selenium deficiency, Poultry Sci., 62, 164, 1983.

281. Combs, G. F., Jr., and Saroka, J. M., unpublished research, 1985.

282. Chen, J., Human selenosis in China, presented at Workshop on Strategies for the Development of Selenium Compounds as Cancer Chemopreventive Agents, Nat. Cancer Inst., Feb. 7,8, 1985.

283. Sakurai, H., and Tsuchiya, K., A tentative recommendation for maximum daily intake of selenium, Environ. Physiol. Biochem., 5, 107, 1975.

284. Committee on Dietary Allowances, Food and Nutrition Board, National Research Councik, National Academy of Sciences, *Recommended Dietary Allowances*, Ninth Revised Edition, National Academy of Sciences, Washington, D. C., 1980.

285. Medinsky, M. A., Cuddihy, R. G., Griffith, W. C., Weissman, S. H., and McClellar, R. O., Projected uptake and toxicity of selenium compounds from the environment, Environ. Res., 36, 181, 1985.

286. Presser, T. S., and Barnes, I., Selenium concentrations in waters tributary to and in the vicinity of the Kesterson National Wildlife Refuge, Fresno and Merced Counties, California, Water Resources Investigation Rep. 84-4122, U. S. Geological Survey, Washington, D. C., 1984.

287. U. S. Environmental Protection Agency, *National Interim Primary Drinking Water Regulations*, Environmental Protection Agency, Office of Water Supply, EPA- 57019-76-003, 1977.

288. Lafond, M. G., and Calabrese, E. J., Is the selenium drinking water standard justified? Med. Hypoth., 5, 877, 1979.

Index

D

E